LABORATORY
&
DIAGNOSTIC
TESTS

with Nursing Implications

LABORATORY & DIAGNOSTIC TESTS

with Nursing Implications

sixth edition

Joyce LeFever Kee, MSN, RN
Associate Professor Emerita
College of Health and Nursing Science
University of Delaware
Newark, Delaware

Prentice
Hall

Upper Saddle River, New Jersey 07458

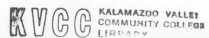

Library of Congress Cataloging-in-Publication Data

Kee, Joyce LeFever.
    Laboratory & diagnostic tests with nursing implica-
tions / Joyce LeFever Kee. — 6th ed.
        p. ; cm.
    Includes bibliographical references and index.
    ISBN 0-13-030519-7
    1. Diagnosis, Laboratory.   2. Nursing.   I. Title: Lab-
oratory and diagnostic tests with nursing implications.
II. Title.
        [DNLM: 1. Laboratory Techniques and Proce-
dures—Nurses' Instruction. QY 4 K26L 2002]
    RT48.5 .K44 2002
    616.07'56—dc21
                                          2001031505

Notice: The authors and the publisher of this volume have taken care to make certain that the
doses of drugs and schedules of treatment are correct and compatible with the standards generally
accepted at the time of publication. Nevertheless,
as new information becomes available, changes in
treatment and in the use of drugs become necessary. The reader is advised to carefully consult the
instruction and information material included in
the package insert of each drug or therapeutic
agent before administration. This advice is especially important when using, administering, or
recommending new or infrequently used drugs.
The authors and publisher disclaim all responsi-
bility for any liability, loss, injury, or damage in-
curred as a consequence, directly or indirectly,
of the use and application of any of the contents
of this volume.

Publisher: Julie Alexander
Executive Editor: Maura Connor
Acquisitions Editor: Nancy Anselment
Editorial Assistant: Sarah Caffrey
**Director of Manufacturing
  and Production:** Bruce Johnson
Managing Editor: Patrick Walsh
Production Editor: Pine Tree Composition, Inc.
Production Liaison: Cathy O'Connell
Manufacturing Buyer: Pat Brown
Design Director: Cheryl Asherman
Senior Designer: Maria Guglielmo
Cover Design: Joseph Sengotta
Composition: Pine Tree Composition, Inc.
Printing and Binding: R. R. Donnelley & Sons
  Company

Pearson Education Ltd., *London*
Pearson Education Australia Pty, Limited, *Sydney*
Pearson Education Singapore, Pte. Ltd.
Pearson Education North Asia Ltd., *Hong Kong*
Pearson Education Canada, Ltd., *Toronto*
Pearson Education de Mexico, S.A. de C.V.
Pearson Education—Japan, *Tokyo*
Pearson Education Malaysia, Pte. Ltd.
Pearson Education, Upper Saddle River, New Jersey

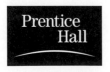

10 9 8 7 6 5
ISBN 0-13-030519-7

This book
I dedicate in
loving memory of
my mother and father
Esther Baker LeFever and **Samuel Herr LeFever**
for their years of
love, encouragement, and support

CONTENTS

PREFACE

Each day hundreds of thousands of laboratory and diagnostic tests are performed and thus nursing responsibilities are forever increasing. Nurses should understand laboratory and diagnostic tests and should provide nursing implications through nursing assessment, judgment, implementation, teaching, and interaction.

Laboratory and Diagnostic Tests with Nursing Implications, Sixth Edition is designed to provide nurses and other health professionals with the necessary information regarding laboratory and diagnostic tests and corresponding nursing implications. It gives quick, pertinent information about the tests, emphasizing the purposes, procedure, and nursing implications with rationale. Reference values are given for adults and children. The tests (laboratory and diagnostic) are arranged in alphabetic order which provides the user with a quick access to the tests.

This text is appropriate for students in various types of nursing programs, including students in masters, baccalaureate, associate degree, diploma, and practical nursing programs. This book should be most valuable to the registered nurse and licensed practical nurse in hospital settings, including specialty areas such as the ICU and emergency room, clinics, health care provider offices, and in independent nursing practice.

The sixth edition

The sixth edition lists more than 400 laboratory and diagnostic tests with approximately 28 new tests added to this edition. Major additions and revisions made include:

- Selected new laboratory tests: High sensitivity C-reactive protein (hs CRP) helpful in detecting risk for coronary artery disease (CAD); amyloid beta protein precursor that aids in the diagnosis of Alzheimer's disease; viral cultures using various specimens; hematologic tests such as fetal hemoglobin (Hb F), methemoglobin, D-Dimer test to aid in the detection of disseminated intravascular coagulation (DIC), Heinz Bodies for detecting hemoglobinopathies, platelet antibody test to detect thrombocytopenia that may be drug-induced; and antibody tests such as parvovirus B 19 antibody, antismooth muscle antibody, antiscleroderma antibody, and antiparietal cell antibody tests.

- Selected new diagnostic tests: Bone densitometry, corneal staining, cystometry, fetal nonstress test, fetoscopy, electronystagmography, laparoscopy, sleep studies, and thoracoscopy.
- Latest tests (antigen and antibodies) for human immunosuppressive virus-type (HIV-1 and HIV-2) and hemoglobin A_1c updated.
- Latest updated data for diagnostic tests: magnetic resonance imaging (MRI), computed tomography (CT), angiography, cardiac catheterization, nuclear scans, Pap smear, mammography, various gastrointestinal tests, various stress tests, positron emission tomography (PET), echocardiography, Holter monitoring, pulmonary function tests, and ultrasonography.
- Additional Therapeutic Drug Monitoring (TDM) information.
- Updated Laboratory Test Groups (Appendix B).
- Updated Laboratory Test Values for Adults and Children that are listed according to the laboratory departments (Appendix C).

Organization

Each test is discussed in seven subsections in the following sequence: (1) reference values/normal findings, (2) description, (3) purpose, (4) clinical problems, (5) procedure, (6) factors affecting laboratory or diagnostic results, and (7) nursing implications with rationale. Following the name and initials for each test, there may be names of other closely associated tests. **Reference values/normal findings** are given for children and adults, including the elderly. The **description** focuses on background data and pertinent information related to the test. The general **purpose** for each test is listed. **Clinical problems** include disease entities, drugs, and foods that cause or are associated with abnormal test results. The **procedure** is explained with a rationale for the test and with appropriate steps that the nurse and other health professionals can follow. **Factors affecting laboratory or diagnostic results** alert the nurse to factors that could cause an abnormal test result. The last subsection and most valuable information for each test concerns the **nursing implications with rationale.** For most diagnostic tests, nursing implications are given as "pretest" and "posttest."

There are four parts in the text. Part 1, Laboratory Tests; Part 2, Diagnostic Tests; Part 3, Laboratory/Diagnostic Assessments of Body Function; and Part 4, Therapeutic Drug Monitoring (TDM). There is a list of laboratory tests with page numbers at the beginning of Part I and a list of diagnostic tests with page numbers at the beginning of Part II. In addition, general information appears in the Introduction to the book including the importance of **specimen collection** with detailed information about all types of specimen collection. The **Instructions for Laboratory and Diagnostic Tests** section explains the information that will be found under the eight major subheadings for each test and gives basic information that relates to most of the laboratory and diagnostic tests.

Part 3, **Laboratory/Diagnostic Assessments of Body Function,** should be most valuable to both the practicing nurse and the student. The section consists of 12 categories related to organ system and clinical conditions. These are: **Cardiac Function; Respiratory Function; Renal Function; Liver, Gallbladder, Pancreatic Functions; Gastrointestinal Function; Neurologic and Musculoskeletal Functions; Endocrine Function; Reproductive Function; Arthritic and Collagen Conditions; Shock; Neoplastic Conditions;** and **Hematologic Conditions.** Each category contains numerous laboratory and diagnostic tests ordered to assist in the diagnosis of disease entities and to determine organ function. These tests are briefly discussed with reference values as they relate to the organ or condition of that category. A few of the same tests (e.g., enzyme tests) can be found in more than one category (cardiac, muscle, liver). The nurse could determine if the test is more specific for one category or the other. **The nursing process with nursing diagnosis, nursing implications, and nursing evaluation** are found at the end of each category.

Part 4, **Therapeutic Drug Monitoring (TDM),** lists drugs that are monitored frequently by serum and urine for the purposes of achieving and maintaining therapeutic drug effects and for preventing drug toxicity. The TDM section includes 120 drugs and their therapeutic range, peak time, and toxic level.

There are three appendices: **Abbreviations, Laboratory Test Groups** (laboratory profiles ordered for diagnosing clinical problems), and **Laboratory Test Values for Adults and Children.** The detailed index should be most helpful for locating the page of a test when the test name is different from the alphabetic listing used.

ACKNOWLEDGMENTS

I wish to extend my sincere thanks and deep appreciation to the following people: Linda S. Farmer, Laboratory Specialist, Dade-Behring, Delaware, for updating the reference values, procedures, instructions for laboratory and diagnostic tests, and Appendix B, Laboratory Test Groups; David C. Sestili, Pulmonary Laboratories Manager, Medical Center of Delaware, Christiana Hospital, Newark, Delaware, for his contribution on pulmonary function tests; Ronald J. LeFever, Pharmacist, Pharmacy Services, Medical College of Virginia, Richmond, Virginia, for correcting and adding drugs to the TDM section; Jane Purnell Taylor, Associate Professor, Neumann College, Aston, Pennsylvania, for updating the HIV test, and adding fetal nonstress test and fetoscopy; Judith Fullhart, Gastroenterologic Nursing Manager, Veterans Affairs Medical Center, Wilmington, Delaware, for contributing and updating the various gastrointestinal tests; Frank DiGregorio, Jr., Supervisor, Community Imaging Center, Wilmington, Delaware, for updating the various stress tests, Echocardiography, Holter Monitoring, Nuclear Scans, Positron Emission Tomography, and Ultrasonography; Heiddy DiGregorio, Christiana Care Health Services for updating selected nursing implications for diagnostic tests; Ellen K. Boyda, Family Nurse Practitioner, Boothwyn, Pennsylvania, for updating Acid-Base Balance and Pap Smear; Timothy J. Cole, Assistant Professor of Radiology, Medical College of Virginia, Richmond, Virgina, for updating Magnetic Resonance Imaging and Computed Tomography; Virginia L. Edwards, Assistant Clinical Professor, School of Medicine, Medical College of Virginia, Richmond, Virgina, for updating Angiography and Cardiac Catheterization; Susan Summerton, Radiologist, and Diane Arbaugh, Registered Mammographer, Papastavros Associates, Wilmington, Delaware, for checking mammography; and Helen Tang-Yates, Health Center, University of Delaware, Newark, Delaware, for her contribution to the Importance of Specimen Collection.

My sincere appreciation also goes to Don Passidomo, librarian at the Veterans Affairs Medical Center, for his suggestions and help with library research; Nancy Anselment, Editor, Nursing, Prentice Hall Health, for her guidance; and Mary Ellen Ruitenberg, Assistant Editor, for her assistance. To my husband, I give my love and appreciation for his support and help.

INTRODUCTION

The importance of specimen collection

Nurses participate actively in laboratory testing protocols for clients. Some believe that nurses simply order laboratory tests, either on requisition slips or electronically. This is not the case. Nursing input is critical to obtaining valid and reliable laboratory test results. In the role of caregiver and teacher, the nurse must communicate with the client, physician, and laboratory personnel to obtain information that might affect test results. Nursing responsibilities include explaining the laboratory test, ensuring that both the client and staff follow the procedure, assessing clinical findings with laboratory test results, noting pertinent information on the laboratory requisition slip (e.g., drugs the patient is taking that might affect test results), and collecting the specimen.

Collection of specimens is the focus of this section. The following paragraphs present an overview of the various aspects of specimen collection: the types of specimens, the collection sites, the effect of the client's position and activity on test results, the importance of the time of collection, drug interference, labeling and handling of specimens, types of collection tubes, and the types of reported laboratory measurement.

Types of Specimens: Blood, urine (random or 24-hour collection), cerebrospinal fluid (CSF), feces, sputum, and synovial, pleural, peritoneal, and wound exudate are the types of specimens that are used for laboratory studies. Because blood is the most frequently analyzed specimen, its collection will be outlined below.

When blood is withdrawn, it clots. The fluid that can be separated from the clotted blood is called *serum*. The term *plasma* is often used interchangeably with serum; however, plasma contains the protein *fibrinogen,* a component that is converted to the substance that composes the clot, *fibrin*.

Most tests (e.g., electrolyte levels) use serum from clotted blood. If a laboratory test requires plasma or whole blood, the tube used to collect the blood must contain an anticoagulant so that the blood will not clot. The stoppers of the collection tubes are color-coded to indicate whether they contain serum (red top) or plasma (lavender, green, gray, or blue top).

Site of Collection: Because blood is most commonly drawn from a vein, the venous source does not have to be indicated on the laboratory slip; however, if the blood is drawn from an artery or capillary, this should be recorded on the slip. The legs and feet are not used for venipuncture because of the risk of exacerbating circulatory conditions.

When collecting the blood sample, the tourniquet should not be left on for longer than a minute. It can cause fluid shift from the vessel to the tissue spaces, leading to hemoconcentration and resulting in erroneous results. After collection, the blood specimen should be gently inverted several times to mix with the anticoagulant if in the tube. Shaking the tube can damage the red blood cells (RBCs) (hemolysis) and possibly cause an inaccurate test result.

Client Position and Activity: Standing or recent ambulation causes body fluid to shift from the vascular to the tissue spaces. Vascular hemoconcentration could result, affecting the concentration of proteins, enzymes, albumin, globulin, cholesterol, triglycerides, calcium, and iron. It takes 20 to 30 minutes for fluid levels to reestablish equilibrium after this shift in position. Exercise just prior to specimen collection can also cause false results; this is especially true with enzyme testing.

Time of Collection: A time for routine blood collection needs to be established. Early morning before breakfast is the best time for blood collection because food and fluid will not affect test results. Fasting, however, is required only for a few laboratory tests, such as glucose, triglyceride, cholesterol, potassium, Vitamin B_{12}, folate, and thyroid studies. For fasting specimens, the client is requested to fast for 8 to 12 hours.

Drug Interference: Due to the growing number of drugs taken by clients, there is an increased chance that the laboratory results will be affected. This is especially true if drugs are taken over a period of time and at high doses. Drugs affecting test results should be noted on the laboratory slip. Drugs with a short half-life are withheld until the blood is drawn and thereby do not affect adversely the laboratory test result.

Labeling and Handling: The laboratory requisition slip should include the following information: the client's full name, age, sex, room location, and possible diagnosis; the physician's name; the test being requested (indicated by a check mark); the date; the time of collection; and any special notation (such as drugs). Another type of identification, such as the client's Social Security number or medical record number, may be required. In computerized laboratories, a bar-code label may be applied.

Proper handling and prompt transport of the specimen to the laboratory is vitally important. Fresh specimens provide more accurate test results. When a blood specimen is not processed promptly, hemolysis can occur, causing inaccurate results; when a urine specimen sits longer than 30 minutes, the pH of the urine becomes alkaline as a result of bacterial growth.

Collection Tubes: Tubes have color-coded stoppers that indicate the type of additive in the tube. The additives include anticoagulants such as oxalates, citrates, ethylenediaminetetraacetic acid (EDTA), and heparin. Blood-serum specimens are obtained in a red-top tube that does not contain an additive. Examples of the laboratory groups and color-top tubes follow.

Red: No additive, clotted blood. Serum is obtained from the clotted blood mass. Laboratory test groups that use red-top tubes are chemistries (electrolytes, proteins, enzymes, lipids, hormones), drug monitoring, radioimmunoassay (RIA) methods, serology, and blood banking. Hemolysis should be avoided.

Lavender: The additive is EDTA. This color is used to identify plasma and blood specimens. Laboratory test groups that use lavender-top tubes are hematologic tests (complete blood cell count [CBC], platelet count) and certain chemistries.

Green: The additive is heparin. This color is used to identify blood-plasma specimens. Laboratory test groups that use green-top tubes are arterial blood gases and the lupus erythematosus (LE) test; electrolyte and hormone levels are usually obtained from serum (red-top tube), but sometimes require a green-top tube.

Blue: The additive is citrate. Blue is used to identify blood-plasma specimens. Laboratory test groups that use blue-top tubes are coagulation studies (prothrombin time [PT], activated partial thromboplastin time [APTT], partial thromboplastin time [PTT]), and hemoglobin levels.

Gray: The additive is sodium fluoride. Gray is used for blood-plasma specimens. The laboratory test for glucose uses gray-top tubes. The additive is used to prevent glycolysis and thus preserve the glucose concentration in the in vivo state.

Types of Reported Laboratory Measurements

International System of Units: The World Health Organization (WHO) recommends that the medical and scientific community throughout the world adopt the Système International d'Unités (SI units) in order to establish a common international language for communicating laboratory measurements. Most clinical laboratories in Canada, Australia, and western Europe, and some in the United States, are now using SI units. Currently, both metric and SI units are usually reported.

Reference Values: Reference values (expected values) are based on "apparently healthy" individuals and the equipment and methods used in laboratories. Due to differences in the methods and equipment used, reference values may vary among institutions.

Critical (Panic) Values: At times a client's test results may fall outside the range of reference values, and a decision must be made as to whether the physician should be notified. Most laboratories have a list of critical values. When a client's results exceed the values on this list, the physician or charge nurse must be notified immediately. The critical-value policy and list are specific to each institution.

Instructions for laboratory and diagnostic tests

This sixth edition of *Laboratory and Diagnostic Tests with Nursing Implications* includes new and additional laboratory and diagnostic tests. Statements made in the **procedure** section, such as "there is no food or fluid restriction," will not be repeated in the **nursing implications** section. With all laboratory and diagnostic tests, the nurse needs to explain the purpose and procedure of the test, both of which can be obtained from the **description** and **procedure** section. The following headings for laboratory and diagnostic tests help to clarify the changes.

Reference Values: Laboratory (norm) values can differ somewhat among institutions. The values given in this text are comparable to the reference values given in most institutions; however, nurses need to check the reference values at their institution.

Description: General information, such as the indications for a test or the pharmacology of a drug, are included in the description. Much of this information should be included when discussing the purpose of the test with the client.

Purpose: The general purpose is given for each laboratory and diagnostic test. If there is more than one purpose, only the most common ones are provided.

Clinical Problems: The disease entities that are associated with decreased and elevated test results are listed according to decreasing frequency of occurrence. Drugs that influence test results are given for both decreased and elevated levels. Drugs taken by client that can affect test results should be listed on the laboratory requisition slip.

Procedure: The procedure is an important part of the test, and the nurse must discuss the procedure, step by step, with the client. Most of the procedures for laboratory and diagnostic tests are similar among institutions. The following are helpful suggestions applicable to most tests.

Laboratory Tests

1. Follow institutional policy and procedure.
2. Collect the recommended amount of specimen (blood, urine, etc.).
3. Avoid using the arm/hand with an intravenous (IV) line for drawing venous blood.
4. Label clearly the specimen container with client's identifying information.
5. Note significant drug data on the label or laboratory requisition slip, or both.
6. Avoid hemolysis; do not shake blood specimens.
7. Observe strict aseptic technique when collecting and handling each specimen. Use OSHA guidelines as adopted by each institution (e.g., universal precautions).

8. Enforce food and fluid restriction only when indicated.
9. Collect 24-hour urine specimens:
   a. Have the client void prior to test, discard urine, and then save all urine for the specified time, such as 24 hours.
   b. Instruct the client to urinate into a sterile container, usually provided by the laboratory, then pour the urine into the large 24-hour container.
   c. Instruct the client to avoid contaminating the urine specimen with toilet paper or feces.
   d. Refrigerate the 24-hour urine or keep it on ice, unless preservatives are added or unless otherwise indicated.
   e. Label the urine collection bottle/container with the client's name, date, and exact time of collection (e.g., 6/21/04, 7 AM to 6/22/04, 7:01 AM).
10. List drugs and food the client is taking that could affect test results.
11. When possible, withhold medications and foods that could cause false test results until after the test. Before withholding drugs, check with the health care provider. This may not be practical or possible; however, if the client takes medication and the laboratory test is abnormal, this should be brought to the health care provider's attention.
12. Promptly send the specimen to the laboratory.

Diagnostic Tests

1. A signed consent form is usually requested.
2. Food and fluid restriction is frequently ordered. Check with the procedure.
3. Institutional policies must be followed.

Factors Affecting Laboratory and Diagnostic Tests.

Factors that affect test results should be identified and avoided when possible. When test results are abnormal, determine if factors identified could be contributing to the test results, and report to health care provider.

Nursing Implications

1. Be knowledgeable about laboratory and diagnostic tests.
2. Explain the purpose(s) and procedure of each test to the client and family.
3. Provide time, and be available, to answer questions. Be supportive to the client and family.
4. Follow the procedure that is stated for each test. Label specimens with client information.
5. Relate test findings to clinical problems and drugs. The test may be repeated to confirm a suspected problem.
6. Report abnormal results to the health care provider.
7. Compare test results with other related laboratory and/or diagnostic tests.
8. Encourage clients to keep medical appointments for follow-up.
9. Provide health teaching related to the clinical problem.

10. With diagnostic tests:
   a. Have the client void before premedication or before the test, or both.
   b. Obtain a history of allergies to iodine or seafood. Observe for severe allergic reaction to contrast dye.
   c. Obtain baseline vital signs. Monitor vital signs as indicated following the test.
   d. If a sedative is used, instruct the client not to drive home.

Joyce LeFever Kee
Helen Tang-Yates
Linda S. Farmer

CONTRIBUTORS, CONSULTANTS, AND REVIEWERS

Diane Arbaugh, RT
Registered Mammographer
Papastavros Associates
Wilmington, Delaware

Mammography

Ellen K. Boyda, RN, MS, CRNP
Family Nurse Practitioner
Pulmonary Clinical Nurse Specialist
Independent Practice
Boothwyn, Pennsylvania

Acid-Base Balance
Papanicolaou Smear

Frank DiGregorio, Jr, CNMT, RDMS
Supervisor
Community Imaging Center
Wilmington, Delaware

Stress Tests (Thallium, Persantine,
*   Dobutamine)*
Echocardiography
Holter Monitoring
Nuclear Scans
Positron Emission Tomography (PET)
Ultrasonography

Heiddy M. DiGregorio, RMC
Christiana Care Health Services
Newark, Delaware

Updated selected nursing implications
*   for diagnostic tests*

Virgina L. Edwards, RN, MS, FNP
Assistant Clinical Professor
Division of Cardiology
School of Medicine
Medical College of Virginia
Richmond, Virginia

Angiography
Cardiac Catheterization

Linda S. Farmer, MT, ASCP
Laboratory Manager
St. Francis Hospital
Wilmington, Delaware

All Laboratory Tests

Judith Fullhart, MS, RN, CGRN
Gastroenterologic Nursing Manager
Veterans Affairs Medical Center
Wilmington, Delaware

Cholangiography Tests
Colonoscopy
Endoscopic Retrograde
*   Cholangiopancreatography*
Esophageal Studies
Esophagogastroduodenoscopy
Gastric Analysis
Gastrointestinal Series

Ronald J. LeFever, BS, RPh
Pharmacist
Pharmacy Services

Medical College of Virginia
Richmond, Virginia

Therapeutic Drug Monitoring (TDM)

David C. Sestili, CRTT, RPFT
Pulmonary Laboratories Manager
Medical Center of Delaware
Christiana Hospital
Newark, Delaware

Pulmonary Function Tests

Susan Summerton, MD
Radiologist
Papastavros Associates
Wilmington, Delaware

Mammography

Jane Purnell Taylor, RN, MS
Associate Professor
Division of Nursing and Health
    Sciences
Neumann College
Aston, Pennsylvania

Human Immunodeficiency Virus-Type 1
    (HIV-1)
Fetal Nonstress Tests
Fetoscopy

Helen Tang-Yates, BS, MT (ASCP), CLS
Health Center
University of Delaware
Newark, Delaware

Importance of Specimen Collection

Other Reviewers

Betteanne Riegle, RN, MS, CCHN
University at Buffalo
State University of New York
Buffalo, NY

Sue Elster, PhD, RN
Assistant Professor
Northern Illinois University School of
    Nursing
DeKalb, IL

PART ONE

Laboratory Tests

1

Acetaminophen (serum)

Tylenol, Tempra, Datril, Liquiprin, Paracetamol, Panadol, Aceta

Reference Values

Adult: *Therapeutic:* 5–20 μg/ml, 31–124 μmol/l (SI units). *Toxic:* >50 μg/ml, 305 μmol/l (SI units), >200 μg/ml possible hepatotoxicity.

Child: *Therapeutic:* Same as adult. *Toxic:* Similar to adult.

Description

Acetaminophen has a similar antipyretic and nonnarcotic analgesic effect to that of aspirin. Unlike salicylates (e.g., aspirin), acetaminophen does not inhibit platelet aggregation, does not produce gastric distress and bleeding, and has only a weak antiinflammatory response.

Overdose of acetaminophen can be dangerous, since it can lead to hepatotoxicity. It is metabolized in the liver to active metabolites and is absorbed rapidly from the gastrointestinal (GI) tract. Peak time occurs in ½ to 2 hours after oral ingestion. When there is an accumulation of acetaminophen in the body from massive dose(s) or chronic use, one of its metabolites tends to cause hepatotoxicity. Actually, a single dose of 10 g or 30 tablets (325 mg each) could cause liver damage. The half-life of acetaminophen is about 3 hours. If the half-life is >4 hours, hepatic injury is likely to occur. After ingestion of a large amount of acetaminophen, either accidentally (children) or in a suicide attempt, serum concentrations are plotted on a semilogarithmic scale. If the serum value is 200 μg/ml (1240 μmol/l) in 4 hours, or 50 μg/ml (310 μmol/l) in 12 hours after ingestion, hepatotoxicity could occur 3 to 6 days later. The antidote to acetaminophen toxicity is *N*-acetylcysteine. It must be administered soon after acetaminophen ingestion. Liver function tests (i.e., AST [SGOT], ALT [SGPT]), bilirubin, prothrombin time (PT), and electrolytes should be closely monitored.

Purposes

- To determine if the therapeutic acetaminophen dose is within therapeutic range.
- To check for acetaminophen toxicity.

Clinical Problems

Decreased Level: High-carbohydrate meal.

Elevated Level: Acetaminophen overdose, liver disease. *Drug Influence:* Phenobarbital.

Procedure

- Collect 3 to 5 ml of venous blood in red-top tube.
- Record the dose and the time the drug was taken on the laboratory requisition slip.
- There is no food or fluid restriction.

Factors Affecting Laboratory Results

- None known.

NURSING IMPLICATIONS WITH RATIONALE

- Explain to the client that the purpose of the test is to monitor the therapeutic level or the toxic level of acetaminophen (give trade name).
- Suggest to the health care provider that liver function tests be ordered periodically for clients on long-term acetaminophen therapy. Liver damage could result when the drug is taken for weeks and/or months.
- Keep the acetaminophen bottle tightly closed and away from light.

Elevated Level

- Recognize that liver disease and acetaminophen overdose could result in hepatotoxicity.
- Observe for signs and symptoms of acetaminophen toxicity (i.e., anorexia, nausea, vomiting, lethargy, generalized weakness, epigastric or abdominal pain).
- Observe for signs and symptoms of liver damage (i.e., vomiting, jaundice, right upper quadrant tenderness, abnormal liver function tests).

Client Teaching

- Inform the client about the need to take the prescribed dosage. An overdose or chronic use of acetaminophen could cause liver damage. Usually the drug should not be taken for more than 10 days at a time unless prescribed by the health care provider (HCP).
- Inform the client who consumes large amounts of alcohol of the need to consult his or her HCP before taking acetaminophen products. This person could be prone to liver damage, and ingestion of acetaminophen would compound the liver problem.
- Instruct the client to keep acetaminophen products out of the reach of children. If a child ingests large amounts of the drug, the poison center should be called immediately, syrup of ipecac given if indicated by the center, and the child taken to the emergency room. Acetylcysteine (Mucomyst) has been used as an antidote for adults within 16 hours after drug overdose.

Acetone, ketone bodies (serum or plasma)

Reference Values

Adult: *Acetone:* Semiquantitative: Negative (<1 mg/dl); quantitative: 0.3–2.0 mg/dl, 51.6–344.0 μmol/l (SI units). *Ketones:* 0.5–4 mg/dl.

Child: *Newborn to 1 Week:* Slightly higher than adult. *Over 1 Week:* Same as adult.

Description

Ketone bodies are composed of three compounds—acetone, acetoacetic (diacetic) acid, and betahydroxybutyric acid—which are products of fat metabolism and fatty acids. Ketone bodies result from uncontrolled diabetes mellitus and starvation, causing increased fat catabolism instead of carbohydrate metabolism. In diabetic ketoacidosis, the serum acetone is >50 mg/dl.

Ketones are small and excretable in the urine. However, the elevation is first apparent in the plasma or serum, then in the urine. Serum acetone (as ketones) is useful in monitoring acidosis caused by uncontrolled diabetes or starvation, since the serum level will decrease toward normal before the urine test (acetest) does.

Purposes

- To detect the presence of ketone bodies.
- To identify the occurrence of diabetic ketoacidosis.

Clinical Problems

Elevated Level: Diabetic ketoacidosis, starvation/malnutrition, vomiting and diarrhea, heat stroke, exercise.

Procedure

- Collect 3 to 5 ml of venous blood in a red-top tube.
- There is no food or fluid restriction.

Factors Affecting Laboratory Results

- Contamination can cause false-positive results.

> ### NURSING IMPLICATIONS WITH RATIONALE
>
> Elevated Level
>
> ■ Relate elevated serum acetone levels to diabetes acidosis and starvation. Many of the diet programs call for high-protein and low-carbohydrate intake. Daily carbohydrate intake of <100 g can result in ketosis (excess ketone bodies) caused by the substitution of fat metabolism for energy.
> ■ Obtain a history from the client concerning his or her diet. If the client is on a reducing diet, the elevated serum level (ketosis) could be caused by a low-carbohydrate diet.
> ■ Assess for signs and symptoms of diabetic ketoacidosis, such as rapid, vigorous breathing; restlessness; confusion; sweet-smelling breath; and a serum acetone level >50 mg/dl.
> ■ Check the urine for ketone bodies. An acetest is usually performed and is positive.

Acid phosphatase (ACP) (serum)

Prostatic Acid Phosphatase (PAP)

Reference Values

Adult: <2.6 ng/ml; 0–5 U/l range, varies according to the method used; 0.2–13 IU/l (SI units).

Description

The enzyme acid phosphatase (ACP) is found in the prostate gland and in semen in high concentration. It is found in lesser extent in bone marrow, red blood cells (RBCs), liver, and spleen. The highest rise in serum ACP occurs in prostatic cancer. In benign prostatic hypertrophy (BPH), the level is also above normal. A markedly elevated alkaline phosphatase level may cause a falsely high serum ACP level.

Purpose

■ To compare the ACP test with other laboratory values for diagnosing prostatic cancer or BPH.

Clinical Problems

Decreased Level: Down syndrome. *Drug Influence:* fluorides, oxalates, phosphates, alcohol.

Elevated Level: Carcinoma of the prostate, multiple myeloma, Paget's disease, cancer of the breast and bone, BPH, sickle cell anemia, cirrhosis, chronic renal failure, hyperparathyroidism, osteogenesis imperfecta, myocardial infarction. *Drug Influence:* Androgens in females, clofibrate (Atromid-S).

Procedure

- Collect 3 to 7 ml of venous blood in a red-top tube.
- Hemolysis should be prevented, and the specimen should be taken to the laboratory immediately. ACP is heat- and pH-sensitive. If the specimen is exposed to air and left at room temperature, there will be a decrease in activity after 1 hour.
- There is no food or fluid restriction.

Factors Affecting Laboratory Results

- Hemolysis of the blood sample can cause an inaccurate test result.
- Certain drugs can decrease the serum ACP level *(see Drug Influence, above)*.
- Exposure of the blood specimen to air and room temperature for longer than 1 hour can cause a decrease in the ACP level.

NURSING IMPLICATIONS WITH RATIONALE

Decreased Level

- Know which drugs can cause a decreased serum ACP level.

Elevated Level

- Recognize clinical problems associated with an elevated serum ACP level. A high serum ACP level occurs with metastasized prostatic cancer.
- Indicate on the laboratory slip if the client had a prostate examination 24 hours before the test. Prostatic massage or extensive palpation of the prostate can elevate the serum ACP.
- Check the serum ACP following treatment for carcinoma of the prostate gland. With surgical intervention, the serum level should drop in 3 to 4 days; following estrogen therapy (when the treatment is successful), it should drop in 3 to 4 weeks. If serum ACP has not been ordered, a reminder or suggestion to the physician may be necessary.
- Notify the laboratory before the serum ACP is drawn so that immediate attention will be given to the specimen.
- Encourage the client to express concerns about the prostate problem.

Activated partial thromboplastin time (APTT)
See Partial Thromboplastin Time

Adenovirus antibody (serum)

Reference Values

Adult and Child: Negative. **Positive:** Fourfold titer increase.

Description

The adenovirus is frequently present among school-aged children and military recruits; many may be asymptomatic. Adenovirus can be responsible for upper respiratory tract disease, cystitis (hemorrhagic), and keratoconjunctivitis. Transmission may be by direct or indirect contact.

Purpose

- To determine the cause of upper respiratory tract disease and pharyngitis.

Clinical Problems

Positive: Adenovirus infections of the upper respiratory tract, hemorrhagic cystitis, keratoconjunctivitis, pharyngitis.

Procedure

- There is no food or fluid restriction.
- Collect 3 to 5 ml of venous blood in a red-top tube. Avoid hemolysis. A second blood specimen is usually obtained 2 to 3 weeks later to determine the acute and convalescent titers. The blood specimen should be marked either acute or convalescent phase.
- A swab of the drainage from the infected area (e.g., the throat, eye, urethra) may be obtained for immunofluorescence testing to determine the presence of an adenoviral infection. The swab specimen should be labeled and taken immediately to the laboratory for testing.

Factors Affecting Laboratory Testing

- Hemolysis of the blood specimen.
- Inaccurate labeling of the blood sample.

NURSING IMPLICATIONS WITH RATIONALE

- Obtain a history from the client or family concerning the infected area involved. List symptoms the client may have (such as drainage and its color).
- Check with the client about contact with other persons who have described similar symptoms.

Client Teaching

- Explain to the client the procedure for laboratory testing. There will most likely be a second blood sample taken 2 to 3 weeks after the first blood specimen.
- If there is a swab specimen to be obtained, explain to the client that a swab will be taken of the infected area.
- Answer the client's or family's questions or refer to appropriate health care providers.

Adrenocorticotropic hormone (ACTH) (plasma)

Corticotropin, Corticotropin-Releasing Factor (CRF)

Reference Values

7 AM to 10 AM: 8–80 pg/ml; highest levels occur in early morning.

4 PM: 5–30 pg/ml.

10 PM to Midnight: <10 pg/ml; lowest levels occur at bedtime.

Description

Adrenocorticotropic hormone (ACTH), or corticotropin, is stored and released from the anterior pituitary gland (adenohypophysis) under the influence of corticotropin-releasing factor (CRF—from the hypothalamus) and the plasma cortisol from the adrenal cortex. The negative-feedback mechanism controls ACTH release; when plasma cortisol is low, ACTH is released, and when plasma cortisol is increased, ACTH release is inhibited. Stress caused by surgery, infections, and physical and emotional trauma increases the ACTH level. The ACTH level follows a diurnal pattern: peaks in the early morning and ebbs in the late evening or at bedtime.

A plasma ACTH is performed to determine whether a decreased plasma cortisol level is due to adrenal cortex hypofunction or pituitary hypofunction. Two tests, ACTH suppression and ACTH stimulation, may be ordered to identify the origin of the clinical problem, either the adrenal cortex or the pituitary gland.

ACTH Suppression Test: For the ACTH suppression test, a synthetic potent cortisol, dexamethasone (Decadron), is given to suppress the production of ACTH. If an extremely high dose is needed for ACTH suppression, the cause is of pituitary origin, such as pituitary tumor producing an excess of ACTH secretion. If the plasma cortisol continues to be high with ACTH suppression, the cause could be adrenal cortex hyperfunction (Cushing's syndrome). Suppressing pituitary release of ACTH will not affect a hyperactive adrenal gland.

ACTH Stimulation Test: For the ACTH stimulation test, ACTH (cosyntropin) is administered and the plasma cortisol level should double in 1 hour. If the plasma cortisol level remains the same or is lower, adrenal gland insufficiency (Addison's disease) is the cause.

To check for pituitary hypofunction, the drug metyrapone (Metopirone) is given to block the production of cortisol, thus causing an increase in ACTH secretion. If the ACTH level does not increase, the problem is pituitary insufficiency.

Purposes

- To determine if a decreased plasma cortisol level is due to adrenal cortex hypofunction or pituitary hypofunction.
- To evaluate the ACTH suppression test results for health problem of pituitary origin.
- To check for adrenal or pituitary hypofunction.
- To utilize the ACTH stimulation test to determine the presence of adrenal gland insufficiency.

Clinical Problems

Decreased Level: Adrenocortical hyperplasia, cancer of the adrenal gland, hypopituitarism. *Drug Influence:* Steroids (cortisone, prednisone, dexamethasone), estrogen, amphetamines, alcohol.

Elevated Level: Stress (trauma, physical or emotional), Addison's disease (adrenal hypofunction), pituitary neoplasm, surgery, pyrogens, pregnancy. *Drug Influence:* Metyrapone, vasopressin, insulin.

Procedure

- Food and fluid may be restricted. A low-carbohydrate diet may be requested for 24 hours prior to the test.
- Collect 5 to 7 ml of venous blood in a lavender-top *plastic* tube or prechilled purple-top tube. Pack the tube in ice *immediately* and send it to the laboratory. Blood should not come in contact with glass. If a glass tube is used, centrifuge and transfer to a plastic vial *as soon as possible* (ASAP). Additional testing may be needed because a single plasma value may be misleading.
- If adrenal hypofunction is suspected, the blood sample is taken at the peak time, which is early morning. When adrenal hyperfunction is suspected, the blood sample is usually taken at low time, which is in the evening.

- Note on the laboratory label the time the blood specimen was drawn. If the test is to be repeated the next morning, the blood sample should be drawn at the same time as the first specimen.
- Restrict activity and stress (if possible) for 8 to 12 hours before the test. When possible, restrict drugs such as cortisone until after the test.

Factors Affecting Laboratory Results

- Certain drugs *(see Drug Influence for decreased and elevated levels).*
- Stress and physical activity.
- Collection of the blood sample in a glass tube.
- Collection of the blood samples at different times of the day and not noting this on the laboratory slip.

NURSING IMPLICATIONS WITH RATIONALE

- Obtain a history of the client's clinical symptoms and drug regimen. Steroids increase the ACTH secretion.
- Compare elevated plasma ACTH levels with plasma cortisol if ordered. With adrenal gland insufficiency or a pituitary tumor, ACTH secretion will be increased.

Client Teaching

- Explain to the client undergoing ACTH suppression with dexamethasone or ACTH stimulation with ACTH or metyrapone that these drugs are used to confirm the cause of the hormonal imbalance.
- Encourage the client to avoid stress and physical exercise, for they could increase plasma ACTH levels.
- Be supportive of the client and the family. Allow time for the client to ventilate his/her fears.

AIDS *virus*

See Human Immunodeficiency Virus (HIV)

Alanine aminotransferase (ALT) (serum)

Serum Glutamic Pyruvic Transaminase (SGPT)

Reference Values

Adult: 10–35 U/l; 4–36 U/l at 37°C (SI units). *Male:* Levels may be slightly higher. Child: *Infant:* Could be twice as high as adult. *Child:* Similar to adult. Elderly: Slightly higher than adult.

Description

Alanine aminotransferase (ALT)/serum glutamic pyruvic transaminase (SGPT) is an enzyme found primarily in the liver cells and is effective in diagnosing hepatocellular destruction. It is also found in small amounts in the heart, kidney, and skeletal muscle.

Serum ALT levels can be higher than levels of its sister transferase (transaminase), aspartate aminotransferase (AST)/serum glutamic oxatoacetic transaminase (SGOT), in cases of acute hepatitis and liver damage from drugs and chemicals, with its serum levels reaching to 200 to 4000 U/l. ALT is used for differentiating between jaundice caused by liver disease and hemolytic jaundice. With jaundice, the serum ALT levels of liver origin can be higher than 300 units; from causes outside the liver, the levels can be <300 units. Serum ALT levels usually elevate before jaundice appears.

ALT/SGPT levels are frequently compared with AST/SGOT levels for diagnostic purposes. ALT is increased more markedly than AST in liver necrosis and acute hepatitis, while AST is more markedly increased in myocardial necrosis (acute myocardial infarction), cirrhosis, cancer of the liver, chronic hepatitis, and liver congestion. ALT levels are normal or slightly elevated in myocardial necrosis. The ALT levels return more slowly to normal range than AST levels in liver conditions.

Purpose

- To detect the presence of a liver disorder.

Clinical Problems

Decreased Level: Exercise. *Drug Influence: Salicylates.*

Elevated Level: *Highest Increase:* Acute (viral) hepatitis, necrosis of the liver (drug or chemical toxicity). *Slight or Moderate Increase:* Cirrhosis, cancer of the liver, congestive heart failure, acute alcohol intoxication. *Drug Influence:* Antibiotics (carbenicillin, clindamycin, erythromycin, gentamicin, lincomycin, mithramycin, spectinomycin, tetracycline), narcotics (meperidine [Demerol], morphine, codeine), antihypertensives (methyldopa, guanethidine), digitalis preparations, indomethacin (Indocin), salicylates, rifampin, flurazepam (Dalmane), propranolol (Inderal), oral contraceptives (progestin-estrogen), lead, heparin.

Procedure

- Collect 3 to 5 ml of venous blood in a red-top tube. Avoid hemolysis, because RBCs have a high concentration of ALT.
- There is no food or fluid restriction.
- Drugs administered to the client that can cause false-positive levels should be listed on the laboratory slip along with the date last given.

Factors Affecting Laboratory Results

- Hemolysis of the blood specimen may cause false test results.
- Aspirin can cause a decrease or increase of serum ALT.
- Certain drugs can increase the serum ALT level *(see Drug Influence above)*.

NURSING IMPLICATIONS WITH RATIONALE

Elevated Levels

- Relate the client's serum ALT/SGPT to clinical problems. A high serum elevation (>2000 U) can indicate liver necrosis from toxic agents or from acute viral hepatitis.
- Compare ALT and AST levels if both have been ordered. ALT is a better indicator of acute liver damage and will be at higher levels than AST in liver necrosis and acute hepatitis.
- Check for signs of jaundice. ALT levels rise several days before jaundice begins if it is related to liver damage. However, if jaundice is present and serum ALT levels are normal or slightly elevated, the liver may not be the cause of the jaundice.

Client Teaching

- Instruct the client to report signs of jaundice, such as yellow color in the sclera of the eyes.

Albumin (serum)

Reference Values

Adult: 3.5–5.0 g/dl; 52% to 68% of total protein.

Child: *Newborn:* 2.9–5.4 g/dl. *Infant:* 4.4–5.4 g/dl. *Child:* 4.0–5.8 g/dl.

Description

Albumin, a component of proteins, makes up more than half of plasma proteins. Albumin is synthesized by the liver. It increases osmotic pressure (oncotic pressure), which is necessary for maintaining the vascular fluid. A decrease in serum albumin will cause fluid to shift from within the vessels to the tissues, resulting in edema.

The *A/G ratio* is a calculation of the distribution of two major protein fractions, albumin and globulin. The reference value of A/G ratio is >1.0, which is the albumin value divided by globulin value (albumin ÷ globulin). A high ratio value is considered insignificant; low ratio value occurs in liver and renal diseases. Protein electrophoresis is more accurate and has replaced the A/G ratio calculation.

Purpose

- To detect an albumin deficit.

Clinical Problems

Decreased Level (Hypoalbuminemia): Cirrhosis of the liver, acute liver failure, severe burns, severe malnutrition, preeclampsia, renal disorders, certain malignancies, ulcerative colitis, prolonged immobilization, protein-losing enteropathies, malabsorption. *Drug Influence:* Penicillin, sulfonamides, aspirin, ascorbic acid.

Elevated Level (Hyperalbuminemia): Dehydration, severe vomiting, severe diarrhea. *Drug Influence:* Heparin.

Procedure

- Collect 3 to 5 ml of venous blood in a red-top tube.
- There is no food or fluid restriction.

Factors Affecting Laboratory Results

- Certain drugs could cause false negatives and false positives *(see Drug Influence above)*.

NURSING IMPLICATIONS WITH RATIONALE

- Check for peripheral edema and ascites when serum albumin is low. A low serum albumin decreases the oncotic pressure; thus fluid shifts from the vascular fluid to the tissue spaces, causing edema.
- Assess for skin integrity if pitted edema or anasarca is present. Implement measures to avoid skin breakdown.
- Offer foods high in protein (i.e., meats, cheese, beans).

Client Teaching
- Teach the client the importance of maintaining an adequate amount of protein in the diet with health care provider's approval. Protein should increase the serum albumin level and decrease peripheral edema unless the client has cirrhosis of the liver.

Alcohol (ethyl or ethanol) (serum or plasma)

Reference Values

No Alcohol: 00.0% *No Significant Alcohol Influence:* <0.05% or 50 mg/dl. *Alcohol Influence Present:* 0.05%–0.10% or 50–100 mg/dl. *Reaction Time Affected:* 0.10%–0.15% or 100–150 mg/dl. *Indicative of Alcohol Intoxication:* >0.15% or >150 mg/dl. *Severe Alcohol Intoxication:* >0.25% or 250 mg/dl. *Comatose:* >0.30% or 300 mg/dl. *Fatal:* >0.40% or 400 mg/dl.

Description

The ethyl alcohol (ethanol) level in the blood is a frequently requested laboratory test for medical and legal reasons. In most states an alcohol level >0.10% or 100 mg/dL is considered by law to be proof of alcohol intoxication. However, some states consider 0.08% or 80 mg/dl as proof of alcohol toxicity. On an empty stomach, plasma alcohol peaks in 40 to 70 minutes.

Serum/plasma alcohol may be used as a screening test on an unconscious client. Nurses should check for any legal ramifications (state laws) in reference to drawing blood for plasma alcohol levels.

Purpose

- To detect the percentage of alcohol in the blood stream and to determine whether the client was DUI (driving under the influence).

Clinical Problems

Elevated Level: Moderate to severe alcohol intoxication, chronic alcohol consumption, cirrhosis of the liver, malnutrition, folic acid deficiency, leukopenia, acute pancreatitis, gastritis, hypoglycemia, hyperuricemia. *Drug Influence:* Alcohol–drug interactions: (1) increases the effects of sedatives, hypnotics, narcotics, and tranquilizers (especially chlordiazepoxide [Librium] and diazepam [Valium]), depressing the central nervous system response; (2) antagonizes the action of warfarin (Coumadin) and phenytoin (Dilantin).

Procedure

- Obtain a consent form if required by law.
- Cleanse the venipuncture area with benzalkonium, and then wipe the solution off with a sterile swab or sponge. *Do not use* alcohol or tincture to cleanse the area.
- Collect 3 to 5 ml of venous blood in a red-top tube. A green-, lavender-, or blue-top tube can be used. Avoid hemolysis.
- Write on the specimen and laboratory slip the date and time the blood specimen was drawn. The signatures of the collector and a witness may be included on the tube (only for legal cases).

Factors Affecting Laboratory Results

- Methyl alcohol (wood alcohol) and isopropyl alcohol (rubbing alcohol) can cause elevated serum alcohol levels and are very toxic.
- Cleansing the venipuncture site with alcohol or tincture can cause inaccurate results.
- Alcohol–drug interactions can affect results *(see Drug Influence above)*.

NURSING IMPLICATIONS WITH RATIONALE

Elevated Level (>.0.10% or 100 mg/dl)

- Provide safety measures to prevent physical harm to the client when the serum alcohol level is greatly increased. Side rails may be needed while the client is sleeping off the effects of alcohol.
- Follow legal ramifications in your state for drawing plasma alcohol level.

Client Teaching

- Instruct the client not to consume alcoholic beverages when taking sedatives, hypnotics, narcotics, tranquilizers (Valium, Librium), anticonvulsants (Dilantin), and anticoagulants (Coumadin). Alcohol and tranquilizers can depress respirations and might cause respiratory arrest.
- Encourage the client to attend Alcoholics Anonymous (AA) meetings for chronic alcoholism. Listen to the client's concerns.

Aldolase (ALD) (serum)

Reference Values

Adult: <6 U/l, 3–8 U/dl (Sibley-Lehninger), 22–59 mU/l at 37°C (SI units).

Child: *Infant:* 12–24 U/dl (four times). *Child:* 6–16 U/dl (two times).

Description

Aldolase is an enzyme present most abundantly in the skeletal and cardiac muscles. This enzyme is used to monitor skeletal muscle diseases such as muscular dystrophy, dermatomyositis, and trichinosis. It is not elevated in muscle disease of neural origin, such as multiple sclerosis, poliomyelitis, and myasthenia gravis.

Serum aldolase is helpful in diagnosing early cases of Duchenne's muscular dystrophy before clinical symptoms appear. Progressive muscular dystrophy may cause elevated serum aldolase levels 10 to 15 times greater than normal. In late stages of muscular dystrophy, the enzyme level may return to normal or below normal. Serum aldolase is not the most effective diagnostic test for myocardial infarction (MI), because there is only a slight rise. Following an acute MI, it peaks (two times normal) in 24 hours and returns to normal in 4 to 7 days.

Purpose

- To aid in the diagnosis of skeletal muscle diseases, such as muscular dystrophy.

Clinical Problems

Decreased Level: Late muscular dystrophy.

Elevated Level: Early and progressive muscular dystrophy; trichinosis; dermatomyositis; acute MI; acute hepatitis; cancer of gastrointestinal tract, prostate, and liver; lymphosarcoma; leukemia. *Drug Influence:* Alcohol, cortisone, narcotics.

Procedure

- Collect 3 to 5 ml of venous blood in a red-top tube. Unhemolyzed serum must be used when measuring for aldolase.
- There is no food or fluid restriction.

Factors Affecting Laboratory Results

- Hemolysis causes false-positive results.

NURSING IMPLICATIONS WITH RATIONALE

Elevated Level

- Recognize the purpose of monitoring aldolase levels. This is a useful test for diagnosing muscular disorders.
- List on the laboratory slip any drugs the client is receiving that can elevate the serum aldolase level.
- Check serum aldolase results, and plan your nursing care according to symptoms present and psychologic needs.

Aldosterone (serum)

Reference Values

Adult: <16 ng/dl (fasting); 4–30 ng/dl (sitting position).

Child (3–11 years): 5–70 ng/dl.

Pregnancy: 2 to 3 times higher than adult.

Description

Aldosterone is the most potent of all mineralocorticoids produced by the adrenal cortex. Its major function is to regulate sodium, potassium, and water balance according to body needs. Aldosterone promotes sodium reabsorption from the distal tubules of the kidney and potassium and hydrogen excretion. With sodium reabsorption, water is retained. Eighty to 90% of aldosterone is inactivated in the liver.

This hormone responds to various changes in the body. When there is a sodium loss and a water loss, aldosterone is secreted for reestablishing sodium and water balance. Renin promotes aldosterone secretion, which causes more sodium and water to be retained and body fluid to be increased. Stress will increase aldosterone secretion. Hypernatremia (serum sodium excess) inhibits aldosterone secretion.

Serum aldosterone is not the most reliable test, because there can be fluctuations caused by various influences. If the client is in a supine position, serum aldosterone will be lower than if he or she were in a sitting or standing position. A 24-hour urine test is considered more reliable than a random serum aldosterone collection. Several serum aldosterone levels may be requested.

Purposes

- To detect deficit or excess of aldosterone.
- To compare serum and urine aldosterone levels with other laboratory tests for determining overhydration with elevated sodium level and adrenal hypo- or hyperfunction.

Clinical Problems

Decreased Level: Overhydration with increased sodium, severe hypernatremia (sodium excess), high-sodium diet, adrenal cortical hypofunction, diabetes mellitus, licorice ingestion (excessive), glucose caused by excess infusion.

Elevated Level: Dehydration, hyponatremia (sodium deficit), low-sodium diet, essential hypertension, adrenal cortical hyperfunction, cancer of the adrenal gland, cirrhosis of the liver, emphysema, severe congestive heart failure (CHF). *Drug Influence:* Diuretics (furosemide [Lasix] and others), hydralazine (Apresoline), diazoxide (Hyperstat), nitroprusside.

Procedure

- Collect 5 ml of venous blood in a red-top tube. A green-top tube (heparinized) may also be used.
- The client should be in a supine position for at least 1 hour before the blood is drawn.
- Write the date and time on the specimen. Aldosterone levels exhibit circadian rhythm, with peak levels occurring in the morning and lower levels in the afternoon.
- Food and fluids are not restricted, but excess salt and interfering substances (licorice) should not be consumed before the test. Normal salt intake is suggested.

Factors Affecting Laboratory Results

- A high- or low-salt diet can affect test results.
- Prolonged use of potent diuretics affects test results.
- Excessive licorice and glucose ingestion may decrease test results.
- Sitting or standing when blood is drawn may cause false-positive results.

NURSING IMPLICATIONS WITH RATIONALE

- Assess the client for signs and symptoms of dehydration when the serum aldosterone is elevated, such as poor skin turgor, dry mucous membranes, and shocklike symptoms, and for hyponatremia when the serum aldosterone is elevated.
- Compare the serum aldosterone and the 24-hour urine aldosterone results if both have been ordered.
- Record vital signs on the client. A rapid pulse and later a drop in blood pressure could be indicative of hypovolemia (fluid volume deficit).

Client Teaching

- Instruct the client to remain in a supine position for at least 1 hour before blood is drawn to prevent false test results.

Aldosterone (urine)

Reference Values

Adult: 6–25 µg/24 hours

Description

(See the Description for Aldosterone [Serum].)

Aldosterone causes sodium reabsorption and potassium excretion from the distal tubules of the kidney. Aldosterone secretion from the adrenal cortex influences sodium retention, fluid retention, fluid volume, and blood pressure.

A 24-hour urine aldosterone level has an advantage over a serum aldosterone level, because fluctuation levels can be eliminated. Both urine and serum aldosterone will be increased by hyponatremia, a low-salt diet, and hyperkalemia. Likewise, hypernatremia, a high-salt diet, and hypokalemia will decrease urine and serum aldosterone. A urine sodium test may be ordered for comparison purposes.

Purposes

See Aldosterone (Serum).

Clinical Problems

Decreased Level: Same as for serum aldosterone.

Elevated Level: Tumors of the adrenal cortex or primary aldosteronism, same as for serum aldosterone.

Procedure

- Collect a 24-hour urine specimen in a large container with an acidic preservative.
- Have the client void, and discard the urine before the test begins.
- Label the container with the exact date and time for the test (e.g., 4/9/04, 7:35 AM to 4/10/04, 7:35 AM).

Factors Affecting Laboratory Results

- Failure to place all urine collected in a 24-hour period in the urine container can cause false results.
- Toilet paper and feces in the urine affect test results.

NURSING IMPLICATIONS WITH RATIONALE

- Check at specified times to determine whether the urine collection is being properly obtained.

Client Teaching

- Instruct the client on how to collect the 24-hour urine specimen. All urine should be saved after the initial urine is discarded. The urine may be kept on ice or refrigerated if indicated. Toilet paper or feces should not be in the urine.
- Answer the client's questions concerning the test and the collection procedure.

Alkaline phosphatase (ALP) with isoenzyme (serum)

Reference Values

Adult: 42–136 U/l; ALP[1]: 20–130 U/l; ALP[2]: 20–120 U/l.

Child: *Infant and child (aged 0–12 years):* 40–115 U/l. *Older child (13–18 years):* 50–230 U/l.

Elderly: Slightly higher than adult.

Description

Alkaline phosphatase (ALP) is an enzyme produced mainly in the liver and bone; it is also derived from the intestine, kidney, and placenta. The ALP test is useful for determining liver and bone diseases. In cases of mild liver-cell damage, the ALP level may be only slightly elevated, but it could be markedly elevated in acute liver disease. Once the acute phase is over, the serum level will promptly decrease, whereas the serum bilirubin will remain increased. For determining liver dysfunction, several laboratory tests are performed (i.e., bilirubin, leucine aminopeptidase [LAP], 5'-nucleotidase [5'-NT], and gamma-glutamyl transpeptidase [GGTP]).

With bone disorders, the ALP level is increased because of abnormal osteoblastic activity (bone cell production). In children it is not abnormal to find high levels of ALP before and during puberty because of bone growth.

Isoenzymes of ALP are used to distinguish between liver and bone diseases, ALP[1] indicating disease of liver origin, and ALP[2], bone origin.

Purposes

- To determine the presence of a liver or bone disorder.
- To compare ALP results with other laboratory tests for confirmation of a liver or bone disorder.

Clinical Problems

Decreased Level: Hypothyroidism, malnutrition, scurvy (vitamin C deficit), hypophosphatasia, pernicious anemia, placental insufficiency. *Drug Influence:* Fluoride, oxalate, propranolol (Inderal).

Elevated Level: Obstructive biliary disease (jaundice), cancer of the liver, hepato-cellular cirrhosis, hepatitis, hyperparathyroidism, leukemia, cancer of the bone (breast and prostate), Paget's disease, osteitis deformans, healing fractures, multiple myeloma, osteomalacia, late pregnancy, rheumatoid arthritis (active), ulcerative disease. *Drug Influence:* IV albumin, antibiotics (erythromycin, lincomycin, oxacillin, penicillin), colchicine, methyldopa (Aldomet), allopurinol, phenothiazine tranquilizers, indomethacin (Indocin), procainamide, oral contraceptives (some), tolbutamide, isoniazid (INH), paraaminosalicylic acid (PAS).

Procedure

- Collect 3 to 5 ml of venous blood in a red-top tube. Avoid hemolysis.
- There is no food or fluid restriction. For ALP isoenzymes, fasting overnight might be indicated.
- Withhold for 8 to 24 hours drugs that can elevate the ALP level, with health care provider's permission.
- List the client's age and drugs that may affect test results on the laboratory slip.

Factors Affecting Laboratory Results

- Certain drugs that increase or decrease the serum ALP levels may cause false results *(see Drug Influence above).*
- Administered IV albumin can elevate the serum ALP to 5 to 10 times its normal value.
- Age of the client (i.e., youth and old age cause a serum increase).
- Late pregnancy to 3 weeks postpartum, which could cause a serum ALP elevation.

NURSING IMPLICATIONS WITH RATIONALE

- Know factors that can elevate serum ALP levels, such as drugs, IV albumin (can elevate serum ALP 5 to 10 times its normal value), age of client (elevated in children and elderly), late pregnancy to 3 weeks postpartum, and blood drawn 2 to 4 hours after a fatty meal.
- Record pertinent information from the procedure on the laboratory slip.
- Assess for clinical signs and symptoms of liver or bone disease.
- Check the results of other ordered liver tests to determine the significance of the elevated serum ALP in liver disease.

Client Teaching

- Inform the client that other enzyme tests may be ordered to verify diagnosis.

Alpha-1-antitrypsin (α-1-AT) (serum)

Alpha-1-Trypsin Inhibitor

Reference Values

Adult: 78–200 mg/dl, 0.78–2.0 g/l.

Child: *Newborn:* 145–270 mg/dl. *Infant:* Similar to adult range.

Description

Antitrypsin (α-1-AT), or trypsin inhibitor, is a protein produced by the liver. It inhibits specific proteolytic enzymes that are released in the lung by bacteria or by phagocytic cells. A deficiency of homozygous antitrypsin (heredity linked) permits proteolytic enzymes to damage lung tissue, thus causing emphysema.

With inflammatory conditions, α-1-AT serum level can be increased. Following the inflammatory insult that could result from a surgical wound, the serum α-1-AT increases in 2 to 3 days and can remain elevated for 1 to 2 weeks. The serum level then returns to normal.

Purposes

- To determine if chronic obstructive pulmonary disease is caused by a deficiency of α-1-AT.
- To detect the presence of α-1-AT deficiency.

Clinical Problems

Decreased Level: Chronic obstructive lung disease (pulmonary emphysema), severe liver damage, malnutrition, severe protein-losing (nephrotic) syndrome.

Elevated Level: Acute and chronic inflammatory conditions, infections (selected), necrosis, late pregnancy, exercise (returns to normal in 1 day). *Drug Influence:* Oral contraceptives.

Procedure

- Collect 3 to 5 ml of venous blood in a red-top tube.
- Keep the client NPO, except for water, for 8 hours before drawing blood.
- Hold oral contraceptives for 24 hours before the test, with the health care provider's permission. Any oral contraceptive taken should be listed on the laboratory slip.

Factors Affecting Laboratory Results

- Oral contraceptives can increase the α-1-AT level.

- Oral intake of food before the test can cause an inaccurate result, especially if the client has an elevated serum cholesterol or serum triglyceride level.

NURSING IMPLICATIONS WITH RATIONALE

Decreased Level

- Recognize clinical problems that are associated with α-1-AT deficiency (e.g., emphysema).

Client Teaching

- Explain to the client that the test is ordered to determine whether there is an antitrypsin (protein) deficiency that can cause a lung disorder (disease). A non-smoker with an α-1-AT deficiency can have emphysema. Antitrypsin inhibits proteolytic enzymes from destroying lung tissue; with a lack of this protein, the alveoli are damaged.
- Instruct the client that he or she should have nothing by mouth except water for 8 hours before the blood test; this restriction before the blood test may vary among health care providers (HCP).
- Instruct the client with an α-1-AT deficit to use preventive methods in protecting his or her lungs (i.e., avoid persons with upper respiratory infection [URI], seek medical care when having a respiratory infection).
- Encourage the client to stop smoking and to avoid areas having highly polluted air. Air pollution can cause respiratory inflammation and can promote chronic obstruction lung disease.

Elevated Level

- Check the serum α-1-AT level 2 to 3 days after extensive surgery. Inflammation can markedly increase the serum level. A baseline serum level may be ordered before surgery for several reasons (e.g., for determining lung disease and the effects of surgery).
- Report if the serum α-1-AT remains elevated 2 weeks after surgery.
- Note that serum α-1-AT can be markedly elevated during late pregnancy.

Alpha fetoprotein (AFP) (serum and amniotic fluid)

Reference Values

Nonpregnancy: <15 ng/ml.

Pregnancy:

SERUM		AMNIOTIC FLUID	
Weeks of Gestation	ng/ml	Weeks of Gestation	ng/ml
8–12	0–39	14	11.0–32.0
13	6–31	15	5.5–31.0
14	7–50	16	5.7–31.5
15	7–60	17	3.8–32.5
16	10–72	18	3.6–28.0
17	11–90	19	3.7–24.5
18	14–94	20	2.2–15.0
19	24–112	21	3.8–18.0
20	31–122		
21	19–124		

Description

Serum alpha fetoprotein (AFP), a screening test, is usually done between 16 and 20 weeks' gestation to determine the probability of twins, or to detect low birth weight or serious birth defects, such as open neural-tube defect. If a high serum AFP level occurs, the test should be repeated one week later. Ultrasound and amniocentesis may be performed to confirm elevated serum levels and to diagnose neural-tube defects in the fetus.

Purpose

- To identify the probability of neural-tube defects, fetal death, or other anomalies in pregnancy *(see Clinical Problems)*.

Clinical Problems

Decreased Level: Down's syndrome, absence of pregnancy.

Elevated Level: *Nonpregnant:* Cirrhosis of the liver (not liver metastasis), hepatitis, germ-cell tumor of gonads, such as testicular cancer, metastases to liver. *Pregnant:* Neural-tube defects (spina bifida, anencephaly, myelomeningocele), fetal death, fetal distress, Turner's syndrome, other anomalies (duodenal atresia, tetralogy of Fallot, hydrocephalus, trisomy 13), severe Rh immunization.

Procedure

- Collect 5 to 7 ml of venous blood in a red-top tube. Avoid hemolysis.
- There is no food or fluid restriction.

Factors Affecting Laboratory Results

- Fetal blood contamination could cause an elevated amniotic AFP level.
- Inaccurate recording of gestation week could affect results.
- Multiple pregnancy or fetal death could cause a false-positive test.
- Hemolysis of blood sample could affect results.
- Body weight may be a factor (although not definitely confirmed). A heavier female tends to have a lower serum AFP level.

NURSING IMPLICATIONS WITH RATIONALE

- Explain that the test is for screening purposes. If the test is positive, genetic counseling might be necessary.
- Be supportive of individuals and family.

Client Teaching

- Instruct the client that it is essential to give the correct gestation date of the pregnancy, if known, to avoid a laboratory test error. Inform the client that the test might be repeated in a week.
- If an ultrasound is performed, instruct the client that it is usually done to confirm gestational age or to confirm the positive serum AFP and amniocentesis result(s).

Alzheimer's disease markers

See Amyloid Beta Protein Precursor (CSF)

Amino acid (urine)

Reference Values

Normal values are age dependent; 200 mg/24 h.

Description

This test screens for elevated levels of amino acid in the urine (aminoaciduria), which can indicate inborn errors of metabolism. With abnormal metabolism there can be an excess in one or more amino acids in the plasma and urine. The test is performed when genetic abnormalities are suspected. The amino acid screening test is postive when there is an increase in amino acid or its metabolites in the urine.

Aminoaciduria disease can include phenylketonuria, maple-syrup urine disease, cystinuria, and tyrosinemia. Further testing would be needed to confirm the metabolic disorder.

Purposes

- To screen for renal aminoacidurias.
- To detect inborn errors of metabolism.

Clinical Problems

Elevated Level: Mental retardation, retarded growth, cystinuria, severe brain damage, oasthouse urine disease, phenylketonuria, tyrosinosis, ketosis. *Drug Influence:* Penicillins, valproic acid.

Procedure

- There is no food or fluid restriction.
- Collect a clean random urine specimen. A 24-hour urine specimen may be requested.
- Pack the specimen in ice and send immediately to the laboratory. Refrigeration can be used.

Factors Affecting Laboratory Results

- Lack of protein ingestion in 48 hours can affect test results.
- Failure to ice or refrigerate the specimen.

NURSING IMPLICATIONS WITH RATIONALE

- Obtain a history of health problems that may relate to the abnormal metabolism disorder.

■ Check the drug history; notify the health care provider if the client is taking a penicillin derivative.

■ Allow the client and family time to express their concerns.

Ammonia (plasma)

Reference Values

Adult: 15–45 μg/dl, 11–35 μmol/l (SI units).

Child: *Newborn:* 64–107 μg/dl. *Child:* 29–70 μg/dl; 29–70 μmol/l (SI units).

Description

Ammonia, a by-product of protein metabolism, is formed from the bacterial action in the intestine and from metabolizing tissues. Most of the ammonia is absorbed into the portal circulation and is converted in the liver to urea. With severe liver decompensation or when blood flow to the liver is altered, the plasma ammonia level remains elevated.

Elevated plasma ammonia is best correlated with hepatic failure; however, other conditions that interfere with liver function (congestive heart failure [CHF], acidosis) may cause a temporary elevation of plasma ammonia.

Purpose

■ To detect a liver disorder from the inability of the liver to convert ammonia to urea.

Clinical Problems

Decreased Level: Renal failure, malignant hypertension, essential hypertension. *Drug Influence:* Antibiotics (neomycin, tetracycline, kanamycin), monoamine oxidase inhibitors, diphenhydramine (Benadryl), potassium salts, sodium salts.

Elevated Level: Hepatic failure, hepatic encephalopathy or coma, portacaval anastomosis, Reye's syndrome, erythroblastosis fetalis, cor pulmonale, CHF, pulmonary emphysema, high-protein diet with liver failure, acidosis, exercise. *Drug Influence:* Ammonia chloride, diuretics (thiazides, furosemide [Lasix], ethacrynic acid [Edecrin]), ion exchange resin, isoniazid (INH).

Procedure

■ Collect 5 ml of venous blood in a green-top tube. The blood sample should be delivered immediately in packed ice to the laboratory. Ammonia levels increase rapidly after blood is drawn.

- Minimize use of tourniquet for drawing blood.
- There is no food or fluid restriction unless indicated by the laboratory. Smoking should be avoided before the test.
- List drugs the client is taking that could affect test results.

Factors Affecting Laboratory Results

- Failure to place the blood sample on ice and to analyze it immediately can result in a false test.
- A high- or low-protein diet can cause false test result.
- Exercise might increase the plasma ammonia level.
- Certain antibiotics (neomycin and tetracycline) decrease the ammonia level.

NURSING IMPLICATIONS WITH RATIONALE

Elevated Level

- Identify clinical problems and drugs that can increase the plasma ammonia level.
- Notify the laboratory personnel when a plasma ammonia level is drawn so that it can be analyzed immediately to avoid false results.
- List antibiotics on the laboratory slip. Certain antibiotics (such as neomycin and tetracycline) can decrease the ammonia level, causing a false result.
- Observe for signs and symptoms of hepatic failure, especially when the plasma ammonia is elevated. There are many neurologic changes, such as behavioral and personality changes, lethargy, confusion, flapping tremors of the extremities, twitching, and, later, coma.
- Recognize that exercise may be a cause of an elevated plasma-ammonia level.
- Know various treatments used in decreasing the plasma ammonia level. A few of these are a low-protein diet, antibiotics (such as neomycin) to destroy intestinal bacteria, enemas, cathartics (such as magnesium sulfate) to prevent ammonia formation, and sodium glutamate and L-arginine in IV dextrose solution to stimulate urea formation.

Client Teaching

- Explain to the client why he or she may be NPO 8 hours before the test: Foods containing protein may cause a higher ammonia level.

Amylase with isoenzymes (serum)

Reference Values

Adult: 60–160 Somogyi U/dl, 30–170 U/l (SI units).

Pregnancy: Slightly increased.

Child: Not usually done.

Elderly: Slightly higher than adult.

Serum Isoenzymes: S (salivary) type: 45–70%. P (pancreatic) type: 30–55%. Values may differ with method used.

Description

Amylase is an enzyme that is derived from the pancreas, the salivary glands, and the liver. Its function is to change starch to sugar. In acute pancreatitis, serum amylase is increased to twice its normal level. Its level begins to increase 2 to 12 hours after onset, peaks in 20 to 30 hours, and returns to normal in 2 to 4 days. Acute pancreatitis is frequently associated with inflammation, severe pain, and necrosis caused by digestive enzymes (including amylase) escaping into the surrounding tissue.

Increased serum amylase can occur after abdominal surgery involving the gallbladder (stones or biliary duct) and stomach (partial gastrectomy). Following abdominal surgery, some surgeons order a routine serum amylase for 2 days to determine whether the pancreas has been injured.

The urine amylase level is helpful in determining the significance of a normal or slightly elevated serum amylase, especially when the client has symptoms of pancreatitis. Amylase levels can also be obtained from abdominal fluid, ascitic fluid, pleural effusion, and saliva.

There are two types of amylase isoenzymes, P type (pancreatic origin) and S type (salivary origin). P-type elevation occurs more frequently in acute pancreatitis. Elevated S type can occur as a result of parotitis, and ovarian and bronchogenic tumors. Amylase isoenzymes are usually ordered to rule out a nonpancreatic source of the elevated serum amylase level. A pancreatic isoenzyme kit is commercially available.

Purpose

- To assist in the diagnosis of acute pancreatitis and other health problems *(see Clinical Problems)*.

Clinical Problems

Decreased Level: Intravenous 5% dextrose in water (IV D$_5$W), advanced chronic pancreatitis, acute and subacute necrosis of the liver, chronic alcoholism, toxic hepatitis, severe burns, severe thyrotoxicosis. *Drug Influence:* Glucose (IV D$_5$W), citrates, fluorides, oxalates.

Increased Level: Acute pancreatitis, chronic pancreatitis (acute onset), partial gastrectomy, peptic ulcer performation, obstruction of pancreatic duct, acute cholecystitis, cancer of the pancreas, diabetic acidosis, diabetes mellitus, acute alcoholic intoxication, mumps, renal failure, benign prostatic hypertrophy, burns, pregnancy. *Drug Influence:* Meperidine (Demerol), codeine, morphine, bethanechol chloride (Urecholine), pentazocine (Talwin), ethyl alcohol (large amounts), ACTH, guanethidine, thiazides, salicylates, tetracycline.

Procedure

- Obtain 3 to 5 ml of venous blood in a red-top tube.
- Restrict food for 1 to 2 hours before the blood sample is drawn. If the client has eaten or has received a narcotic 2 hours before the test, the serum results could be invalid.
- List on the laboratory slip drugs that could cause a false amylase level.

Factors Affecting Laboratory Results

- Narcotic drugs can cause false-positive levels.
- IV fluids with glucose can result in false-negative levels.
- Contamination of the specimen with saliva can occur through coughing, sneezing, or talking when the tube is opened. This could cause false-positive results.

NURSING IMPLICATIONS WITH RATIONALE

Decreased Level

- Know that D$_5$W administered intravenously can decrease the serum amylase level, causing a false-negative result.
- Identify drugs that give false-negative levels.
- Determine when the client has ingested food or sweetened fluids. Blood should not be drawn until 2 hours after eating because sugar can decrease the serum amylase level.

Elevated Level

- Know the disease entities related to increased levels, especially acute pancreatitis, abdominal surgery (partial gastrectomy, biliary resection), diabetes mellitus, cancer of the pancreas, acute alcoholic intoxication, and benign prostatic hypertrophy.
- Label the laboratory slip (for serum amylase) with the drugs the client is receiving or has received in the last 24 hours. Morphine, meperidine, codeine, pentazocine, aspirin, and hydrochlorothiazide can cause a false-positive serum amylase level.

- Check serum amylase levels for several days after abdominal surgery. Surgery of the stomach or gallbladder might cause trauma to the pancreas and cause excess amylase to be released.
- Report symptoms of severe pain when pancreatitis is suspected. The health care provider may want to draw a serum amylase level before a narcotic is given. An elevated level may indicate an acute pancreatitis.
- Explain to the client that blood is drawn for determining whether the severe pain is due to a pancreatic problem or to another cause.
- Ask the client if he or she has had pancreatitis before and has taken narcotic analgesics. A report should be given to the health care provider.
- Report elevated serum amylase results occurring beyond 3 days. If the serum amylase levels remain elevated beyond 3 days (72 hours), pancreatic cell destruction could still be occurring.

Client Teaching

- Instruct the client to assume adequate health practices, such as controlling alcohol intake and increasing protein and carbohydrates in the diet.

Amylase (urine)

Reference Values

Adult: 4–37 U/l/2 h.

Description

(See Amylase [Serum].)

Amylase is an enzyme that is produced by the pancreas, salivary glands, and liver and is excreted by the kidneys. When there is an inflammation of the pancreas or salivary gland, more amylase goes into the blood and more amylase is excreted in the urine. The urine levels of amylase could remain elevated for a week, whereas the serum amylase level tends to remain elevated for a short time (peaks in 24 hours and returns to normal in 48 to 96 hours).

The urine amylase test is ordered at 1-hour, 2-hour, or 24-hour timed intervals, with the 2-hour urine specimen the most commonly ordered. A 24-hour specimen may be within normal range, whereas a 2-hour specimen shows an increase.

One drawback of urine amylase as well as of serum amylase values is their relation to renal function. A diminished renal function could lead to a decrease in urine amylase and increased serum amylase.

Purpose

See Amylase (Serum).

Clinical Problems

Decreased Level: Diminished renal function. *See Amylase (Serum).*

Increased Level: Acute pancreatitis, choledocholithiasis. *See Amylase (Serum).*

Procedure

- A timed urine collection is required; thus the exact beginning and end of the urine collection should be recorded (date, hour, and minute; e.g., 2/10/04, 9:02 AM to 2/10/04, 11:05 AM). First the client voids and the urine is discarded.
- The urine specimen should be refrigerated or kept on ice. No preservative is needed.

Factors Affecting Laboratory Results

- Fecal material or toilet paper contamination can affect test results.
- Diminished urine output affects test results.
- Drugs that increase or decrease amylase levels are listed at drug influence.
- Prolonged urine collection time affects test results.

NURSING IMPLICATIONS WITH RATIONALE

Decreased Level

- Check urinary output for 8 hours and 24 hours, blood urea nitrogen (BUN), and serum creatinine levels. A decrease in urine output and an increase in BUN and serum creatinine levels indicate poor kidney function. A decreased urine output could result in a decreased urine amylase.

Client Teaching

- Explain to the client the importance of collecting urine at a specified time. The client should use a urinal or bedpan and should be instructed that all urine should be saved.
- Encourage the client to drink water during the test unless water intake is restricted for medical reasons. A decreased urine output could result in no 2-hour specimen or a possible false result.

Increased Level

- Check urinary output and give fluids if the urine output is decreased. Encouraging fluids during the test should help in securing a urine specimen.
- Check the serum amylase level(s) and compare with the urine amylase level. A low serum amylase level and an increased urine amylase level could indicate that the acute problem is no longer present.

- List on the laboratory slip the drugs the client is receiving that can increase amylase levels (e.g., narcotics).
- Notify the health care provider when the client is having severe abdominal pain. The health care provider may want to order a 2-hour or 24-hour urine specimen the next day.

Amyloid beta protein precursor (CSF)

Alzheimer's Disease Marker

Reference Values

Normal: 450 units/l cerebrospinal fluid (CSF)

Description:

A CSF test that can aid in diagnosing Alzheimer's disease is amyloid beta protein precursor test. It is found that the amyloid beta protein is present in the senile plaques within the brain. Amyloid can also be found in the meningeal blood vessels of clients with Alzheimer's disease. It is believed that this type of protein may have neurotoxic effects on the brain cells. Small amounts of amyloid can be found in the CSF of most healthy persons; however, a higher value occurs in the CSF of clients with Alzheimer's, and a somewhat slightly higher value than normal may occur in an aged client with senile dementia.

Purpose

- To aid with the diagnosis of Alzheimer's disease.

Clinical Problems

Elevated Level: Alzheimer's disease, senile dementia.

Procedure

- A consent form should be signed.
- There is no food or fluid restriction.
- The bladder should be emptied.
- The client's position for the procedure is lying on his/her side in a "fetal" or a sitting position.
- The client should remain relaxed and still during the procedure. Taking deep breaths may help the client to relax.
- Collect at least 2 ml of CSF and place the fluid specimen in a sterile tube.

Factors Affecting Laboratory Results

- Blood in the spinal fluid can cause false test results.

NURSING IMPLICATIONS WITH RATIONALE

Client Teaching

- Explain to the client and family the test procedure. A family member may wish to be with the client during the test procedure.
- Answer the client or family member's questions, and if unknown, refer the questions to the appropriate health professional.

Posttest

- Place client in a reclining position for 8 to 12 hours; the client can turn side to side. The client's head should not be raised to avoid "spinal" headache, which could occur from leaking of spinal fluid at the needle insertion site.
- Report any numbness or tingling in the extremities.
- Encourage the client to increase fluid intake for the next 24 hours.

Angiotensin-converting enzyme (ACE) (serum)

Angiotensin-1-Converting Enzyme

Reference Values

Adult >20 yrs: 8–67 U/l.

Child and Adult <20 yrs: Test is NOT performed because they normally have elevated ACE levels.

Description

Angiotensin-converting enzyme (ACE) is found primarily in the lung epithelial cells and to a lesser extent in blood vessels and renal cells. The purpose of ACE is to regulate arterial blood pressure by converting angiotensin I to the vasoconstrictor angiotensin II, which increases blood pressure and stimulates the adrenal cortex to release aldosterone (sodium-retaining hormone). However, this test has little value for diagnosing hypertension.

High serum ACE levels are found primarily with active sarcoidosis. This test should not be performed for clients who are under 20 years of age because they normally have elevated ACE levels. Approximately 5% of the population has an elevated ACE level. The purpose for the ACE test is to diagnose and determine the severity of pulmonary sarcoidosis. Seventy to 90% of clients with active sarcoidosis have elevated serum ACE levels. Other conditions that have elevated ACE levels include Gaucher's disease (disorder of fat metabolism), leprosy, alcoholic cirrhosis, active histoplasmosis, tuberculosis, pulmonary embolism, hyperthyroidism, and Hodgkin's disease.

Purposes

- To assist in diagnosing various healh problems, such as pulmonary sarcoidosis, related to an elevated serum ACE level.
- To compare the results of serum ACE levels with other laboratory tests for diagnosing a health problem.

Clinical Problems

Decreased Level: Therapy for sarcoidosis, diabetes mellitus, hypothyroidism, respiratory distress syndrome, severe illness. *Drug Influence:* Steroids (prednisone, cortisone).

Elevated Level: Sarcoidosis, Gaucher's disease, leprosy, alcoholic cirrhosis, histoplasmosis, tuberculosis, pulmonary embolism, hyperthyroidism, Hodgkin's disease, myeloma, non-Hodgkin's lymphoma, idiopathic pulmonary fibrosis, scleroderma.

Procedure

- The client should be NPO for 12 hours prior to the test.
- Collect 7 ml of venous blood in a red-top (preferred) or green-top tube. Check with the laboratory concerning which tube to use, the clotted blood (red-top) or heparinized (green-top) tube. Avoid hemolysis. Deliver the blood sample immediately to the laboratory.
- Record the client's age on the laboratory slip.

Factors Affecting Laboratory Results

- Hemolysis of the blood sample affects test results. A delay in testing the blood could cause a low serum ACE level.
- Persons under 20 years of age usually have an elevated serum ACE level; thus the test could be false-positive.
- Steroids (cortisone preparations) can decrease the serum ACE level.

NURSING IMPLICATIONS WITH RATIONALE

- Check blood pressure. This test is not used to determine the cause of hypertension; however, ACE indirectly contributes to increase in blood pressure.
- Record the age of the client on the laboratory slip. Rarely is this test ordered for a client under 20 years of age.
- Suggest that the test be canceled or postponed if the client is under 20 years old.

Client Teaching

- Instruct the client that he or she should have nothing by mouth for 12 hours prior to the test. This would most likely be NPO after dinner.
- Answer questions or concerns the client may have about the test or health problems. If necessary, refer questions to other health care providers.

Anion gap

Reference Values

Adult: 10–17 mEq/l (values differ from 7 to 20 mEq/L).

Description

The anion gap is the difference between electrolytes, the positive ions (cations), sodium and potassium, and the negative ions (anions), chloride and bicarbonate (serum CO_2) to determine if an acid–base imbalance is present. Unmeasured anions in the serum such as phosphates, sulfates, lactates, ketone bodies, and other organic acids contribute to metabolic acid–base imbalances (metabolic acidosis and alkalosis). Actually, the difference between the milliequivalents of cations and anions is referred to as the *anion gap*.

Serum levels of the cations, sodium and potassium, and the anions, chloride and bicarbonate, are applied to the formula:

$$\text{Anion gap} = (\text{sodium} + \text{potassium}) - (\text{chloride} + CO_2 \text{ [bicarbonate]})$$

An elevated anion gap (>17 mEq/l) indicates metabolic acidosis; a decreased anion gap (<10 mEq/l) indicates metabolic alkalosis.

Purpose

- To determine the presence of acidosis.

Clinical Problems

Decreased Level (<10 mEq/l): High electrolyte values such as sodium, calcium, magnesium; multiple myeloma, nephrosis. *Drug Influence:* Lithium, diuretics, chlorpropamide.

Elevated Level (>17 mEq/l): Lactic acidosis, ketoacidosis (uncontrolled diabetes mellitus, starvation, anorexia nervosa), severe salicylate intoxication, renal failure, severe dehydration, antifreeze ingestion, paint thinner. *Drug Influence:* Penicillin and carbenicillin in high doses, salicylates, paraldehyde, diuretics (thiazides and loop diuretics), methanol ingestion.

Normal Level Occurring in Metabolic Acidosis: Diarrhea, renal tubular acidosis, ureterosigmoidostomy, hyperalimentation, small bowel fistula, pancreatic drainage.

Procedure

- Obtain serum electrolyte values of sodium (Na), potassium (K), chloride (Cl), and CO_2 (bicarbonate determinant) from the laboratory slip. If not available, collect 7 to 10 ml of venous blood in a red-top tube.
- There is no food or fluid restriction.

Factors Affecting Laboratory Results

- *See Drug Influence under decreased and elevated levels.*
- Hemolysis of blood sample increases potassium and bicarbonate levels.

NURSING IMPLICATIONS WITH RATIONALE

- Calculate the anion gap from recently obtained electrolyte values of sodium, potassium, chloride, and serum CO_2. Use the formula given in "Description" above.
- Observe for signs and symptoms of metabolic acidosis (i.e., rapid, vigorous breathing [Kussmaul's breathing], increased pulse rate, flushed skin).

Antibiotics/aminoglycosides (serum)

Amikacin (Amikin), Gentamicin (Garamycin), Tobramycin (Nebcin)

Reference Values

Adult:

	THERAPEUTIC RANGE		
Drug Name	**Peak**	**Trough**	**Toxic Level**
Amikacin	15–30 μg/ml	<10 μg/ml	>35 μg/ml
Gentamicin	6–12 μg/ml	<2 μg/ml	>12 μg/ml
Tobramycin	5–10 μg/ml	<2 μg/ml	>12 μg/ml

Child: Same as adult.

Description

Aminoglycosides are broad-spectrum antibiotics that are effective against gram-negative microorganisms. These agents are not well absorbed from the gastrointestinal tract and so are given parenterally. Peak action after intramuscular (IM) injection is $\frac{1}{2}$ to $1\frac{1}{2}$ hours and after 30-minute IV infusion is $\frac{1}{2}$ hour. Half-life is about 2 hours. Aminoglycosides cross the placental barrier but do not cross the blood-brain barrier. They are excreted mostly unchanged by the kidneys.

Ototoxicity and nephrotoxicity can result from overdose of aminoglycoside or from long-term administration. Renal function tests (i.e., creatinine, creatinine clearance, and urinalysis) should be assessed periodically while the client is receiving these agents. If clients with renal insufficiency receive any of these drugs, dosage should be adjusted (decreased). Drug half-life is usually 24 to 96 hours in clients having renal damage.

Purpose

- To assess clients receiving aminoglycosides for therapeutic effect and possible toxic effect by monitoring urinary output, blood urea nitrogen (BUN), and serum creatinine levels.

Clinical Problems

Elevated Levels: Overdose of aminoglycoside, renal insufficiency or failure.

Drug Influence: Diuretics, cephalosporins (increase chance of nephrotoxicity).

Procedure

- Collect 3 to 5 ml of venous blood in a red-top tube.
- Collect specimen during steady state, usually 24 to 36 hours after drug is started.
- Record on the laboratory requisition slip the dose, route (IM or IV), and last time drug was administered.
- There is no food or fluid restriction.

Factors Affecting Laboratory Results

- Renal insufficiency or failure could cause an elevated serum aminoglycoside level.

NURSING IMPLICATIONS WITH RATIONALE

- Check serum aminoglycoside (amikacin, gentamicin, tobramycin) results, and report nontherapeutic levels to health care provider immediately.
- Assess intake and output. Notify the health care provider if urine output has greatly decreased. This could be a sign of aminoglycoside toxicity.

■ Suggest renal function tests for clients receiving long-term aminoglycoside therapy and especially for those with renal insufficiency.

■ Recognize that diuretics and cephalosporins coadministered with an aminoglycoside could enhance the risk of nephrotoxicity.

■ Assess hearing status of the client. Any hearing impairment (loss of high tone) while the client is receiving aminoglycoside could indicate ototoxicity.

Elevated Level

■ Recognize that overdose of aminoglycoside or renal insufficiency could cause an elevated serum aminoglycoside level.

■ Observe for signs and symptoms of nephrotoxicity (i.e., proteinuria, elevated creatinine, elevated BUN, decreased creatinine clearance test).

■ Observe for signs and symptoms of ototoxicity (i.e., nausea and vomiting with motion, dizziness, headache, tinnitus, decrease in ability to hear high-pitched tones).

Antibiotic susceptibility (sensitivity)

Reference Values

Adult: Organism is sensitive or intermediate or resistant to antibiotics.

Child: Same as adult.

Description

(See Cultures.)

It is important to identify not only the organism responsible for the infection but also the antibiotic(s) that will inhibit the growth of the bacteria. The health care provider orders a culture and sensitivity test (C and S) when a wound infection, urinary tract infection, or other types of infected secretions are suspected. The choice of antibiotic depends on the pathogenic organism and its susceptibility to the antibiotics.

There are two methods employed to test antibiotic susceptibility: tube dilution and disk diffusion (also called agar diffusion), with the latter being the most commonly used method. A filter paper containing small antibiotic disks is placed in a Petri dish streaked with the single type of bacteria. If bacteria surround the disk, the organism is resistant to the antibiotic. If the bacteria growth around the disk is inhibited, the organism is susceptible to the antibiotic. Recently, the term *minimal inhibitory concentration* (MIC) has been used to express (in µg/ml) the lowest concentration of the antibiotics that will prevent visible growth of a cultured microorganism.

With the tube dilution method, bacteria are cultured in several tubes having various concentrations of antibiotic. The lowest concentration of antibiotic that inhibits the growth of the organism is the choice of antibiotic concentration for the client.

Purpose

- To check the effectiveness of selected antibiotics on a specific bacteria from a culture.

Clinical Problems

Resistant (R): The antibiotic is noneffective against the organism.

Intermediate (I): Bacterial growth retardation is inconclusive.

Sensitive (S): The antibiotic is effective against the organism.

Procedure

- It takes approximately 24 hours for bacterial growth and 48 hours for the test results.
- The specimen for C and S should be taken to the laboratory within 30 minutes of collection or else refrigerated.
- The specimen should be handled with care, preventing contamination and bacterial transmission. *(See Culture Procedure.)*

Factors Affecting Laboratory Results

- Antibiotics and sulfonamides could cause a false-negative reaction.

NURSING IMPLICATIONS WITH RATIONALE

- Collect specimen for C and S before preventive antibiotic therapy is started. Antibiotic therapy started before specimen collection could cause an inaccurate result.
- Record on the laboratory slip the antibiotic(s) the client is receiving, the dosages, and how long the antibiotic(s) has (have) been taken.
- Check laboratory report for C and S result. If the client is receiving an antibiotic and the report shows the organism is resistant to that antibiotic, the nurse should notify the health care provider.

Client Teaching

- Inform the client that the culture test results will be available in 48 hours.

Anticardiolipin antibodies (ACA) (serum)

Antiphospholipid Antibodies (APA); Cardiolipin Antibodies (aCl);
IgG Cardiolipin Antibodies and IgM Cardiolipin Antibodies

Reference Value

Negative.

Description

Anticardiolipin antibodies (ACA) are autoantibodies found in some clients with systemic lupus erythematosus (SLE). They occur in 45% of clients with SLE and less than 7% of clients without SLE. These antibodies were originally found in clients with SLE and were called *lupus anticoagulants* (LA). Later it was determined that these antibodies did not act as anticoagulants and that they were found in health problems other than lupus. ACA and LA are members of the antiphospholipid (APA) family of immunoglobulins active against phospholipids. ACA may also be present in clients having thrombocytopenia, spontaneous or recurrent thrombosis, and fetal loss.

Purposes

- To aid in the diagnosis of SLE, especially in clients who have thrombocytopenia and repeated fetal loss.
- To detect ACA syndrome in clients with other health problems.

Clinical Problems

Elevated Level: SLE, thrombocytopenia, thrombosis, fetal loss, infection, severe hemorrhage (rare), malignancy, acquired immunodeficiency syndrome (AIDS).
Drug Influence: Chlorpromazine, procainamide, quinidine, penicillin, various antibiotics, phenytoin.

Procedure

- There is no food or fluid restriction.
- Collect 3 to 5 ml of venous blood in a red-top tube. Avoid hemolysis; send the specimen immediately to the laboratory.

Factors Affecting Laboratory Results

- Hemolysis of the blood specimen may cause a false test result.

NURSING IMPLICATIONS WITH RATIONALE

- Obtain a history of the client's health problem with current symptoms.
- Observe for signs and symptoms of SLE; i.e., fatigue, fever, rash butterfly over nose, leukopenia.

Client Teaching

- Instruct the client to have daily rest periods, which help to decrease symptoms.
- Explain to the client the purpose of oral anticoagulant or platelet inhibitor therapy for thrombocytopenia or recurrent thrombosis if these treatments are ordered.
- Listen to the client's concerns; answer questions or refer them to other health care providers.

Anticonvulsants (blood, serum, plasma)

Carbamazepine (Tegretol), Ethosuximide (Zarontin), Phenytoin (Dilantin) (see Phenytoin), Primidone (Mysoline), Valproic Acid (Depakene)

Reference Values

Adult:

Drug Name	THERAPEUTIC RANGE		TOXIC LEVEL	
	µg/ml	µmoL/l	µg/ml	µmoL/l
Carbamazepine	4–12	16.9–50.8	>12–15	>50.8–69
(Child)	(Same as adult)		(Same as adult)	
Ethosuximide	40–100	283–708	>100	>708
(Child)	(2–4 per 1 mg/kg/day)		(Same as adult or higher)	
Phenytoin	10–20	39.6–79.3	>20	>79.3
Primidone	5–12	23–55	>12–15	>55–69
(Child <5 years)	(7–10)	(30–45)	(>12)	(>55)
Valproic acid	50–100	347–693	>100	>693
(Child)	(Same as adult)		(Same as adult)	

Description

The drugs listed as anticonvulsant agents are given to control or to alleviate grand mal, psychomotor, and/or petit mal seizures. Most of them have different therapeutic ranges, peak levels, and half-life.

Carbamazepine (Tegretol): This agent is used for grand mal seizures. Peak serum level occurs 4 to 8 hours after oral dose; half-life is about 10 to 26 hours in adults and 8 to 20 hours in children. Steady state is reached in 2 weeks. When carbamazepine is administered with phenytoin, phenobarbital, ethosuximide, primidone, or valproic acid, serum level of the drug might decrease. A serious side effect is bone marrow depression.

Ethosuximide (Zarontin): This agent is used for petit mal seizures. Peak serum level occurs 3 to 5 hours after oral dose; half-life is about 60 hours in adults and 30 hours in children. Steady state is reached in 7 to 10 days. When administered with carbamazepine or valproic acid, ethosuximide's serum level might decrease or increase. Side effects include anorexia, nausea, vomiting, and lupus erythematosus-like syndrome.

Phenytoin (Dilantin): *(See separate listing.)*

Primidone (Mysoline): This agent is used for grand mal and psychomotor seizures. Peak serum level occurs 7 to 8 hours after oral dose; half-life varies from 8 to 48 hours (shorter half-life with primidone and longer with the two active metabolites, phenobarbital and phenylethylmalonamide [PEMA]). Steady state is rapidly reached. When primidone is administered with carbamazepine, its serum level may increase. Side effects include sedation, nausea, dizziness, and visual disturbance.

Valproic Acid: This agent is used alone or with other anticonvulsants for grand mal and petit mal seizures. Peak serum level occurs 1 to 4 hours after oral dose; half-life is 8 to 15 hours. Valproic acid inhibits phenobarbital metabolism. If primidone or phenobarbital are given with valproic acid, its dosage needs to be adjusted (lowered). Valproic acid can elevate ethosuximide and phenytoin levels when coadministered. It can cross the placenta. Valproic acid therapy may cause a false-positive urine ketone test. Side effects include anorexia, nausea, vomiting, fatigue, and altered liver function tests.

Purposes

- To monitor specific anticonvulsant serum levels.
- To detect the toxic level of a specific anticonvulsant.

Clinical Problems

Decreased Level: *Carbamazepine: Drug Influence:* Barbiturates, benzodiazepines, ethosuximide, phenytoin, primidone, valproic acid.

Ethosuximide: Drug Influence: Carbamazepine, valproic acid.

Valproic Acid: Drug Influence: Carbamazepine, phenytoin, phenobarbital, primidone.

Elevated Level: *Carbamazepine:* Overdose of carbamazepine, liver disease, cardiovascular disease, bone marrow disease. *Drug Influence:* Phenytoin, barbiturates, propoxyphene (Darvon), erythromycin.

Ethosuximide: Overdose of ethosuximide, liver disease. *Drug Influence:* Carbamazepine, valproic acid.

Primidone: Overdose of primidone, liver disease. *Drug Influence:* Phenobarbital.

Procedure

- Collect 5 to 7 ml of venous blood in a red-top tube (valproic acid, carbamazepine), gray-top tube (primidone), or green-top tube (ethosuximide). *Check with laboratory for preferred collecting tube.*
- Record the name of drug, dose, route, and last time drug was administered on the laboratory requisition slip. Trough serum levels (drawn before next dose) are usually requested. List drugs the client is taking that might interfere with test results on requisition slip.
- There is no food or fluid restriction.

Factors Affecting Laboratory Results

- Drugs *(see Drug Influence above)* that the client is taking could increase or decrease test results.

NURSING IMPLICATIONS WITH RATIONALE

- Administer valproic acid with meals to reduce gastrointestinal distress.
- Monitor serum drug levels (weekly, monthly, yearly) during long-term drug therapy.
- Monitor complete blood count (CBC) and platelet count prior to carbamazepine (Tegretol) therapy and at regular intervals (weekly, monthly). Bone marrow depression is rare; however, it could occur as a result of long-term carbamazepine therapy.
- Assess liver function tests (i.e., aspartate aminotransferase [AST], serum glutamic-oxaloacetic acid [SGOT], alanine aminotransferase [ALT], serum glutamic-pyruvic transaminase [SGPT], bilirubin, alkaline phosphatase) while the client is receiving long-term anticonvulsant therapy. Compare test findings with base line levels. These drugs are metabolized in the liver, and hepatic damage could result.
- Assess serum amylase level while client is receiving long-term valproic acid (Depakene) therapy. Pancreatitis could result.

Client Teaching

- Inform the client not to discontinue prescribed anticonvulsant agent abruptly without the health care provider's permission. Withdrawal of any anticonvulsant drugs could precipitate seizures.
- Inform the client that photosensitivity reaction could occur when taking anticonvulsants. While in the sun, sunglasses and sunscreen lotion should be used.

Elevated Level

- Relate clinical conditions and drugs *(see Clinical Problems above)* that could elevate serum and anticonvulsant levels.
- Observe for signs and symptoms of common side effects from anticonvulsant therapy (i.e., anorexia, nausea, vomiting, fatigue, lethargy, dizziness, headache).

- Inform the diabetic client on valproic acid therapy that the drug could cause a false-positive urine ketone test.
- Report immediately symptoms of carbamazepine and primidone toxicity (i.e., diplopia, blurred vision) to the health care provider.
- Report lupus erythematosus-like symptoms resulting from long-term ethosuximide therapy.
- Assess for bleeding or bruising (petechiae, ecchymosis, epistaxis, melena) while receiving valproic acid. Report findings to the health care provider. Check the CBC for a low platelet count and blood count.

Antidepressants (tricyclics) (serum)

Amitriptyline, Desipramine, Doxepin, Imipramine, Nortriptyline

Reference Values

Adult:

Drug Name	THERAPEUTIC RANGE ng/ml	TOXIC LEVEL ng/ml
Amitriptyline HCl (Elavil)	75–225	>500
Desipramine HCl (Norpramin)	125–300	>500
Doxepin HCl (Sinequan)	150–300	>500
Imipramine HCl (Tofranil)	150–300	>500
Nortriptyline HCl (Aventyl)	75–150	>300

Description

Antidepressants are used primarily for unipolar and endogenous depressive disorders which are characterized by loss of interest in work or home, inability to complete tasks, and deep depression. There are three groups of antidepressants: tricyclic antidepressants (TCAs), second-generation antidepressants (newest group), and monoamine oxidase (MAO) inhibitors. Anticholinergic symptoms are common side effects of tricyclic antidepressants. With second-generation antidepressants, extrapyramidal symptoms (EPS) are common. Clients taking MAO inhibitors should avoid foods rich in tyramine (cheese, cream, chocolate, bananas, beer, red wines). Hypertensive crisis could occur when foods rich in tyramine and MAO inhibitors are eaten.

Purposes

- To regulate the tricyclic drug level for obtaining a therapeutic drug level.
- To monitor the tricyclic drug dose.
- To avoid a toxic drug level.

Clinical Problems

Decreased Level: Mild, reactive, unipolar, and/or atypical depression. *Drug Influence:* Barbiturates, chloral hydrate.

Elevated Level: Toxic tricycle antidepressant. *Drug Influence:* Hydrocortisone, neuroleptics, cimetidine, oral contraceptives.

Procedure

- No food or fluid restriction is required.
- Collect 7 ml of venous blood in a red-top tube. Deliver blood container immediately to the laboratory.
- Obtain blood specimen 2 hours before the next drug dose.

NURSING IMPLICATIONS WITH RATIONALE

- Assess client's history related to depression.
- Record drugs that the client presently is taking. Central nervous system depressants and alcohol, if taken with antidepressants, could cause respiratory depression and hypotension.
- Monitor vital signs and urinary output. Report abnormal findings.
- Check serum tricyclic level of the drug the client is taking. Report if the level is NOT within therapeutic range.
- Assess the client's compliance to drug therapy. Report changes.
- Discuss the importance of drug compliance with the client. This is important to maintain a therapeutic drug level and possibly to avoid toxic level if the drug is taken in excess.
- Discuss possible side effects such as dry mouth, blurred vision, fatigue, urinary retention, postural hypotension, and gastrointestinal disturbances, and report any of these to the health care provider.
- Discuss foods to avoid if the client is taking an MAO inhibitor *(see Description)*.

Antidiuretic hormone (ADH) (plasma)

Vasopressor

Reference Values

Adult: 1–5 pg/ml; 1–5 ng/l.

Description

Antidiuretic hormone (ADH) is produced by the hypothalamus and stored in the posterior pituitary gland (neurohypophysis). The primary function of ADH is in water reabsorption from the distal renal tubules in response to the serum osmolality. *Antidiuretic* means "against diuresis." There is more ADH secreted from the posterior pituitary gland when the serum osmolality is increased to >295 mOsm/kg (concentrated body fluids). More water reabsorption occurs, which dilutes the body fluid. When the serum osmolality is decreased to <280 mOsm/kg, less ADH is secreted, and thus more water is excreted via kidneys.

Syndrome (secretion) of inappropriate ADH (SIADH) is an excess secretion of ADH that is not influenced by the serum osmolality level. SIADH causes excess water retention. Stress, surgery, pain, and certain drugs (narcotics, anesthetics) contribute to SIADH.

Purposes

- To detect a deficit or excess in ADH secretion.
- To identify the presence of body fluid deficit or excess.

Clinical Problems

Decreased Level: Diabetes insipidus, psychogenic polydipsia, nephrotic syndrome. *Drug Influence:* Alcohol, lithium, demeclocycline, phenytoin (Dilantin).

Elevated Level: SIADH, brain tumor, cancer (ectopic ADH), pulmonary tuberculosis, pain, IPPB (intermittent positive pressure breathing), surgery, pneumonia. *Drug Influence:* Anesthetics, narcotics, estrogens, oxytocin, antineoplastic (anticancer) drugs, thiazides, antipsychotics, tricyclic antidepressants.

Procedure

- The client should be NPO for 12 hours and should avoid strenuous exercise for 12 hours. Stress should be decreased or avoided.
- Collect 5 to 7 ml of venous blood in a lavender-top *plastic* tube or plastic syringe. A glass container can cause degradation of the ADH. If blood is drawn in glass, prechill the glass and separate immediately.
- Deliver the blood specimen immediately (within 10 minutes) to the laboratory.

Factors Affecting Laboratory Results

- Certain drugs *(see Drug Influence),* food, fluids, stress, pain, and exercise can affect test results.
- Using a glass container for blood specimen collection can cause ADH degradation.
- If the blood specimen is taken at night or if the client is in a standing position, the ADH level will be increased.
- A delay in the delivery of the blood specimen will affect test results. Serum should be separated from the clot within 10 minutes.

NURSING IMPLICATIONS WITH RATIONALE

- Check to determine if drugs that may affect test results should be withheld for 12 hours before the test. Drugs that must be taken before the test should be recorded on the laboratory slip.
- Record in the client's chart and on the laboratory slip if the client is having undue stress or pain. This could increase the ADH secretion and plasma level.
- Check that the blood specimen is taken immediately to the laboratory. The serum should be separated from the clot within 10 minutes.

Client Teaching

- Explain to the client the need to avoid stress and exercise before the test.
- Instruct the client to have nothing by mouth after dinner meal.
- Listen to the client's concerns.

Antiglomerular basement membrane antibody (Anti-GBM, AGBM) (serum)

Glomerular Basement Membrane Antibody

Reference Values

Negative or none detected.

Description

This test is performed to detect circulating glomerular basement membrane (GBM) antibodies that can damage the GBMS in the glomeruli. The beta-hemolytic streptococcus can cause an antibody response in the renal glomeruli.

Glomerulonephritis, caused by anti-GBM, is usually severe and rapidly progressive. Pulmonary hemorrhage often occurs because of cross-reactivity of anti-GBM with pulmonary vascular basement membrane.

Purpose

- To detect GBM antibodies that could cause or are causing renal disease.

Clinical Problems

Positive Result: Anti-GBM nephritis, tubulointerstitial nephritis, pulmonary capillary basement membranes.

Procedure

- Collect 5 to 7 ml of venous blood in red-top tube. The test should be run immediately; if there will be a delay the blood should be frozen.
- There is no food or fluid restriction.
- Tissue from kidney biopsy might be the specimen. Tissue should be frozen after collection.

Factors Affecting Laboratory Results

- Improper care of the specimen can result in inaccurate test results.

NURSING IMPLICATIONS WITH RATIONALE

- Obtain a history of a streptococcal throat infection.
- Monitor urine output. Because the glomeruli are damaged, oliguria usually occurs.
- Assess for signs and symptoms of renal (glomerular) disease (i.e., edema of the extremities, shortness of breath, proteinuria, hematuria, increased blood pressure, elevated serum blood urea nitrogen and creatinine, decreased urine output).

Client Teaching

- Instruct the client to follow a medical regimen of diet, drugs, and rest.

Antimitochondrial antibody (AMA) (serum)

Reference Values

Negative: At a 1:5 dilution.
Intermediate Level: 1:20–1:80.

Strongly Suggestive of Primary Biliary Cirrhosis: >1:80.

Positive for Primary Biliary Cirrhosis: >1:160.

Description

The antimitochondrial antibody (AMA) test is used to differentiate between primary biliary cirrhosis and other liver diseases. Eighty to 90% of clients with primary biliary cirrhosis have a positive titer for AMAs. A positive test result would usually rule out extrahepatic biliary obstruction and acute infectious hepatitis. To confirm biliary cirrhosis, other liver tests should be performed, such as AST/SGOT, ALT/SGPT, alkaline phosphatase, serum bilirubin, and GGT.

This test is usually performed in conjunction with antismooth muscle antibodies (ASMA, ASTHMA) test. ASMA titer is elevated with biliary cirrhosis and chronic active hepatitis. Like AMA, ASMA is seldom elevated with extrahepatic biliary obstruction. The antibodies may also be associated with autoimmune disease.

Purposes

- To aid in the diagnosis of biliary cirrhosis.
- To compare the test result with that of other liver tests.

Clinical Problems

Positive Titer: Primary biliary cirrhosis, chronic hepatitis, autoimmune disorders such as systemic lupus erythematosus (SLE), rheumatoid arthritis, pernicious anemia.

Procedure

- The client should be NPO for 8 hours prior to the test.
- Collect 3 to 5 ml of venous blood in a red-top tube.
- Avoid hemolysis. The blood specimen should be delivered to the laboratory immediately.

Factors Affecting Laboratory Results

- Hemolysis of the blood specimen can affect test results.

NURSING IMPLICATIONS WITH RATIONALE

- Assess for the presence of jaundice.
- Check other liver tests and compare test results. If the health care provider suspects biliary cirrhosis, AMA and ASMA/ASTHMA tests are usually ordered.

Client Teaching

- Instruct the client to have nothing by mouth after midnight or 8 hours prior to the test.
- Listen to the client's concerns. Answer appropriate questions.

Antimyocardial antibody (serum)

Reference Values

Negative: None detected.

Positive: Titer levels.

Description

Antimyocardial antibody develops in response to a specific antigen in the heart muscle that can cause autoimmune damage to the heart. This antibody may be detected in the blood prior to or soon after heart disease. The antibody may be present after cardiac surgery, myocardial infarction, streptococcal infection, or rheumatic fever. This test may be used to monitor therapeutic response to treatment.

Purpose

- To identify the presence of AMA as the cause of the cardiac condition.

Clinical Problems

Elevated Titer: Myocardial infarction, myocarditis, pericarditis, following cardiac surgery, acute rheumatic fever, chronic rheumatic diseases, streptococcal infections, idiopathic cardiomyopathy, endomyocardial fibrosis, thoracic injury, systemic lupus erythematosus.

Procedure

- There is no food or fluid restriction.
- Collect 3 to 5 ml of venous blood in a red-top tube. Send to the laboratory immediately.

Factors Affecting Laboratory Results

- None known.

NURSING IMPLICATIONS WITH RATIONALE

- Obtain a history of heart disease.
- Check cardiac enzyme levels, (creatine phosphokinase [CPK], aspartate aminotransferase [AST], and lactate dehydrogenase [LDH]). If elevated, heart disease is likely.
- Observe for signs and symptoms of heart disease, such as chest pain, dyspnea, diaphoresis, and indigestion.
- Listen to the client's concerns.

Antinuclear antibodies (ANA) (serum)

Anti-DNA Antibody, Anti-DNP Antibody

Reference Values

Adult: Negative at 1:20 dilution.

Description

The antinuclear antibodies (ANA) test is a screening test for diagnosing systemic lupus erythematosus (SLE) and other collagen diseases. ANAs are immunoglobulins (IgM, IgG, IgA) that react with the nuclear part of leukocytes. They form antibodies against deoxyribonucleic acid (DNA), ribonucleic acid (RNA), and others. Two ANAs, anti-DNA and anti–D-nucleoprotein (Anti-DNP), are almost always present with SLE. Anti-DNA will fluctuate according to the disease process, with remission, and with exacerbation. It is normally present (95%) in lupus nephritis.

The total ANA level can also be elevated in scleroderma, rheumatoid arthritis, cirrhosis, leukemia, infectious mononucleosis, and malignancy. For diagnosing lupus, the ANA test should be compared with other tests for lupus.

Purpose

- To compare the ANA test with other laboratory tests for diagnosing SLE or other collagen diseases.

Clinical Problems

Elevated—Positive (>1:20): SLE (most frequent cause), progressive systemic sclerosis, scleroderma, leukemia, rheumatoid arthritis, cirrhosis of the liver, infectious mononucleosis, myasthenia gravis, malignancy. *Drug Influence:* Antibiotics (penicillin, streptomycin, tetracycline), antihypertensives (hydralazine [Apresoline], methyldopa [Aldomet]), anti-TB (para-aminosalicylic acid [PAS], isoniazid [INH]), diuretics (acetazolamide [Diamox], thiazides [hydrochlorothiazide]), oral contraceptives, procainamide (Pronestyl), trimethadione (Tridione), phenytoin (Dilantin).

Procedure

- Collect 3 to 5 ml of venous blood in a red-top tube. Take to the laboratory immediately.
- There is no food or fluid restriction.
- List drugs the client is taking that could cause false-positive test results.

Factors Affecting Laboratory Results

- Certain drugs cause false-positive results *(see Drug Influence above)*.
- The aging process can cause a slight positive ANA titer.

NURSING IMPLICATIONS WITH RATIONALE

Elevated—Positive Titer

- Relate clinical problems and drugs to positive ANA results. With SLE, the ANA titer may fluctuate according to the severity of the disease.
- Compare test result with other tests for lupus.
- Assess for signs and symptoms of SLE (i.e., skin rash over the cheeks and nose, joint pain).
- Promote rest during an acute phase.
- Listen to the client's concerns.

Antiparietal cell antibody (APCA) (blood)

Parietal Cell Antibody

Reference Values

Negative: to <1:120 titer.
Positive: 1:180 titer.

Description

Parietal cells in the stomach secrete hydrochloric acid (HCl), which is needed for protein catabolism. Parietal cell antibody is frequently caused by an autoimmune response.

Antiparietal cell antibody (APCA) at approximately 80 to 90% is sensitive for detecting pernicious anemia (PA). The APCA titer may decrease during the duration of PA. Also this test helps in differentiating between autoimmune chronic gastritis and that of pernicious anemia. Intrinsic factor (IF) antibodies may also be found in pernicious anemia because of the disruption of the IF production caused by the autoimmune process. PA may have a genetic tendency that is not caused by an autoimmune response.

An elevated APCA may be present in other autoimmune disorders such as myasthenia gravis, Type I diabetes mellitus or insulin dependent diabetes mellitus (IDDM). APCA titer level may increase with age. It should not be the only test used for diagnosing pernicious anemia.

Purposes

- To screen for the presence of pernicious anemia (PA).
- To rule out the occurrence of other autoimmune disorders, for example, myasthenia gravis, Type I diabetes mellitus.

Clinical Problems

Elevated Titer Level: Pernicious anemia, chronic gastritis, gastric ulcer, Type I diabetes mellitus, gastric cancer, myasthenia gravis, thyroid disease.

Procedure

- There is no food or fluid restriction.
- Collect 7 to 10 ml of venous blood in a red-top or gray-top tube.

Factors Affecting Laboratory Results

- None known.

NURSING IMPLICATIONS WITH RATIONALE

- Obtain a history from the client related to the present health complaint. Clinical manifestations of pernicious anemia may include weakness, orthopnea, burning sensation of the tongue, dyspnea, lightheadedness, sensitivity to temperature changes.

Client Teaching

- Encourage the client to have a balanced diet high in protein, vitamins, and iron. Foods rich in fish, red meat, eggs, and milk help to increase the daily Vitamin B_{12} intake.
- Inform the client other tests may be necessary to confirm the diagnosis (especially if pernicious anemia is suggestive).

Antiphospholipid antibodies (APA)

See Anticardiolipin Antibodies (ACA)

Antiscleroderma antibody (Scl-70) (serum)

Antibodies to Scl-70 Antigen

Reference Values

Negative: Borderline: 20–25 units.

Positive: >25 units.

Description

Antiscleroderma antibodies occur in 40 to 70% of clients with advanced or diffuse cutaneous scleroderma, interstitial pulmonary fibrosis, and peripheral vascular disease. The presence of antibodies to Scl-70 antigen is seldom present in other rheumatic disorders such as systemic lupus erythematosus (SLE), rheumatoid arthritis.

A negative test result does not indicate the absence of sclerodermal disease. Scleroderma is considered an autoimmune collagen disorder.

Purpose

■ To assist in the diagnosis of scleroderma.

Clinical Problems

Elevated Levels: Scleroderma, CREST syndrome, progressive systemic sclerosis.
Drug Influence: Aspirin, diphenylhydantoin (Benadryl), isoniazid, methyldopa, ethosuximide, penicillin, tetracycline, streptomycin.

Procedure

■ Collect 5 ml of venous blood in a red-top tube.
■ There is no food or fluid restriction.

Factors Affecting Laboratory Results

■ See drug list that can cause a false positive test result.

NURSING IMPLICATIONS WITH RATIONALE

■ Obtain a history of health problems. Record if client has any physical symptoms such as a rash. There can be localized or systemic forms of scleroderma.

Client Teaching

■ Explain to the client that other tests may be requested by the health care provider.

- If the client is diagnosed with systemic scleroderma, the nurse may inform the client that most systemic forms of scleroderma progress very slowly.
- Tell the client to dress warmly, including gloves, because cold weather may increase discomfort and pain.

Antismooth muscle antibody (ASMA, ASTHMA) (serum)

Reference Values

Negative: Or <1:20.
Positive: >1:20.

Description

Antismooth muscle antibody (ASMA, ASTHMA) is associated primarily with autoimmune chronic active hepatitis (CAH). With CAH, the titer level is usually >1:160. The titer elevation of ASTHMA occurs in more than 70% of clients with CAH, and most of the clients are females. CAH is frequently referred to as an autoimmune disease. Clients with primary biliary cirrhosis may have a slight titer elevation. Lower titer levels may be present in other conditions such as cancer, viral infections, and acute viral hepatitis. The antimitochondrial antibody (AMA) test and antinuclear antibody (ANA) tests may be prescribed with the ASTHMA test to differentiate the cause of the liver disorder. An elevated AMA titer is more prevalent with biliary cirrhosis, whereas ASTHMA and ANA elevations occur with chronic active hepatitis, which is referred to as lupoid hepatitis. With CAH, the ASTHMA is usually higher than the ANA.

Purpose

- To assist with the diagnosis of CAH.

Clinical Problems

Elevated Levels: *High titers:* Chronic active hepatitis. *Low titers:* Primary biliary cirrhosis, cancer of the liver, infectious mononucleosis, multiple sclerosis (MS), rheumatoid arthritis, acute viral hepatitis, intrinsic asthma.

Procedure

- Collect 5 to 7 ml of venous blood in a red-top tube.

- Apply pressure to the venipuncture site to decrease bleeding. Clients with liver dysfunction tend to bleed more readily.
- There is no food or fluid restriction.

Factors Affecting Laboratory Results

- None known.

NURSING IMPLICATIONS WITH RATIONALE

- Obtain a history from the client related to the health problem. Jaundice may be present. Record drugs that the client is taking which may be a contributing cause of CAH.

Client Teaching

- Explain to the client that other laboratory tests may be performed, for example, ANA, AMA, bilirubin, and a liver biopsy may be requested to assure the diagnosis.
- If steroids are prescribed for CAH, explain how the steroid drug should be taken, such as with food. If steroid drugs are discontinued, the daily dose should be tapered over a period of days to avoid adverse effects.
- Listen to the client's concerns. Refer questions to other health professionals as needed.

Antistreptolysin O (ASO) (serum)

Reference Values

Upper limit of normal varies with age, season, and geographic area.

Adult: <100 IU/ml; <160 Todd U/ml.

Child: *Newborn:* Similar to mother's. *2 to 5 years:* <100 IU/ml. *12 to 19 years:* <200 IU/ml; <200 Todd U/ml.

Description

The beta-hemolytic streptococcus secretes an enzyme known as streptolysin O, which is capable of lysing red blood cells (RBCs). Streptolysin O acts as an antigen and stimulates the immune system to develop antistreptolysin O (ASO) antibodies. A high titer of ASO indicates that streptococci are present and may cause rheumatic fever or acute glomerulonephritis. Increased serum ASO levels can also indicate a recent streptococcal infection.

The ASO antibodies appear approximately 1 to 2 weeks after an acute streptococcal infection, peak 3 to 4 weeks after onset, and could remain elevated for months. Many school-aged children have a higher ASO titer level than do preschool children or adults.

Other streptococcal antigens are antideoxyribonuclease (ADNase—titer >10) and antistreptococcal hyaluronidase (ASH—titer >128).

Purposes

- To identify clients who are susceptible to specific autoimmune disorders (e.g., collagen disease).
- To aid in determining the effect of the beta-hemolytic streptococcus in secreting the enzyme streptolysin O.

Clinical Problems

Decreased Level: *Drug Influence:* Antibiotics.

Elevated Level: Acute rheumatic fever, acute glomerulonephritis, streptococcal upper respiratory infections, rheumatoid arthritis (mildly elevated), hyperglobulinemia with liver disease, collagen disease (mildly elevated).

Procedure

- Collect 3 to 5 ml of venous blood in red-top tube. Avoid hemolysis.
- There is no food or fluid restriction.
- Repeated ASO testing (once or twice a week) is advisable to determine the highest level of increase.

Factors Affecting Laboratory Results

- Antibiotic therapy decreases the antibody response.
- An increased level may occur in healthy persons (carriers).

NURSING IMPLICATIONS WITH RATIONALE

- Note that antibiotic therapy could decrease antibody response.

Elevated Level

- Check serum ASO levels when the client is complaining of joint pain in the extremities. A high elevated level could be indicative of acute rheumatic fever, and a slight elevation could be indicative of rheumatoid arthritis.
- Check the urinary output when the serum ASO is elevated. A urinary output of less than 600 ml/24 hours may be associated with acute glomerulonephritis.

Client Teaching

- Instruct the client and family that when the client has a sore throat he or she should have a throat culture taken to check for beta-hemolytic streptococcus. A throat culture might need to be repeated if the sore throat persists.

Arterial blood gases (ABGs) (arterial blood)

Blood Gases

Reference Values

Adult: pH: 7.35–7.45; $PaCO_2$: 35–45 mm Hg; PaO_2: 75–100 mm Hg; SaO_2: >95%; SvO_2: >70%; HCO_3: 24–28 mEq/l; base excesses (BE): +2 to −2 mEq/l.

Child: pH: 7.36–7.44. Other measurements are same as adult.

Description

Arterial blood gases (ABGs) are usually ordered to assess disturbances of acid–base (A-B) balance caused by a respiratory disorder and/or a metabolic disorder. The basic components of ABGs include the pH, $PaCO_2$, PaO_2, SO_2, HCO_3, and BE.

pH: The pH, the negative logarithm of the hydrogen ion concentration, determines the acidity or alkalinity of body fluids. A pH less than 7.35 indicates acidosis, either respiratory acidosis or metabolic acidosis. A pH greater than 7.45 indicates alkalosis, either respiratory or metabolic alkalosis.

$PaCO_2$: The partial pressure of carbon dioxide ($PaCO_2$) reflects the adequacy of alveolar ventilation. When there is alveolar damage, carbon dioxide (CO_2) cannot escape. Carbon dioxide combines with water to form carbonic acid ($H_2O + CO_2 = H_2CO_3$), causing an acidotic state. When the client has alveolar hypoventilation, the $PaCO_2$ is elevated, and respiratory acidosis results. Chronic obstructive lung disease is a major cause of respiratory acidosis. When the client has alveolar hyperventilation (blowing off CO_2 by rapid deep breathing), the $PaCO_2$ is decreased, and respiratory alkalosis results.

PaO_2: The partial pressure of oxygen (PaO_2) determines the amount of oxygen available to bind with hemoglobin. The pH affects the combining power of oxygen and hemoglobin, and with a low pH, there will be less oxygen in the hemoglobin. The PaO_2 is decreased in respiratory diseases, such as emphysema, pneumonia, and pulmonary edema; in the presence of abnormal hemoglobin (CO Hb, Meth Hb, Sulfa Hb); and in polycythemia.

SO_2: The oxygen saturation (SO_2) is the percentage of oxygen in the blood that combines with hemoglobin. It is measured indirectly by calculation of the PaO_2 and pH or measured directly by co-oximetry. The combination of oxygen saturation, partial pressure of oxygen, and hemoglobin indicates tissue oxygenation.

HCO_3 and BE: Bicarbonate ion (HCO_3) is an alkaline substance that comprises over half of the total buffer base in the blood. When there is a deficit of bicarbonate and other bases or an increase in nonvolatile acid such as lactic acid, metabolic acidosis occurs. If a bicarbonate excess is present, then metabolic alkalosis results. The bicarbonate plays a very important role in maintaining a pH of 7.35 to 7.45.

The base excess (BE) value is frequently checked with the HCO_3 value. A base excess of less than -2 is acidosis and greater than $+2$ is alkalosis.

Acid–Base Imbalances: To determine the type of A-B imbalance, the pH, $PaCO_2$, HCO_3, and BE are checked. The $PaCO_2$ is a respiratory determinant, and the HCO_3 and BE are metabolic determinants. The $PaCO_2$, HCO_3, and BE values are compared to the pH. A pH of less than 7.35 is acidosis and one of greater than 7.45 is alkalosis.

1. If the pH is <7.35, the $PaCO_2$ is >45 mm Hg, and the HCO_3 and BE are normal, the A-B imbalance is respiratory acidosis.
2. If the pH is >7.45, the $PaCO_2$ is <35 mm Hg, and the HCO_3 and BE are normal, the A-B imbalance is respiratory alkalosis.
3. If the pH is <7.35, the $PaCO_2$ is normal, the HCO_3 and BE are <24 mEq/l and <-2, the A-B imbalance is metabolic acidosis.
4. If the pH is >7.45, the $PaCO_2$ is normal, the HCO_3 and BE are >28 mEq/l and $>+2$, the A-B imbalance is metabolic alkalosis.

Acid–Base (A-B) Imbalance	pH	PaCO$_2$	Hco$_3$	BE
Respiratory acidosis	↓	↑	N	N
Respiratory alkalosis	↑	↓	N	N
Metabolic acidosis	↓	N	↓	↓
Metabolic alkalosis	↑	N	↑	↑

Purposes

- To detect metabolic acidosis or alkalosis, or respiratory acidosis or alkalosis.
- To monitor blood gases during an acute illness.

Clinical Problems

Respiratory Acidosis (pH <7.35; PaCO$_2$ >45 mm Hg): Chronic obstructive lung disease (emphysema, chronic bronchitis, severe asthma), acute respiratory distress syndrome (ARDS), Guillain-Barré syndrome, anesthesia, pneumonia. *Drug Influence:* Narcotics, sedatives.

Respiratory Alkalosis (pH >7.45; PaCO$_2$ <35 mm Hg): Salicylate toxicity (early phase), anxiety, hysteria, tetany, strenuous exercise (swimming, running), fever, hyperthyroidism, delirium tremens, pulmonary embolism.

Metabolic Acidosis (pH <7.35; HCO$_3$ <24 mEq/l): Diabetic ketoacidosis, severe diarrhea, starvation/malnutrition, shock, burns, kidney failure, acute myocardial infarction.

Metabolic Alkalosis (pH >7.45; HCO$_3$ >28 mEq/l): Severe vomiting, gastric suction, peptic ulcer, potassium loss, excess administration of bicarbonate, hepatic failure, cystic fibrosis. *Drug Influence:* Sodium bicarbonate, sodium oxalate, potassium oxalate.

Procedure

- There is no food or fluid restriction.
- If the client is receiving anticoagulant therapy or taking aspirin, the laboratory, nurse, or pulmonary technician drawing the blood should be notified.
- Collect 1–5 ml of arterial blood in a heparinized needle and syringe, remove the needle, make sure there is no air in the syringe, and apply an airtight cap over the tip of the syringe.
- Place the syringe with arterial blood in an ice-water bag (to minimize the metabolic activity of the sample) and deliver it immediately to the laboratory. Ice water is colder than ice.
- Indicate on the laboratory slip whether the client is receiving oxygen and the flow rate, type of O_2 administration device (e.g., cannula, mask), and the client's current temperature.
- Apply pressure to the puncture site for 5 minutes, longer for persons on anticoagulants or streptokinase therapy.

Factors Affecting Laboratory Results

- Improper handling of the blood sample, such as not using ice water, exposure of specimen to air, and not expelling all the heparin out of the collection syringe, causes inaccurate results.
- Hemolysis of the blood sample causes false results.
- Narcotics and sedatives can contribute to the respiratory acidotic state, and sodium bicarbonate could cause metabolic alkalosis.
- Inaccurate results can occur as a result of suctioning, changes in O_2 therapy, and ventilator use; exposure to carbon monoxide or nitrate; and blood transfusion.

NURSING IMPLICATIONS WITH RATIONALE

Respiratory Acidosis

- Assess for signs and symptoms of respiratory acidosis, such as dyspnea, headache, disorientation, and increased $PaCO_2$ (>45 mm Hg).
- Perform chest clapping to break up bronchial and alveolar secretions. Carbon dioxide can be trapped in the lungs because of excess secretions and mucous plugs.
- Administer oxygen at a low concentration (2 to 3 l) when emphysema is present.
- Check for metabolic compensatory mechanism with respiratory acidosis—HCO_3 would be elevated, >28 mEq/l.

Client Teaching

- Teach the client breathing exercises to enhance CO_2 excretion from the lungs.
- Instruct the client on how to properly use the incentive spirometer device or mini-nebulizer if ordered.

- Demonstrate the postural drainage procedure, if not contraindicated, by lowering the head of the bed or having the client lie over the side of the bed. Secretions are mobilized and excreted by gravity.

Respiratory Alkalosis

- Relate a low $PaCO_2$ value to clinical problems associated with tachypnea (rapid respiratory rate). Anxiety, hysteria, nervousness, and strenuous physical exertion can cause tachypnea. With rapid breathing, an excess of CO_2 is lost.
- Assess for signs and symptoms of respiratory alkalosis, such as tachypnea, dizziness, tingling of fingers, tetany spasms, and a $PaCO_2$ <35 mm Hg.

Client Teaching

- Instruct the client to breathe slowly and deeply. Breathing into a paper bag will help to decrease hyperventilation.

Metabolic Acidosis

- Relate decreased values of HCO_3 and BE to metabolic acidosis. When there is tissue breakdown from shock, malnutrition, and such, acid metabolites (e.g., lactic acid) are released. Another cause of metabolic acidosis is the presence of ketone bodies (fatty acid) from diabetic ketoacidosis.
- Assess for signs and symptoms of metabolic acidosis, such as rapid, vigorous breathing (Kussmaul's breathing), flushed skin, restlessness, decreased bicarbonate (HCO_3) value of <24 mEq/l, and decreased BE < -2.
- Check for respiratory compensatory mechanism with metabolic acidosis: $PaCO_2$ would be decreased, <35 mm Hg. The lung compensates by blowing off CO_2 through hyperventilation to decrease carbonic acid in the blood and thereby decreasing the acidotic state.

Metabolic Alkalosis

- Relate elevated HCO_3 and BE values to metabolic alkalosis. With severe vomiting and gastric suction, hydrogen and chloride (hydrochloric acid) are lost, causing an alkalotic state. Drugs containing sodium bicarbonate taken in excess or over a long period of time could cause metabolic alkalosis.
- Assess for signs and symptoms of metabolic alkalosis, such as shallow breathing, vomiting, elevated HCO_3 value of >28 mEq/l, and elevated BE value of $> +2$.
- Stop nasogastric drainage or decrease amount of vomiting as necessary.

Client Teaching

- Instruct the client not to ingest large quantities of antacids containing base substances like bicarbonate. An alkalotic state could result.

Ascorbic acid (Vitamin C) (plasma and serum)

Reference Values

Adult: 0.6–2.0 mg/dl (plasma), 34–114 μmol/l (SI units, plasma), 0.2–2.0 mg/dl (serum), 12–114 μmol/l (SI units, serum).

Child: 0.6–1.6 mg/dl (plasma).

Description

(See Ascorbic Acid Tolerance.)

Ascorbic acid (Vitamin C) is a water-soluble vitamin found in fresh fruits and vegetables. Deficiencies of Vitamin C still occur, but the severe deficiency known as scurvy is rare.

Vitamin C is important for the formation of collagen substances and certain amino acids, in wound healing, and in withstanding the stresses of injury and infection. Because Vitamin C is vitally important to the body's defense mechanisms in dealing with stress caused by injury and disease, the client's ascorbic acid level should be known. This test can also be used to determine whether the ascorbic acid therapy is adequate. Excess ingestion of Vitamin C is not considered toxic, as is excess ingestion of Vitamins A and D, because excess Vitamin C is water-soluble and is excreted in the urine.

Purpose

- To determine if the ascorbic acid therapy is adequate.

Clinical Problems

Decreased Level (<0.6 mg/dl): Scurvy, low Vitamin C diet, malabsorption, pregnancy, infections, cancer, severe burns.

Elevated Level: Excess Vitamin C ingestion. *Causes of False-Positive Readings:* Clinitest, serum creatinine, serum uric acid, serum bilirubin, serum ALT and AST, blood glucose, serum cholesterol. *Causes of False-Negative Readings:* Test for occult blood in stool, serum triglycerides.

Procedure

- Collect 7 ml of venous blood in a gray-top tube (plasma) or a red-top tube (serum).
- There is no food or fluid restriction.

Factors Affecting Laboratory Results

- High doses of ascorbic acid can cause inaccurate results.

NURSING IMPLICATIONS WITH RATIONALE

- Recognize the functions of ascorbic acid in maintaining the state of wellness. Ascorbic acid has been taken by persons in large doses (>1 g) to prevent colds. This has not been medically proven effective.
- Answer the client's questions concerning the importance of Vitamin C. It helps with the healing process.

Decreased Level

- Relate Vitamin C deficit to certain clinical problems (e.g., infections, burns). Vitamin C is lost during severe infections and burns.

Client Teaching

- Teach the client to eat foods rich in Vitamin C (e.g., oranges, grapefruits, strawberries, cantaloupe, pineapple, broccoli, cabbage, spinach, kale, turnips—all excellent to good sources). Approximately 25% of the population has an ascorbic acid deficit in the body.

Elevated Level

- Record on the client's chart habitual use of high doses of Vitamin C. High doses of ascorbic acid can cause false-positive laboratory results.

Ascorbic acid tolerance (plasma and urine)

Vitamin C Tolerance

Reference Values

Adult: *Plasma:* >2.0 mg/dl. *Urine:* 4-, 5-, or 6-hour sample. *Oral:* 10% of administered amount. IV: 30%–40% of administered amount.

Child: Not usually done.

Description

The ascorbic acid tolerance test is useful for determining the degree of ascorbic acid deficiency. Clients having severe burns, infections, or malignancy frequently have an ascorbic acid deficiency even when they are receiving Vitamin C or have a diet adequate in Vitamin C. With an ascorbic acid deficit, wound healing and recovery are prolonged.

The blood and urine tests are normally done together.

A ■ LABORATORY TESTS

Purpose
- To detect Vitamin C deficiency.

Clinical Problems
Decreased Level: Infections, burns, cancer.

Elevated Level: Excess Vitamin C administration.

Procedure
- Foods high in ascorbic acid (i.e., fruits and vegetables) should be omitted for 24 hours before the test. Water can be given.
- Have the client void, and discard the urine before beginning the test.
- Administer ascorbic acid orally (11 mg/kg of body weight in a glass of water) or intravenously (10 mg/kg of body weight in saline solution).
- Collect 7 ml of venous blood in a gray-top tube 4 to 6 hours after the ascorbic acid is administered.
- Collect a 4-, 5-, or 6-hour urine specimen in a bottle containing acetic acid. The bottle should be kept on ice or refrigerated and taken to the laboratory immediately at the end of the specified time.

Factors Affecting Laboratory Results
- Oral high-potency vitamin supplements cause false test results.
- Ascorbic acid in IV fluids cause false test results.
- Inaccurate urine collection time and inaccurate labeling result in false test results.

NURSING IMPLICATIONS WITH RATIONALE
- Explain to the client that the purpose of the test is to determine whether there is a Vitamin C deficiency in the body.
- Explain to the client that for 24 hours he or she should not eat foods high in ascorbic acid (i.e., oranges or orange juice, grapefruit, strawberries, or green vegetables). Drinking water is permissible.
- Have the client void, and discard the urine.
- Administer ascorbic acid orally or intravenously according to body weight.
- Instruct the client that all urine should be saved for 4, 5, or 6 hours (according to the order or laboratory policy) in a bottle kept on ice or refrigerated.

Following collection time, the urine specimen should be taken immediately to the laboratory.

- Explain to the client that blood will be drawn 4 to 6 hours after the ascorbic acid is administered.
- Post the time for urine collection on the chart or Kardex or by the bedside. Visitors should not discard the client's urine.

Aspartate aminotransferase (AST) (serum)

Serum Glutamic Oxaloacetic Transaminase (SGOT)

Reference Values

Adult: *Average range:* 8–38 U/l; 5–40 U/ml (Frankel), 4–36 IU/l, 16–60 U/ml at 30°C (Karmen), 8–33 U/l at 37°C (SI units). Female values may be slightly lower than those of males. Exercise tends to increase values (values can vary among institutions).

Child: *Newborns:* Four times the normal level. *Child:* Similar to adults. *Elderly:* Slightly higher than adults.

Description

Aspartate aminotransferase/serum glutamic oxaloacetic transaminase (AST/SGOT) is an enzyme found mainly in the heart muscle and liver, with moderate amounts in skeletal muscle, the kidneys, and the pancreas. Its concentration is low in the blood except when there is cellular injury, and then large amounts are released into the circulation.

High levels of serum AST are found following an acute myocardial infarction (MI) and liver damage. Six to 10 hours after an acute MI, AST leaks out of the heart muscle and reaches its peak in 24 to 48 hours after the infarction. The serum AST level returns to normal 4 to 6 days later if there is no additional infarction. Serum AST is usually compared with other cardiac enzymes (creatine kinase [CK], lactate dehydrogenase [LDH]).

In liver disease, the serum level increases by 10 times or more and remains elevated for a longer period of time.

Purposes

- To detect an elevation of serum AST, an enzyme found mainly in the heart muscle and liver that increases during an acute MI and liver damage.
- To compare AST results with CK and LDH for diagnosing an acute MI.

Clinical Problems

Decreased Level: Pregnancy, diabetic ketoacidosis. *Drug Influence:* Salicylates.

Elevated Level: Acute MI, hepatitis, liver necrosis, musculoskeletal diseases and trauma, acute pancreatitis, cancer of the liver, severe angina pectoris, strenuous exercise, IM injections. *Drug Influence:* Antibiotics (ampicillin, carbenicillin, clindamycin, cloxacillin, erythromycin, gentamicin, lincomycin, nafcillin, oxacillin, polycillin, tetracycline), vitamins (folic acid, pyridoxine, vitamin A), narcotics (codeine, morphine, meperidine [Demerol]), antihypertensives (methyldopa

[Aldomet], guanethidine), mithramycin, digitalis preparation, cortisone, flurazepam (Dalmane), indomethacin (Indocin), isoniazid (INH), rifampin, oral contraceptives, salicylates, theophylline.

Procedure

- Collect 3 to 5 ml of venous blood in a red-top tube. Avoid hemolysis.
- Draw blood before drugs are given. The enzyme will remain stable for 4 days, refrigerated.
- List on the laboratory slip drugs the client is taking that can cause false-positive levels, with the date and time last given.
- There is no food or fluid restriction.

Factors Affecting Laboratory Results

- IM injections could increase serum AST levels.
- Hemolysis of the blood specimen could affect laboratory results.
- Drugs increasing the serum AST level *(see Drug Influence above)* could affect test results.
- Salicylates may cause false-positive or -negative serum levels.

NURSING IMPLICATIONS WITH RATIONALE

Elevated Level

- Hold drugs causing an elevated serum AST level for 24 hours prior to the blood test, with the physician's permission. Drugs that should not be withheld should be listed on the laboratory slip and charted.
- Compare serum AST levels with other cardiac enzyme results. Check serum ALT levels to determine if liver damage could be responsible for the abnormal value.
- Do not administer IM injections before the blood test; IM injections can increase the serum AST level. Few medications (e.g., morphine) can be given intravenously without affecting the serum level.
- Assess the client for signs and symptoms of MI (e.g., chest and arm pain, dyspnea, or diaphoresis). Changes should be reported and charted.
- Listen to the client's concerns. Answer questions or refer questions to appropriate health professionals.

Client Teaching

- Instruct the client to report symptoms of chest and arm pain, nausea, or diaphoresis immediately—day or night.

Aspirin

See Salicylates

Atrial natriuretic factor (ANF)

See Atrial Natriuretic Hormone (ANH)

Atrial natriuretic hormone (ANH) (plasma)

Atrial Natriuretic Factor (ANF), Atrionatriuretic Peptides

Reference Values

20–77 pg/ml; 20–77 ng/l (SI units).

Description

Atrial natriuretic hormone (ANH) is secreted from the atria of the heart and acts as an antagonist to renin and aldosterone. It is released during expansion of the atrium, produces vasodilation, and increases glomerular filtration rate. It counteracts the renin-angiotensin system by inhibiting the action of angiotensin II, thus promoting a decrease in blood pressure. ANH reduces renal reabsorption of sodium, blocks renin release by the kidney, and blocks aldosterone secretion from the adrenal glands, and thus has an antihypertensive effect. With the physiologic effects of ANH, preload, afterload, and blood volume are reduced. An elevated ANH level can be used as a diagnostic tool to detect cardiovascular disease, early asymptomatic left ventricular disorder, and congestive heart failure (CHF). However, with chronic level CHF, the ANH is decreased; whereas, with acute congestive heart failure, the ANH level is elevated.

Purposes

- To detect an elevated ANH level.
- To confirm cardiovascular disease, particularly CHF.

Clinical Problems

Decreased Level: Chronic CHF. *Drug Influence:* Prazosin, urapidil.

Elevated Level: Acute CHF, paroxysmal atrial tachycardia, early cardiovascular disease, subarachnoid hemorrhage.

Procedure

- The client is NPO for 8 to 12 hours to the test.
- Withhold cardiac drugs such as beta-blockers, calcium blockers, diuretics, vasodilators, and digoxin until after the blood sample has been taken. Some health care providers want these drugs withheld for 24 hours.
- Collect 5 ml of venous blood in a lavender-top tube. Ice the tube and take it immediately to the laboratory.

Factors Affecting Laboratory Results

- Cardiac drugs *(see Procedure)*.
- Improper care of the blood sample.

NURSING IMPLICATIONS WITH RATIONALE

- Obtain a health and drug history from the client. List drugs that the client is currently taking. Certain cardiac drugs should be withheld until after the test because they could affect the ANH level, causing an inaccurate lab result *(see Procedure)*.
- Take vital signs. Compare findings to baseline readings.
- Answer the client's questions. Be supportive of the client.

Client Teaching

- Instruct the client to keep health care appointments.
- Inform the client to notify his or her health care provider if difficulty in breathing, shortness of breath, chest pain, and/or indigestion occurs.

Barbiturate (blood)

Reference Values

Adult:

Barbiturate	Action	Therapeutic	Toxic
Secobarbital (Seconal)	Short acting	1–5 µg/ml	>8 µg/ml
Pentobarbital (Nembutal)	Short acting	1–5 µg/ml	>8 µg/ml
Amobarbital (Amytal)	Intermediate acting	5–14 µg/ml	>20 µg/ml
Phenobarbital	Long acting	10–30 µg/ml 20–40 µg/ml (seizure control)	>60 µg/ml

Child: *Phenobarbital: Therapeutic:* 15–30 µg/ml; *Toxic:* >35 µg/ml.

Description

Barbiturate toxicity is a frequent cause of unconsciousness resulting from accidental or intentional barbiturate overdose. Barbiturates have different effects, and those that are short acting tend to be more potent and toxic than the long-acting types. Phenobarbital tends to be least toxic; however, this depends on the amount taken. This long-acting barbiturate peaks in 12 to 18 hours, and its serum half-life is 48 to 96 hours.

Alcohol and tranquilizers can intensify the effects of barbiturates. Blood barbiturate levels are usually measured on unconscious/comatose clients when the cause of unresponsiveness is unknown.

Purposes

- To monitor specific barbiturate serum level.
- To detect a high serum barbiturate level.

Procedure

- Collect 5 ml of venous blood in a red-top (preferred) or lavender-top tube.
- There is no food or fluid restriction.
- Urine and gastric contents may be examined for barbiturates.

Factors Affecting Laboratory Results

- Alcohol and tranquilizers cause false results.
- Drugs: antipyrine and theophylline can elevate the barbiturate level.

NURSING IMPLICATIONS WITH RATIONALE

- Observe for signs and symptoms of barbiturate toxicity (i.e., depressed respirations, bradycardia, and loss of consciousness).
- Obtain a history from the family or a friend to determine whether the client has been taking a barbiturate and, if so, which type. Report the drug history.
- Monitor the urinary output. Renal dysfunction caused by renal ischemia and tubular damage can prolong recovery. Diuretics, especially osmotic, have been used for correcting the effects of long-lasting barbiturates.
- Report if the client is taking tranquilizers and barbiturates. The combination of these two drugs could cause respiratory distress.

Client Teaching

- Inform the client that it is important to keep medical appointments when taking barbiturates so that the health care provider can evaluate the effects of the drug and have the blood barbiturate levels checked.
- Instruct the client not to combine alcohol with barbiturates. Alcohol intensifies the effects of barbiturates, and respiratory distress could result.

Bilirubin (indirect) (serum)

Van Den Bergh Test

Reference Values

Adult: 0.1–1.0 mg/dl, 1.7–17.1 μmol/l (SI units).

Child: Same as adult.

Description

(See Bilirubin [Total and Direct].)

Indirect-reacting or unconjugated bilirubin is protein bound and is associated with increased destruction of red blood cells (hemolysis).

Elevated indirect bilirubin can occur in autoimmune- or transfusion-induced hemolysis, in hemolytic processes caused by sickle cell anemia, in pernicious anemia, and with malaria and septicemia. Internal hemorrhage into soft tissues and the body cavity can cause the bilirubin to rise in 5 to 6 hours. With certain clinical problems, congestive heart failure (CHF), and severe liver damage, both indirect and direct bilirubin levels will increase. Indirect bilirubin frequently increases because the damaged liver cells cannot conjugate normal amounts, which leads to increased, unconjugated bilirubin.

Levels of indirect serum bilirubin may increase in hemolytic disease, such as erythroblastosis fetalis, in newborns. The newborn's liver is immature, and when extremely high levels of bilirubin occur, irreversible neurologic damage, referred to as kernicterus, could result.

Purpose

- To detect the presence of unconjugated bilirubin due to hemolytic disease or liver disease.

Clinical Problems

Decreased Level: *Drug Influence: See Bilirubin (Total and Direct).*

Elevated Level: Erythroblastosis fetalis, sickle cell anemia, transfusion reaction, pernicious anemia, malaria, septicemia, hemolytic anemias, CHF, decompensated cirrhosis, hepatitis. *Drug Influence:* Aspirin, rifampin, phenothiazines. *(See Bilirubin [Total and Direct].)*

Procedure

- There is no laboratory test for indirect bilirubin. Indirect bilirubin is calculated by subtracting direct bilirubin from the total bilirubin:

Total bilirubin − Direct bilirubin = Indirect bilirubin

In newborn infants, only the total is determined, and this represents the indirect bilirubin only.

Factors Affecting Laboratory Results

- *See Bilirubin (Total and Direct).*

NURSING IMPLICATIONS WITH RATIONALE

Elevated Levels

- Check the client's indirect serum bilirubin level, and compare it with the direct bilirubin result. If the indirect bilirubin is elevated and the direct is not, then the cause is a hemolytic problem.

Client Teaching

- Instruct the client not to eat before blood is drawn. Carrots, yams, or foods high in fat should not be eaten the night before.

Bilirubin (total and direct) (serum)

Reference Values

Adult: *Total:* 0.1–1.2 mg/dl, 1.7–20.5 µmol/l (SI units). *Direct (conjugated):* 0.1–0.3 mg/dl, 1.7–5.1 µmol/l (SI units).

Child: *Newborn: Total:* 1–12 mg/dl, 17.1–205 µmol/l (SI units). *Child:* 0.2–0.8 mg/dl.

Description

Bilirubin is formed from the breakdown of hemoglobin by the reticuloendothelial system and is carried in the plasma to the liver, where it is conjugated (directly) to form bilirubin diglucuronide and is excreted in the bile. There are two forms of bilirubin in the body: the conjugated, or direct-reacting (soluble), and the unconjugated, or indirect-reacting (protein bound). If the total bilirubin is within normal range, direct and indirect bilirubin levels do not need to be analyzed. If one value of bilirubin is reported, it represents the total bilirubin.

Direct or conjugated bilirubin is frequently the result of obstructive jaundice, either extrahepatic (from stones or tumor) or intrahepatic in origin. Conjugated bilirubin cannot escape in the bile into the intestine and thus backs up and is absorbed into the blood stream. Damaged liver cells cause a blockage of the bile sinusoid, increasing the serum level of direct bilirubin. With hepatitis and decompensated cirrhosis, both direct and indirect bilirubin may be elevated.

Serum bilirubin (total) in newborns can be as high as 12 mg/dl; the panic level is >15 mg/dl. Jaundice is frequently present when serum bilirubin levels are >3 mg/dl.

Purposes

- To monitor bilirubin levels associated with jaundice.
- To suggest the occurrence of a liver disorder.

Clinical Problems

Decreased Level: Iron-deficiency anemia. *Drug Influence:* Barbiturates, salicylates (aspirin)—large amounts, penicillin, caffeine.

Elevated Level: Obstructive jaundice caused by stones or neoplasms, hepatitis, cirrhosis of the liver, infectious mononucleosis, liver metastasis (cancer), Wilson's disease. *Drug Influence:* Antibiotics (amphotericin B, clindamycin, erythromycin, gentamicin, lincomycin, oxacillin, tetracyclines), sulfonamides, antituberculosis drugs (para-aminosalicylic acid, isoniazid [INH]), allopurinol, diuretics (acetazolamide [Diamox], ethacrynic acid [Edecrin]), mithramycin, dextran, diazepam (Valium), barbiturates, narcotics (codeine, morphine, meperidine [Demerol]), flurazepam (Dalmane), indomethacin (Indocin), methotrexate, methyldopa (Aldomet), papaverine, procainamide (Pronestyl), steroids, oral contraceptives, tolbu-tamide (Orinase), Vitamins A, C, and K.

Procedure

- Collect 3 to 5 ml of venous blood in a red-top tube. Avoid hemolysis.
- Keep the client NPO except for water.
- Hold medications that would increase the serum bilirubin for 24 hours, with the health care provider's approval. If medications are given, list the drugs on the laboratory slip and the time they were last given.
- *Caution:* Whenever blood is drawn for liver function tests, avoid self-contamination to prevent possible infection (such as hepatitis). Use isolation technique. Protect the blood specimen from sunlight and artificial light, as light will reduce the bilirubin content. Blood should be sent to the laboratory immediately so that separation of serum from the cells can be performed as soon as possible to avoid hemolysis. Infants can have the blood taken from the heel of the foot. Two blood microtubes should be filled.

Factors Affecting Laboratory Results

- A high-fat dinner prior to the test may affect bilirubin levels.
- Carrots and yams may increase the serum bilirubin level.
- Hemolysis of the blood specimen can give inaccurate results. The tube should not be shaken.
- A blood specimen exposed to sunlight or artificial light will degrade the bile pigment. Certain drugs *(see Drug Influence)* can increase or decrease the serum bilirubin level.

NURSING IMPLICATIONS AND RATIONALE

Elevated Level

- Check the serum bilirubin (total), and if it is elevated, check the direct and indirect bilirubin levels.
- Check the sclera of the eyes and the inner aspects of the arm for jaundice.

Client Teaching

- Instruct the client that he or she should have nothing by mouth except water before the test. If his or her medications are withheld, an appropriate explanation should be given. The nurse should emphasize that fats, carrots, and yams should not be eaten the night before the blood test.
- Inform the mother whose baby is jaundiced that the bilirubin level will be closely monitored until the level is in normal range.

Bilirubin and bile (urine)

Reference Values
Adult: *Negative:* 0.02 mg/dl.

Description
Bilirubin is not normally present in urine; however, a very small quantity could be present without being detected by routine test methods. Bilirubin is formed from the breakdown of hemoglobin and is transported to the liver, where it is conjugated and is excreted as bile. Conjugated or direct bilirubin is water soluble and is excreted in the urine when there is an increased serum level. Unconjugated or indirect bilirubin is fat-soluble and cannot be excreted in the urine.

Bilirubinuria (bilirubin in urine) indicates liver damage or biliary obstruction (e.g., stones), and a large amount has a characteristic dark-amber color. When the amber-colored urine is shaken, it produces a yellow foam. It can frequently be tested by the floor nurse with a dipstick or reagent tablet.

Purpose
- To compare the urine bilirubin level with the serum bilirubin level and other liver enzyme tests to detect liver disorder.

Clinical Problems
Elevated Level: Obstructive biliary disease, liver disease (hepatitis, toxic agents), CHF with jaundice, cancer of the liver (secondary). *Drug Influence:* Phenothiazines—chlorpromazine (Thorazine), acetophenazine (Tindal); chlorprothixene (Taractan); phenazopyridine (Pyridium); chlorzoxazone (Paraflex).

Procedure
- Use either urine dipstick or Ictotest reagent tablets for the bilirubinuria test. The bili-Labstix is dipped in urine and after 20 seconds is compared to a color chart on the bottle. For urine dipstick and Ictotest tablets, follow the directions on the bottle.
- Test urine bilirubin within 1 hour. Keep urine away from ultraviolet light.
- There is no food or fluid restriction.

Factors Affecting Laboratory Results
- Certain drugs can give a false-positive result *(see Drug Influence above)*.
- Exposure of urine to light for 1 hour will cause deterioration of bile pigments.

NURSING IMPLICATIONS WITH RATIONALE

Elevated Level

- Check the serum bilirubin—total and direct—and report if it is elevated. Test the urine for bilirubinuria. Compare urine and serum findings.
- Assess the color of the urine. If it is dark-amber in color, shake the urine specimen and note whether a yellow foam appears.
- Record the results of a urine dipstick and the urine color on the client's chart or Kardex.
- Notify the health care provider of amber urine with yellow foam and of test results.

Bleeding time (blood)

Reference Values

Adult: *Ivy Method:* 3–7 minutes. *Duke Method:* 1–3 minutes. SI units for the Ivy and Duke methods are the same. (Duke method is seldom performed.)

Description

Two methods, Ivy and Duke, are used to determine whether bleeding time is normal or prolonged. Bleeding time is lengthened in thrombocytopenia (decreased platelet count, <50,000). The test is frequently performed when there is a history of bleeding (easy bruising), familial bleeding, or preoperative screening. The Ivy technique, in which the forearm is used for the incision, is the most popular method. Aspirin and anti-inflammatory medications can prolong the bleeding time.

Purpose

- To check bleeding time for various health problems.

Clinical Problems

Decreased Rate: Hodgkin's disease.

Prolonged Rate: Thrombocytopenic purpura, platelet abnormality, vascular abnormalities, leukemia, severe liver disease, disseminated intravascular coagulation (DIC), aplastic anemia, factor deficiencies (V, VII, XI), Christmas disease, hemophilia. *Drug Influence:* Salicylates (aspirin, others), dextran, mithramycin, warfarin (Coumadin), streptokinase (streptodornase; fibrinolytic agent).

Procedure

Ivy Method

- Cleanse the volar surface of the forearm (below the antecubital space) with alcohol and allow it to dry. Inflate the blood pressure cuff to 40 mm Hg, and leave it inflated during the test. Puncture the skin 2.5 mm deep on the forearm; start timing with a stopwatch. Blot blood drops carefully every 30 seconds until bleeding ceases. The time required for bleeding to stop is recorded in seconds.
- The test should *not* be performed while the client is taking anticoagulant or aspirin; withhold medications for 3 to 7 days.

Duke Method

- The area used is the earlobe.
- There is no food or fluid restriction.

Factors Affecting Laboratory Results

- Method used; improper technique—the puncture wound might be deeper than required. Blotting the incision area and not the blood drops can break off fibrin particles, prolonging the bleeding time.
- Aspirin and anticoagulants increase the bleeding time.

NURSING IMPLICATIONS WITH RATIONALE

Prolonged Rate

- Relate prolonged bleeding time to clinical problems and drugs. The nurse should be familiar with the methods used to obtain the bleeding time.
- Obtain a drug history of the last time (date) the client took aspirin or anticoagulants. Aspirin prevents platelet aggregation, and bleeding can be prolonged by taking only one aspirin tablet (5 grains, or 325 mg) 3 days prior to test. A history of taking "cold medications" should be recorded, because many cold remedies contain salicylates.
- Note whether the client has been consuming alcohol. Alcohol increases bleeding time, and the bleeding may be difficult to stop.
- Apply a dressing to the puncture wound site (Ivy method) to stop the bleeding.

Client Teaching

- Instruct the client not to take aspirin and over-the-counter cold remedies for 3 days before the test. If the client takes aspirin or anticoagulants, the laboratory should be notified and the drug names should be written on the laboratory slip.
- Explain to the client how the test is performed. In the Ivy method the forearm is used, and in the Duke method the earlobe is used. The step-by-step method of the procedure should be explained *(see Procedure above)*. The nurse should check with the laboratory for changes in procedure.
- Listen to the client's concerns.

Blood gases

See Arterial Blood Gases

Blood urea nitrogen (BUN) (serum)

Reference Values

Adult: 5–25 mg/dl.

Child: *Infant:* 5–15 mg/dl. *Child:* 5–20 mg/dl.

Elderly: Could be slightly higher than adult.

Description

Urea is formed as an end product of protein metabolism and is excreted by the kidneys. An elevated blood urea nitrogen (BUN) level could be an indication of dehydration, prerenal failure, or renal failure. Dehydration from vomiting, diarrhea, and/or inadequate fluid intake can cause an increase in the BUN (up to 35 mg/dl). With dehydration, the serum creatinine level would most likely be normal or high normal. Once the client is hydrated, the BUN should return to normal; if it does not, prerenal or renal failure would be suspected. Nephrons (kidney cells) tend to decrease during the aging process, and so older persons may have a higher BUN. Digested blood from gastrointestinal (GI) bleeding is a source of protein and can cause the BUN to elevate. A low BUN value usually indicates overhydration (hypervolemia).

The **BUN/Creatinine Ratio** is a calculation with reference value of 10:1 to 15:1. A decreased BUN/creatinine ratio occurs with malnutrition, liver disease, low-protein diet, excessive IV fluids, dialysis, or overhydration. An elevated BUN/creatinine ratio, >15:1, is found in renal disease, inadequate renal perfusion, shock, dehydration, GI bleeding, and drugs such as steroids and tetracyclines. See separate listing for BUN/creatinine.

Purpose

■ To detect a renal disorder or dehydration associated with increased BUN levels.

Clinical Problems

Decreased Level: Severe liver damage, low-protein diet, overhydration, malnutrition (negative nitrogen balance), IV fluids (glucose). *Drug Influence:* Phenothiazines.

Increased Level: Dehydration; high-protein intake; GI bleeding; prerenal failure (low renal blood supply caused by congestive heart failure, diabetes mellitus, acute myocardial infarction, renal insufficiency/failure from shock, sepsis, kidney diseases [glomerular nephritis, pyelonephritis]), licorice (excessive ingestion). *Drug Influence:* Nephrotoxic drugs; diuretics (hydrochlorothiazide [Hydrodiuril], ethacrynic acid [Edecrin], furosemide [Lasix], triamterene [Dyrenium]); antibiotics, (bacitracin, cephaloridine [high doses], gentamicin, kanamycin, chloramphenicol [Chloromycetin], methicillin, neomycin, vancomycin); antihypertensive agents (methyldopa [Aldomet], guanethidine [Ismelin]); sulfonamides; propranolol; morphine; lithium carbonate; salicylates.

Procedure

- Collect 3 to 5 ml of venous blood in a red-top tube. Avoid hemolysis.
- It is preferable to have the client remain NPO for 8 hours.

Factors Affecting Laboratory Results

- The hydration status of the client should be known. Overhydration can give a false-low BUN level, and dehydration can give a false-high BUN level.
- Drugs (i.e., antibiotics, diuretics, and antihypertensive agents) raise the BUN level.

NURSING IMPLICATIONS WITH RATIONALE

- Compare serum BUN and serum creatinine results. If both BUN and creatinine are elevated, kidney disease should be highly suspected.

Decreased Level

- Assess the client's dietary intake. A low-protein intake and a high-carbohydrate intake can decrease the BUN level.
- Report on clients receiving continuous dextrose intravenously without protein intake.
- Check the client for signs and symptoms of overhydration (irritated cough, dyspnea, neck-vein engorgement, and chest rales) when the BUN is decreased. Overhydration (hypervolemia) causes hemodilution, diluting the urea in the blood.

Elevated Level

- Report urinary output <25 ml/hour or 600 ml/day. Urea is excreted by the kidneys, and with a decreased urine output, urea accumulates in the blood.
- Check vital signs. A fast pulse, decreased blood pressure, and increased respiration could indicate dehydration and, if severe enough, could lead to shock.
- Determine the hydration status of the client. If dehydration is present, the elevated BUN may be attributed to hemoconcentration. Hydrating with IV fluids should correct the problem.

- Avoid overhydration with IV fluid. Rapid administration of IV fluids can overload the vascular system, especially in the aged, in children, and in heart patients, resulting in hypervolemia. This can lead to pulmonary edema.
- Assess the client's dietary intake. A high-protein diet will increase the serum BUN. Individuals on a high-protein diet for dieting purposes will have an elevated BUN level unless adequate fluids are taken.
- Recognize drugs that increase the BUN (i.e., antibiotics, diuretics, antihypertensive agents, and others; *see Drug Influence*).

Client Teaching

- Instruct clients with a slightly elevated BUN to increase fluid intake. Care should be taken in forcing fluids in clients with heart and kidney problems.

Blood urea nitrogen/creatinine ratio (serum)

Urea Nitrogen/Creatinine Ratio

Reference Values

Adult: 10:1 to 20:1 (BUN:creatinine). *Average:* 15:1.

Description

The blood urea nitrogen (BUN)/creatinine ratio is an effective test primarily for determining renal function. BUN level can increase because of dehydration as well as renal dysfunction. The creatinine level does not increase with dehydration but definitely increases with renal dysfunction. This ratio test is more sensitive to the relationship of BUN to creatinine than separate tests of BUN and creatinine. However, liver function, dietary protein intake, and muscle mass may affect test result.

A decreased ratio can occur from acute renal tubular necrosis and low protein intake. The ratio may be increased because of reduced renal perfusion, glomerular disease, obstructive uropathy, or high protein intake.

Purpose

- To determine renal function.

Clinical Problems

Decreased Ratio: Acute renal tubular necrosis, low protein intake, malnutrition, pregnancy, liver disease, hemodialysis (urea loss). *Drug Influence:* Phenacemide.

Elevated Ratio: Reduced renal perfusion (dehydration, heart failure), glomerular disease, tissue or muscle destruction, high protein intake, obstructive uropathy, azotemia. *Drug Influence:* Tetracycline, corticosteroids.

Procedure

- No food or fluid restriction is required.
- Collect 5 to 7 ml of venous blood in a red-top tube.

Factors Affecting Laboratory Results

- Variations in protein intake; liver disease.

NURSING IMPLICATIONS WITH RATIONALE

- Assess the client's renal function, including urine output, BUN, and serum creatinine level. Urine output should be at least 600 ml per day.
- Place a note in client's chart or Kardex that urine needs to be measured.
- Assess the client's dietary intake. Record increase or decrease in protein intake.
- Check his or her hydration status. Dehydration may cause increase in the BUN/creatinine ratio.

Client Teaching

- Instruct the client that urine needs to be measured and to urinate in a urinal or bedpan. Inform the health care personnel after each voiding so that urine can be measured. Tell the client not to put toilet paper in the urine.

Blood volume

Reference Values

Adult: *Total Blood Volume:* 55–80 ml/kg. Male: 7.5% body weight. Female: 6.5% body weight. *Red Cell Volume:* Male: 25–35 ml/kg. Female: 20–30 ml/kg. *Plasma Volume:* Male: 32–46 ml/kg. Female: 30–45 ml/kg.

Description

The blood volume determination is commonly used to determine the total blood, red blood cell (RBC), and plasma volumes. Two radioactive substances can be used for measurement: Cr-51–tagged red cells for RBC volume and I-131– or I-125–tagged human serum albumin for plasma volume. The client's blood is mixed with the radioactive substance.

This test is useful for monitoring blood loss during surgery, evaluating gastrointestinal (GI) or uterine bleeding, determining the cause of hypotension, determining the blood component lost (i.e., RBCs, plasma) for replacement therapy, and diagnosing polycythemia vera.

Purposes

- To determine total blood volume (RBC and plasma).
- To monitor blood loss during surgery.
- To evaluate GI or uterine bleeding

Clinical Problems

Decreased Volume: Dehydration (total and plasma volume), hypovolemic shock, hemorrhaging.

Elevated Volume: Dehydration (RBC volume), polycythemia vera, overhydration (total volume).

Procedure

- Obtain the height and weight of the client.
- Obtain a blood sample.
- Personnel from the nuclear medicine laboratory will obtain a blood sample and mix a radioisotope (radionuclide, i.e., I-131, I-125, Cr-51) with the blood. After 15 to 30 minutes, the blood containing the radioactive substance will be reinjected into the client.
- Collect another blood sample in 15 minutes.

Factors Affecting Diagnostic Results

- IV fluids can affect the test results.
- Prolonged time for blood sample collection can affect results. If I-131–tagged albumin is used, it will leave the plasma (intravascular fluid compartment) after 15 minutes and enter the extravascular fluid compartment.

NURSING IMPLICATIONS WITH RATIONALE

- Explain the procedure to the client.
- Start IV therapy, if ordered, after the blood volume determination test has been completed.
- Explain to the client that the radioactive substance he or she will receive is of low amount and should be harmless.
- Answer the client's questions, or refer him or her to the appropriate health professionals.
- Observe for signs and symptoms of dehydration (i.e., dry mucous membrane, poor skin turgor, and shocklike symptoms).
- Observe for signs and symptoms of shock (i.e., tachycardia; tachypnea; pale, cold, clammy skin; and later a drop in blood pressure).

Bromide (serum)

Reference Values

Adult: Toxic levels: >100 mg/dl.

Child: Same as adult.

Description

The use of bromides as a prescription drug for depression and sedation is seldom ordered; however, today many bromide-containing compounds in patent medicines are available to the public. Because of the cumulative effect of bromides, chronic bromide intoxication is becoming a common occurrence. Acute bromide intoxication is rare, since bromide can cause gastrointestinal irritation.

The half-life of bromide is 12 days. Bromide is slowly excreted by the kidney, and the treatment for chronic bromide intoxication is to accelerate urinary excretion by chloride administration and mercurial diuretics.

Purpose

- To check for possible bromide toxicity.

Procedure

- Collect 5 ml of venous blood in a green-top tube.
- There is no food or fluid restriction.
- A colorimetric test using gold chloride is an old but still useful test. The gold chloride reacts with the bromide in the plasma/serum, forming a yellow/red/orange color, depending on the bromide concentration.

Factors Affecting Laboratory Results

- An extremely high bromide level will cause a decreased chloride level, because both are anions.

NURSING IMPLICATIONS WITH RATIONALE

- Observe for signs and symptoms of chronic bromide intoxication (i.e., anorexia, fever, skin rash, motor incoordination, tremors, delirium, impaired intellectual function, constipation, and weight loss).
- Obtain a history of over-the-counter drugs taken: when, for how long, and the daily quantity taken. If the bottle is available, read the label of the ingredients contained in the medicine.
- Check urine output. Bromides are excreted slowly by the kidneys, so "good" kidney function is extremely important.

Client Teaching

- Teach clients to read labels on patent medicines. Explain the importance of contacting a health care provider before taking most patent medicines.

Calcitonin (hCT) (serum)

Reference Values

Adult: *Male:* <40 pg/ml, <40 ng/l (SI units). *Female:* <25 pg/ml, <25 ng/l (SI units).

Child: *Newborn:* usually higher than in adults.

Child: <70 pg/ml, <70 ng/l (SI units).

Description

Calcitonin, a potent hormone secreted by the C cells of the thyroid gland, aids in maintaining normal serum calcium and phosphorus levels. This hormone is secreted in response to an elevated serum calcium level. It inhibits calcium reabsorption by the osteoclasts and osteocytes of the bones and increases calcium excretion by the kidneys. Calcitonin acts as an antagonist to the parathyroid hormone (PTH) and Vitamin D, lowering serum calcium levels to maintain calcium balance in the body.

Excess calcitonin secretion occurs in medullary carcinoma of the thyroid. A serum calcitonin level is frequently ordered to aid in the diagnosis of thyroid medullary carcinoma (>500–2000 pg/ml [probable] and >2000 pg/ml [definite]) and ectopic calcitonin-producing tumors of the lung and breast. Monitoring calcitonin levels after medullary carcinoma removal will help predict if the tumor recurs.

When the serum calcitonin level is slightly to moderately elevated (100–500 pg/ml), a *calcitonin stimulation test* might be performed in diagnosis of thyroid medullary carcinoma. This test consists of either a 4-hour calcium infusion or a 10-second pentagastrin infusion with measurement of serum calcitonin before and after the infusion.

Purpose

- To aid in the diagnosis of thyroid medullary carcinoma or parathyroid hyperplasia or adenoma.

Clinical Problems

Elevated Level: Medullary carcinoma of the thyroid, carcinoma of the lung or breast, chronic renal failure, parathyroid hyperplasia or adenoma, pernicious anemia, Zollinger-Ellison syndrome, acute or chronic thyroiditis, islet cell tumors, pheochromocytoma.

Procedure

- The client should be NPO after midnight. A small amount of water could be given if needed.
- Collect 5 to 7 ml of venous blood in a green- or lavender-top tube or in a chilled red-top tube (preferred). Avoid hemolysis. Send the blood specimen immediately to the laboratory for analysis or freeze to avoid deterioration.

Calcitonin Stimulation Test

- Draw serum calcitonin level before administering IV calcium or IV pentagastrin.
- Administer IV calcium (15 mg/kg) over 4 hours to provoke calcitonin secretion.

OR

- Administer IV pentagastrin (0.5 μg/kg) over 5 to 10 seconds.
- After IV calcium infusion, draw serum calcitonin level 3 to 4 hours postinfusion. After pentagastrin infusion, draw serum calcium level at 2 minutes, 5 minutes, and 10 minutes.

Factors Affecting Laboratory Results

- Hemolysis could increase serum calcitonin level.
- Levels may be increased during pregnancy and lactation.

NURSING IMPLICATIONS WITH RATIONALE

- Obtain a history of familial thyroid carcinoma. Record and report a positive history.
- Observe for signs and symptoms of hypercalcemia (i.e., lethargy, headaches, weakness, muscle flaccidity, nausea and vomiting, and anorexia).

Client Teaching

- Instruct the client to remain NPO after midnight.
- Explain the calcitonin stimulating test (if ordered) to the client. Refer to the procedure.
- Inform the client that test results may take several days.

Calcium (Ca) and ionized calcium (serum)

Reference Values

Adult Total Ca: 4.5–5.5 mEq/l, 9–11 mg/dl, 2.3–2.8 mmol/l (SI units). *Ionized Ca:* 4.25–5.25 mg/dl, 2.2–2.5 mEq/l, 1.1–1.24 mmoL/l.

Child: *Newborn:* 3.7–7.0 mEq/l, 7.4–14.0 mg/dl. *Infant:* 5.0–6.0 mEq/l, 10–12 mg/dl. *Child:* 4.5–5.8 mEq/l, 9–11.5 mg/dl.

Description

Calcium is found most abundantly in the bones and teeth. Approximately 50% of the calcium is ionized, and only ionized calcium can be used by the body. Protein and albumin in the blood bind with calcium, thus decreasing the amount of free, ionized calcium. The ionized calcium level can be determined by using formulas that estimate the ionized calcium from total calcium. These formulas have been disputed. Only a few laboratories have the equipment to perform serum-ionized calcium levels. In acidosis, more calcium is ionized, regardless of the serum level, and in alkalosis, most of the calcium is protein bound and cannot be ionized.

The *serum-ionized calcium* (iCa) level is not affected by changes in serum protein/albumin concentration, and it reflects calcium metabolism better than total calcium values. A decrease in ionized calcium, <2.2 mEq/l or <4.25 mg/dl, might lead to neuromuscular irritability or tetany symptoms (tingling, twitching, spasmodic contractions).

Calcium is necessary for the transmission of nerve impulses and contraction of the myocardium and skeletal muscles. It causes blood clotting by converting prothrombin into thrombin. It strengthens capillary membranes. With a calcium deficit, there is an increased capillary permeability, which causes fluid to pass through the capillary.

A low serum-calcium level is called *hypocalcemia,* and an increased level is called *hypercalcemia.* Calcium imbalances require immediate attention, for serum calcium deficit can cause tetany symptoms, unless acidosis is present, and serum calcium excess can cause cardiac dysrhythmias.

Purposes

- To check for serum calcium excess or deficit.
- To monitor calcium levels.
- To detect calcium imbalance.

Clinical Problems

Decreased Level: Diarrhea, malabsorption of calcium from the gastrointestinal (GI) tract, extensive infections, burns, lack of calcium and Vitamin D intake, hypoparathyroidism, chronic renal failure caused by phosphorous retention, alcoholism, pancreatitis. *Drug Influence:* Cortisone preparations, antibiotics (gentamicin, methicillin), magnesium products (antacids), laxatives (excessive use), heparin, insulin, mithramycin, acetazolamide (Diamox).

Elevated Level: Hypervitaminosis D; hyperparathyroidism; malignant neoplasm of the bone, lung, breast, bladder, or kidney; multiple myeloma; prolonged immobilization; multiple fractures; renal calculi; exercise; alcoholism (alcoholic binge); milk-alkali syndrome. Drug Influence: Alkaline antacids, estrogen preparations, calcium salts, Vitamin D.

Procedure

- Collect 3 to 5 ml of venous blood in a red-top tube.
- There is no food or fluid restriction, unless SMA12 or similar group test is ordered.

Factors Affecting Laboratory Results

- Drugs *(see Drug Influence)* can cause calcium excess or deficit.
- A diet low in calcium or high in calcium and Vitamin D can affect results.
- IV saline (NaCl) solution can promote calcium loss.

NURSING IMPLICATIONS WITH RATIONALE

Decreased Level

- Observe for signs and symptoms of hypocalcemia (i.e., tetany symptoms: muscular twitching and tremors, spasms of the larynx, parathesia [tingling in and numbness of fingers], facial spasms, and spasmodic contractions).
- Check serum calcium values, and report abnormal results to the health care provider, especially if tetany symptoms are present.
- Assess for positive Chvostek's and Trousseau's signs of hypocalcemia. To test for positive Chvostek's sign, tap the area in front of the ear and observe for spasms of the cheek and the corner of the lip. To test for positive Trousseau's sign, inflate the blood pressure cuff for several minutes and observe for carpal spasms.
- Administer oral calcium supplements before or 1 to 1$\frac{1}{2}$ hours after meals.
- Observe for symptoms of hypocalcemia when the client is receiving massive transfusions of citrated blood. Citrates prevent calcium ionization. The serum calcium level may be affected.
- Monitor the pulse regularly if the client is receiving a digitalis preparation and calcium supplements. Calcium excess enhances the action of digitalis and can cause digitalis toxicity (nausea, vomiting, anorexia, bradycardia—arrhythmias).
- Administer IV fluids with 10% calcium gluconate slowly. Calcium should be administered in 5% dextrose in water and not in a saline solution, since sodium promotes calcium loss. Calcium should not be added to solutions containing bicarbonate because rapid precipitation will occur.

- Monitor the electrocardiogram during hypocalcemia for prolonged ST segments and lengthened QT intervals.

Client Teaching

- Instruct the client to avoid overuse of antacids and to prevent the chronic laxative habit. Excessive use of certain antacids could cause alkalosis, decreasing calcium ionization. In addition, many antacids contain magnesium, which could lower the serum calcium level. Many laxatives contain phosphates (phosphorous), which have an opposing effect on calcium, causing calcium loss. Chronic use of laxatives will decrease calcium absorption from the GI tract. Suggest fruits for improving bowel elimination.
- Encourage the client to consume foods high in calcium, in milk and milk products, and/or in protein. Protein is needed to enhance calcium absorption.
- Teach the client with hypocalcemia to avoid hyperventilation and crossing his or her legs, which could cause tetany symptoms.

Elevated Level

- Observe for signs and symptoms of hypercalcemia (i.e., lethargy, headaches, weakness, muscle flaccidity, heart block, anorexia, nausea, and vomiting).
- Promote active and passive exercises for bedridden clients. This will prevent calcium loss from the bone.
- Identify symptoms of digitalis toxicity when the client has an elevated serum calcium level and is receiving a digitalis preparation.
- Notify the health care provider if the client is receiving a thiazide diuretic, because this will inhibit calcium excretion and promote hypercalcemia.
- Check the urine pH. Calcium salts are more soluble in acid urine (pH <6.0) than in alkaline.
- Handle clients with long-standing hypercalcemia and bone demineralization gently to prevent pathologic fractures.

Client Teaching

- Instruct the client to avoid foods high in calcium, to be ambulatory when possible, and to increase oral fluid intake. Increased fluid intake dilutes calcium in the serum and urine and prevents calculi formation.
- Encourage the client to eat acid-ash foods, such as cranberry juice, meats, fish, poultry, eggs, cheese, and cereals, to keep the urine acidic.

Calcium (Ca) (urine)

Reference Values

Adult: *24-Hour:* Low-calcium diet: <150 mg/24 hours, <3.75 mmol/24 hours (SI units); average-calcium diet: 100–250 mg/24 hours, 2.50–6.25 mmol/24 hours; high-calcium diet: 250–300 mg/24 hours, 6.25–7.50 mmol/24 hours.

Child: Same as adult.

Description

Urine calcium reflects the dietary intake of calcium, the serum calcium level, and the effects of disease entities (hypo- or hyperparathyroidism, multiple myeloma, bone tumors, etc.). Hypercalciuria (increased calcium levels in the urine) usually accompanies an increased serum calcium level. Calcium excretion fluctuates and is lowest in the morning and highest after meals.

A 24-hour urine specimen for calciuria is useful for determining parathyroid gland disorders. In hyperparathyroidism, hyperthyroidism, and osteolytic disorders, the urinary calcium excretion is usually increased; it is decreased in hypoparathyroidism.

Purpose

See Calcium (Serum).

Clinical Problems

Decreased Level: Hypoparathyroidism, Vitamin D deficiency, hypothyroidism, chronic renal failure, malabsorption syndrome. *Drug Influence:* Thiazide diuretics.

Elevated Level: Hyperparathyroidism, osteoporosis, hyperthyroidism, malignancies (bone, breast, bladder), multiple myeloma, leukemias, hypervitaminosis D, amyotrophic lateral sclerosis (ALS), renal calculi acid–base imbalance. *Drug Influence:* Cholestyramine resin, sodium- and magnesium-containing drugs, parathyroid injection, Vitamin D.

Procedure

- Label the bottle with the exact date and the times that the urine collection started and ended.
- Acidic preservatives are required by most laboratories.
- Indicate on the laboratory slip whether the client's calcium intake has been limited in the last 3 days or whether the client has had an average or high calcium intake.

Factors Affecting Laboratory Results

- Discarded urine. All urine should be saved for the 24-hour urine collection.
- High or low calcium content of diet may affect test results.
- Thiazide diuretics can decrease the urine calcium level, and drugs containing sodium and magnesium can elevate the urine calcium level.

NURSING IMPLICATIONS WITH RATIONALE

Decreased Level

- Observe for tetany symptoms if the client's urine calcium level is low. *(See Calcium [Serum] for tetany symptoms.)*
- Have available a 10% solution of calcium gluconate for emergencies. When administered, IV calcium should be diluted in 5% dextrose in water and not in saline solution.
- *(See Calcium [Serum] for other nursing implications.)*

Elevated Level

- Observe clients for symptoms of renal calculi, especially if there is a history of renal calculi. Strain the urine, if indicated, and report severe low-back pain.
- Prevent the possibility of a pathologic fracture by moving the client gently. The client should be encouraged to do active exercises.
- *(See Calcium [Serum] for other nursing implications.)*

Client Teaching

- Instruct the client and family members that urine is to be saved. Tell the client not to put toilet paper or feces in the urine.

Calcium channel blockers (serum)

Verapamil (Calan, Isoptin), Nifedipine (Procardia), Diltiazem (Cardizem)

Reference Values

Adult:

Drug Name	Therapeutic Range	Toxic Level
Verapamil	100–300 ng/ml; 0.08–0.3 µg/ml	300 ng/ml; 0.3 µg/ml
Nifedipine	50–100 ng/ml	100 ng/ml
Diltiazem	50–200 ng/ml	200 ng/ml

Note: Dosage is calculated according to mg/kg.

Description

Calcium channel blockers inhibit slow-channel calcium influx into the myocardial cells and vascular smooth muscle. As the result of these actions, a decrease in myocardial contraction and myocardial oxygen consumption and coronary and systemic vasodilation can occur. The calcium channel blockers were commercially available in the United States in the late 1970s for treating ischemic heart disease, or angina pectoris. Of the three calcium channel blockers, nifedipine (Procardia) is the most potent vasodilator, then verapamil (Calan, Isoptin), and, least, diltiazem (Cardizem). Calcium channel blockers are being prescribed more frequently for their antianginal actions.

Verapamil (Calan, Isopotin): This agent can be administered orally or intravenously. Verapamil has a negative inotropic effect and should be used with caution in clients with heart failure. Ninety percent is bound to plasma proteins; 70% of the metabolized drug is excreted in the urine, 15% is excreted in feces, and 4% to 5% is excreted unchanged in the urine. The peak serum level is 5 hours for an oral dose and 10 to 15 minutes for an IV bolus. The half-life is 3 to 7 hours and after chronic therapy, 8 to 10 hours.

Nifedipine (Procardia): This agent has potent coronary and peripheral vasodilator effects. Ninety percent of the drug is absorbed and bound to plasma proteins. About 75% of the metabolized drug is excreted in the urine and 15% through the gastrointestinal (GI) tract. The peak serum level is 2 hours after the oral dose. The half-life is 4 to 5 hours.

Diltiazem (Cardizem): This calcium channel blocker is not as potent as verapamil or nifedipine. It is absorbed rapidly in the GI tract, and 80% is bound to plasma protein. Metabolites of diltiazem are excreted in the urine and feces. The peak serum level is 2 hours.

Purposes

- To monitor a specific calcium channel blocker level for maintaining a therapeutic range.
- To detect the toxic level for a specific calcium channel blocker, such as verapamil, nifedipine, or diltiazem

Clinical Problems

Elevated Level: Overdose of verapamil, nifedipine, or diltiazem; liver or renal diseases. *Drug Influence:* Beta-blockers (e.g., propranolol [Inderal]).

Procedure

- Collect 3 to 5 ml of venous blood in a red-top tube. Check with your laboratory for the preferred collecting tube.
- Record on the laboratory requisition slip the name of the drug, and the dose, route, and last time administered.
- There is no food or fluid restriction.

Factors Affecting Laboratory Results

- None known.

NURSING IMPLICATIONS WITH RATIONALE

- Check the client's pulse rate and blood pressure (BP) before each administered dose. The vasodilation effect of verapamil and diltiazem lowers pulse rate and BP. Nifedipine can decrease BP substantially without decreasing pulse rate.
- Observe for signs and symptoms related to calcium channel blocking agents (i.e., nausea, abdominal distress, headache, dizziness, lightheadedness, flushing hypotension, bradycardia).
- Monitor BP every 15 minutes for 1 hour after administering an IV bolus of verapamil. Transient asymptomatic hypotension could occur.
- Monitor urine output. Decreased output could indicate renal insufficiency; toxicity could result.
- Recognize that a calcium channel blocker administered with a beta-blocker could cause severe hypotension.

Client Teaching

- Teach the client how to take a radial pulse. Inform the client that the pulse rate should be checked before each dose and changes reported to the health care provider.
- Instruct the client not to abruptly discontinue a calcium channel blocking agent. Withdrawal symptoms (e.g., severe hypotension) could result.

- Instruct a client having constipation (verapamil induced) to eat foods high in fiber or to take a mild laxative.
- Instruct a client having palpitations and/or peripheral ankle or leg edema (nifedipine induced) to rest and to elevate the leg(s). Report changes to the health care provider.

Candida antibody test

Reference Values

Negative

Positive: >1:8 titer.

Description

This antibody test is to identify systemic candidiasis most often caused by *Candida albicans,* a yeast infection. Candidiasis frequently occurs in the immunocompromised person, and if untreated, the condition can become life-threatening. *Candida* sp infection accounts for approximately 80% of all major systemic fungal infections. It is the fourth most common organism found in bloodstream infections. Nosocomial candidiasis has increased about fivefold in the 1980s, which contributes to the prolongation of hospitalization.

Vulvovaginal candidiasis may result from prolonged use of potent broad-spectrum antibiotics (oral or intravenously administered) and glucocorticoid therapy. This type of candidiasis is associated with debilitating diseases, uncontrolled diabetes mellitus, and pregnancy. If untreated, it can lead to systemic candidiasis. Usually candidiasis occurs to the skin and mucous membrane.

Purpose

- To diagnose systemic candidiasis that cannot be determined by culture or by tissue specimen.

Clinical Problems

Elevated Level: Systemic candidiasis.

Procedure:

- Collect 5 ml of venous blood in a red-top tube. Avoid hemolysis by not shaking the tube.
- There is no food or fluid restriction.

Factors Affecting Laboratory Results

- Hemolysis of the blood specimen.

NURSING IMPLICATIONS WITH RATIONALE

- Obtain a history of the client's health complaint. Determine if the client is immunocompromised because of HIV or a debilitating disease.
- Record the drugs that the client is taking.
- Check vital signs. Report abnormal findings.

Client Teaching

- Instruct the client to remain on the drug treatment regimen for candidiasis. Stopping the therapy could cause a relapse.
- Listen to the client's concerns. Answer questions, and if unknown, refer the client to other health professionals.

Carbon dioxide combining power (serum or plasma)

CO_2 Combining Power

Reference Values

Adult: 22–30 mEq/l, 22–30 mmol/l (SI units).

Panic Range: <15 mEq/l and >45 mEq/l.

Child: 20–28 mEq/l.

Description

The serum carbon dioxide (CO_2) test, usually included with the electrolyte test, is performed to determine metabolic acid–base abnormalities. The serum CO_2 acts as a bicarbonate (HCO_3) determinant. When serum CO_2 is low, HCO_3 is lost, and acidosis results (metabolic acidosis). With an elevated serum CO_2, HCO_3 is conserved and alkalosis results (metabolic alkalosis).

Purpose

- To check for the presence of metabolic acidosis or alkalosis.

Clinical Problems

Decreased Level: Metabolic acidosis, diabetic ketoacidosis, starvation, severe diarrhea, dehydration, shock, acute renal failure, salicylate toxicity, exercise. *Drug Influence:* Diuretics (chlorothiazide [Diuril], hydrochlorothiazide [Hydrodiuril], triamterene [Dyrenium]), antibiotics (methicillin, tetracycline), nitrofurantoin (Furadantin), paraldehyde.

Elevated Level: Metabolic alkalosis, severe vomiting, gastric suction, peptic ulcer, hypothyroidism, potassium deficit, emphysema (hypoventilation). *Drug Influence:* Barbiturates, steroids (hydrocortisone, cortisone), diuretics (mercurial agents, ethacrynic acid [Edecrin]).

Procedure

- Collect 3 to 5 ml of venous blood in a green-top tube. A tourniquet should be used for a short time.
- There is no food or fluid restriction.

Factors Affecting Laboratory Results

- Drugs that can increase or decrease the serum CO_2 level *(see Drug Influence above)*.

NURSING IMPLICATIONS WITH RATIONALE

Decreased Level

- Know that a decreased serum CO_2 level is related to an acidotic state. Whenever there is excess acid in the body and the kidneys cannot excrete it, metabolic acidosis results. There are many causes of acidosis *(see Clinical Problems above)*.
- Assess for signs and symptoms of metabolic acidosis when the client's serum CO_2 level is decreased, especially when it is <15 mEq/l. Symptoms include deep, vigorous breathing (Kussmaul's breathing) and flushed skin.
- Report clinical findings of metabolic acidosis to the health care provider.

Elevated Level

- Know that an increased serum CO_2 level is related to an alkalotic state. Whenever there is an excess of HCO_3 in the body or a loss of acid, metabolic alkalosis occurs. There are many causes of alkalosis *(see Clinical Problems above)*.
- Assess for signs and symptoms of metabolic alkalosis when the client has been vomiting or has undergone gastric suctioning for several days. Signs and symptoms include shallow breathing, a serum CO_2 level >30 mEq/l, and a base excess >+2.

Carbon monoxide, carboxyhemoglobin (blood)

Reference Values

Adult: *Nonsmoker:* <2.5% of hemoglobin. **Smoker:** 4%–5% saturation of hemoglobin. *Heavy Smoker:* 5%–12% saturation of hemoglobin. **Toxic:** >15% saturation of hemoglobin.

Child: Similar to adult nonsmoker.

Description

Carbon monoxide (CO) combines with hemoglobin to produce carboxyhemoglobin, which can occur 200 times more readily than the combination of oxygen with hemoglobin (oxyhemoglobin). When CO replaces oxygen in the hemoglobin in excess of 25%, CO toxicity occurs.

Carbon monoxide is formed from incomplete combustion of carbon-combining compounds, as in automobile exhaust, fumes from improperly functioning furnaces, and cigarette smoke. Continuous exposure to CO, increasing carboxyhemoglobin by >60%, leads to coma and death. The treatment for CO toxicity is to administer a high concentration of oxygen.

Purpose

- To determine the percentage of CO in the hemoglobin; if high, it could be fatal.

Clinical Problems

Elevated Level: Smoking and exposure to smoking, automobile exhaust fumes, defective gas-burning appliances.

Procedure

- Collect 7 ml of venous blood in a lavender-top tube.
- The most common method of analysis is performed with an IL CO oximeter, a direct-reading instrument.
- There is no food or fluid restriction.

Factors Affecting Laboratory Results

- Heavy smoking.

NURSING IMPLICATIONS WITH RATIONALE

- Determine from the client's history (obtained from the client, family, or friends) whether CO inhalation could have occurred.

- Assess for mild to severe CO toxicity. Symptoms of mild CO toxicity are headache, weakness, malaise, dizziness, and dyspnea with exertion. Symptoms of moderate to severe toxicity are severe headache, bright-red mucous membranes, and cherry-red blood. When carboxyhemoglobin exceeds 40%, the blood's residue is brick red.
- Identify individuals who might be a candidate for CO poisoning. Persons complaining of continuous headaches or who are living (24 hours a day) in a house with an old heating system in the winter should have a blood CO test performed.

Carcinoembryonic antigen (CEA) (serum, plasma)

Reference Values

Adult: *Nonsmokers:* <2.5 ng/ml. *Smokers:* <5 ng/ml. *Acute Inflammatory Disorders:* >10 ng/ml. *Neoplasms:* >12 ng/ml.

Child: Not normally done; assumed to be low (level) after the child is several months old.

Description

Carcinoembryonic antigen (CEA) has been found in the GI epithelium of embryos and has been extracted from tumors in the adult gastrointestinal (GI) tract. Originally the CEA test was to detect colon cancer, especially adenocarcinoma. Elevated levels might occur when inflammation and tissue destruction are present. CEA should never be used as the sole criterion for diagnosis.

The CEA test is a nonspecific test; however, elevated levels have been found in approximately 70% of clients with known cancer of the large intestine and pancreas. The primary role of the CEA test is to monitor the treatment of colon and pancreatic carcinoma; it is also used for follow-up studies once cancer has been diagnosed. If the levels fall after treatment, the cancer is most likely under control. A CEA test may be ordered at 30- to 90-day intervals, and if a significant CEA level recurs, the physician may resume chemotherapy treatments or consider another form of therapy.

Purposes

- To monitor the treatment for colon or pancreatic carcinoma.
- To compare with other laboratory tests for diagnosing an inflammatory condition, or GI or pancreatic cancer.

Clinical Problems

Elevated Level: *Cancer:* GI tract (esophagus, stomach, small and large intestine, rectum), liver, pancreas, lung, breast, cervix, bladder, testes, kidney, leukemia; pulmonary emphysema; cirrhosis of the liver; bacterial pneumonia; chronic ischemic heart disease; acute pancreatitis; acute renal failure; ulcerative colitis; chronic cigarette smoking; neuroblastoma; inflammatory diseases; surgical trauma.

Procedure

- Collect 5 to 7 ml of venous blood in a red-top or lavender-top tube (preferred). Avoid hemolysis.
- Heparin should not be administered for 2 days before the test, since it interferes with the results.
- There is no food or fluid restriction.

Factors Affecting Laboratory Results

- Heparin interferes with the result of the CEA test.
- Hemolysis can affect test results.

NURSING IMPLICATIONS WITH RATIONALE

Elevated Level

- Relate clinical problems to elevated CEA levels. CEA levels >2.5 ng/ml do not always indicate cancer, nor do levels <2.5 ng/ml indicate an absence of cancer. The CEA test is useful for management of cancer treatment.
- Be supportive of client and family while awaiting test results.
- Hold heparin injections for 2 days before the test, with the health care provider's permission. If heparin is given, this fact should be noted on the laboratory slip.

Cardiolipin antibodies (IgG, IgM) (serum)

See Anticardiolipin Antibodies

Carotene (serum)

Reference Values

Adult: 60–300 μg/dl, 0.74–3.72 μmol/l (SI units) (varies with diet).

Child: 40–130 μg/dl.

Description

Carotene is a fat-soluble vitamin found in yellow and green vegetables and fruits. After absorption from the intestine, carotene is stored in the liver and can be converted to Vitamin A, according to body needs. When fat absorption is decreased, the serum carotene level is decreased, which is indicative of fat malabsorption syndrome. Causes of serum carotene deficit include poor diet, malabsorption, high fever, and pancreatic insufficiency.

Purpose

- To determine the cause of malabsorption syndrome or liver disease.

Clinical Problems

Decreased Level: Malabsorption syndrome, pancreatic insufficiency, protein malnutrition, febrile illness, severe liver disease, cystic fibrosis.

Elevated Level: Hyperlipidemia, diabetes mellitus, chronic nephritis, hypothyroidism, diet high in carrots, hypervitaminosis A (slight elevation), pregnancy, hypocholesterolemia.

Procedure

- Collect 7 to 10 ml of venous blood in a red-top tube. Protect from light.
- Foods rich in carotene—yellow and green vegetables, vegetable juice, and fruits—should be omitted for 2 to 3 days before the test (check laboratory procedure). If the health care provider wishes to check the serum carotene level for determining the absorption ability, a diet high in carotene will be ordered for several days. Water is permitted.
- NPO, a diet low in carotene, or a diet high in carotene should be recorded on the laboratory slip.

Factors Affecting Laboratory Results

- Mineral oil will interfere with carotene absorption.
- Foods rich in carotene can affect the serum results.

NURSING IMPLICATIONS WITH RATIONALE

Client Teaching

- Explain to the client that diet will be high or low in carotene, depending on the health care provider's clinical assumptions and orders. Drinking water is permitted.
- Explain to the client that the test is to determine whether there is a vitamin (carotene) deficiency.
- Answer the client's questions concerning what foods to avoid or to eat before the test. Vegetables and fruits are rich in carotene.

Catecholamines (plasma)

Reference Values

Epinephrine: *Supine:* <50 pg/ml. *Sitting:* <60 pg/ml. *Standing:* <90 pg/ml.

Norepinephrine: *Supine:* 110–410 pg/ml. *Sitting:* 120–680 pg/ml. *Standing:* 125–700 pg/ml.

Dopamine: *Supine and Standing:* <87 pg/ml.

Pheochromocytoma: *Total Catecholamines:* >1000 pg/ml.

Description

The three main catecholamines are epinephrine (adrenaline), norepinephrine, and dopamine, which are hormones secreted by the adrenal medulla. These catecholamines respond to stress, fear, hypoxia, hemorrhage, and strenuous exercise by increasing the blood pressure (BP). Catecholamines can be measured from plasma or by a 24-hour urine collection specimen. Catecholamine levels can vary according to time of day, body posture, and stress. The 24-hour urine catecholamine collection has the advantage of determining the daily secretion of hormones. A single plasma catecholamine level could be misleading because of catecholamine fluctuation, but it is considered 75% effective in diagnosing pheochromocytomas. Incorrect collection of a plasma catecholamine level can cause an inaccurate test result.

Fractional analysis of catecholamine levels (epinephrine, norepinephrine, dopamine) is helpful for identifying certain adrenal medullary tumors suspected in hypertensive clients. A comparison of the plasma catecholamine level with a 24-hour urine catecholamine test can aid in diagnosing pheochromocytoma.

Purpose

- To assist in the diagnosis of the health problem related to the abnormal amount of catecholamines in the plasma and urine.

Clinical Problems

Decreased Level: *Norepinephrine:* Anorexia nervosa, orthostatic hypotension. *Dopamine:* Parkinsonism.

Elevated Level: *Epinephrine and Norepinephrine:* Pheochromocytoma (continuous elevation with epinephrine); ganglioblastoma, ganglioneuroma, and neuroblastoma (higher elevations with norepinephrine); diabetic ketoacidosis; kidney disease; shock; thyrotoxicosis; acute myocardial infarction (MI); strenuous exercise. *Drug Influence:* Epinephrine, norepinephrine, bronchodilators, amphetamines, selected beta-adrenergics.

Procedure

- Foods rich in amines, such as chocolate, cocoa, wine, beer, tea, aged cheese, nuts (especially walnuts), and bananas, should be avoided 2 days prior to test.
- Selected drugs, such as over-the-counter cold medications that contain sympathomimetics, diuretics, antihypertensives, should be avoided for 2 days prior to the test.
- Strenuous exercise and smoking should be avoided prior to the test.
- NPO (food and fluids) 12 hours prior to the test.
- An indwelling venous catheter may be inserted for collection of blood samples. Having an IV in place helps to avoid a surge in catecholamine release when a venipuncture is performed during collection of the blood sample. The test may require a blood sample while the client is in a supine position and a sample while in a standing position. Blood should be collected early in the morning.
- Collect 7 to 10 ml of venous blood in a green- or lavender-top tube. Place the blood sample immediately in an ice bath and take to the laboratory. The laboratory should be notified when the specimen is obtained because the test should be run within 5 to 10 minutes after being drawn.

Factors Affecting Laboratory Results

- Not following the test procedure.
- Not putting the blood sample on ice or not running the test immediately.
- Plasma catecholamine levels decrease rapidly if red blood cells are not separated from the plasma within 5 to 10 minutes.

NURSING IMPLICATIONS WITH RATIONALE

- Monitor the client's BP. Report BP that remains elevated and responds poorly to drug therapy.
- Check urine output. Report abnormal decreases in urine output.
- Ascertain if the client is extremely apprehensive or has given indications of stressful situation(s). Catecholamine levels are increased during stressful conditions.
- Alert the laboratory of the order for plasma catecholamine. This is necessary so that the test can be processed in the laboratory within 5 minutes after the blood sample is obtained.

Client Teaching

- Explain the procedure to the client. An explanation should be given at least 24 hours before the test (most cases 48 hours). Writing the procedure for the client may be helpful in relieving anxiety.
- Emphasize the importance of not exercising or smoking before the test. Encourage the client to relax as much as possible prior to the test.
- Listen to the client's concerns. Refer questions to other health care providers as needed.

Catecholamines (urine)

Reference Values

Adult: <100 µg/24 hours (higher with activity), <0.59 µmol/24 hours (SI units), 0–14 µg/dl (random), epinephrine <20 ng/24 hours, norepinephrine <100 ng/24 hours.

Child: Level less than adult because of weight differences.

Description

Catecholamines are hormones (epinephrine and norepinephrine) secreted by the adrenal medulla. Catecholamine production increases after strenuous exercise; however, urinary levels are 3 to 100 times greater than normal in cases of pheochromocytoma (tumor of the adrenal medulla). In some psychiatric clients, the urine catecholamine level increases only slightly. In children, this test may be used to diagnose malignant neuroblastoma.

Certain drugs, coffee, and bananas cause elevated catecholamine levels. The urine catecholamine test is considered a more reliable test than a serum catecholamine test.

Purposes

See Catecholamines (Plasma).

Clinical Problems

Elevated Level: Pheochromocytoma, severe stress (septicemia, shock, burn, peritonitis), malignant neuroblastoma, acute myocardial infarction (first 48 hours), chronic ischemic heart disease, cor pulmonale, carcinoid syndrome, manic-depressive disorder, depressive neurosis, strenuous exercise. *Drug Influence:* Antibiotics (ampicillin, demeclocycline, erythromycin, tetracyclines), antihypertensives (methyldopa [Aldomet], hydralazine [Apresoline]), vitamins (ascorbic acid

[Vitamin C], B complex), chlorpromazine (Thorazine), quinine, quinidine, isoproterenol (Isuprel) or epinephrine by inhalation.

Procedure

- Collect urine for 24 hours in a large container with a preservative (10 ml of concentrated hydrochloric acid), and keep the bottle refrigerated. The pH of the
  urine collection should be below 3.0.
- Drugs, chocolate, coffee, and bananas should not be taken for 3 to 7 days before
  the test. The number of days may vary among laboratories.
- Food and fluids other than those already mentioned are not restricted.
- Label the large container with the client's name and the dates and exact times
  of the 24-hour urine collection (e.g., 4/10/04, 7:30 AM to 4/11/04, 7:30 AM).

Factors Affecting Laboratory Results

- Foods such as bananas, coffee, chocolate, and vanilla, could cause an inaccurate test
  result.
- Certain drugs can affect test results *(see Drug Influence above)*.

NURSING IMPLICATIONS WITH RATIONALE

Client Teaching

- Explain to the client and family that all urine should be saved in the refrigerated container. Inform the client that toilet paper and feces should not be put in the urine.
- Explain to the client that there is a strong acid that acts as a preservative in the
  urine container and that he or she should not urinate directly into the container.
- Explain that fasting can increase catecholamine levels. Foods are not restricted
  except for those in the procedure.

Elevated Level

- Recognize the causes of an elevated urine catecholamine level other than
  pheochromocytoma. These include severe stress, strenuous exercise, and acute
  anxiety and other psychiatric disorders. The highest levels occur in pheochromocytoma.
- Check vital signs and report rising blood pressure readings.
- Report if the client has been involved in strenuous activity or has suffered from severe anxiety.

Cerebrospinal fluid (CSF)

(Color, Pressure, Cell Count, Protein, Chloride, Glucose, Culture)
Spinal Fluid

Reference Values

	Color	Pressure (mm H$_2$O)	Cell Count (Leukocytes) (mm^3, μl)	Protein (mg/dl)	Chloride (mEq/l)	Glucose (mg/dl)
Adult	Clear, colorless	75–175	0–8	15–45	118–132	40–80
Child	Clear, colorless	50–100	0–8	14–45	120–128	35–75
Premature infant			0–20	<400		
Newborn 1–6 months	Clear		0–15	30–200 30–100	110–122	20–40

Description

Cerebrospinal fluid (CSF), also known as spinal fluid, circulates in the ventricles of the brain and through the spinal cord. Of the 150 ml of CSF, approximately 100 ml are produced by the blood in the brain ventricles and are reabsorbed back into circulation daily.

Spinal fluid is obtained by a lumbar puncture (spinal tap) performed in the lumbar sac at L3–4, or at L4–5. First CSF pressure is measured, then fluid is aspirated and placed in sterile test tubes. Data from the analysis of the spinal fluid are important for diagnosing spinal cord and brain diseases.

The analysis of spinal fluid usually includes color, pressure, cell count (leukocytes, or white blood cells [WBCs]), protein, chloride, and glucose. In addition, the pH of the CSF is usually checked; it is usually slightly lower, about one tenth (0.1) of a point, than the pH of the serum. The CSF protein and glucose levels are lower than the blood levels; however, the CSF chloride level is higher than the serum chloride level. Normally a culture is done to detect any organism present in the fluid.

Purpose

- To detect color, pressure, leukocyte count, protein, glucose, and presence of bacteria in the CSF.

Clinical Problems

CSF	Decreased Level	Elevated Level	Comments
Color		Abnormal color: 1. Pink or red—subarachnoid or cerebral hemorrhage; traumatic spinal tap 2. Xanthochromia (yellow color)—previous subarachnoid hemorrhage	Yellow color indicates old blood (4 to 5 days after a cerebral hemorrhage), mixture of bilirubin and blood, or extremely elevated protein levels; fluid discoloration normally remains for 3 weeks.
Pressure	Dehydration, hypovolemia	Intracranial pressure due to meningitis, subarachnoid hemorrhage, brain tumor, brain abscess, encephalitis	Slight elevation can occur with holding breath or tensing of muscles.
Cell count (lymphocytes)		<500 mm^3 (μl): viral infections—poliomyelitis, aseptic meningitis; syphilis of CNS; multiple sclerosis; brain tumor; abscess; subarachnoid hemorrhage (40% or more monocytes) >500 mm^3 (μl): ↑ granulocytes, purulent infection	WBC differential count may be ordered to identify the types of leukocytes.
Protein		Meningitis: tuberculosis, purulent, aseptic Guillain-Barré syndrome Subarachnoid hemorrhage Brain tumor Abscess Syphilis Drug influence: anesthetics acetophenetidin (phenacetin) chlorpromazine (Thorazine) salicylates (aspirin) streptomycin sulfonamides	Protein and cell counts usually increase together.

CSF	Decreased Level	Elevated Level	Comments
Chloride	Tubercular meningitis Bacterial meningitis		IV saline or electrolyte infusion could cause an inaccurate result. Syphilis, brain tumors and abscess, and encephalitis do not affect the CSF chloride level.
Glucose	Purulent meningitis Presence of fungi, protozoa, or pyogenic bacteria Subarachnoid hemorrhage Lymphomas Leukemia	Cerebral trauma Hypothalamic lesions Diabetes (hyperglycemia)	Brain abscess or tumor and degenerative diseases have little effect on the CSF glucose. The CSF glucose is usually two thirds of the blood glucose. The blood glucose level is determined for comparative reasons.
Culture		Meningitis	Generally done when meningitis is suspected

Procedure

- Collect a sterile lumbar puncture tray, an antiseptic solution (i.e., providone-iodine or iodine), a local anesthetic (i.e., lidocaine), sterile gloves, and tape.
- Place the client in a "fetal" position, with the back bowed, the head flexed on the chest, and the knees drawn up to the abdomen.
- Label the three test tubes 1, 2, and 3.
- The physician checks the spinal fluid pressure, using a manometer attached to the needle. The physician collects a total of 9 to 12 ml of spinal fluid—3 ml in a no. 1 tube, 3 ml in a no. 2 tube, and 3 ml in a no. 3 tube. The first tube could be contaminated (with blood from the spinal tap) and should *not* be used for cell count, culture, or protein determination.
- Label the tubes with the client's name and room number, and the date. Take the test tubes immediately to the laboratory.
- There is no food or fluid restriction.

Queckenstedt Procedure: The Queckenstedt procedure is performed during a lumbar puncture when spinal block is suspected. Temporary pressure is applied to the jugular veins while the CSF pressure is monitored. Normally the CSF pressure will rise when the jugular veins are compressed. In partial or total CSF block, the pressure fails to rise with jugular vein compression, or it takes 15 to 30 seconds for CSF pressure to drop after compression is released.

Factors Affecting Laboratory Results

- Refrigeration may affect the results of the culture.
- A traumatic spinal tap could cause the presence of blood in the fluid specimen, which could be mistaken for a clinical problem.

- Certain drugs could cause a false, increased, CSF protein level (*see Clinical Problems: Drug Influence above*).
- IV fluid containing chloride could invalidate the CSF chloride level determination.
- Hyperglycemia could increase the CSF glucose level.

NURSING IMPLICATIONS WITH RATIONALE

- Explain the procedure for the lumbar puncture to the client by giving a step-by-step detailed explanation.
- Collect the specimen in numerical order of tubes. Do not mix the numbers. The first tube may have some red blood cells because of the needle insertion. For culture, the second or third test tube is used. For protein and cell count, the third specimen tube is used.
- Check the vital signs before the procedure and afterward at specified times (i.e., ½, 1, 2, and 4 hours).
- Assess for changes in the neurologic status after the procedure (i.e., increased temperature, increased blood pressure, irritability, numbness and tingling in the lower extremities, and nonreactive eye pupils).
- Administer an analgesic as ordered to relieve a headache if it occurs.
- Be supportive of the client before, during, and after the lumbar puncture.

Client Teaching

- Instruct the client to relax and to take deep and slow breaths with his or her mouth open. Hold the client's hand to give reassurance, unless this is opposed by the client.
- Instruct the client to remain flat in bed in the prone or supine position for 4 to 8 hours following the lumbar puncture. Headaches are common because of spinal fluid leaking from the site of the lumbar puncture, which can occur if the client is in an upright position.

Ceruloplasmin (Cp) (serum)

Reference Values

Adult: 18–45 mg/dl, 180–450 mg/l (SI units).

Child: *Infant:* <23 mg/dl, or may be normal. *Child:* 30–65 mg/dl.

Description

Ceruloplasmin (Cp) is a copper-containing glycoprotein known as one of the alpha-2-globulins in the plasma. Ceruloplasmin is produced in the liver and binds with copper. The principal role of ceruloplasmin is not clearly understood, except that when there is a serum deficit, there is an increased urinary excretion of copper and increased depositing of copper on the cornea, brain, liver, and kidney, causing damage and destruction of the organs. A deficit of ceruloplasmin or hypoceruloplasmin can result in Wilson's disease (hepatolenticular degeneration), commonly seen between the ages of 7 and 15 and in early middle age.

Purpose
- To detect Wilson's disease or a liver disorder.

Clinical Problems

Decreased Level: Wilson's disease (hepatolenticular degeneration), protein malnutrition, nephrotic syndrome, newborns and early infancy.

Elevated Level: Cirrhosis of the liver; hepatitis; pregnancy; Hodgkin's disease; cancer of the bone, stomach, lung; myocardial infarction; rheumatoid arthritis; infections and inflammatory process; exercise. *Drug Influence:* Oral contraceptives, estrogen drugs.

Procedure
- Collect 3 to 5 ml of venous blood in a red-top tube.
- There is no food or fluid restriction.
- Withhold drugs containing estrogen for 24 hours before the blood test, with the health care provider's permission.

Factors Affecting Laboratory Results
- Estrogen therapy, pregnancy, and exercise could cause an elevated serum ceruloplasmin level.
- In Wilson's disease with severe liver damage, a normal serum level could result.

NURSING IMPLICATIONS WITH RATIONALE

Decreased Level
- Relate hypoceruloplasmin (serum ceruloplasmin deficit) to Wilson's disease; serum level below 15 mg/dl after the age of 7.
- Assess for signs and symptoms of Wilson's disease (i.e., abnormal muscular rigidity [dystonia], tremors of the fingers, dysarthria, and mental disturbances).
- Check the cornea of the eye for a discolored ring (Kayser-Fleischer ring) from copper deposits.

Elevated Level
- Relate clinical problems of liver disorders, cancer, infections, inflammations, and drugs to hyperceruloplasmin (serum ceruloplasmin excess).
- Note whether the client has been exercising in the last 24 hours, because a slight elevation could be due to strenuous exercise.

Chlamydia (serum and tissue smear or culture)

Reference Values

Normal Titer: <1:16.

Positive Titer: ≥1:64.

Description

Chlamydia is a bacterialike organism and has some features of a virus. There are two species of chlamydia: *C. psittaci,* which can cause psitticosis in birds and humans, and *C. trachomatis,* which appears in three types (lymphogranuloma venereum [LGV, venereal disease], genital and other infections, and trachoma [eye disorder]).

The occurrence of *C. psittaci* is more common in persons working in pet stores who may have contact with infected birds such as parakeets, and in those working in the poultry industry who may come in contact with infected turkeys. A respiratory infection may result and could cause chlamydial pneumonia. Serologic testing or tissue culture may be performed for diagnosis.

The *C. trachomatis* strain, LGV, is transmitted through sexual intercourse. It can occur in both males and females, causing enlargement of the inguinal and pelvic lymph nodes. Pregnant women can pass chlamydia infection to the newborn during birthing. This can cause trachoma ophthalmia neonatorum in the infant, which may lead to blindness later if untreated. Untreated genital infections caused by *C. trachomatis* could lead to sterility.

With psitticosis and LGV, the serum titer level is >1:64 (more than four times the reference value). The titer level for genital infection caused by *C. trachomatis* is usually between 1:16 and 1:64. Normally the general population has a titer level of <1:16. Tissue culture may be used to confirm test results with the titer level. Tetracycline and erythromycin not penicillin, are usually the antibiotics used to treat chlamydia.

Purpose

- To identify the presence of a chlamydial infection, *C. psittaci or C. trachomatis.*

Clinical Problems

Positive Titer: Psitticosis; LGV; genital infections—pelvic inflammatory disease (PID), endometriosis, salpingitis; trachoma ophthalmia neonatorum; chlamydial pneumonia.

Negative Titer: Antibiotic therapy.

Procedure

- Collect 3 to 5 ml of venous blood in a red-top tube. Avoid hemolysis.
- Tissue smear or culture may be obtained from the cervix or other areas.
- There is no food or fluid restriction.

Factors Affecting Laboratory Results

- Hemolysis of the blood specimen.
- Antibiotic therapy taken before tests could cause negative test results.

NURSING IMPLICATIONS WITH RATIONALE

- Obtain a history from the client of any contact with birds that may be infected with *C. psittaci*. Clients who work in pet shops or the poultry industry may be infected with *C. psittaci* and have psitticosis.
- Check for signs and symptoms of psitticosis, which include a nonproductive or slightly productive cough, chills, fever, headache, gastrointestinal symptoms, bradycardia, and mental changes.
- Assess if the woman is pregnant and has enlargement of the pelvic or inguinal lymph nodes. Genital infection from chlamydia could be passed to the infant during vaginal birthing process. Prenatal screening of pregnant women for chlamydial infection is being considered. Symptoms can be vague. The incidence of chlamydial infection in infants is 28 out of 1,000 live births.

Client Teaching

- Encourage the client with *C. trachomatis* infection to give name(s) of sexual partner(s). Certain antibiotic therapies can eliminate the organism and prevent passing the infection to others. The sexual partner(s) may also need treatment.
- Explain to the mother with a chlamydial infection that the infant should be checked.
- Inform clients with a titer <1:16 that an acute chlamydial infection is unlikely.
- Listen to the client's concerns. Respond to questions and/or refer to other health professionals as needed.

Chlordiazepoxide (serum)

Librium, Librax

Reference Values

Adult: *Therapeutic Range:* 1.0–5.0 µg/ml. *Peak Time:* 1–3 hours. *Toxic Level:* >5 µg/ml.

Description

Chlordiazepoxide (Librium), a benzodiazepine and anxiolytic, is used mostly for the treatment of anxiety and alcohol withdrawal effects. It also suppresses seizure activity.

Purposes

- To monitor chlordiazepoxide levels for the treatment of anxiety or alcohol withdrawal.
- To detect a chlordiazepoxide toxic level.

Clinical Problems

Decreased Level: *Drug Influence:* Phenothiazine drug group.
Elevated Level: Overdose of chlordiazepoxide.

Procedure

- Collect 7 ml of venous blood in a red-top tube.
- There is no food or fluid restriction.

Factors Affecting Laboratory Results

- Phenothiazines and taking other benzodiazepines with chlordiazepoxide could cause central nervous system depression.

NURSING IMPLICATIONS WITH RATIONALE

- Observe for side effects of chlordiazepoxide (i.e., lethargy, drowsiness, slurred speech, tremors, transient hypotension, dizziness, bradycardia, dry mouth).

Client Teaching

- Instruct the client to report side effects. Many of the side effects will disappear after taking the drug for a few days.
- Advise the client that if dizziness occurs he or she should rise slowly from a lying position.
- Inform the client to avoid heavy smoking, because it could cause side effects. Heavy smoking can enhance the effect of chlordiazepoxide.
- Explain to the client that antacids might delay absorption of Librium. Inform the health care provider if the client is taking antacids.

Chloride (Cl) (serum)

Reference Values

Adult: 95–105 mEq/l, 95–105 mmol/l (SI units).
Child: *Newborn:* 94–112 mEq/l. *Infant:* 95–110 mEq/l. *Child:* 98–105 mEq/l.

Description

Chloride is an anion found mostly in the extracellular fluid. Chloride plays an important role in maintaining body water balance, osmolality of body fluids (with sodium), and acid–base balance. It combines with hydrogen ion to produce the acidity (hydrochloric acid [HCl]) in the stomach.

For maintaining acid–base balance, chloride competes with bicarbonate for sodium. When the body fluids are more acidic, the kidneys excrete chloride and sodium, and bicarbonate is reabsorbed. In addition, chloride shifts in and out of red blood cells in exchange with bicarbonate.

Most of the chloride ingested is combined with sodium (sodium chloride [NaCl] or "salt"). The daily required chloride intake is 2 g. *Hypochloremia* means serum chloride deficit; *hyperchloremia* means serum chloride excess.

Purpose

- To check the chloride level in relation to potassium, sodium, and acid-base balance.

Clinical Problems

Decreased Level: Vomiting, gastric suctioning, diarrhea, hypokalemia (decreased potassium), hyponatremia (decreased sodium), low-sodium diet, continuous IV 5% dextrose in water (D_5W), gastroenteritis, colitis, adrenal gland insufficiency (Addison's disease), diabetic acidosis, heat exhaustion, hyperaldosteronism, acute infections, burns, excessive diaphoresis (sweating/perspiration), metabolic alkalosis. *Drug Influence:* Diuretics (mercurials, thiazides, loop), bicarbonates.

Elevated Level: Dehydration, hypernatremia (increased sodium), hyperparathyroidism, cancer of the stomach, multiple myeloma, adrenal gland hyperactivity, head injury, eclampsia, cardiac decompensation, excessive IV saline (0.9% NaCl), kidney dysfunction (glomerulonephritis, acute renal failure, pyelonephritis), hyperventilation, metabolic acidosis. *Drug Influence:* Acetazolamide, ammonium chloride, boric acid, cortisone preparations, ion exchange resins, prolonged use of triamterene (Dyrenium).

Procedure

- Collect 3 to 5 ml of venous blood in a red- or green-top tube.
- There is no food or fluid restriction. This test may be combined with other tests (e.g., for serum electrolytes), so the client may be NPO. Check with the laboratory.

Factors Affecting Laboratory Results

- Drugs *(see Drug Influence above)*.

NURSING IMPLICATIONS WITH RATIONALE

Decreased Level

- Assess for signs and symptoms of hypochloremia (hyperexcitability of the nervous system and muscles, tetany [twitching, tremors], slow and shallow breathing, and decreased blood pressure resulting from fluid and chloride loss).
- Inform the health care provider when the client is receiving IV D$_5$W continuously. If no other solutes are given, the body fluids will be diluted, and the client will not receive the daily required chloride intake.
- Check the serum potassium and sodium levels. Chloride is frequently lost with sodium and potassium (plentiful in the gastrointestinal tract). With vomiting, potassium, hydrogen, and chloride are lost, causing hypokalemic-hypochloremic alkalosis. Both potassium and chloride must be replaced, for if potassium is given and not chloride, hypokalemic alkalosis will persist.
- Observe for symptoms of overhydration when the client is receiving several liters of normal saline (0.9% NaCl) for sodium and chloride replacement. Sodium holds water, and if there is a history of a heart or kidney disorder, water accumulation could occur. Symptoms of overhydration include a constant, irritated cough; dyspnea; neck and hand vein engorgement; and chest rales.

Client Teaching

- Instruct the client *not* to drink only plain water if there is a serum chloride deficit. Encourage the client to drink fluids containing sodium and chloride (e.g., broth, tomato juice, cola drinks).
- Instruct the client to drink and eat foods rich in chloride (i.e., broth, seafoods, milk, meats, eggs, and table salt).

Elevated Level

- Assess for signs and symptoms of hyperchloremia (similar to acidosis)—weakness, lethargy, and deep, rapid, vigorous breathing.
- Notify the health care provider if the client is receiving IV fluids containing normal saline. Check for symptoms of overhydration.
- Monitor daily weights and intake and output to determine whether fluid retention is present because of sodium and chloride excess.

Client Teaching

- Instruct the client to avoid drinking or eating salty foods. Encourage the client not to use the salt shaker and some salt substitutes.
- Instruct the client to read labels, because some salt substitutes contain calcium chloride or potassium chloride.

Chloride (sweat)

Screening (Silver Nitrate); Iontophoresis (Pilocarpine)

Reference Values

Adult: <60 mEq/l.

Child: <50 mEq/l; marginal: 50–60 mEq/l; abnormal: >60 mEq/l (possible cystic fibrosis).

Description

Sodium and chloride concentrations in sweat are higher in persons with cystic fibrosis, even though there usually is not an increased amount of sweat. Sweat chloride is considered more reliable than sweat sodium for diagnostic purposes. Some falsely negative sweat sodium levels have been reported in persons with cystic fibrosis.

Two types of sweat chloride tests are used: (1) screening tests, which use silver nitrate on agar or filter (special) paper and require contact with the hand (palm or fingers), and (2) iontophoresis, in which pilocarpine is placed on the forearm to increase sweat gland secretion. A positive screening test is usually validated with iontophoresis, because the chloride level in the palm of the hand is usually higher than anywhere else. Some health care providers believe that the screening should be routine in all children; however, others disagree.

Purpose

■ To aid in the detection of cystic fibrosis.

Clinical Problems

Elevated Level: Cystic fibrosis, asthma.

Procedure

Screening Test (Silver Nitrate)

■ Wash the child's hand and dry it. For 15 minutes, keep the hand from contacting any other part of the body.
■ Moisten the test paper containing silver nitrate compound with distilled water (not saline).
■ Press the child's hand on the paper for 4 seconds.
■ A positive result occurs when the excess chloride combines with the silver nitrate to form white silver chloride on the paper.
■ A heavy hand imprint is left by the child with cystic fibrosis.

119

Iontophoresis (Pilocarpine): Usually performed by laboratory personnel.

- Electrodes are placed on the skin of the forearm to create a small electric current for transporting pilocarpine (a stimulating drug) into the skin to induce sweating.
- Sweat is collected and weighed. Chloride is measured.
- There is no food or fluid restriction.

Factors Affecting Laboratory Results

- Unwashed hands for the screening test affect test results.
- Use of saline solution to moisten the test paper causes inaccurate test results.

NURSING IMPLICATIONS WITH RATIONALE

- Explain the procedures (screening or iontophoresis or both) to the child and family. Answer questions if possible, or refer them to appropriate health professionals.
- Explain to the child and family that the tests are not painful.
- Remain with the child during the procedure. Give comfort and reassurance as needed.

Elevated Level

- Associate an elevated sweat chloride level with cystic fibrosis. With cystic fibrosis, sweat chloride levels could be two to five times greater than normal.
- Obtain a familial history of cystic fibrosis, when indicated.
- Determine whether the child has washed and dried his or her hands before the screening test is performed. Dried sweat can leave a chloride residue, thus causing a false-positive result.

Cholesterol (serum)

Reference Values

Adult: *Desirable Level:* <200 mg/dl. *Moderate Risk:* 200–240 mg/dl. *High Risk:* >240 mg/dl. *Pregnancy:* High risk levels but a return to prepregnancy values 1 month after delivery.

Child: *Infant:* 90–130 mg/dl. *Child (2–19 years); Desirable Level:* 130–170 mg/dl. *Moderate Risk:* 171–184 mg/dl. *High Risk:* >185 mg/dl.

Description

Cholesterol is a blood lipid synthesized by the liver and is found in red blood cells, cell membranes, and muscles. About 70% of cholesterol is esterified (combined with fatty acids), and 30% is in the free form. Cholesterol is used by the body to form bile salts for fat digestion and for the formation of hormones by the adrenal glands, ovaries, and testes. Thyroid hormones and estrogen decrease the concentration of cholesterol, and an oophorectomy increases it.

Serum cholesterol is used as an indicator of atherosclerosis and coronary artery disease. Hypercholesterolemia causes plaque deposits in the coronary arteries, thus contributing to myocardial infarction. High serum cholesterol levels can be due to a familial (hereditary) tendency, biliary obstruction, and/or dietary intake. Approximately one third of Americans have a serum cholesterol level below 200 mg dL, which is desirable.

Purposes

- To check the client's cholesterol level.
- To monitor cholesterol levels.

Clinical Problems

Decreased Level: Hyperthyroidism, Cushing's syndrome (adrenal hormone excess), starvation, malabsorption, anemias, acute infections. *Drug Influence:* Antilipids (Zocor, Mevacor, Lipitor), thyroxine, antibiotics (kanamycin, neomycin, parmomycin, tetracycline), nicotinic acid, estrogens, glucagon, heparin, salicylates (aspirin), colchicine, oral hypoglycemic agents.

Elevated Level: Acute myocardial infarction; atherosclerosis; hypothyroidism; biliary obstruction; biliary cirrhosis; cholangitis; familial hypercholesterolemia; uncontrolled diabetes mellitus; nephrotic syndrome; pancreatectomy; pregnancy (third trimester); types II, III, and V hyperlipoproteinemia; heavy stress periods; high-cholesterol diet (animal fats). *Drug Influence:* Aspirin, corticosteroids, steroids (anabolic agents and androgens), oral contraceptives, epinephrine and norepinephrine, bromides, phenothiazines (chlorpromazine [Thorazine], trifluoperazine [Stelazine], vitamins A and D, sulfonamides, phenytoin (Dilantin).

Procedure

- Keep the client NPO (food, fluids, and medications) for 12 hours. The client may have water.
- Collect 3 to 5 ml of venous blood in a red-top tube. Avoid hemolysis.
- List drugs the client is taking that are not withheld on the laboratory slip.

Factors Affecting Laboratory Results

- Aspirin and cortisone could cause decreased or elevated serum cholesterol levels.

- A high-cholesterol diet before the test could cause elevated serum cholesterol levels.
- Severe hypoxia could increase the serum cholesterol level.
- Hemolysis of the blood specimen may cause an elevation of the serum cholesterol level.

NURSING IMPLICATIONS WITH RATIONALE

Elevated Level

- Relate clinical problems and drugs to hypercholesterolemia. An elevated cholesterol level can indicate liver disease as well as coronary artery disease.
- Hold drugs that could increase the serum level for 12 hours before the blood is drawn, with the health care provider's permission.

Client Teaching

- Explain to the client and family what is considered a normal serum cholesterol level and the effects of an elevated cholesterol level.
- Encourage the client to lose weight if overweight and hypercholesterolemic. Losing weight if obese can decrease serum cholesterol level.
- Instruct the client with hypercholesterolemia to decrease the intake of foods rich in cholesterol (i.e., bacon, eggs, butter, fatty meat, certain seafood, coconut, and chocolate).
- Teach the client with severe hypercholesterolemia to keep medical appointments for follow-up care.

Cholinesterase (blood [RBCs] or plasma)

Acetylcholinesterase (True Cholinesterase of Blood Nerve Tissue—RBC);
Pseudocholinesterase (Serum)

Reference Values

Adult: 0.5–1.0 U (RBC), 3–8 U/ml (plasma), 6–8 IU/l (RBC), 8–18 IU/l at 37°C (plasma).

Child: Similar to adult.

Description

There are two different cholinesterases (CHS): *acetylcholinesterase* (true cholinesterase), found in the red blood cells (RBCs; erthyrocytes) and nerve tissue, and *pseudocholinesterase,* or serum cholinesterase (PCHE). Cholinesterase is an enzyme that breaks down acetylcholine at the nerve synapse and neuromuscular junction.

Decreased cholinesterase levels may indicate insecticide poisoning caused by excessive exposure to organic phosphate agents, liver disorders (hepatitis and cirrhosis), or an acute infection. This test is not used for assessment of liver function.

Purpose

- To detect a decrease in plasma cholinesterase level due to insecticide poisoning or other health problems.

Clinical Problems

Decreased Level: Insecticide poisoning, liver disorders (hepatitis, cirrhosis, obstructive jaundice), malnutrition, acute infections, anemias, carcinomatosis.

Elevated Level: Nephrotic syndrome.

Procedure

- Collect 5 to 7 ml of venous blood in a green- or lavender-top tube.
- There is no food or fluid restriction.

Factors Affecting Laboratory Results

- Nonheparinized tube for cholinesterase-RBC test affects test result.

NURSING IMPLICATIONS WITH RATIONALE

Decreased Level

- Obtain a history of the client's exposure to insecticides—kind, length of time, and amount. Excessive exposure to organic phosphate can cause acute or chronic toxicity, and the acetylcholinesterase level would be decreased.
- Report if the client has not been eating or has an acute infection.

Clot retraction (blood)

Reference Values

Adult: 1–24 hours (retraction of clot).

Child: Similar to adult.

Description

The clot retraction (shrunken clot) test is useful in determining whether bleeding disorders are due to a decreased platelet count. In this simple test, the rate and degree of contraction of a blood clot are measured; the clot of blood in the test tube will diminish in size as fluid (serum) separates from the red cells. Platelets are responsible for the shrinkage of the blood clot. Frequently, when there is a platelet deficit, clot retraction will be slower and the clot formation will be softer.

In 1 hour the clot should be one half its original size (volume). The retraction should be near completion in 4 hours and definitely completed in 24 hours.

Purpose

- To determine if the bleeding disorder is due to a decreased platelet count.

Clinical Problems

Decreased Clot Formation: Thrombocytopenia (decreased platelets), thrombasthenia (abnormal platelets), anemia (pernicious, folic acid, aplastic), Waldenström's macroglobulinemia.

Procedure

- Collect 5 ml of venous blood in a red-top tube.
- There is no food or fluid restriction.

Factors Affecting Laboratory Results

- A high hematocrit can cause poor clot retraction.
- Decreased fibrinogen can cause RBCs to spill out of the serum when retraction begins, resulting in poor cell retraction.
- Anticoagulants can inhibit clot formation.

NURSING IMPLICATIONS WITH RATIONALE

Decreased or Poor Clot Formation

- Report to the health care provider if bleeding time is prolonged.
- Note when the blood clot begins to separate from the tube wall. This usually begins to happen within 30 minutes to 1 hour. Note the length of time required for clot retraction (clot shrinking and fluid release).
- Check the consistency of the clot. Soft clots and shapeless clots may be due to abnormal or decreased platelets.
- Check the client's hemoglobin, hematocrit, and platelet count. A high hematocrit resulting from hemoconcentration or polycythemia may cause decreased clot retraction. Clot retraction is influenced by the number of functional platelets and not necessarily by the total count.

Coagulation factors (plasma)

See Factor Assay

Cold agglutinins (serum)

Cold Hemagglutinin

Reference Values

Adult: 1:8 antibody titer, >1:16 significantly increased, >1:32 definitely positive.

Child: Similar to adult.

Elderly: Values are increased more than adults.

Description

Cold agglutinins (CAs) are antibodies that agglutinate red blood cells at temperatures between 0°C and 10°C. Elevated titers (>1:32) are found frequently in clients with primary atypical pneumonia or with other clinical problems, such as influenza, pulmonary embolism, and cirrhosis. The cold agglutinins test is often done during the acute and convalescence phases of illness.

Purposes

- To determine the presence of an increased antibody titer, significant for atypical pneumonia, influenza, or leukemia.
- To compare test results with other laboratory tests.

Clinical Problems

Elevated Level: Primary atypical pneumonia, influenza, cirrhosis of the liver, lymphatic leukemia, multiple myeloma, pulmonary embolism, acquired hemolytic anemias, malaria, infectious mononucleosis, frostbite, viral infections (cytomegalovirus), tuberculosis.

Procedure

- Collect 5 to 7 ml of venous blood in a red-top tube. Keep the specimen warm. Take it immediately to the laboratory. The blood sample should not be refrigerated.
- The laboratory may rewarm the sample for 30 minutes before the serum is separated from the cells.

125

■ There is no food or fluid restriction.

Factors Affecting Laboratory Results

■ Antibiotic therapy may cause inaccurate results.
■ Elevated cold agglutinins may interfere with typing and cross matching.
■ Improper blood collection procedure may affect results.

NURSING IMPLICATIONS WITH RATIONALE

Elevated Level

■ Relate elevated cold agglutinin levels to clinical problems, particularly primary atypical pneumonia.
■ Answer the client's questions concerning the significance of the test. Answers might include "most persons have an antibody titer level, but some have higher levels, such as older adults and those with viral infections; high titers may persist for years, and the test may be repeated at a later date."

Complement: total (serum)

CH_{50}

Reference Values

Adult: 75–160 U/ml; 75–160 kU/l (SI units).

Description

Total complement plays an important role in the immunologic enzyme system reacting to an antigen–antibody response. The complements make up about 10% of the serum globulins. The complement system has over 20 components; 9 major components numbering C1 to C9. C3 and C4 are the most abundant complements and are discussed separately in the text. The total complement may be referred to as *total hemolytic complement,* or CH_{50}. CH_{50} assesses the function of the complement system. When the complement system is stimulated, it increases phagocytosis, lysis, or destruction of bacteria, and produces an inflammatory response to infection.

Most assays for CH_{50} are most sensitive to changes in C2, C4, and C5. Assay should be used as a screen for overall complement function and not as a quantitative measure of C1 activation during the course of disease states.

Purposes

- To identify the effects of the immunologic enzyme system regarding the presence of inflammatory condition(s) or tissue rejection.
- To compare serum complement tests with serum immunoglobulins to determine the cause of the health problem.

Clinical Problems

Decreased Level: Allograft rejection, hypogammaglobulinemia, acute poststreptococcal glomerulonephritis, acute serum sickness, systemic lupus erythematosus, lupus nephritis, hepatitis, subacute bacterial endocarditis, hemolytic anemia, rheumatic fever, multiple myeloma, advanced cirrhosis.

Elevated Level: Acute rheumatic fever, rheumatoid arthritis, acute myocardia infarction, ulcerative colitis, diabetes mellitus, thyroiditis, Wegener's granulomatosis, obstructive jaundice.

Procedure

- There is no food or fluid restriction.
- Collect 3 to 5 ml of venous blood in a red-top tube. Allow it to clot at room temperature. Spin at 4°C. Transfer the serum and freeze immediately. This test may be sent to a large reference laboratory.

Factors Affecting Laboratory Results

- Hemolysis of the blood sample caused by rough handling.

NURSING IMPLICATIONS WITH RATIONALE

- Obtain a history from the client of an infectious process or abnormal response to infection. Complement deficiency may occur to those persons susceptible to infection and with certain autoimmune diseases.
- Assess the client's vital signs and urine output. Report abnormal findings.
- Compare total complement results with serum immunoglobulins. Complement results give information about the client's immune system.

Complement C3 (serum)

C3 Component of the Complement System

Reference Values

Adult: *Male:* 80–180 mg/dl, 0.8–1.8 g/l (SI units). *Female:* 76–120 mg/dl, 0.76–1.2 g/l (SI units).

Child: Usually not performed.

Description

Complement C3 is the most abundant component of the complement system (a group of 11 proteins). The complement system has an important role in the immunologic system and the complements' components are activated when IgG and IgM antibodies are combined with their specific antigens.

The total complement system and C3 are decreased in systemic lupus erythematosus (SLE), glomerulonephritis, and acute renal transplant rejection. Following onset of an acute or chronic inflammatory process or acute tissue destruction (necrosis), the total complement may be temporarily elevated. C3 and C4 of the complement system are best known, and the others (C1, C2, and C5 to C9) are still under study and intense research.

Purposes

- To assist in the detection of acute inflammatory disease (e.g., rheumatoid arthritis) and other health problems (elevated level), and SLE, glomerulonephritis (decreased level); *see Clinical Problems.*
- To compare the test results with other laboratory data to determine health problem.

Clinical Problems

Decreased Level: Systemic lupus erythematosus, glomerulonephritis, acute poststreptococcal glomerulonephritis, acute renal transplant rejection, cirrhosis of the liver, multiple sclerosis (slightly lower), protein malnutrition, anemias (pernicious, folic acid), septicemia (gram-negative), bacterial endocarditis.

Elevated Level: Acute rheumatic fever, rheumatoid arthritis, early SLE, and malignant neoplasms of the esophagus, stomach, colon, rectum, pancreas, lungs, breast, cervix, ovary, prostate, and bladder.

Procedure

- Collect 3 to 5 ml of venous blood in a red-top tube.
- Take the blood sample to the laboratory immediately.
- There is no food or fluid restriction.

Factors Affecting Laboratory Results

- Heat can destroy complement components.
- C3 is unstable, and the serum value may decrease if the sample is left standing for 1 to 2 hours at room temperature.

NURSING IMPLICATIONS WITH RATIONALE

- Compare the serum C3 and C4 results.
- Be supportive of client and family.

Decreased Level

- Relate a decreased C3 level to clinical problems such as SLE and kidney disorders.
- Check the serum C3 value with other laboratory studies that are ordered and related to the disease process.

Elevated Level

- Relate an elevated C3 level to an acute or chronic inflammatory process and tissue necrosis, such as rheumatic fever, rheumatoid arthritis, and malignancies with metastasis.

Complement C4 (serum)

C4 Component of the Complement System

Reference Values

Adult: 15–45 mg/dl; 0.15–0.45 g/l or 150–450 mg/l (SI units).

Child: Usually not performed.

Description

(See Complement C3.)

Complement C4 is the second most abundant component of the complement system. A decrease in the C4 as well as the C3 levels is commonly found in diseases such as systemic lupus erythematosus (SLE), glomerulonephritis, and renal transplant rejection.

An elevated serum C4 level is indicative of an acute inflammatory process; however, a well (healthy) person may have an elevated C4 level. With cancer, the C4 level is usually increased (with links to the stage of the disease), but the serum level drops significantly in the terminal phase of the malignancy.

Purposes

See Complement C3 (Serum).

Clinical Problems

Decreased Level: Lupus nephritis, SLE (C4 decreased time is longer than C3 decreased time), acute poststreptococcal glomerulonephritis (C4 level usually lower than C3 level), cirrhosis of the liver, bacterial endocarditis.

Elevated Level: Rheumatoid spondylitis; juvenile rheumatoid arthritis; cancer of the esophagus, stomach, colon, rectum, pancreas, lung, breast, cervix, ovary, prostate, and bladder.

Procedure

- Collect 3 to 5 ml of venous blood in a red-top tube.
- Take the blood sample to the laboratory immediately.
- There is no food and fluid restriction.

Factors Affecting Laboratory Results

- Heat will decrease the complement C4 level.
- C4 is unstable and the serum level will decrease if it remains at room temperature for more than 1 to 2 hours.

NURSING IMPLICATIONS WITH RATIONALE

Decreased Level

- Relate a decreased serum C4 level to clinical problems. With lupus nephritis and poststreptococcal glomerulonephritis, the serum C4 level is extremely low.
- Compare the serum C3 and C4 results to determine which component of the complement system is involved.

Coombs direct (blood [RBCs])

Direct Antiglobulin Test

Reference Values

Adult: Negative.

Child: Negative.

Description

The direct Coombs test detects antibodies attached to red blood cells (RBCs) that may cause cellular damage. This test can identify a weak antigen–antibody reaction even when there is no visible RBC agglutination. A positive Coombs test reveals antibodies present in RBCs, but the test does not identify the antibody responsible.

This test is useful for diagnosing early erythroblastosis fetalis (hemolytic disease of newborns), autoimmune hemolytic anemia, hemolytic transfusion reaction, and some drug sensitizations (i.e., to levodopa and methyldopa).

The direct Coombs test is also known as the direct antiglobulin test, a method of detecting in vivo sensitization of RBCs.

Purpose

- To detect antibodies on RBCs.

Clinical Problems

Positive (+1 to +4): Erythroblastosis fetalis, acquired hemolytic anemia (auto-immune), transfusion reactions (blood incompatibility), leukemias (lymphocytic, myelocytic), systemic lupus erythematosus. *Drug Influence:* Antibiotics (cephaloridine [Loridine], cephalothin [Keflin], penicillin, streptomycin, tetracycline), chlorpromazine (Thorazine), phenytoin (Dilantin), ethosuximide (Zarontin), hydralazine (Apresoline), isoniazid (INH), levodopa (Dopar), methyldopa (Aldomet), procainamide (Pronestyl), quinidine, rifampin (Rifadin), sulfonamides.

Procedure

- Collect 5 to 7 ml of venous blood in a lavender-top tube. A red-top tube could be used, but a serum separator tube should not be used. Venous blood from the umbilical cord of a newborn may be used. Avoid hemolysis.
- There is no food or fluid restriction.

Factors Affecting Laboratory Results

- Certain drugs may cause a positive test result *(see Drug Influence above).*

NURSING IMPLICATIONS WITH RATIONALE

Positive Test

- Report the drugs the client is receiving that could produce a positive direct Coombs test (i.e., antibiotics, phenytoin, sulfonamides, chlorpromazine, methyldopa, and others *(see Drug Influence above).*
- Observe for signs and symptoms of whole-blood transfusion reactions (i.e., chills, fever [slight temperature elevation], and rash).
- Observe the newborn for symptoms of erythroblastosis fetalis, especially if the condition is suspected. The main symptom is jaundice of the skin, nails, and sclerae.

Coombs indirect (serum)

Reference Values

Adult: Negative.

Child: Negative.

Description

The Coombs indirect test can detect free circulating antibodies in the client's serum. This test is done in cross matching blood for transfusions to prevent transfusion reaction to incompatible blood caused by minor blood-type factors. As a result of previous transfusions, a recipient's blood may contain specific antibody (antibodies) that could cause a transfusion reaction.

The indirect Coombs test is also known as the indirect antiglobulin test, a method of detecting in vitro sensitization of red blood cells (RBCs).

Purpose

- To check the recipient's and the donor's blood for antibodies prior to blood transfusion.

Clinical Problems

Positive (+1 to +4): Incompatible cross-matched blood, specific antibody (previous transfusion), anti-Rh antibodies (detected during pregnancy), acquired hemolytic anemia. *Drug Influence:* Same as for the direct Coombs test (*see Coombs Direct*).

Procedure

- Collect 5 to 7 ml of venous blood in a red-top tube. Do not use a serum separator tube. The blood bank will use the serum from the recipient's blood and select the compatible blood for proper transfusion.
- There is no food or fluid restriction.

Factors Affecting Laboratory Results

- Certain drugs can cause positive results. (*See Clinical Problems: Drug Influence under Coombs Direct.*)

NURSING IMPLICATIONS WITH RATIONALE

- Obtain a history of previous transfusions and report any previous transfusion reactions.

- Report any drugs the client is receiving that could cause a positive result. Record drug information on the client's chart in the nurse's notes or progress notes.

Client Teaching

- Explain to the client that the donor's and the recipient's blood is checked for antibodies prior to a blood transfusion to avoid a transfusion reaction.

Copper (Cu) (serum)

Reference Values

Adult: *Male:* 70–140 μg/dl, 11–22 μmol/l (SI units). *Female:* 80–155 μg/dl, 12.6–24.3 μmol/l (SI units). *Pregnancy:* 140–300 μg/dl.

Child: *Newborn:* 20–70 μg/dl. *Child:* 30–190 μg/dl. *Adolescent:* 90–240 μg/dl.

Description

Copper is required for hemoglobin synthesis. Approximately 90% of the copper is bound to α_2-globulin, referred to as ceruloplasmin, which is the means of copper transportation in the body. In hepatolenticular disease (Wilson's disease), the serum copper level is <20 μg/dl, and the urinary copper level is >100 μg/24 hours. There is a decrease in copper metabolism with Wilson's disease, and excess copper is deposited in the brain (basal ganglia) and liver, causing degenerative changes. A low-copper diet and D-penicillamine will promote copper excretion.

Hypercupremia (excess copper) can be observed during pregnancy, anemias, leukemia, collagen disease, and thyroid diseases. Serum copper and serum ceruloplasmin tests are frequently ordered together and compared. Both show decreased levels with Wilson's disease.

Purposes

- To detect if there is a serum copper excess or deficit.
- To aid in the diagnosis of Wilson's disease (hepatolenticular disease).

Clinical Problems

Decreased Level: Hepatolenticular disease (Wilson's disease), protein malnutrition, chronic ischemic heart disease.

Elevated Level: Cancer (bone, stomach, large intestine, liver, lung), Hodgkin's disease, leukemias, hypothyroidism, hyperthyroidism, anemias (pernicious and iron deficiency), rheumatoid arthritis, systemic lupus erythematosus, pregnancy, cirrhosis of the liver. *Drug Influence:* Oral contraceptives.

Procedure

- Collect 5 ml of venous blood in a red-top tube or a royal blue-top tube (used for trace metal).
- There is no food or fluid restriction.
- *Note:* A test for urinary copper may be requested simultaneously with the blood test.

Factors Affecting Laboratory Results

- A diet low or high in copper before the blood test may cause inaccurate results.
- Metallic contamination of collection tubes or equipment affects test results.

NURSING IMPLICATIONS WITH RATIONALE

Decreased Level

- Assess for signs and symptoms of hepatolenticular disease (Wilson's disease— i.e., rigidity, dysarthria, dysphagia, incoordination, and tremors).
- Check for a Kayser-Fleischer ring (dark ring) around the cornea. This is a copper deposit that the body has not been able to metabolize.
- Compare the serum copper level with the serum ceruloplasmin level if both have been ordered. If hepatolenticular disease is present, the serum levels will be decreased.

Client Teaching

- Explain to the client with Wilson's disease that foods rich in copper (i.e., organ meats, shellfish, mushrooms, whole-grain cereals, bran, nuts, and chocolate) should be avoided. Canned foods should be omitted. A low-copper diet and D-penicillamine promote copper excretion.

Cortisol (plasma)

Hydrocortisone, Compound F

Reference Values

Adult: 8 AM–10 AM: 5–23 µg/dl, 138–635 nmol/l (SI units). 4 PM–6 PM: 3–13 µg/dl, 83–359 nmol/l (SI units).

Child: 8 AM–10 AM: 15–25 µg/dl. 4 PM–6 PM: 5–10 µg/dl.

Description

Cortisol is a potent glucocorticoid release from the adrenal cortex in response to ACTH stimulation. Cortisol affects carbohydrate, protein, and lipid metabolism; acts as an anti-inflammatory agent; helps with maintenance of blood pressure; inhibits insulin action; and stimulates glucogenesis in the liver.

Levels of plasma cortisol are higher in the morning and lower in the afternoon. When there is adrenal or pituitary dysfunction, the diurnal variation in cortisol function ceases.

Purposes

- To determine the presence of an elevated or decreased plasma cortisol level.
- To associate a decreased cortisol level with an adrenocortical hypofunction.

Clinical Problems

Decreased Level: Anterior pituitary hypofunction, adrenal cortical hypofunction (Addison's disease), respiratory distress syndrome (low-birth-weight newborns), hypothyroidism, exercise (slight decrease). *Drug Influence:* Androgens, phenytoin (Dilantin).

Elevated Level: Cancer of the adrenal gland, benign tumor on the adrenal cortex, adrenal cortical hyperfunction (Cushing's syndrome), stress, pregnancy, obesity, acute myocardial infarction, acute alcohol intoxication, diabetic acidosis, hyperthyroidism. *Drug Influence:* Oral contraceptives, estrogens, spironolactone (Aldactone), triparanol.

Procedure

- Collect 5 to 7 ml of venous blood in a red-top or green-top (heparinized) tube.
- Write the date and time the blood was drawn on the laboratory slip. If the client has taken estrogen or oral contraceptives in the last 6 weeks, the drug(s) should be listed on the laboratory slip. *Recommendation:* Stop medication 2 months before test.
- Advise the client to rest in bed for 2 hours before the blood is drawn.
- There is no food or fluid restriction.

Factors Affecting Laboratory Results

- Certain drugs can affect cortisol levels *(see Drug Influences).*
- Physical activity prior to the blood test might decrease the cortisol level.
- Obesity can cause an elevated serum level.
- Inaccurate labeling of the blood specimen (i.e., with the wrong time) can affect results.

NURSING IMPLICATIONS WITH RATIONALE

- Obtain a history of drugs taken prior to hospital admission or the test. Oral contraceptives and estrogen taken within 6 weeks of the test can cause false-positive results.

Decreased Level

- Observe for signs and symptoms of Addison's disease (adrenal cortical insufficiency). Symptoms are anorexia, vomiting, abdominal pain, fatigue, dizziness, trembling, and diaphoresis.

Elevated Level

- Observe for signs and symptoms of Cushing's syndrome (excess adrenal cortical hormone). Symptoms are fat deposits in the face (moonface), neck, and back of the chest; irritability; mood swings; bleeding under the skin; muscle wasting; and weakness.

Client Teaching

- Instruct the client that he or she should be on bed rest for 2 hours prior to the test. Physical activity affects the cortisol level.

C-reactive protein (CRP) (serum)

N High Sensitivity CRP (hs CRP)

Reference Values

Adult: Not usually present: *Qualitative:* >1:2 titer, positive. *Quantitative:* 20 mg/dl.

Child: Not usually present.

N High Sensitivity CRP

Adult: <0.175 mg/l.

Description

C-Reactive protein (CRP) appears in the blood 6 to 10 hours after an acute inflammatory process and tissue destruction, and it peaks within 48 to 72 hours. CRP is a nonspecific test ordered for diagnostic reasons similar to those for the erythrocyte sedimentation rate (ESR) test, but CRP precedes an increase in the ESR during inflammation and necrosis and returns to normal sooner. Serum CRP is also found in many body fluids (i.e., pleural, peritoneal, and synovial).

The CRP test is used to monitor acute inflammatory phases of rheumatoid arthritis and rheumatic fever so that early treatment can be initiated before progressive tissue damage occurs. CRP elevates during bacterial infections but not viral infections.

N High Sensitivity CRP (hs CRP) is a highly sensitive test for detecting the risk of cardiovascular and peripheral vascular diseases. This test is frequently combined with cholesterol screening. Approximately one-third of the population who has had a heart attack have normal cholesterol levels and normal blood pressure. A positive hs CRP may indicate that the client is at a high risk for coronary artery disease (CAD). This test can detect an inflammatory process occurring that is caused by the built-up of plaque (atherosclerosis) in the arterial system, particularly coronary arteries. Positive hs CRP values are much lower than the standard serum CRP, which makes it a more value test for predicting coronary heart disease.

Purposes

- To associate an increased CRP titer with an acute inflammatory process.
- To detect the risk of coronary heart disease (hs CRP).
- To compare test results with other laboratory tests (e.g., antistreptolysin O test).

Clinical Problems

Normal Level: *Drug Suppression:* Steroids (cortisone, prednisone), salicylates (aspirin).

Elevated Level: Rheumatoid arthritis, rheumatic fever, acute myocardial infarction, peripheral vascular disease of the brain, kidney and extremities, cancer (breast and with metastasis), inflammatory bowel disease, Hodgkin's disease, systemic lupus erythematosus, bacterial infections, late pregnancy, intrauterine contraceptive devices. *Drug Influence:* Oral contraceptives.

Procedure

- Collect 3 to 5 ml of venous blood in a red-top tube. Avoid heat, because CRP is thermolabile.
- Keep the client NPO except for water for 8 to 12 hours before the test. Laboratory policies on NPO could vary and should be checked.

Factors Affecting Laboratory Results

- Pregnancy (third trimester) could elevate the CRP level.
- Oral contraceptives and intrauterine contraceptive devices might elevate the CRP level.

NURSING IMPLICATIONS WITH RATIONALE

Elevated Level

- Recognize that an elevated serum CRP level is associated with an active inflammatory process and tissue destruction (necrosis). The CRP test is nonspecific; however, the CRP is elevated during acute rheumatic fever, rheumatoid arthritis, and acute myocardial infarction.
- Assess for signs and symptoms of an acute inflammatory process, such as pain and swelling in joints, heat, redness, or increased body temperature.
- Notify the health care provider (HCP) of a recurrence (exacerbation) of an acute inflammation. The HCP may wish to order a serum CRP test or serum hs CRP level.
- Assess for signs and symptoms of chest pain that may be caused by coronary heart disease.
- Check the results of the serum CRP level. If the titer is decreasing, the client is responding to treatment and/or the acute phase is declining. The CRP titer may be compared to the ESR. The serum CRP level will elevate and return to normal faster than the ESR.
- Compare the serum hs CRP with serum cholesterol and serum lipoprotein tests. An elevated hs CRP and serum cholesterol profile may indicate a high risk of coronary artery disease.

Creatine phosphokinase (CPK) (serum), CPK isoenzymes (serum)

Creatine Kinase (CK)

Reference Values

Adult: *Male:* 5–35 μg/ml, 30–180 IU/l, 55–170 U/l at 37°C (SI units). *Female:* 5–25 μg/ml, 25–150 IU/l, 30–135 U/l at 37°C (SI units).

Child: *Newborn:* 65–580 IU/l at 30°C. Child: *Male:* 0–70 IU/l at 30°C. *Female:* 0–50 IU/l at 30°C.

CPK Isoenzymes:

CPK-MM:	94%–100%	(muscle)
CPK-MB:	0%–6%	(heart)
CPK-BB:	0%	(brain)

Most labs have replaced CPK isoenzymes with CPK-MB fraction only.

Description

Creatine phosphokinase (CPK), also known as creatine kinase (CK), is an enzyme found in high concentration in the heart and skeletal muscles and in low concentration in the brain tissue. Serum CPK/CK is frequently elevated by skeletal muscle disease, acute myocardial infarction (MI), cerebrovascular disease, vigorous exercise, intramuscular (IM) injections, and electrolyte imbalance-hypokalemia. CPK/CK has two types of isoenzymes: M, associated with muscle, and B, associated with the brain. Electrophoresis separates the isoenzymes into three subdivisions: MM (in skeletal muscle and some in the heart), MB (in the heart), and BB (in brain tissue). When CPK/CK is elevated, a CPK electrophoresis is done to determine which group of isoenzymes is elevated. Increased isoenzyme CPK-MB could indicate damage to the myocardial cells.

Serum CPK/CK and CPK-MB rise within 4 to 6 hours after an acute MI, reach a peak in 18 to 24 hours (>6 times the normal value), and then return to normal within 3 to 4 days, unless new necrosis or tissue damage occurs. If medication for acute MI has to be given parenterally (for instance, morphine), it would be better to give it intravenously than intramuscularly so that mild muscle injury (from IM) would not elevate the CPK level; however, injections have little or no effect on CPK-MB. Draw blood for a serum CPK/CK level before giving an IM injection.

Purposes

- To suggest myocardial or skeletal muscle disease.
- To compare test results with aspartate aminotransferase/serum glutamic oxaloacetic transaminase (AST/SGOT) and lactate dehydrogenase (LDH) levels to determine myocardial damage.

Clinical Problems

Elevated Level: Acute myocardial infarction (AMI), skeletal muscle disease, cerebrovascular accident (CVA), and with all, elevated CPK isoenzymes. *Drug Influences:* IM injections, dexamethasone (Decadron), furosemide (Lasix), aspirin (high doses), ampicillin, carbenicillin, clofibrate.

CPK-MM Isoenzyme: Muscular dystrophy, delirium tremens, crush injury/trauma, surgery and postoperative state, vigorous exercise, IM injections, hypokalemia, hemophilia, hypothyroidism.

CPK-MB: Acute MI, severe angina pectoris, cardiac surgery, cardiac ischemia, myocarditis, hypokalemia, cardiac defibrillation.

CPK-BB: CVA, subarachnoid hemorrhage, cancer of the brain, acute brain injury, Reye's syndrome, pulmonary embolism and infarction, seizures.

Procedure

- Collect 5 to 7 ml of venous blood in a red-top tube. Avoid hemolysis.

- Note on the laboratory slip the number of times the patient has received IM injections in the last 24 to 48 hours.
- There is no food or fluid restriction.

Factors Affecting Laboratory Results

- IM injections can cause an elevated serum level of total CPK/CK.
- Vigorous exercise elevates the levels.
- Trauma and surgical intervention elevate serum levels.

NURSING IMPLICATIONS WITH RATIONALE

- Avoid giving IM injections until after blood is drawn for CPK.

Elevated Level

- Relate elevated serum (CPK/CK and isoenzymes [CPK-MM, CPK-MB, and CPK-BB]) to clinical problems. The CPK-MB is useful in making the differential diagnosis of myocardial infarction.
- Indicate whether the client has received an IM injection in the last 24 to 48 hours on the laboratory slip, and chart.
- Assess the client's signs and symptoms of an acute MI. Symptoms include pain; dyspnea; diaphoresis (excess perspiration); cold, clammy skin; pallor; cardiac dysrhythmia.
- Check the serum CPK/CK level at intervals, and notify the physician of serum level changes. The serum CPK/CK may be repeated every 6 to 8 hours during the acute phase. When the CPK/CK and CPK-MB are highly elevated, there may be extensive muscle damage to the myocardium. For acute MI, also check results of the AST (SGOT) and LDH tests.
- Compare serum AST/SGOT and LDH levels with CPK and CPK-MB.
- Provide measures for alleviating pain.

Creatinine (serum)

Reference Values

Adult: 0.5–1.5 mg/dl; 45–132.3 µmol/l (SI units). Females may have slightly lower values because of their lesser muscle mass.

Child: *Newborn:* 0.8–1.4 mg/dl. Infant: 0.7–1.7 mg/dl. *Child (2–6 years):* 0.3–0.6 mg/dl, 27–54 µmol/l (SI units). *Older Child:* 0.4–1.2 mg/dl, 36–106 µmol/l (SI units). Values increase slightly with age relative to muscle mass.

Elderly: May have decreased values relative to decreased muscle mass and decreased creatinine production.

Description

Creatinine, a by-product of muscle catabolism, is derived from the breakdown of muscle creatine phosphate. The amount of creatinine produced is proportional to the muscle mass. Creatinine is filtered by the glomeruli and it is excreted in the urine.

Serum creatinine is considered a more sensitive and specific indicator of renal disease than blood urea nitrogen (BUN). It rises later and is *not influenced by diet or fluid intake.* A slight BUN elevation could be indicative of hypovolemia (fluid volume deficit); however, a serum creatinine of 2.5 mg/dl could be indicative of renal impairment. BUN and creatinine are frequently compared. If BUN increases and serum creatinine remains normal, dehydration (hypovolemia) is present; and if both increase, then renal disorder is present. Serum creatinine is especially useful in evaluation of glomerular function.

Purpose

- To diagnose renal dysfunction.

Clinical Problems

Decreased Level: Pregnancy, eclampsia.

Elevated Level: Acute and chronic renal failure, shock (prolonged), systemic lupus erythematosus, cancer (intestine, bladder, testes, uterus, prostate), leukemias, Hodgkin's disease, essential hypertension, acute myocardial infarction, diabetic nephropathy, congestive heart failure (long standing), diet rich in creatinine (i.e., beef [high], poultry and fish [minimal] effect). *Drug Influence:* Amphotericin B, cephalosporins (cefazolin [Ancef], cephalothin [Keflin]), gentamicin, kanamycin, methicillin, ascorbic acid, barbiturates, lithium carbonate, mithramycin, methyldopa (Aldomet), glucose, protein, ketone bodies (increased), triamterene (Dyrenium).

Procedure

- Collect 3 to 5 ml of venous blood in a red-top tube.
- List any drugs the client is taking that could elevate the serum level on the laboratory slip.
- There is no food or fluid restriction. Red meats should be avoided the night before the test.

Factors Affecting Laboratory Results

- Certain drugs *(see Drug Influence)* may increase the serum creatinine level.
- Red meat consumed in large quantities may affect results.

NURSING IMPLICATIONS WITH RATIONALE

- Relate the elevated creatinine levels to clinical problems. Serum creatinine may be low in clients with small muscle mass, in amputees, and in clients with muscle disease. Older clients may have decreased muscle mass.
- Hold medications (see Drug Influence) for 24 hours before the test, with the health care provider's permission. Certain medications that cannot be withheld should be listed on the laboratory slip and noted on the client's chart.
- Check the amount of urine output in 24 hours. Less than 600 ml/24 hours can indicate renal insufficiency. Creatinine is excreted by the kidneys, and a continuous decrease in urine output could result in an increased serum creatinine level.
- Compare the BUN and creatinine levels. If both are increased, the problem is most likely kidney disease.

Client Teaching

- Instruct the client to eat less beef, poultry, and fish if the serum creatinine level is extremely elevated. Normally food does not have an effect on the serum creatinine level.

Creatinine clearance (urine)

Creatinine (Urine)

Reference Values

Adult: 85–135 ml/min. Females may have somewhat lower values.

Child: Similar to adult.

Elderly: Slightly decreased values than adult due to decreased glomerular filtration rate (GFR) caused by reduced renal plasma flow.

Urine Creatinine: 1–2 g/24 hours.

Description

Creatinine is a metabolic product of creatine phosphate in skeletal muscle, and it is excreted by the kidneys. Creatinine clearance is considered a reliable test for estimating GFR. With renal insufficiency, the GFR is decreased, and the serum creatinine is increased. GFR decreases with age, and with the older adult, the creatinine clearance may be diminished to as low as 60 ml/minute.

The creatinine clearance test consists of a 12- or 24-hour urine collection and a blood sample.

The formula for calculating creatinine clearance test is:

$$\text{Creatinine clearance} = \frac{\text{Urine creatinine (mg/dl)} \times \text{Urine volume (dl)}}{\text{Serum creatinine (mg/dl)}}$$

A creatinine clearance <40 ml/minute is suggestive of moderate to severe renal impairment.

Purposes

- To detect renal dysfunction.
- To monitor renal function.

Clinical Problems

Decreased Level: Mild to severe renal (kidney) impairment, hyperthyroidism, progressive muscular dystrophy, amylotrophic lateral sclerosis. *Drug Influence:* Phenacetin, steroids (anabolic), thiazides.

Elevated Level: Hypothyroidism, hypertension (renovascular), exercise. *Drug Influence:* Ascorbic acid, steroids, levodopa, methyldopa (Aldomet), phenolsulfon-phthalein (PSP) test.

Procedure

- Hydrate client before test.
- Instruct the client to avoid meats, poultry, fish, tea, and coffee for 6 hours before the test and during test, with the health care provider's permission.
- List drugs the client is taking that could affect test results on the laboratory slip.

Blood: Collect 3 to 5 ml of venous blood in a red-top tube the morning of the test.

Urine: Have the client void and discard the urine before the test begins. Note the time. Save all urine during the specified time (12 hours or 24 hours) in a urine container, without any preservative, that is refrigerated or kept on ice.

- Encourage water intake hourly during the test to have sufficient urine output.
- Label the container with the exact time and date the urine collection started and ended.

Factors Affecting Laboratory Results

- Phenacetin decreases the creatinine clearance.
- Toilet paper and feces will contaminate the urine.

NURSING IMPLICATIONS WITH RATIONALE

- Inform the health care provider of medications the client is receiving that could cause false test results.

Client Teaching

- Explain to the client the procedure for blood and urine collection. Blood is drawn in the morning. The client voids and the urine is discarded. Then all urine is saved for 12 hours or 24 hours in a urine container. Toilet paper and feces should not be in the urine.
- Instruct the client not to eat meats, poultry, fish, tea, or coffee for 6 hours before the test or during the test, according to the health care provider's orders.
- Encourage water intake throughout the test—approximately 100 ml/hour.
- Instruct client not to do strenuous exercise during the test.

Cross matching (blood)

Blood Typing Tests, Compatibility Test for RBCs, Type and Cross Match

Reference Values

Adult: Compatibility; absence of agglutination (clumping) of cells.

Child: Same as adult.

Description

The four *major* blood types (A, B, AB, and O) belong to the ABO blood group system. Red blood cells (RBCs) have either antigen A, B, AB, or none on the surface of the cells. Type A has A antigen, B has B antigen, AB has A and B antigens, and O does not contain an antigen. These antigens are capable of producing antibodies. The AB blood person is the universal recipient (can accept all blood), because there are no antibodies; the O blood person is the universal donor (can give blood to all types).

ABO blood type and Rh factor are first determined, then the compatibility of donor and recipient blood is determined by major cross match. The major cross match is between the donor's RBCs and the recipient's serum, and the test is performed to determine if the recipient has any antibodies to destroy the donor's RBCs.

Purpose

- To determine blood type.

Procedure

- Collect 7 to 10 ml of venous blood in a red-top tube (not a serum separator tube).
- There is no food or fluid restriction.

Factors Affecting Laboratory Results

■ Previously received incompatible blood can make blood cross matching difficult.

NURSING IMPLICATIONS WITH RATIONALE

■ Observe the client for signs and symptoms of fluid volume deficit (hypovolemia), such as tachycardia (pulse >100), tachypnea (rapid breathing), pale color, clammy skin, and low blood pressure (late symptoms). Crystalloid solutions (saline, lactated Ringer's) might be given rapidly to replace fluid volume until a transfusion can be administered. Usually 15 to 45 minutes are required to type and cross match blood.
■ Check the date of the unit of blood. Usually blood should be used within 28 days. Blood that is older than 28 days should not be given to a client having hyperkalemia.
■ Monitor the recipient's vital signs before and during transfusions. Signs and symptoms of transfusion reaction include temperature >1.1°C, chills and dyspnea.
■ Start the blood transfusion at a slow rate for the first 15 minutes; stay with the client and observe for adverse reactions.
■ Flush the transfusion set with normal saline if other IV solutions are ordered to follow the blood.

Cryoglobulins (serum)

Reference Values

Adult: ≤6 mg/dl.
Child: Negative.

Description

Cryoglobulins are serum globulins (protein) that precipitate from the plasma at 4°C and return to a dissolved status when warmed. They are present in IgG and IgM groups and are usually found in such pathologic conditions as leukemia, multiple myeloma, systemic lupus erythematosus (SLE), rheumatoid arthritis, and hemolytic anemia.

Purposes

■ To aid in the diagnosis of leukemia, SLE, and hemolytic anemia (see Clinical Problems).
■ To compare the test result with other laboratory tests.

Clinical Problems

Elevated Level: SLE, rheumatoid arthritis, polyarteritis nodosa, Hodgkin's disease, lymphocytic leukemia, multiple myeloma, acquired hemolytic anemias (autoimmune), cirrhosis (biliary), Waldenström's macroglobulinemia.

Procedure

- Collect 3 to 5 ml of venous blood in a red-top tube.
- The blood sample should not be refrigerated before it is taken to the laboratory.
- There is no food or fluid restriction.

Factors Affecting Laboratory Results

- None reported.

NURSING IMPLICATIONS WITH RATIONALE

Elevated Level

- Recognize that the increased presence of cryoglobulins might be caused by autoimmune diseases, collagen diseases, or leukemia.
- Observe for signs and symptoms of SLE (i.e., "butterfly" rash [erythematosus rash on the cheeks and the bridge of the nose], arthritis, and urinary insufficiency).
- Observe for signs and symptoms of rheumatoid arthritis (i.e., pain and stiffness in the joints [especially in the morning]; swollen, red, tender joints; joint deformities; and inability to make a fist and flexion contractures).
- Compare serum cryoglobulins with other laboratory tests.

Cultures (blood, sputum, stool, throat, wound, urine)

Reference Values

Adult: Negative or no pathogen.

Child: Same as adult.

Description

(Also see Antibiotic Susceptibility.)

Cultures are taken to isolate the microorganism that is causing the clinical infection. Most culture specimens are obtained using sterile swabs with medium (solid or broth), a sterile container (cup) with a lid, and a sterile syringe with a sterile bottle of liquid medium. The culture specimen should be taken immediately to the laboratory after collection (no longer than 30 minutes), because some organisms will die if not placed in the proper medium and incubated.

Most specimens for culture are either blood, sputum, stool, throat secretions, wound exudate, or urine. It usually takes 24 to 36 hours to grow the organisms and 48 hours for the growth and culture report.

Purpose

- To isolate the microorganism in body tissue or body fluid.

Clinical Problems

Specimen	Clinical Condition or Most Commonly Isolated Organism
Blood	Bacteremia, septicemia, postoperative shock, fever of unknown origin
Sputum	Pulmonary tuberculosis, bacterial pneumonia, chronic bronchitis, bronchiectasis
Stool	*Salmonella* species, *Shigella* species, enteropathogenic *Escherichia coli, Staphylococcus* species, *Yersinia*
Throat	Beta-hemolytic streptococci (rheumatic fever), thrush (*Candida* species), tonsillar infection, *Staphylococcus aureus*
Wound	*Staphylococcus* species: *S. aureus, Pseudomonas aeruginosa, Proteus* species, *Bacteroides* species, *Klebsiella* species, *Serratia* species
Urine	*Escherichia coli, Klebsiella* species, *Pseudomonas aeruginosa, Serratia* species, *Shigella* species, Yeasts: *Candida* species

Procedure

- Hand washing is essential before and after collection of the specimen.
- Send the specimen for culture to the laboratory *immediately* after collection.
- Obtain the specimen before antibiotic therapy is started. If the client is receiving antibiotics, the drug(s) should be listed on the laboratory slip.
- Collection containers or tubes should be sterile. Aseptic technique should be used during collection. Contamination of the specimen could cause false-positive results and/or transmission of the organisms.
- Check with the laboratory for specific techniques used.

Blood: Cleanse the client's skin according to the institution's procedure. Usually the skin is scrubbed first with povidone-iodine (Betadine). Iodine can be irritating to the skin, so it is removed and an application of benzalkonium chloride or alcohol is applied. Cleanse the top(s) of the culture bottle(s) with iodine and leave it or them to dry. The bottle(s) should contain a culture medium. Collect 5 to 10 ml of venous blood and place in the sterile bottle. Special vacuum tubes containing a culture medium for blood may be used instead of a culture bottle.

Sputum: *Sterile Container or Cup:* Obtain sputum for culture early in the morning, before breakfast. Instruct the client to give several deep coughs to raise sputum. Tell the client to avoid spitting saliva secretion into the sterile container. Saliva and postnasal drip secretions can contaminate the sputum specimen. Keep a lid on the sterile container. The container *should not* be completely filled and should be taken immediately to the laboratory. The sputum sample should not remain for hours by the client's bedside unless one needs a 24-hour sputum specimen (in this case, an extra sterile container should be left). *Acid-Fast Bacilli (TB Culture):* Follow the instructions on the container. Collect 5 to 10 ml of sputum, and take the sample immediately to the laboratory or refrigerate the specimen. Three sputum specimens may be requested, one each day for 3 days. Check for proper labeling.

Stool: Collect an approximately 1-inch-diameter feces sample. Use a sterile tongue blade and place the stool specimen in a sterile container with a lid. The suspected disease or organism should be noted on the laboratory slip. The stool specimen should not contain urine. The client should not be given barium or mineral oil, which can inhibit bacteria growth.

Throat: Use a sterile cotton swab or a polyester-tipped swab. The sterile culture kit could be used. Swab the inflamed or ulcerated tonsillar and/or posphryngeal areas of the throat. Place the applicator in a culturette tube with its culture medium. Take the throat culture specimen immediately to the laboratory. Do *not* give antibiotics before taking the culture.

Wound: Use a culture kit containing a sterile cotton swab or a polyester-tipped swab and a tube with culture medium. Swab the exudate of the wound and place the swab in the tube containing a culture medium. Wear sterile gloves when there is an excess amount of purulent drainage.

Urine: *Clean-Caught (Midstream) Urine Specimen:* Clean-caught urine collection is the commonest method for collecting a urine specimen for culture. There are noncatheterization kits giving step-by-step instructions. Catheterizing for urine culture is seldom ordered. Usually the client collects the urine specimen for culture, so a detailed explanation should be given, according to the instructions. The penis or vulva should be well cleansed. At times, two urine specimens (2 to 10 ml) are requested to verify the organism and in case of a possible contamination of the urine specimen. Collect a midstream urine specimen early in the morning, or as ordered, in a sterile container. The lid should fit tightly on the container and the urine specimen should be taken immediately to the bacteriology laboratory or refrigerated. Label the urine specimen with the client's name, the date, and the exact time of collection (e.g., 7/22/04 @ 8:00 am). List any antibiotics or sulfonamides the client is taking on the laboratory slip.

Factors Affecting Laboratory Results

- Contamination of the specimen causes inaccurate results.
- Antibiotics and sulfonamides may cause false-negative results.
- Urine in the stool collection may cause false test results.

NURSING IMPLICATIONS WITH RATIONALE

- Explain the procedure for obtaining the culture specimen. Answer questions. If the client participates in the collection of the specimen (e.g., urine), the procedure should be reviewed several times.

- Hold antibiotics or sulfonamides until after the specimen has been collected. These drugs could cause false-negative results. If these drugs have been given, they should be listed on the laboratory slip and recorded on the client's chart.
- Deliver all specimens immediately to the laboratory or refrigerate the specimen.
- Handle the specimen(s) with extreme care. Aseptic technique should be used. Prevent contamination of the specimen(s) or transmission of the organism to other clients or yourself. Observe strict aseptic techniques.
- Keep lids on sterile specimen containers. Sputum cups should not be uncovered by the bedside.
- Suggest a culture if a pathogenic organism is suspected. Check the client's temperature.

Cytomegalovirus (CMV) antibody (serum)

Reference Values

(Enzyme immunoassay (EIA) for IgG and IgM)

Adult or Child: Negative to <0.30: no CMV IgM Ab detected. 0.30–0.59: weak positive for CMV IgM Ab (suggestive of a recent infection in neonates. Significance of this low level in adults is not determined). >0.60: positive for CMV IgM Ab.

Description

Cytomegalovirus (CMV) belongs to the herpes virus family and causes the most common congenital infection in infants. CMV can be found in most body secretions (saliva, cervical secretions, urine, breast milk, and semen). If the pregnant woman is infected with CMV, it crosses the placenta, infecting the fetus. In infants, this virus can cause cerebral tissue malformation and damage. Urine specimens for CMV bodies or throat swabs may be used to detect CMV, but they frequently are not as helpful in detection as the serology test.

Many adults have been exposed to the virus and have developed immunity to CMV. Transmission of the CMV virus to immunocompromised persons such as persons with the aquired immunodeficiency syndrome (AIDS) is serious, because these people tend to acquire this virus readily. Also, transmission of CMV can be via blood transfusions from CMV-seropositive donors. Serologic studies (CMV-IgM antibodies and CMV-IgG antibodies) yield results in a shorter period than by culture. Cultures may be used to confirm the findings.

149

Purpose

- To identify the CMV of possible infected childbearing or pregnant women, infants, or immunocompromised persons.

Clinical Procedure

Elevated: Prone to CMV-infected childbearing women, infants, persons with AIDS or other immune deficiency, posttransplant organ recipients, following open heart surgery, hepatitis syndromes.

Procedure

- There is no food or fluid restriction.
- Collect 5 to 7 ml of venous blood in a red-top tube. Two blood samples are usually requested; the first is drawn during the acute phase, and 10 to 14 days later the second specimen is drawn for the convalescent phase.

Factors Affecting Laboratory Results

- A false-positive test result may occur to those with the rheumatoid factor in the serum or those exposed to the Epstein-Barr virus.
- Serum CMV test performed on infants who are younger than 6 months old. These infants could have the maternal CMV antibodies in their blood.

NURSING IMPLICATIONS WITH RATIONALE

- Obtain a history from the client of possible herpeslike viral infection.
- Assess the client for chronic respiratory infection or changes in vision. CMV retinitis can occur, which may result in blindness. Antiviral drugs may be used to treat CMV.
- Use aseptic technique when caring for clients infected with CMV.

Client Teaching

- Explain to the client that a blood sample is taken during the acute phase and again in approximately 2 weeks during the convalescent phase to determine the effectiveness of the treatment.
- Listen to the client's concerns about the possible effects of this virus on self or infant. Refer questions to appropriate health professionals as necessary.

D-Dimer test (blood)

Fragment D-Dimer, Fibrin Degradation Fragment

Reference Values

Negative for D-Dimer fragments: >250 ng/ml: >250 µg/l (SI units).

Description

D-dimer, a fibrin degradation fragment, occurs through fibrinolysis. This test measures the amount of fibrin degradation that occurs. It confirms the presence of fibrin split products (FSPs) and is more specific for diagnosing disseminated intravascular coagulation (DIC) than FSPs. However, both D-dimer and FSP tests are frequently used to determine DIC in a client.

D-dimer levels are increased when a fibrin clot is broken down by the thrombolytic drug, tissue plasminogen activator (tPA), streptokinase.

Purpose

- To detect the presence of DIC in a client.

Clinical Problems

Elevated Levels: Disseminated intravascular coagulation (DIC); pulmonary embolism; arterial, coronary, and venous thrombosis; possibly myocardial infarction; neoplastic disease, surgery up to post 2nd day; late pregnancy, sickle cell crisis.

Procedure

- Collect 7 ml of venous blood in a blue-top tube. Avoid hemolysis; invert tube gently, do not shake the tube.
- Apply pressure to the venapuncture site especially if the client has a bleeding tendency. Pressure may need to be applied for up to 5 minutes.
- Blood specimen should be taken to the laboratory within 4 hours.
- There is no food or fluid restriction.

Factors Affecting Laboratory Results

- Hemolysis of the blood specimen.

NURSING IMPLICATIONS WITH RATIONALE

- Obtain a history of unexplained bleeding or any condition that is included in the Clinical Problems.

- Note signs of sweating, cold and mottled fingers and toes, petechiae and bleeding. Report adverse signs and symptoms immediately.
- Check and monitor vital signs.

Client Teaching

- Explain to the client and family the purposes of the test.

Dexamethasone suppression test (DST)

ACTH Suppression Test

Reference Values

>50% reduction of plasma cortisol and urine 17-hydroxycorticosteroids (17-OHCS).

Rapid or Overnight Screening Test: Plasma cortisol: 8 AM <10 μg/dl; 4 PM <5 μg/dl. Urine 17-OHCS (5-hour specimen): <4 mg/5 hours.

Increased Dexamethasone Dose: *Low Dose:* Plasma cortisol: one half of client's base-line level. Urine 17-OHCS: <2.5 mg/24 hours/second day. *High Dose:* Plasma cortisol; one-half of client's baseline level. Urine 17-OHCS: one half of client's baseline level.

Note: The high dose test is done if results do not change with a low dose of dexamethasone.

Description

Dexamethasone (Decadron) is a potent glucocorticoid. The dexamethasone suppression test distinguishes between adrenal hyperplasia and adrenal tumor as the cause of adrenal hyperfunction, and is used to diagnose and to manage depression.

When given dexamethasone, there is a reduction (suppression) in adrenocorticotropin hormone (ACTH) secretion (negative feedback), thus causing a lower plasma and urine cortisol. Low-dose and high-dose dexamethasone are used to distinguish between adrenal hyperplasia and adrenal tumor (nonsuppress at low or high doses). Adrenal hyperplasia will suppress at high doses but not at low doses.

In psychiatry the test is useful in diagnosing affective diseases, such as endogenous depression (melancholia). In approximately 50% of these clients, suppression of plasma cortisol does not occur.

The test could be a rapid or overnight screening test or a 2-day test (8 doses of dexamethasone) with low and/or high doses of the drug.

Purpose

- To distinguish between adrenal hyperplasia and adrenal tumor as the cause of adrenal hyperfunction.

Clinical Problems

No Plasma Cortisol or Urine 17-OHCS: Adrenal adenoma (tumor), ectopic ACTH-producing tumor, bilateral adrenal hyperplasia (except with high steroid doses).

Procedure

- Obtain a baseline plasma cortisol and urine 17-OHCS level 24 hours before the test.
- Avoid tea, caffeinated coffee, chocolates. No other food or fluid restriction is required.
- Refrigerate urine for 17-OHCS levels.

Rapid or Overnight Screening Test

- NPO after midnight. Check with laboratory policy.
- Give dexamethasone 1 mg or 5 μg/kg PO at 11 PM.
- Obtain baseline plasma cortisol and urine 17-OHCS levels. Draw blood at 8 AM for plasma cortisol level. Obtain a urine OHCS level at 12 noon.

Increased Dexamethasone Dose: Two days of low or high doses of dexamethasone (Decadron).

Low Dose

- Give dexamethasone 0.5 mg every 6 hours for 2 days (total of 4 mg).
- Obtain a plasma cortisol level at 8 AM, 4 PM, and 11 PM and a 24-hour urine 17-OHCS level after a 2-day low-dose test. If no suppression is found, the high-dose test may be recommended.

High Dose

- Give dexamethasone 2 mg every 6 hours for 2 days (total of 16 mg).
- Obtain a plasma cortisol level at 8 AM, 4 PM, and 11 PM and a 24-hour urine 17-OHCS level after a 2-day high-dose test.

Factors Affecting Laboratory Results

- Ingestion of excess coffee, tea, and chocolates could increase steroid release.
- Not refrigerating urine for 17-OHCS test could affect results.

NURSING IMPLICATIONS WITH RATIONALE

- Report anxiety, stress, fever, or infection to the health care provider.
- Obtain baseline plasma cortisol and urine 17-OHCS levels 24 hours before the test. For the screening test, a plasma cortisol level should be obtained at 8 AM

and a urine 17-OHCS level at 12 noon. For the 2-day dexamethasone test, a plasma and urine level should be obtained after 2 days of low or high dexamethasone dosage.

- Administer dexamethasone at specified times *on time*. Milk or antacids may be required to decrease gastric irritation.
- Provide ample time for the client to ask questions. Refer unknown answers to appropriate health professionals.
- Assess for side effects of dexamethasone resulting from high doses (i.e., weight gain, gastric discomfort).
- Monitor electrolytes during the test. Steroid causes serum potassium loss and serum sodium excess.
- Check blood glucose with Chemstrip bG for hyperglycemia while the client is taking high doses of dexamethasone. This drug is a glucocorticosteroid and can elevate blood glucose levels.
- Be supportive to client and family members during the test. This is a time-consuming test procedure. Cooperation from client and family members is needed for accurate results.

Client Teaching

- Instruct the client to avoid caffeinated coffee, tea, and chocolate.

Diazepam (serum)

Valium

Reference Values

Therapeutic: *Adult:* 0.5–2.0 mg/l, 400–600 ng/ml.
Toxic: *Adult:* 3 mg/l, >3000 ng/ml.

Description

Diazepam (Valium), a benzodiazepine, has been one of the most commonly prescribed antianxiety agents in the United States. The clinical uses of diazepam include treatment of status epilepticus; alcohol withdrawal; induction of anesthesia for minor surgical procedures, endoscopic procedures; cardioversion; and muscle relaxation, especially in paraplegia, cerebral palsy, and tetanus.

Diazepam is absorbed from the gastrointestinal tract and is metabolized in the liver to a large number of metabolites. The peak blood level occurs 1 to 2 hours after the oral dose. After a single oral dose of 10 to 15 mg, peak value level usually is 200 to 300 ng/ml. Half-life is 10 to 40 hours (40 hours with continuous use). The major metabolite, *N*-desmethyldiazepam, has a half-life of 50 to 90 hours. Onset of action is 30 to 60 minutes after oral dose, 15 to 30 minutes after IM injection, and 1 to 5 minutes after IV dose. Diazepam is excreted in the urine as metabolites. This drug can cross the placenta and might cause teratogeny (birth defects).

A steady state for the serum diazepam level may take 1 to 2 weeks to attain. Monitoring the serum diazepam level should be continued once the steady state is reached, and especially when daily dose is changed.

Purposes

- To monitor diazepam levels.
- To detect toxic levels of diazepam.

Clinical Problems

Decreased Level: Smoking.

Elevated Level: Diazepam overdose, liver disease, alcohol. *Drug Influence:* Cimetidine (Tagamet), isoniazid (INH), valproic acid (Depakene).

Procedure

- Collect 3 to 5 ml of venous blood in a red-top tube 2 hours after an oral dose or at trough level (before the next dose).
- Record the dose, route, and last-administered dose on the laboratory requisition slip.
- There is no food or fluid restriction.

Factors Affecting Laboratory Results

- Drugs *(see Drug Influence above)* might cause an increased diazepam level.
- Taking other benzodiazepines (i.e., chlordiazepoxide [Librium], chlorazepate dipotassium [Tranxene]) along with diazepam will interfere with correct test results, because these agents contain many of the same active metabolites.

NURSING IMPLICATIONS WITH RATIONALE

- Record the dose, route, and last time the drug was given on the requisition slip. Usually the blood specimen is drawn 2 hours after taking diazepam.
- Elicit from a female client if she is pregnant or intends to become pregnant before giving diazepam. This drug may have teratogenic effects.
- Monitor frequently serum diazepam levels in children, in the elderly, and in debilitated adults. Small doses of diazepam should be given to these individuals to avoid diazepam toxicity.
- Recognize that erratic absorption of diazepam could result from IM administration. Diazepam toxicity could occur after numerous injections.

Decreased Level

- Recognize that smoking can decrease the diazepam level.
- Avoid administering diazepam in IV fluids. This drug could precipitate in the fluids or adhere to the IV bag or tubing, thus decreasing prescribed dosage.

Elevated Level

- Recognize that diazepam overdose, liver disease, or alcohol could elevate the serum diazepam level.
- Check for signs and symptoms of diazepam toxicity (i.e., drowsiness, ataxia, confusion, headache, slurred speech, tremors, hypotension, tachycardia, and circulatory collapse).

Client Teaching

- Instruct the client not to ingest alcohol or other central nervous system depressants while taking diazepam. The effects of taking these substances together could cause severe drowsiness, respiratory distress, or respiratory arrest.
- Explain to the client that diazepam should never be abruptly discontinued. Diazepam is tapered to lower doses over 1 to 2 weeks to avoid withdrawal symptoms (i.e., confusion, tremors, paranoia, ataxia, visual hallucinations, sweating, and abdominal and muscle cramps).

Differential white blood cell (WBC) count

See WBC Differential

Digoxin (serum)

Lanoxin

Reference Values

Therapeutic: *Adult:* 0.5–2 ng/ml; 0.5–2 nmol/l (SI units). *Infants:* 1–3 ng/ml. *Child:* Same as adult.

Toxic: *Adult:* >2 ng/ml; >2.6 nmol/l (SI units). *Infants:* >3.5 ng/ml. *Child:* Same as adult.

Description

Digoxin, a form of digitalis, is a cardiac glycoside agent given to increase the force and velocity of myocardial contraction. More than 75% to 95% of the drug is absorbed through the gastrointestinal (GI) tract, and a large amount of digoxin is excreted unchanged through the kidneys. The half-life of digoxin is 35 to 40 hours, with a shorter half-life in neonates and infants and a longer time in short-term infants/premature infants.

Serum plateau levels of digoxin occur 6 to 8 hours after an oral dose, 2 to 4 hours after IV administration, and 10 to 12 hours after IM administration. The most frequent routes used for administering digoxin are by mouth (oral) and IV.

Electrolyte imbalance (hypokalemia or hypomagnesemia), acid–base disturbances, and certain drugs predispose the person to digitalis toxicity. Common signs and symptoms of digitalis toxicity include pulse rate <60 per minute, anorexia, nausea, vomiting, headaches, and visual disturbance.

Purpose

- To monitor digoxin levels.

Clinical Problems

Decreased Level: Decreased GI absorption, decreased GI motility. *Drug Influence:* Antacids, Kaopectate, metoclopramide (Reglan), barbiturates, cholestyramine (Questran), spironolactone (Aldactone).

Elevated Level: Digoxin overdose, renal disease, liver disease. *Drug Influence:* Amphotericin B, diuretics (ethacrynic acid [Edecrin], furosemide [Lasix], thiazides), chlorthalidone (Hygroton), quinidine, reserpine (Serpasil), succinylcholine, sympathomimetics, corticosteroids.

Procedure

- Collect 3 to 5 ml of venous blood in a red-top tube.
- Obtain a blood sample 6 to 10 hours after administration of oral digoxin, or, frequently preferred, take sample prior to next dose.
- There is no food or fluid restriction.

Factors Affecting Laboratory Results

- Administering digoxin intramuscularly might cause the absorption rate to be erratic, especially in a debilitated or elderly person with poor tissue perfusion.
- A low serum potassium or magnesium level could cause digitalis toxicity, and a high serum calcium level could cause digitalis toxicity.
- Hypothyroidism, severe heart disease, and renal function abnormalities may predispose a client to digitalis toxicity.

NURSING IMPLICATIONS WITH RATIONALE

- Do not confuse digoxin with other digitalis glycosides (e.g., digitoxin). Digitoxin has a longer half-life and cumulative effect.
- Check serum digoxin results and report nontherapeutic levels to the physician immediately.
- Keep the digoxin bottle away from light.
- Obtain a blood sample for serum digoxin determination during predicted plateau levels for oral, IV, and IM administration.
- Take the apical pulse for 1 minute prior to administering digoxin. If the pulse rate is <60 per minute, do not give the digoxin, and notify the health care provider.

Decreased Level

- Associate GI disturbance and certain drugs (i.e., antacids, Kaopectate, barbiturates, cholestyramine, spironolactone) with a decreased therapeutic serum digoxin level. The digoxin dose might need to be increased if those drugs are being taken. If the digoxin dose has been increased while the client is on the drug(s) and later the drug has been discontinued, the digoxin dosage should be decreased.
- Inform the health care provider which drugs the client is taking that might decrease the effectiveness of the prescribed digoxin dose.

Elevated Level

- Check serum potassium, magnesium, and calcium levels. Hypokalemia, hypomagnesemia, and hypercalcemia enhance the action of digoxin and could cause digitalis toxicity.
- Observe for signs and symptoms of digitalis toxicity (i.e., pulse rate <60 per minute, anorexia, nausea, vomiting, headache, visual disturbance).

Client Teaching

- Instruct the client to take his or her pulse before taking digoxin and to call the health care provider if the rate is <60 per minute in adults; in children a rate of <70 per minute should be reported.

Dilantin

See Phenytoin

D-xylose absorption test (blood and urine)

Reference Values

Adult: *Blood D-xylose:* 25–40 mg/dl/2 hours. *Urine D-xylose:* Urine excretion: >3.5 g/5 hours; >5 g/24 hours.

Child: *Blood D-xylose:* 30 mg/dl/1 hour.

Description

The D-xylose absorption test determines the absorptive capacity of the small intestine. After ingestion of D-xylose, a pentose sugar, serum and urine D-xylose levels are measured. Usually a low serum D-xylose level (<25 mg/dl) and a low urine D-xylose level (<3 g) are indicative of malabsorption syndrome.

Abnormal test results occur in celiac disease, small-bowel ischemia, Whipple's disease, Zollinger-Ellison syndrome, enteritis, massive intestinal resection, and intestinal bacterial overgrowth.

Various clinical problems such as vomiting, hypomotility, dehydration, alcoholism, rheumatoid arthritis, severe congestive heart failure, ascites, and poor renal function could cause low urine D-xylose levels that are not secondary to intestinal malabsorption. Endoscopic examination and biopsy frequently are necessary to confirm the diagnosis of malabsorption.

Purpose

- To aid in the diagnosis of gastrointestinal disturbance/disorder.

Clinical Problems

Decreased Level: Celiac disease, small-bowel ischemia, Whipple's disease, Zollinger-Ellison syndrome, radiation enteritis, multiple jejunal diverticula, diabetic neuropathy, diarrhea, lymphoma, amyloidosis, scleroderma, massive intestinal resection, bacterial overgrowth.

Procedure

- Restrict foods for 8 hours for adults and for 4 hours for children prior to test. Foods that contain pentose, such as fruits, jams, jellies, and pastries, should be withheld for 24 hours prior to the test.
- The client ingests 25 g of D-xylose dissolved in 8 oz (240 ml) of water. An additional 8 oz of water should follow the mixture of D-xylose and water. Some institutions use a 5-g dose instead of 25 g. Child dose is based on weight: 0.5 g/kg but not more than 25 g.
- Collect 7 ml of venous blood in a red-top tube. Blood specimens are drawn at 30, 60, and 120 minutes or at 2 hours only after D-xylose ingestion.

- Discard the urine specimen prior to the urine collection. Keep all urine refrigerated; at the end of 5 hours, send the urine collection to the laboratory.
- Check the order for the length of collection time (i.e., 5 hours or 24 hours). Note on the laboratory slip the period of urine collection and the age of the client. Older adults with mild renal impairment can have a decreased 5-hour test result and a normal 24-hour test.
- Indicate on the laboratory slip any drugs the client is taking that could affect test results. Nonsteroidal anti-inflammatory drugs (NSAIDs) such as aspirin, indomethacin (Indocin), and atropine should be withheld for 24 hours. Note the drug dose and the last time it was taken on the laboratory slip.

Factors Affecting Laboratory Results

- Drugs such as aspirin, indomethacin (Indocin), and atropine can decrease intestinal absorption.
- Foods high in pentose (e.g., fruits, jams, jellies, and pastries) can affect serum and urine D-xylose results.
- Hemolysis of the blood sample could cause inaccurate test results.
- Renal impairment or insufficiency could decrease urine output, thus affecting urine test results.
- Vomiting, dehydration, hypomotility, alcoholism, and other conditions *(see Description)* could cause a decreased urine D-xylose level that is not due to malabsorption.

NURSING IMPLICATIONS WITH RATIONALE

- Explain the blood and urine test procedures to the client.
- Assess communications for verbal and nonverbal expressions of anxiety and fear concerning tests or the potential or actual problem.
- Report to the health care provider (HCP) if the client is having severe diarrhea, vomiting, and dehydration. These clinical problems could cause a decreased urine D-xylose level.
- Provide ongoing assessment before, during, and after the procedure. Document and communicate alterations.
- Be supportive to the client and to family members. They might be most anxious about the test procedure and the unknown test results. Client compliance during the procedure is essential for accurate test results.

Client Teaching

- Inform the client that food is restricted, but fluids are not. Inform the client not to eat foods high in pentose (jellies, jams, fruits) for 24 hours before the test.
- Instruct the client to save all urine during the 5- or 24-hour urine test. Refrigerate urine collection.
- Instruct the client to withhold aspirin, indomethacin (Indocin), and atropine or atropine products, with HCP's approval, for 24 hours before the test. Aspirin could decrease D-xylose excretion and indomethacin and atropine could

decrease intestinal absorption. Note on the laboratory slip the last drug dose and dosage that the client received.

- Be prepared to repeat information to the client and family if the anxiety or fear level is determined to be high. Provide written instructions to reinforce verbal instructions.

Encephalitis virus antibody (serum)

Reference Values

Titer: <1:10. Definite confirmation of the virus: a fourfold rise in titer level between the acute and convalescent blood specimens.

Description

Encephalitis is inflammation of the brain tissue, which is frequently due to an arbovirus transmitted by a mosquito after the mosquito has been in contact with an animal host. There are several groups of arbovirus causing encephalitis. The animal host varies according to location.

Eastern Equine Encephalitis Virus: It is mainly found in the eastern United States from New Hampshire to Texas. Transmission is by the mosquito from the animal hosts: birds, ducks, fowl, and horses. Symptoms include fever, frontal headaches, drowsiness, nausea and vomiting, abnormal reflexes, rigidity, and bulging of the fontanelle in infants. The mortality rate of 65% to 75% is one of the highest for viral encephalitis.

California Encephalitis Virus: Incidence is highest in children in the north central United States. It is transmitted by infected mosquitoes and tics. Symptoms include fever, severe headaches, stiff neck, sore throat.

St. Louis Encephalitis Virus: This virus occurs most frequently in the southern, central, and western United States. It is a Group B arbovirus and is transmitted by an infected mosquito. The animal host is the bird. The symptoms of headache, stiff neck, abnormal reflexes may be mild or severe.

Venezuelan Equine Encephalitis Virus: The incidence of this virus is highest in South America, Central America, Mexico, Texas, and Florida. It is a Group A arbovirus and is transmitted by an infected mosquito. The animal hosts are the rodent and horse. Symptoms can be mild such as flulike symptoms or severe such as disorientation, paralysis, seizures, and coma.

Western Equine Encephalitis Virus: Occurrence is primarily west of the Mississippi, particularly California, in the summer months and early fall. The virus is transmitted by infected mosquitoes infected by animal hosts: birds, squirrels, snakes, and horses. Symptoms include sore throat, stiff neck, lethargy, stupor, and coma in severe cases.

Purposes

- To detect the presence of an elevated encephalitis virus antibody titer, which indicates an inflammation of the brain tissue caused by an arboviral infection.
- To screen for an arbovirus.

Clinical Problems

Elevated Titer: Viral encephalitis (identified strain), meningoencephalitis.

Procedure

- There is no food or fluid restriction.
- Collect 3 to 5 ml of venous blood in a red-top tube. Two blood specimens should be taken at least 2 to 3 weeks apart, first during the acute phase of the viral infection and second during the convalescent phase.
- Cerebrospinal fluid can be used to identify the virus.

Factors Affecting Laboratory Results

- Not obtaining a blood sample during both the acute and the convalescent phases.

NURSING IMPLICATIONS WITH RATIONALE

- Obtain a history of the client's contact with mosquitoes. Ascertain when the client first became ill.
- Assess for symptoms associated with encephalitis, such as fever, frontal headaches, sore throat, stiff neck, and lethargy.

Client Teaching

- Explain to the client that there will be two blood samples taken, 2 to 3 weeks apart.
- Listen to the client's concerns. Answer the client's questions or refer to other professional health care providers.

Enterovirus group (serum)

Reference Values

Norm: Negative.

Positive: Fourfold rise in titer between the acute and convalescent periods.

Description

The enterovirus group includes many types of viruses that are found in the alimentary tract. Examples of these serotype viruses include Coxsackie A and B, echovirus, poliomyelitis viruses. Testing for enterovirus group is usually indicated when there is an epidemic outbreak of one of these viruses. Other methods for enteroviral testing include specimens from oropharynx, stool, and cerebrospinal fluid (CSF).

Purpose

- To identify the presence of an enterovirus associated with an epidemic outbreak such as Coxsackie A and B.

Clinical Problem

Positive Titer: Enteroviral infections.

Procedure

- There is no food or fluid restriction.
- Collect 3 to 5 ml of venous blood in a red-top tube. Usually two blood specimens are required; one at the acute phase and the second one during the convalescent phase (2 to 3 weeks between the two phases).

Factors Affecting Laboratory Test

- Not collecting two blood samples, one during the acute phase and one during the convalescent phase.

NURSING IMPLICATIONS WITH RATIONALE

- Obtain a history of an alimentary tract infection. Symptoms may vary, so the client's description of the symptoms should be recorded.
- Assess the client's vital signs. Report abnormal findings.

Erythrocyte osmotic fragility

See Osmotic Fragility

Erythrocyte sedimentation rate (ESR) (blood)

Sedimentation (SED) Rate

Reference Values

Adult: *Westergren Method: Male:* <50 years: 0–15 mm/hour. *Female:* <50 years: 0–20 mm/hour. *Male:* >50 years: 0–20 mm/hour. *Female:* >50 years: 0–30 mm/hour. *Wintrobe Method: Male:* 0–9 mm/hour. *Female:* 0–15 mm/hour.

Child: *Newborn:* 0–2 mm/hour; *4–14 years:* 0–10 mm/hour.

Description

The erythrocyte sedimentation rate (ESR) (known also as the sedimentation rate or SED rate) is the rate at which red blood cells (RBCs) settle in unclotted blood in millimeters per hour (mm/hour). The ESR is nonspecific. The rate can be increased in acute inflammatory process, acute and chronic infections, tissue damage (necrosis), rheumatoid, collagen diseases, malignancies, and physiologic stress situations (e.g., pregnancy). To some hematologists, the ESR is unreliable, because it is nonspecific and is affected by physiologic factors that cause inaccurate results.

The C-reactive protein (CRP) test is considered more useful than the ESR because CRP increases more rapidly during an acute inflammatory process and returns to normal faster than the ESR. The ESR is still an old standby used by many physicians as a rough estimate of the disease process and for following the course of illness. With an elevated ESR, other laboratory tests should be conducted to properly identify the clinical problem.

Purpose

- To compare with other laboratory values for diagnosing inflammatory conditions *(see Clinical Problems)*.

Clinical Problems

Decreased Level: Polycythemia vera, congestive heart failure, sickle cell anemias, infectious mononucleosis, factor V deficiency, degenerative arthritis, angina pectoris. *Drug Influence:* Ethambutol (Myambutol), quinine, salicylates (aspirins), cortisone, prednisone.

Elevated Level: Rheumatoid arthritis, rheumatic fever, acute myocardial infarction, cancer (stomach, colon, breast, liver, kidney), Hodgkin's disease, multiple myeloma, lymphosarcoma, bacterial endocarditis, gout, hepatitis, cirrhosis of the liver, acute pelvic inflammatory disease, syphilis, tuberculosis, glomerulonephritis, systemic lupus erythematosus, hemolytic disease of newborns (erythroblastosis fetalis), pregnancy (second and third trimesters). *Drug Influence:* Dextran, methyldopa (Aldomet), methysergide (Sansert), penicillamine (Cuprimine), procainamide (Pronestyl), theophylline, oral contraceptives, vitamin A.

Procedure

- Collect 7 ml of venous blood in a lavender-top tube. Keep the specimen in a vertical position.
- Take the blood specimen to the laboratory immediately. Blood should not stand, because the ESR could increase.
- If the blood specimen is refrigerated, it should be allowed to return to room temperature before it is tested.
- There is no food or fluid restriction.
- Hold medications that can cause false-positive results for 24 hours before the test, with health care provider's permission.

Factors Affecting Laboratory Results

- Factors increasing the ESR—pregnancy (second and third trimesters); menstruation; drugs *(see Drug Influence);* the presence of cholesterol, fibrinogen, and globulins.
- Factors decreasing the ESR—newborns (decreased fibrinogen level); drugs *(see Drug Influence);* high blood sugar, serum albumin, and serum phospholipids.

NURSING IMPLICATIONS WITH RATIONALE

Elevated Level

- Relate an elevated ESR to clinical problems and drugs. The ESR is a nonspecific test but it can indicate an inflammatory process occurring.
- Answer the client's questions about *the significance* of an increased ESR. An answer could be that other laboratory tests are usually performed in conjunction with the ESR for adequate diagnosis of a clinical problem.
- Compare ESR with CRP test results.

Estetrol (E₄) (plasma and amniotic fluid)

Reference Values

Pregnancy:

PLASMA		AMNIOTIC FLUID	
Week of Gestation	**pg/ml**	**Week of Gestation**	**ng/ml**
20–26	140–210	32+	0.8
30	>350	40+	13.0
36	>900		
40	>1050		

Description

Estetrol (E₄) is an effective indicator of fetal distress during the third trimester of pregnancy. Estetrol increases during gestation. At term, estetrol consists of .05% to 2% of the total unconjugated estrogen.

One test alone should not determine fetal distress. Several values such as estriol (E₃) and human placental lactogen are usually obtained to verify the possible diagnosis.

Purpose

- To detect the occurrence of fetal distress.

Clinical Problems

Decreased Level: Fetal distress, intrauterine fetal death, anencephalic fetus, fetal malformations.

Procedure

- Collect 5 to 7 ml of venous blood in a red-top tube.
- There is no food or fluid restriction.

Factors Affecting Laboratory Results

- Unknown.

NURSING IMPLICATIONS WITH RATIONALE

- Obtain a history of current problems related to the pregnancy.
- Monitor fetal heart rate.
- Compare serum estetrol with estriol and human placental lactogen levels. Report laboratory values to the health care provider.

- Listen to the client's and family's concerns. Refer questions to appropriate health professionals as necessary.

Estradiol (E$_2$) (serum)

Reference Values

Adult: *Female:* Follicular phase: 20–150 pg/ml. Midcycle: 100–500 pg/ml. Luteal phase: 60–260 pg/ml. Postmenopausal: <30 pg/ml. *Male:* 15–50 pg/ml.
Child: 3–10 pg/ml.

Description

Estradiol (E$_2$) evaluates gonadal dysfunction such as amenorrhea syndromes and testicular tumors. It is *not* used to evaluate fetal well-being in pregnant females.

Purposes

- To determine the presence of gonadal dysfunction.
- To evaluate menstrual and fertility problems in the female.

Clinical Problems

Decreased Level: Primary amenorrhea, anorexia nervosa, ovarian failure, pituitary insufficiency (hypopituitarism), menopause.

Elevated Level: Ovarian tumors, testicular tumors, adrenal hyperplasia or tumors.

Procedure

- Collect 5 to 7 ml of venous blood in a red-top tube. In the female the blood sample may be drawn before ovulation occurs or at midcycle in the morning.
- List on the laboratory slip the phase of the menstrual cycle.
- There is no food or fluid restriction.

Factors Affecting Laboratory Results

- Incorrect listing of the menstrual phase could affect the test result.

NURSING IMPLICATIONS WITH RATIONALE

- Obtain the phase of the menstrual cycle from the client. Record on the laboratory slip.
- Ascertain the client's concern about the test result. Be supportive.

167

Estriol (E₃) (serum and urine)

Reference Values

Pregnancy

SERUM		URINE	
Weeks of Gestation	ng/dl	Weeks of Gestation	mg/24 hrs
25–28	25–165	25–28	6–28
29–32	30–230	29–32	6–32
33–36	45–370	33–36	10–45
37–38	75–420	37–40	15–60
39–40	95–450		

Description

Estriol (E_3) is a major estrogenic compound produced largely by the placenta. It increases in maternal serum and urine after 2 months of pregnancy and continues at high levels until term. If toxemia, hypertension, or diabetes is present after 30 weeks of gestation, estriol levels are monitored. A decline in serum or urine estriol levels suggests fetal distress caused by placental malfunction.

Serum estriol is replacing urine estriol because specimen collection is easier and there is no 24-hour waiting period. The advantage of the 24-hour urine estriol is avoidance of estriol value variations that usually occur within the day. A urine estriol averages out the "within-day" fluctuations of estriol. Repeated serum and/or urine estriol are frequently ordered.

Purposes

- To monitor estriol levels.
- To determine fetal distress after 30 weeks' gestation.
- To compare test results with estetrol test results regarding fetal distress.

Clinical Problems

Decreased Level: Fetal distress, placental dysfunction, diabetic pregnancy, pregnancy with hypertension, impending toxemia.

Elevated Level: Urinary tract infection, glycosuria. *Drug Influence:* Antibiotics (ampicillin, neomycin), hydrochlorothiazide (Hydrodiuril), cortisone preparations.

Procedure

- There is no food or fluid restriction.

Serum

- Collect 5 to 7 ml of venous blood in a red-top tube.

Urine

- Collect urine for 24 hours in a large container with preservative.
- Label the client's name, date, and the exact times of collection (e.g., 3/28/04, 8 AM to 3/29/04, 8:03 AM).
- Two 24-hour urine specimens (taken a day apart) are usually ordered for more valid results.

Factors Affecting Laboratory Results

- Multiple pregnancy can increase levels.
- Incorrect gestation week can cause a false test result.
- Glycosuria and urinary tract infection could give false urine estriol results.

NURSING IMPLICATIONS WITH RATIONALE

- Monitor the fetal heart rate, the patient's blood pressure, and sugar in the urine. Hypertension and diabetes could cause placental dysfunction, leading to fetal distress.
- Report glycosuria and urinary tract infection during pregnancy; both could cause a false result.
- Be supportive of the client and family.

Client Teaching

- Inform the client that several blood samples may be taken. If a urine collection is ordered, inform the client that all urine should be saved and that there may be more than one 24-hour urine specimen requested.

Estrogen (serum)

Reference Values

Adult: *Female:* Early menstrual cycle: 60–200 pg/ml. Midmenstrual cycle: 120–440 pg/ml. Late menstrual cycle: 150–350 pg/ml. Postmenopausal: <30 pg/ml. *Male:* 40–115 pg/ml. *Child:* 1–6 years: 3–10 pg/ml; 8–12 years: <30 pg/ml.

Description

Estrogens are produced by the ovaries, adrenal cortex, and testes. There are over

30 estrogens identified in the body, but only three measurable types of estrogens: estrone (E_1), estradiol (E_2), and estriol (E_3). Total serum estrogen reflects estrone, mostly estradiol, and some estriol. For fetal well-being during pregnancy, serum E_3 is used.

Purpose

- To diagnose ovarian dysfunction and other health problems *(see Clinical Problems)*.

Clinical Problems

Decreased Level: Ovarian failure or dysfunction, primary hypogonadism, Turner's syndrome, intrauterine death in pregnancy, pituitary insufficiency, postmenopausal symptoms, anorexia nervosa, psychogenic stress.

Elevated Level: Ovarian tumors, precocious puberty, adrenal hyperplasia or tumors, testicular tumor, cirrhosis of the liver.

Procedure

- Collect 5 to 7 ml of venous blood in a red-top tube. Avoid hemolysis.
- Indicate on the laboratory slip the phase of the client's menstrual cycle.
- There is no food or fluid restriction.

Factors Affecting Laboratory Results

- Oral contraceptives can increase the estrogen level; steroids can affect test results; and clomiphene, an estrogen antagonist, could decrease the estrogen level.
- Shaking the blood sample could cause hemolysis.

NURSING IMPLICATIONS WITH RATIONALE

- Indicate on the laboratory slip if the client is taking steroids, oral contraceptives, or estrogens.
- Note on the laboratory slip the phase of client's menstrual cycle.
- Assess communications for verbal and nonverbal expressions of anxiety and fear concerning tests or the potential or actual problem.
- Encourage ventilation of feelings through provision of a private, calm environment. Use quiet, steady speech patterns when interacting with the client. Employ touch if appropriate.

Decreased Level

- Note and record if the client is postmenopausal.

Elevated Level

- Recognize clinical problems that can increase the estrogen level. Men can have an increased estrogen level caused by adrenal or testicular tumors.

- Assess for signs and symptoms of estrogen excess in men, (i.e., enlarged breasts, voice change).
- Be supportive to clients, female and male, having excessive estrogen levels. Encourage them to express their concerns.

Estrogens (total) (urine—24 hours)

Reference Values

Adult: *Female:* Preovulation: 5–25 µg/24 hours. Follicular phase: 24–100 µg/24 hours. Luteal phase: 22–80 µg/24 hours. Postmenopause: 0–10 µg/24 hours. *Male:* 4–25 µg/24 hours.

Child: <12 years: 1 µg/24 hours. *Postpuberty:* Same as adult.

Description

Estrogens, hormones composed of estrone, estradiol, and estriol, are produced by the ovary, by the adrenal gland, and in pregnancy by the placenta. *(Also see Estriol.)* This 24-hour urine test is useful for diagnosing ovarian disorders and for the analysis of tumor tissue in breast cancer. To evaluate ovarian dysfunction, the age of the client and the phase of the menstrual cycle should be known.

Purpose

See Estrogen (Serum).

Clinical Problems

Decreased Level: Ovarian dysfunction, ovarian agenesis, infantilism, pregnancy (intrauterine death), menopausal and postmenopausal symptoms. *Drug Influence:* Phenothiazines (in some cases), tetracyclines (in some cases), vitamins.

Elevated Level: Adrenocortical tumor, adrenocortical hyperplasia, ovarian tumor, some testicular tumors, pregnancy (gradual increase from the first trimester on). *Drug Influence:* Phenothiazines, tetracyclines, vitamins (in some cases).

Procedure

- Collect a 24-hour urine sample in a refrigerated container. A preservative is usually added.
- There is no food or fluid restriction.
- Label the urine bottle with the client's name, the date, and the exact time of collection (e.g., 5/24/04 7:02 AM to 5/25/04 7:01 AM). Toilet paper or feces should not be in the urine.

■ Record the client's age and phase of the menstrual cycle on the laboratory slip.

Factors Affecting Laboratory Results

■ Certain drugs may cause a decrease or an increase in the estrogen level *(see Drug Influence above)*.
■ Saving only part of the 24-hour urine sample may cause an inaccurate result.

NURSING IMPLICATIONS WITH RATIONALE

■ Check to see that a preservative is in the urine container. If not, notify the laboratory.
■ Inform the client and family that all urine should be saved and placed in the refrigerated container. Toilet paper and feces should not be in the urine.

Decreased Level

■ Obtain a history of menstrual problems and the present menstrual cycle (e.g., 14 days since the last menstrual period). The phase of the menstrual cycle has an influence on the result of the test.

Client Teaching

■ Instruct the client to keep accurate monthly records on the time of menstruation, how long each menstrual period lasts, and the amount of menstrual flow.

Estrone (E_1) (serum and urine)

Reference Values

SERUM	URINE
Adult:	
Female:	Female:
Follicular phase: 30–100 pg/ml	Follicular phase: 4–7 µg/24 hr
Ovulatory phase: >150 pg/ml	Ovulation: 11–30 µg/24 hr
Luteal phase: 90–160 pg/ml	Luteal phase: 10–22 µg/24 hr
Postmenopausal: 20–40 pg/ml	Postmenopausal: 1–7 µg/24 hr
Male: 10–50 pg/ml	
Child (1–10 years old): <10 pg/ml	

Description

Estrone (E$_1$) is a potent estrogen; however, estrone and estriol (E$_3$) are not as potent as estradiol (E$_2$). Estrone is a metabolite of estradiol. During the third trimester of pregnancy, the estrone levels can increase up to 10-fold the level for a nonpregnant female. Estrone is the major estrogen present after menopause. The serum estrone test is frequently ordered with other estrogen tests.

Purposes

- To determine ovarian failure.
- To check occurrence of menopause.
- To compare test results with other laboratory estrogen tests.

Clinical Problems

Decreased Level: Ovarian failure or dysfunction, intrauterine death in pregnancy, menopausal and postmenopausal symptoms. *Drug Influence:* Digoxin, estrogens.

Procedure

- Note on the laboratory slip the phase of the client's menstrual cycle.

Serum

- Collect 7 to 10 ml of venous blood in a red-top tube.
- There is no food or fluid restriction.

Urine

- Collect a 24-hour urine sample in a collection container that contains a boric acid preservative. Before the urine collection begins, the client should urinate and discard that urine.
- Label the urine bottle with the client's name, date, and exact time of collection (e.g., 3/14/04 to 3/15/04, 7 AM). Toilet paper and feces should not be in the urine.

Factors Affecting Laboratory Results

- Feces and toilet paper in the urine collection container will contaminate the specimen.

NURSING IMPLICATIONS WITH RATIONALE

- Obtain a history of signs and symptoms related to the clinical problem.
- Report laboratory value(s) of estrone and other estrogen factors to the health care provider. Compare the serum estrone and/or urine estrone results with the serum total estrogen results.
- Be supportive to the client and family. Refer the client's and family's questions to appropriate health professionals.

Client Teaching
- Instruct the client and/or family to save all urine and place in the container, and to avoid putting toilet paper and feces in the urine specimens and collecting container.

Euglobulin lysis time (plasma)

Reference Values

No lysis in 1 to $1^{1}/_{2}$ hours; normal lysis: 1.5 to 3 hours.

Description

This test measures fibrinogen activity by measuring the interval between clot formation and euglobulin precipitation. Euglobulin is an acid-insoluble fraction of plasma. The time for which the clot is dissolved (lysis) is recorded. If a clot lysis is less than 1 hour, pathologic fibrinolysis is occurring.

Purpose

- To detect abnormal fibrinolysis.

Clinical Problems

Shortened Lysis Time: Disseminated intravascular coagulation (DIC), pathologic fibrinolysis, hemorrhage, cirrhosis, septic abortion, incompatible blood transfusions. *Drug Influence:* Clofibrate, epinephrine, streptokinase, urokinase, tissue plasminogen activator.

Procedure

- There is no food or fluid restriction.
- Do not massage the vein to be used for blood sample.
- Collect 4.5 ml of venous blood in a blue-top tube. Mix thoroughly with the anticoagulant in the tube. A control tube may be requested.
- Pack the blood sample in ice and send it to the laboratory immediately. Blood should be centrifuged within 30 minutes.

Factors Affecting Laboratory Results

- Tourniquet that has been applied over a prolonged time.
- Excess pumping of the fist will shorten lysis time.
- Hemolysis of the blood sample.

- Failure to deliver the blood sample immediately to the laboratory.

NURSING IMPLICATIONS WITH RATIONALE

- Obtain a history of possible abnormal bleeding.
- Notify the laboratory when blood will be drawn so it can be tested immediately.
- Check for bleeding or hematoma at the venipuncture site.
- Be available to answer the client's and/or family's questions. Allow the client time to express his or her concerns.

Client Teaching

- Instruct the client to avoid strenuous physical activity 1 hour before the blood is drawn.

Factor assay (plasma)

Factors I through XIII, Coagulation Factors, Blood Clotting Factors

Reference Values

Factor I (Fibrinogen): 200–400 mg/dl, minimal for clotting 75–100 mg/dl.

Factor II (Prothrombin): Minimal hemostatic level: 10–15% concentration.

Factor III (Thromboplastin): Variety of substances.

Factor IV (Calcium): 4.5–5.5 mEq/l or 9–11 mg/dl.

Factor V (Proaccelerin): 50–150% activity; minimal hemostatic level: 5–10% concentration.

Factor VI: Not used.

Factor VII (Proconvertin stable factor): 65–135% activity; minimal hemostatic level concentration.

Factor VIII (Antihemophilic factor [AHF], VIII-A): 55–145% activity; minimal hemostatic level: 30–35% concentration.

Factor IX (Christmas factor, IX-B): 60–140% activity; minimal hemostatic level: 30% concentration.

Factor X (Stuart factor): 45–150% activity; minimal hemostatic level: 7–10% concentration.

Factor XI (Plasma thromboplastin antecedent [PTA] XI-C): 65–135% activity; minimal hemostatic level: 20–30% concentration.

Factor XII (Hageman factor): Minimal hemostatic level: 0% concentration.

Factor XIII (Fibrin stabilizing factor [FSF]: Minimal hemostatic level: 1% concentration.

Description

Factor assays are ordered for identification of defects in the blood coagulation mechanism because of a lack of one or more of the 12 plasma factors (excluding factor VI). These 12 factors are important for clot formation, and these have been numbered according to the sequence of their discovery. To standardize clotting factors, the International Committee on Nomenclature of Blood Clotting Factors was established in 1954, and 12 clotting (coagulation) factors were given Roman numerals, named, and described.

Purpose

- To identify the blood factor that is causing the bleeding or blood disorder.

FUNCTIONS OF COAGULATION FACTORS

Factor	Name	Source, Function
I	Fibrinogen	Manufactured by the liver; essential plasma protein; split by thrombin to produce fibrin strands necessary for clot formation.
II	Prothrombin	Produced in the liver and requires vitamin K for its synthesis. Prothrombin is converted to thrombin by the action of extrinsic and intrinsic thromboplastin.
III	Thromboplastin	Thromboplastic activity is found in most tissues; this factor converts prothrombin to thrombin.
IV	Calcium	Absorbed in the gastrointestinal tract from food. Inorganic ion is required in all stages of coagulation—thromboplastin generation, enzymatic conversion of prothrombin to thrombin, and stabilization of the fibrin clot.
V	Proaccelerin (labile factor)	Formed by the liver; for acceleration of thromboplastin generation; prompt conversion of prothrombin to thrombin; deteriorates rapidly in plasma at room temperature.
VI		Not used.
VII	Proconvertin (stable factor)	Manufactured in the liver and requires vitamin K for its synthesis; not destroyed or consumed in the clotting process; stable in heat; accelerates the conversion of prothrombin to thrombin. Use of anticoagulants depresses factor VII in the plasma.
VIII	Antihemophilic factor (A)	Produced by the reticuloendothelial cells; unstable at room temperatures; required for the generation of thromboplastin; essential for the conversion of the prothrombin to thrombin; sex linked.

FUNCTIONS OF COAGULATION FACTORS

Factor	Name	Source, Function
IX	Plasma thrombo-plastin compo-nent (PTC) (Christmas factor, antihemophilic factor B)	Manufactured in the liver and requires vitamin K for its synthesis; stable in plasma and serum; not destroyed or consumed in the clotting process; essential for generating thromboplastin; sex linked.
X	Stuart factor	Manufactured in the liver and requires vitamin K for its synthesis; stable in plasma and serum; not consumed in the clotting process; helps produce the thromboplastin-generating system.
XI	Plasma thrombo-plastin antece-dent (PTA) (anti-hemophilic C)	Synthesis unknown; present in serum and plasma; consumed during the clotting process; essential for plasma-thromboplastin formation.
XII	Hageman factor	Synthesis unknown; activated in contact with glass and following injury; activated factor XII stimu-lates factor XI to continue the clotting process; converts plasminogen to plasmin in fibrinolysis.
XIII	Fibrinase (fibrin sta-bilizing factor [FSF])	Synthesis unknown; enzyme (fibrinase) present in blood, tissue, and platelets and helps to stabilize fibrin strands to form a firm clot.

Clinical Problems

A deficiency in one or more factors usually causes bleeding disorders. The associated clinical problems and the causes of these problems are outlined in the following table.

COAGULATION FACTOR DEFICIENCIES

Factor	Clinical Problems (Decreased Levels)	Rationale
I	Hypofibrinogenemia Leukemia Severe liver disease Disseminated intravascular coagulation (DIC)	Deficiency of fibrinogen and fibrinolysis
II	Hypoprothrombinemia Severe liver disease Vitamin K deficiency Drugs: salicylates (excessive), anticoagulants, antibiotics (excessive), hepatotoxic drugs	Impaired liver function, Vitamin K deficit
III	Thrombocytopenia	Low platelet count
IV	Hypocalcemia	Low calcium intake in diet
	Malabsorption syndrome Malnutrition Hyperphosphatemia Multiple transfusions containing citrate	

(continued)

COAGULATION FACTOR DEFICIENCIES

Factor	Clinical Problems (Decreased Levels)	Rationale
V	Parahemophilia (congenital) Severe liver disease DIC	Congenital problem, impaired liver function
VII	Hepatitis Hepatic carcinoma Hemorrhagic disease of newborn Vitamin K deficiency Drugs: antibiotics (excessive), anticoagulants	Impaired liver function, certain drugs affecting the clotting time, Vitamin K deficit
VIII	Hemophilia A von Willebrand's disease Disseminated intravascular coagulation (DIC) Multiple myeloma Lupus erythematosus	Congenital disorder (sex linked) occurring mostly in males; circulating factor VIII inhibitors
IX	Hemophilia B (Christmas disease) Hepatic disease Vitamin K deficiency	Congenital disorder (sex linked) occurring mostly in males; circulating factor IX inhibitors
X	Severe liver disease Hemorrhage disease of newborns DIC Vitamin K deficiency Drugs: anticoagulants	Impaired liver function; Vitamin K deficit
XI	Hemophilia C Congenital heart disease Intestinal malabsorption of vitamin K Liver disease Drugs: anticoagulants	Congenital deficiency in both males and females; circulating factor XI inhibitors
XII	Liver disease	
XIII	Agammaglobulinemia Myeloma Lead poisoning Poor wound healing	Circulating factor XIII inhibitors; mild bleeding tendency

Procedure

- Collect 5 to 7 ml of venous blood in a blue-top tube (tube tops used may differ among laboratories).
- Mix the blood with an anticoagulant solution thoroughly, and avoid air bubbles.
- The tubes should be delivered to the laboratory immediately.
- There is no food or fluid restriction.

Factors Affecting Laboratory Results

- Clotted blood cannot be used for this laboratory test.
- The factor assay results (factors I, V, and VIII) could be affected if the blood samples do not receive immediate attention in the laboratory.

NURSING IMPLICATIONS WITH RATIONALE

- Obtain a familial history of bleeding disorders and a history of the client's bleeding tendency.
- Observe the venipuncture site for seeping of blood. Apply pressure to the site.
- Observe for signs of bleeding (i.e., purpura, petechiae, or frank, continuous bleeding). Report your observations, and record them on the client's chart.

Fasting blood sugar (FBS)

See Glucose—Fasting Blood Sugar

Febrile agglutinins (serum)

Reference Values

Adult (febrile, titers): *Brucella:* <1:20, <1:20–1:80 (individuals working with animals. *Tularemia:* <1:40. *Widal (Salmonella):* <1:40 (nonvaccinated). *Weil-Felix (Proteus):* <1:40.

Child: Same as adult.

Description

Febrile agglutination tests (febrile group) identify infectious diseases causing fever of unknown origin. Isolating the invading organism (pathogen) is not always possible, especially if the client has been on antimicrobial therapy, so indirect methods are used to detect antibacterial antibodies in the serum. Detection of these antibodies is determined by the titer of the serum in highest dilution that will cause agglutination (clumping) in the presence of a specific antigen. The test should be done during the acute phase of the disease (maybe several times) and then done about 2 weeks later. A single agglutination titer is of minimal value. These tests can be used to confirm pathogens already isolated or to identify the pathogen present late in the disease (after several weeks).

Diseases commonly associated with febrile agglutination tests are brucellosis (undulant fever), salmonellosis, typhoid fever, paratyphoid fever, tularemia, and certain rickettsial infections (typhus fever).

Purpose

■ To detect elevated titer caused by febrile agglutinins denoting a specific pathogen.

Clinical Problems

Test	Pathogen(s) Antigen(s)	Elevated Levels
Brucella	*Brucella abortus* (cattle) *B. suis* (hogs) *B. melitensis* (goats)	Brucellosis titer >1:160
Pasteurella (tularemia)	*Pasteurella tularensis*	Tularemia (rabbit fever) titer >1:80
Widal	*Salmonella* O (somatic)	Salmonellosis
	Salmonella H (flagellar)	Typhoid fever
	O and H portions of the organism act as antigens to stimulate antibody production	Paratyphoid fever titer: O antigen— >1:80 suspicious, >1:160 definite; H antigen—>1:40 suspicious, >1:80 definite
	Salmonella vi (capular)	Nonvaccinated or vaccinated over 1 year before
Weil-Felix	*Proteus* X	Rickettsial diseases
	Proteus OX19	Epidemic typhus
		Tickborne typhus (Rocky Mountain spotted fever)
	Proteus OX2	Boutonneuse tick fever
		Queensland tick fever
		Siberian tick fever
	Proteus OXK	Scrub typhus titer—>1:80 significant, >1:60 definite

Procedure

■ Collect 5 to 7 ml of venous blood in a red-top tube. Avoid hemolysis.
■ Draw blood before starting antimicrobial therapy, if possible. If the client is receiving drugs for an elevated temperature, write the names of the drugs on the laboratory slip.
■ There is no food or fluid restriction.
■ The blood sample should be refrigerated if it is not tested immediately or frozen if it is to be kept 24 hours or longer.

Factors Affecting Laboratory Results

■ Vaccination could increase the titer level.
■ Antimicrobial therapy could decrease the titer level.
■ Leukemia, advanced carcinoma, some congenital deficiencies, and general debilitation could cause false-negative results.

NURSING IMPLICATIONS WITH RATIONALE

- Obtain a history of the client's occupation, geographic location prior to the fever, and recent vaccinations. Exposure to animals and ticks could be suggestive of the causative organism.
- Record on the laboratory slip and in the client's chart whether the client has been vaccinated against the pathogen within the last year. Vaccinations can increase the antibody titer.
- Monitor the temperature every 4 hours, when elevated.
- Remind the health care provider (HCP) of the need to repeat the tests when the fever persists and/or when the titer levels are suspicious. Titer levels could rise fourfold in 1 to 2 weeks.
- Check to determine whether the blood sample has been taken before you give antibiotics or other drug agents to combat fever and the suspected organism. Antibiotic therapy could depress the titer level.

Client Teaching

- Instruct the client to keep a record of temperatures and to notify the HCP of changes in body temperature.

Ferritin (serum)

Reference Values

Adult: *Female:* 10–235 ng/ml, 10–235 µg/l (SI units). *Male:* 15–445 ng/ml, 15–445 µg/l (SI units). *Postmenopausal:* 10–310 ng/ml.

Child: *1–16 years:* 8–140 ng/ml. *Infant:* 2–12 months: 30–200 ng/ml; 1 month: 200–550 ng/ml.

Newborn: 20–200 ng/ml.

Description

Ferritin, an iron-storage protein, is produced in the liver, spleen, and bone marrow. The ferritin levels are related to the amount of iron stored in the body tissues. It will release iron from tissue reserve as needed and will store excess iron to prevent damage effects from iron overload. One nanogram per milliliter of serum ferritin corresponds to 8 mg of stored iron.

Serum ferritin level is useful in evaluating the total body storage of iron. It can detect early iron deficiency anemia and anemias due to chronic disease that resemble iron deficiency. Serum ferritin is not affected by hemolysis and drugs.

Purposes

- To evaluate the amount of iron stored in the body.
- To detect early iron deficiency anemia.

Clinical Problems

Decreased Level: Iron deficiency, pregnancy, inflamed bowel disease, gastric surgery.

Elevated Level: Metastatic carcinomas, leukemias, lymphomas, hepatic diseases (cirrhosis, hepatitis, cancer of the liver), iron overload (hemochromatosis), hemosiderosis, anemias (hemolytic, pernicious, thalassemia), acute and chronic infection and inflammation (renal disease, neuroblastoma), tissue damage. *Drug Influence:* Oral or injectable iron drugs.

Procedure

- Collect 3 to 5 ml of venous blood in a red-top tube.
- There is no food or fluid restriction.
- List on the laboratory slip if the client is taking iron preparations.

Factors Affecting Laboratory Results

- None known.

NURSING IMPLICATIONS WITH RATIONALE

- Compare serum ferritin level with serum iron and transferrin percent saturation. Serum ferritin levels tend to be more reliable in determining iron deficiencies than serum iron levels. Serum ferritin levels decrease before iron stores are depleted.

Fetal hemoglobin (Hb F) (blood)

Hemoglobin F

Reference Values

From Total Hemoglobin:

Adult: 0–2%.

Child: *Newborn:* 60–90%; *1–5 mo:* <70%; *6–12 mo:* <5%; *>1yr:* <2%.

Description

For newborns, an elevated Hb F is normally found in the red blood cells (RBCs). By the time the infant is 6 months old, the Hb F should be less than 5%, and the remaining hemoglobin should be comprised of Hb A_1 and Hb A_2. If the Hb F remains elevated after 6 months, hemoglobinopathy should be considered such as minor or major thalassemias.

Purpose

- To diagnose various hemoglobinopathies such as minor or major thalassemia.

Clinical Problems

Elevated Level: Thalassemias (minor or major), sickle cell anemia, acquired aplastic anemia (from drugs, toxins, etc.), hyperthyroidism, acute or chronic leukemia especially juvenile myeloid leukemia, multiple myeloma, hemoglobin H disease, hereditary presence of Hb F.

Procedure

- Collect 7 to 10 ml of venous blood in a lavender- or green-top tube. Fill the tube. Invert the tube gently. Avoid hemolysis (do NOT shake tube).
- Collect capillary blood from a young child in a microcollection tube.
- There is no food or fluid restriction.

Factors Affecting Laboratory Results

- Hemolysis of the blood sample
- Blood specimen that is older than 3 hours may cause a false positive result.

NURSING IMPLICATIONS WITH RATIONALE

Client Teaching

- Explain the test procedure to the client or parent. Blood specimen can be taken from a finger or earlobe.
- Listen to client's concerns. Refer questions to which the answers are unknown to other health care professionals.

Fibrin degradation products (FDP) (serum)

Fibrin or Fibrinogen Split Products (FSP)

Reference Values

Adult: 2–10 µg/ml.

Child: Not usually done.

Description

The fibrin degradation products (FDP) test is usually done in an emergency when the client is hemorrhaging as the result of severe injury, trauma, and/or shock. Thrombin, which initially accelerates coagulation, promotes the conversion of plasminogen into plasmin, which, in turn, breaks fibrinogen and fibrin into FDP. The fibrin degradation (split) products act as anticoagulants, causing continuous bleeding from many sites. A clinical condition resulting from this fibrinolytic (clot-dissolving) activity is disseminated intravascular coagulation (DIC).

Purpose

■ To aid in the diagnosis of disseminated intravascular coagulation (DIC).

Clinical Problems

Decreased Level: Cerebral thrombosis.

Elevated Level: DIC caused by severe injury, trauma, or shock; massive tissue damage; surgical complications; septicemia; obstetric complications (abruptio placentae, preeclampsia, intrauterine death, postcesarean birth), acute myocardial infarction, pulmonary embolism, acute necrosis of the liver, acute renal failure, burns, acute leukemia. *Drug Influence:* Streptokinase, urokinase.

Procedure

■ Collect 5 to 7 ml of venous blood in a blue-top tube. Avoid hemolysis.
■ Draw blood before administering heparin.
■ There is no food or fluid restriction.

Factors Affecting Laboratory Results

■ Hemolysis of the blood sample cause inaccurate test results.

NURSING IMPLICATIONS WITH RATIONALE

Elevated Level

- Monitor vital signs, and report shocklike symptoms, such as tachycardia, hypotension, pallor, and cold, clammy skin.
- Observe and report bleeding sites from the chest, the nasogastric tube, incisional or injured areas, and others.
- Report progressive discoloration of the skin (petechial, ecchymoses).
- Monitor infusion rates of IV fluids—crystalloids, colloids, and blood.
- Check urine output hourly. Report decreased urine output (<25 ml/h) and blood-colored urine.
- Provide comfort and support to the client and family.

Fibrinogen (plasma)

Factor I

Reference Values

Adult: 200–400 mg/dL.

Child: *Newborn*: 150–300 mg/dl. *Child*: Same as adult.

Description

Fibrinogen, a plasma protein synthesized by the liver, is split by thrombin to produce fibrin strands necessary for clot formation. A deficiency of fibrinogen results in bleeding. Low fibrinogen levels may be due to *disseminated intravascular coagulation* (DIC), which usually results from severe trauma or obstetric complications. Markedly prolonged prothrombin time (PT), an activated partial thromboplastin time (APTT), and a low platelet count suggest a fibrinogen deficiency and signs of DIC. Fibrin degradation products (FDPs) are usually measured to confirm DIC.

Purposes

- To check for a deficiency of fibrinogen as a cause of bleeding.
- To compare test results with FDPs in diagnosing DIC.

Clinical Problems

Decreased Level: Severe liver disease, hypofibrinogenemia, DIC, leukemia, obstetric complications.

Elevated Level: Acute infections, collagen diseases, inflammatory disease, hepatitis. *Drug Influence:* Oral contraceptives, heparin.

Procedure

- Collect 5 to 7 ml of venous blood in a blue-top tube. Mix blood well with the anticoagulant in the tube (invert tube several times). Avoid hemolysis by not shaking the tube.
- There is no food or fluid restriction.

Factors Affecting Laboratory Results

- Postoperative surgery and third trimester of pregnancy could cause a false-positive fibrinogen elevation.
- Hemolysis of the blood sample can cause inaccurate results.
- Oral contraceptives and heparin can elevate test results.

NURSING IMPLICATIONS WITH RATIONALE

- Report if client had a blood transfusion within 4 weeks.
- Check laboratory results of PT, APTT, and platelet count. If an FDP level is ordered, check the laboratory result, since it confirms DIC.
- Monitor for signs and symptoms of DIC (petechiae and ecchymoses, hemorrhage, tachycardia, hypotension).
- Notify the health care provider if active bleeding occurs.

Client Teaching

- Instruct the client to inform the health care provider of any current, acute infection or illness that might be contributing to the bleeding.

Fluorescent treponemal antibody absorption (FTA-ABS) (serum)

Reference Values

Adult: Nonreactive (negative).

Child: Nonreactive (negative).

Description

The fluorescent treponemal antibody absorption (FTA-ABS) test uses the treponemal organism to produce and detect these antibodies. This test is most sensitive, specific, and reliable for diagnosing all stages of syphilis. It is more sensitive than the venereal disease research laboratory (VDRL) and rapid plasma reagin (RPR) tests. The FTA-ABS test is useful for confirming or ruling out suspected false-positive serology tests for syphilis. The limitations of this test are that the stage and activity of the disease cannot be identified, the effectiveness of the therapy cannot be measured, and the test for syphilis remains positive even after treatment for a very long time or could remain positive forever.

Purpose

- To aid in the diagnosis of syphilis.

Clinical Problems

Reactive: *Positive:* Primary and secondary syphilis. *False-Positives (rare):* Lupus erythematosus, pregnancy, acute genital herpes.

Procedure

- Collect 3 to 5 ml of venous blood in a red-top tube. Avoid hemolysis.
- There is no food or fluid restriction.
- A borderline FTA-ABS test should be repeated.

Factors Affecting Laboratory Results

- Medical treatment does not eliminate the treponemal antibodies. The test results may remain positive after treatment.

NURSING IMPLICATIONS WITH RATIONALE

- Be supportive of the client and family. Keep conversation and information confidential except for what is required by law.
- Encourage the client to have his or her sexual partner seek medical care if the test is positive.
- Check the results of other serology tests for syphilis. A positive VDRL could be false-positive because of acute or chronic illness. The FTA-ABS test is reliable for syphilis, giving accurate results; however, many laboratories have to send the blood sample out for testing. Ask the client if he or she has received treatment for syphilis. Positive FTA-ABS results can occur after treatment (penicillin, erythromycin) for months or several years or for the rest of the client's life.
- Assess for signs and symptoms of syphilis. The primary stage begins with a small papule filled with liquid, which ruptures, enlarges, and becomes a chancre. With secondary syphilis, a generalized rash (macular and papular) develops and is found mainly on the arms, palms, soles of the feet, and face.

Folic acid (folate) (serum)

Reference Values

Adult: 3–16 ng/ml (bioassay), >2.5 ng/ml (radioimmunoassay [RIA]; serum), 200–700 ng/ml (red blood cells, RBCs).

Child: Same as adult.

Description

Folic acid, one of the B vitamins, is needed for normal red and white blood cell function. Folic acid is present in a variety of foods: milk, eggs, leafy vegetables, beans, liver, fruits (oranges, bananas), and whole wheat bread. Dietary deficiency is the most common cause of a serum folic acid deficit, especially in children, older adults, and persons with chronic alcoholism. With a decreased folic acid intake, it takes approximately 3 to 4 weeks for folic acid deficiency to develop and 18 to 24 weeks before folic acid anemia will occur.

Usually the serum folic acid or folate test is performed to detect folic acid anemia, which is a megaloblastic anemia (abnormally large RBCs). Other causes of serum folic acid deficit are pregnancy (because of dietary deficiency and because the fetal requirement for folic acid is so great), alcoholism, and the aged.

Purposes

- To check for folic acid deficiency during early pregnancy.
- To detect folic acid anemia.

Clinical Problems

Decreased Level: Folic acid anemia (megaloblastic anemia): Vitamin B_6 deficiency anemia; malnutrition; malabsorption syndrome (small intestine); pregnancy; malignancies; liver diseases; celiac sprue disease. *Drug Influence:* Anticonvulsants—phenytoin (Dilantin), primidone (Mysoline); antineoplastic agents—methotrexate (folic acid antagonists); antimalaria agents; oral contraceptives.

Elevated Level: Pernicious anemia.

Procedure

- Collect 7 to 10 ml of venous blood in a red-top tube. Avoid hemolysis. Send blood to the laboratory immediately.
- If an RBC folate determination is requested, collect 7 ml of venous blood in a lavender-top tube. Send this to the laboratory immediately. Ascorbic acid will be added in the laboratory.
- There is no food or fluid restriction. Avoid alcohol.

Factors Affecting Laboratory Results

- Drugs *(see Clinical Problems)*.
- Alcohol—persons who consume large quantities of alcohol usually have poor nutritional intake (folic acid deficiency).

NURSING IMPLICATIONS WITH RATIONALE

- Obtain a dietary history. Collaborate with the dietitian on formulating a diet high in folic acid, and have the dietitian plan the diet with the client.
- Observe for signs and symptoms of folic acid deficiency, such as fatigue, pallor, nausea, anorexia, dyspnea, palpitations, and tachycardia.

Client Teaching

- Encourage the client to eat foods rich in folic acid, such as liver, lean meats, milk, eggs, leafy vegetables, bananas, oranges, beans, and whole-wheat bread.

Follicle-stimulating hormone (FSH) (serum and urine)

Reference Values

Serum: *Adult:* Female: Follicular phase: 4–30 mU/ml. Midcycle: 10–90 mU/ml. Luteal phase: 4–30 mU/ml. Menopause: 40–170 mU/ml. Male: 4–25 mU/ml. *Child (Prepubertal):* 5–12 mU/ml.

Urine: *Adult:* Female: Follicular phase: 2–15 IU/24 h. Midcycle: 8–60 IU/24 h. Luteal phase: 4–20 IU/24 h. Menopause: 50–150 IU/24 h. Male: 4–18 IU/24 h. *Child (Prepubertal):* <10 IU/ml.

Description

Follicle-stimulating hormone (FSH), a gonadotropic hormone produced and controlled by the pituitary gland, stimulates the growth and maturation of the ovarian follicle to produce estrogen in females and to promote spermatogenesis in males. Infertility disorders can be determined by a serum and urine FSH test. Increased and decreased FSH levels can indicate gonad failure due to pituitary dysfunction.

Purposes

- To check for a FSH-producing pituitary tumor.
- To compare serum and urine FSH levels for determining the cause of infertility.

Clinical Problems

Decreased Level: Neoplasms of the ovaries, testes, adrenals; polycystic ovarian disease; hypopituitarism; anorexia nervosa. *Drug Influence:* Estrogens, oral contraceptives, testosterone.

Elevated Level: Gonadal failure such as menopause, precocious puberty, FSH-producing pituitary tumor, Turner's syndrome, Klinefelter's syndrome, orchiectomy, hysterectomy, primary testicular failure.

Procedure

- No food or fluid restriction is required.
- State phase of menstrual cycle or if menopausal on the laboratory slip.
- Note on the laboratory slip if the client is taking oral contraceptives or any type of hormones.

Serum

- Collect 5 to 7 ml of venous blood in a red-top tube. Avoid hemolysis.
- Rest 30 minutes to 1 hour before blood is drawn.

Urine

- Collect a 24-hour urine specimen in a large container with a preservative. The pH of the 24-hour urine specimen should be maintained between 5 and 6.5 (glacial acetic acid or boric acid may be added).
- Avoid feces and toilet paper in the urine.

Factors Affecting Laboratory Results

- Alkaline urine can give an inaccurate test result.

NURSING IMPLICATIONS WITH RATIONALE

- Associate a decreased or increased urine FSH level with clinical problems. The excess production of estrogen with most ovarian tumors will decrease the production of FSH. After menopause, more FSH will be secreted to stimulate estrogen production.

Urine

- Label container with the client's name, the dates, and the exact times of urine collection (e.g., 5/10/04, 8 AM to 5/11/04, 8:01 AM).

Client Teaching

- Answer client questions concerning the test. Be supportive of the client and family.
- Inform the client to rest prior to a serum test, because exercise can increase FSH release.

Fungal organisms: fungal disease, mycotic infections (smear, serum, culture—sputum, bronchial, lesion)

Actinomyces, Histoplasma, Blastomyces, Coccidioides, Cryptococcus, Candida, Aspergillus

Reference Values

Adult: Negative, serum: <1:8.

Child: Same as adult.

Description

There are more than 45,000 species of fungi, but only 0.01%, or 45, are considered pathogenic to humans. Fungal infections are more common today and can be classified as (1) superficial and cutaneous mycoses (tinea pedis [athlete's foot], tinea capitis [ringworm of the scalp], tinea barbae [ringworm of the beard], and tinea cruris [jock itch]), (2) subcutaneous mycoses, and (3) systemic mycoses (histoplasmosis, actinomycosis, and blastomycosis).

Most fungus organisms live in the soil and can be transmitted to humans and animals by way of the lungs or a break in the skin. The persons most susceptible to fungal infections are those with debilitating or chronic diseases (e.g., diabetes) or who are receiving drug therapy, such as steroids, prolonged antibiotics, antineoplastic agents, and oral contraceptives.

Purpose

■ To assist in the diagnosis of selected fungal organisms.

Clinical Problems

Organism	Disease Entity	Comments
Actinomyces israelii	Actinomycosis	A gram-positive, non–acid-fast, anaerobic organism that can produce an abscess.
Histoplasma capsulatum	Histoplasmosis	The most common systemic fungal infection. It is commonly found in the eastern part of the United States and in the Mississippi and Ohio valleys. Usually the organism is carried by birds (e.g., starlings and chickens). In most clients histoplasmosis is a localized pulmonary disease and resembles pulmonary tuberculosis.

(continued)

Organism	Disease Entity	Comments
Blastomyces dermatitidis	Blastomycosis	It causes granulomatous lesions that involve the skin or visceral organs. Histologically it is similar to tuberculosis.
Coccidioides immitis	Coccidioidomycosis	It is commonly found in the Southwest and in the San Joaquin Valley of California. Usually the client has respiratory symptoms and fever of unknown origin. If the infection is overwhelming, it resembles military tuberculosis.
Cryptococcus neoformans	Cryptococcosis Meningitis	Fungal disease usually begins as a pulmonary infection but disseminates to the central nervous system (brain). The organism is usually carried by pigeons. Clients with decreased immunologic resistance (such as those with acute leukemia or Hodgkin's disease or who are receiving steroids or immunosuppressive agents) are susceptible to the disease.
Candida albicans, fungemia	Candidiasis (Moniliasis) Thrush	Clients with debilitating diseases or who are taking steroids, antineoplastic agents, or oral contraceptives are susceptible to this fungus.
Aspergillus fumigatus	Aspergillosis	Aspergillus organisms can cause severe respiratory infection. Fungus balls (aspergilloma) develop in the lung tissue. The sputum is golden brown and contains *Aspergillus hyphae*.

Procedure

Serum

- Collect 5 to 7 ml of venous blood in a red-top tube.
- No food or fluid restriction is required. Suggest NPO for 12 hours. Check with your laboratory.
- Obtain serum antibody test 2 to 4 weeks after exposure to organism.

Culture

- Follow directions from the special laboratory on collection of the specimen.

Organism	Tests
Actinomyces israelii	Smear and culture of lesion Biopsy
Histoplasma capsulatum	Sputum culture Histoplasmin skin test Serum test: complement fixation or latex agglutination
Blastomyces dermatitidis	Culture Smear, wet-mount examination of the material from the lesion Biopsy—histologic examination Skin test Serum test: complement fixation

Organism	Tests
Coccidioides immitis	Culture
	Sputum smears
	Skin test
	Serum test: complement fixation (sensitive), latex agglutination (very sensitive)
Cryptococcus neoformans	Culture of cerebrospinal fluid
	Serum test: latex agglutination (sensitive)
Candida albicans	Smear and culture of the skin, mucous membrane, and vagina
Aspergillus fumigatus	Sputum culture
	Skin test
	Serum IgE level and complement fixation

Factors Affecting Laboratory Results

- Contamination of the specimen affects results.

NURSING IMPLICATIONS WITH RATIONALE

- Associate mycotic infections with high-risk clients (i.e., those clients having chronic illnesses [such as diabetes mellitus] or debilitating diseases [such as cancer] or who are receiving prolonged antibiotics, antineoplastic agents [anticancer chemotherapy], steroids, or oral contraceptives).
- Use aseptic technique when collecting a specimen for culture. Preventing the transmission of the organism is most important. Contamination of the specimen can give inaccurate results.
- Obtain a history from the client—where he or she lives and occupation. Fungus organisms (e.g., *Histoplasma, Coccidioides*) are more prevalent in selected parts of the country. Report if the client works with chickens or pigeons.
- Teach the client to wear a mask when exposed to chicken feces. Explain that the *H. capsulatum* spores are in the feces and can be inhaled.
- Monitor the client's temperature. With many of the fungal diseases, the temperature is elevated.
- Report clinical signs and symptoms of respiratory problems (i.e., coughing up sputum, dyspnea, and chest pain).
- Check the color of the sputum. Certain fungi can be identified by the color of their secretions. Golden brown sputum is characteristic of the *Aspergillus* organism.
- Assess the neurologic status when cryptococcosis is suspected. Report headaches and changes in sensorium, pupil size and reaction, and motor function.

Galactose-1-phosphate uridyl transferase (GPT or GPUT) (blood)

Galactokinase (An enzyme that aids in the metabolism of galactose)

Reference Values

Negative: Quantitative test: 18.5–28.5 U/g in hemoglobin (Hb).

Deficiency of the Enzyme: <5 U/g in Hb; Carrier of the deficiency: 5–18 U/g of Hb.

Description

The enzyme, galactose-1-phosphate uridyl transferase (GPT), is needed to convert galactose to glucose during lactose metabolism. It is usually inherited or can be an acquired disorder that can occur during intrauterine development. If inherited, it is an autosomal recessive transmitted disorder. A deficiency of this enzyme can lead to galactosemia (increase in galactose in the blood due to the inability to metabolize galactose). Screening test to detect the enzyme deficiency is performed at birth in some institutions. If the deficiency exists and is not treated soon after birth, this condition can cause mental retardation, failure to thrive, severe liver disorder, and/or irreversible cataracts due to the lack of brain, liver, or eye development.

Purpose

- To detect galactosemia in infants and carriers of the GPT enzyme deficiency.

Clinical Problems

Decreased Enzyme Level: Galactosemia.

Procedure

- Collect 5–7 ml of venous blood in a green- or lavender-top tube. Chill the tube of blood by placing it on ice. Avoid hemolysis.
- Take blood sample from the umbilical cord at birth or from the heel (heelstick). From the heel place 3 drops of blood on a galactosemia screening filter paper.
- There is no food or fluid restriction.

Factors Affecting Laboratory Results

- Hemolysis from rough handling of blood specimen.
- Not chilling or putting the tube on ice.

NURSING IMPLICATIONS WITH RATIONALE

- Ascertain if the parent(s) is/are carriers of galactosemia. If the institution does not check for GPT deficiency at birth, the health care provider should suggest that the test be performed, especially if a client is a carrier.
- Assess the infant for symptoms suggesting GPT enzyme deficiency, such as vomiting, diarrhea, abdominal distention, liver enlargement, central nervous system changes. A positive indication of galactose is elevated blood and urine levels of galactose and galactose-1 phosphate.

Client Teaching

- Instruct the parent who has an infant lacking the enzyme to avoid giving milk to the infant. A galactose- and lactose-free diet, such as soy-bean milk, is suggested. A lactose-free diet avoids galactose toxicity.
- Inform the parent to report vomiting or diarrhea that continues after lactose-free diet.
- Encourage the parents to seek genetic counseling for a positive test.

Gamma-glutamyl transferase (GGT) (serum)

Gamma-Glutamyl Transpeptidase (GGTP, or GTP; γ-Glutamyl Transpeptidase, γGT)

Reference Values 0–45 U/l (overall average).

Adult: *Male:* 4–23 IU/l, 9–69 U/l at 37°C (SI units). *Female:* 3–13 IU/l, 4–33 U/l at 37°C (SI units). Values differ among institutions and method used.

Elderly: Slightly higher than adult.

Child: *Newborn:* 5 times higher than adult. *Premature:* 10 times higher than adult. *Child:* Similar to adult.

Description

The enzyme gamma-glutamyl transferase (GGT) is found primarily in the liver and kidney, with smaller amounts in the spleen, prostate gland, and heart muscle. GGTP is sensitive for detecting a wide variety of hepatic (liver) parenchymal diseases. The serum level will rise early and will remain elevated as long as cellular damage persists.

High levels of GGT occur after 12 to 24 hours of heavy alcoholic drinking and may remain increased for 2 to 3 weeks after alcohol intake stops. Some alcoholic rehabilitation programs are using the GGTP level as a guide to planning care as they work with the alcoholic individuals.

The GGT test is considered more sensitive for liver dysfunction than the alkaline phosphatase (ALP) test.

Purposes

- To detect the presence of a hepatic disorder.
- To monitor the liver enzyme GGT during the liver disorder and treatment.
- To compare with other liver enzymes for identifying liver dysfunction.

Clinical Problems

Elevated Level: Cirrhosis of the liver, acute and subacute necrosis of the liver, alcoholism, acute and chronic hepatitis, cancer (liver, pancreas, prostate, breast, kidney, lung, brain), infectious mononucleosis, hemochromatosis (iron deposits in the liver), diabetes mellitus, hyperlipoproteinemia (type IV), acute myocardial infarction (fourth day), congestive heart failure, acute pancreatitis, acute cholecystitis, epilepsy, nephrotic syndrome. *Drug Influence:* Phenytoin (Dilantin), phenobarbital, aminoglycosides, warfarin (Coumadin).

Procedure

- Collect 3 to 5 ml of venous blood in a red-top tube. Avoid hemolysis.
- There is no food or fluid restriction.

Factors Affecting Laboratory Results

- Phenytoin and barbiturates can cause a false-positive GGT test.
- Excessive and prolonged alcohol intake will elevate the GGT level.

NURSING IMPLICATIONS WITH RATIONALE

Elevated Level

- Compare GGT with ALP, leucine aminopeptidase (LAP), and alanine aminotransferase (SGPT or ALT). The GGT test tends to be more sensitive for detecting liver dysfunction than the others.
- Report to the health care provider if the client is receiving phenytoin or phenobarbital when the test is ordered. Usually these medications cannot be withheld. Note on the laboratory slip the names of the drugs (affecting GGT levels) and the dosages the client is receiving.
- Assess the client's diet.
- Observe for signs and symptoms of liver damage, such as restlessness, jaundice, twitching, flapping tremors, spider angiomas, bleeding tendencies (nose and rectal bleeding), purpura, ascites, and others.

Client Teaching

- Instruct the client to maintain a well-balanced diet (adequate protein and carbohydrate).
- Encourage clients with an alcohol problem to participate in Alcoholics Anonymous or a rehabilitation program.

Gastrin (serum or plasma)

Reference Values

Adult: *Fasting:* <100 pg/ml. *Nonfasting:* 50–200 pg/ml.
Child: Not usually done.

Description

Gastrin is a hormone, secreted from the pyloric mucosa, that stimulates the secretion of gastric juices—mainly hydrochloric acid (HCl). Normally increased gastrin will cause hypersecretion of HCl, which in turn inhibits gastrin secretion.

This test is usually ordered to aid in the diagnosis of pernicious anemia, Zollinger-Ellison syndrome (a condition caused by a noninsulin-producing tumor of the pancreas that secretes excess amounts of gastrin), and stomach cancer.

Purposes

- To aid in the diagnosis of pernicious anemia.
- To aid in the diagnosis of gastric ulcer.
- To differentiate between Zollinger-Ellison syndrome and hypergastrinemia from other causes.

Clinical Problems

Elevated Level: Pernicious anemia, Zollinger-Ellison syndrome, malignant neoplasm of the stomach, peptic ulcer, chronic atrophic gastritis, cirrhosis of the liver, acute and chronic renal failure. *Drug Influence:* IV calcium gluconate.

Procedure

- Collect 5 to 7 ml of venous blood in a red- or lavender-top tube.
- Food and fluids (except water) are restricted for 12 hours before the test.

Factors Affecting Laboratory Results

- IV infusion of calcium elevates the serum gastrin level.

NURSING IMPLICATIONS WITH RATIONALE

- Inform the client that food and beverages are restricted, with the exception of water, for 12 hours before the test. A fasting blood sample is required, but the length of the NPO time may differ among laboratories.

Elevated Level

- Check the client's serum gastrin value; in Zollinger-Ellison syndrome, the serum level can reach 2,800 to 300,000 pg/ml. High levels are present in pernicious anemia and gastritis.
- Observe for signs and symptoms of pernicious anemia (weakness, sore tongue, pallor of the gums and lips, anorexia, loss of weight, and numbness and tingling in the extremities).

Glucagon (plasma)

Reference Values

Adult: 50–200 pg/ml.

Description

Glucagon is secreted by the alpha cells of the pancreas. It functions as a counter-regulatory hormone to insulin in regulating glucose metabolism. It increases blood glucose by converting glycogen to glucose in response to hypoglycemia.

Very high glucagon levels (500 to 1000 pg/ml) occur in glucagonoma, pancreatic alpha cell tumor.

Purpose

- To detect an increase or deficit in serum glucagon that aids in the regulation of glucose metabolism.

Clinical Problems

Decreased Level: Glucose tolerance test during first hour, idiopathic glucagon deficiency, loss of pancreatic tissue.

Elevated Level: Glucagonoma, acute pancreatitis, severe diabetic ketoacidosis, infections, pheochromocytoma.

Procedure

- Collect 5 to 7 ml of venous blood in a lavender-top tube. Avoid hemolysis. Chill the tube and take to laboratory immediately.
- Food and fluids are restricted for 10 to 12 hours prior to the test.
- Withhold drugs such as insulin, cortisone, growth hormones, and epinephrine, with health care provider's permission, until the test is completed.

Factors Affecting Laboratory Results

- Vigorous exercise, undue stress, trauma, and severe hyperglycemia affect test results.
- Administer steroids and insulin after the test.

NURSING IMPLICATIONS WITH RATIONALE

- Compare serum glucose and insulin levels. Glucose and insulin influence plasma glucagon levels.
- Record on the laboratory slip and report if client has taken large doses of steroids in the last 24 hours.
- Observe for signs and symptoms of hyperglycemia.

Client Teaching

- Instruct the client to relax by lying down for 30 minutes to 1 hour prior to the test. Stress and activity could cause false-positive test results.

Glucose—fasting blood sugar (FBS) (blood)

Reference Values

Adult: *Serum and Plasma:* 70–110 mg/dl. *Whole Blood:* 60–100 mg/dl. *Panic Value:* <40 mg/dl and >700 mg/dl.

Child: *Newborn:* 30–80 mg/dl. *Child:* 60–100 mg/dl.

Elderly: 70–120 mg/dl.

Description

Glucose is formed from dietary carbohydrates and is stored as glycogen in the liver and skeletal muscles. Insulin and glucagon, two hormones from the pancreas, affect the blood glucose level. Insulin is needed for cellular membrane permeability to glucose and for transportation of glucose into the cells. Without insulin, glucose cannot enter the cells. Glucagon stimulates glycogenolysis (conversion of stored glycogen to glucose) in the liver.

A decreased blood sugar level (hypoglycemia) results from inadequate food intake or too much insulin. When elevated blood sugar (hyperglycemia) occurs, there is not enough insulin; this condition is known as diabetes mellitus. A fasting blood sugar level >125 mg/dl usually indicates diabetes, and to confirm the diagnosis when the blood sugar is borderline or slightly elevated, a feasting (postprandial) blood sugar and/or a glucose tolerance test may be ordered.

Dextrostix test is a rapid, simple, semiquantitative test for distinguishing hypoglycemia from hyperglycemia. The results are compared to a color chart with values between 40 and 240 mg/dl. This is a useful test in emergency situations. Chemstrip bG is the preferred method for checking blood sugar by finger stick.

Purposes

- To confirm a diagnosis of prediabetic state or diabetic mellitus.
- To monitor blood glucose levels for diabetic clients taking an antidiabetic agent (insulin or oral hypoglycemic drug).

Clinical Problems

Decreased Level: Hypoglycemic reaction (insulin excess); cancer (stomach, liver, lung), adrenal gland hypofunction, malnutrition, alcoholism, cirrhosis of the liver, strenuous exercise, erythroblastosis fetalis (hemolytic disease), hyperinsulinism. *Drug Influence:* Insulin excess.

Elevated Level: Diabetes mellitus, diabetes acidosis, adrenal gland hyperfunction (Cushing's syndrome), acute myocardial infarction, stress, crushed injury, burns, infections, renal failure, hypothermia, exercise, acute pancreatitis, cancer of the pancreas, congestive heart failure, acromegaly, postgastrectomy (dumping) syndrome, extensive surgery. *Drug Influence:* ACTH; cortisone preparations; diuretics (hydrochlorothiazide [Hydrodiuril], furosemide [Lasix], ethacrynic acid [Edecrin]), anesthesia drugs, levodopa.

Procedure

- Collect 3 to 5 ml of venous blood in a gray-top or red-top tube. Blood is drawn between 7 AM and 9 AM.
- NPO except water for 12 hours before the test.
- Give insulin as ordered and after the blood sample is taken.

Factors Affecting Laboratory Results

- Drugs—cortisone, thiazide, and the "loop" diuretics can cause an increase in blood sugar.
- Trauma—stress can cause an increase in blood sugar.
- The Clinitest for determining urine glucose (glycosuria) may be falsely positive if the client is taking excessive amounts of aspirin, vitamin C, and certain antibi-

otics (cephalosporin), because the test is not specific for glucose but for all reducing substances.

- High doses of vitamin C could cause false-negative results when using urine glucose testing tapes (e.g., Testape).

NURSING IMPLICATIONS WITH RATIONALE

- Hold morning insulin and drugs until the blood specimen is taken.
- Record on the laboratory slip if the client has been taking daily cortisone preparations, thiazides, or loop diuretics.

Decreased Level

- Recognize clinical problems associated with a low blood sugar level. Excessive doses of insulin, skipped meals, and inadequate food intake are the common causes of hypoglycemia.
- Observe for signs and symptoms of hypoglycemia (nervousness, weakness, confusion, cold and clammy skin, diaphoresis, and increased pulse rate).

Client Teaching

- Instruct the client to carry lumps of sugar or candy at all times. Most diabetic persons have warnings when hypoglycemia occurs.
- Teach the client to adhere to the American Dietetic Association (ADA) diet, as prescribed. Explain the Exchange Lists for meal planning.
- Encourage the client to contact the American Diabetic Association for literature and information concerning their meeting dates.
- Explain to the client that strenuous exercise can lower the blood sugar. Carbohydrate or protein intake should be increased before exercise or immediately after exercise; the health care provider should be contacted for food instruction.
- Encourage the client to take insulin ½ to 1 hour before breakfast and to eat meals on time.
- Teach clients with a hypoglycemic problem (blood sugar <50 mg/dl) to eat food high in protein and fat and low in carbohydrate. Too much sugar stimulates insulin secretion.

Elevated Level

- Recognize clinical problems associated with high blood sugar levels. Diabetes mellitus, Cushing's syndrome, and stressful situations (trauma, burns, extensive surgery) are the common causes of hyperglycemia.
- Consider drugs (such as cortisone, thiazides, and "loop" diuretics) as the cause of a slightly elevated blood sugar level. If blood sugar becomes too high, notify the health care provider—drug dosages may need to be decreased or insulin may need to be ordered or increased.
- Observe for signs and symptoms of hyperglycemia (excessive thirst [polydipsia], excessive urination [polyuria], excessive hunger [polyphagia], and weight loss). If

the blood sugar is >500 mg/dl, Kussmaul's breathing (rapid, deep, vigorous breathing) caused by acidosis may be observed.

Client Teaching

- Instruct the client to test his or her blood before meals. Demonstrate how to use Chemstrip bG techniques or others.
- Explain to the client that infections can increase the blood sugar level and that medical advice should be sought.

Glucose—postprandial (feasting blood sugar) (blood)

Two-Hour Postprandial Blood Sugar (PPBS)

Reference Values

Adult: *Serum or Plasma:* <140 mg/dl/2 h. **Blood:** <120 mg/dl/2 h.

Elderly: *Serum:* <160 mg/dl/2 h. **Blood:** <140 mg/dl/2 h.

Child: <120 mg/dl/2 h.

Description

A 2-hour PPBS or feasting sugar test is usually done to determine the patient's response to a high carbohydrate intake 2 hours after a meal (breakfast or lunch). This test is a screening test for diabetes, normally ordered if the fasting blood sugar was high normal or slightly elevated. A serum glucose >140 mg/dl or a blood glucose greater than 120 mg/dl is abnormal, and further tests may be needed.

Purposes

See Glucose—Fasting Blood Sugar.

Clinical Problems

Decreased Level: *See Glucose—Fasting Blood Sugar.*

Elevated Level: *See Glucose—Fasting Blood Sugar.*

Procedure

- A high-carbohydrate meal might be requested at breakfast or lunch.

- Collect 3 to 5 ml of venous blood in a gray- or red-top tube 2 hours after the client finishes eating breakfast or lunch. If the nurse does not draw the blood, the laboratory needs to be notified when the client finished breakfast or lunch.
- Food is restricted for 2 hours after breakfast or lunch before the test, but water is not.

Factors Affecting Laboratory Results

- Smoking may increase the serum glucose level.
- *See Glucose—Fasting Blood Sugar.*

NURSING IMPLICATIONS WITH RATIONALE

- Determine the breakfast foods that the client likes and dislikes and notify the dietary department.

Client Teaching

- If the client is not hospitalized, instruct the person to be at the laboratory ½ to 2 hours after breakfast or lunch.

Elevated Level

- *See Glucose—Fasting Blood Sugar.*

Glucose self-monitoring (self-testing) devices

Glucose Finger-Stick, Glucose Capillary Test

Reference Values

Adult: *Blood:* 60–110 mg/dl, 3.3–6.1 μmol/l (SI units).
Child: *Blood:* 50–85 mg/dl, 2.7–4.7 μmol/l (SI units).
Urine: Negative.

Description

To control blood glucose levels, glucose monitoring devices are available for checking blood glucose levels. The glucose monitoring devices can be used in institutions such as hospitals, and the clients with insulin-dependent (IDDM) or Type I and noninsulin dependent diabetes mellitus (NIDDM) or Type II can use it in their homes for managing diabetes mellitus. The test takes about 2 minutes, and test results are considered reliable.

The new generation of meters have greatly improved accuracy and precision over earlier models. They are less dependent on operator skill, and most have eliminated the need for timing, blotting, and wiping the strip. Though the manufacturers may not agree, most of the newer meters still are not as reliable as a laboratory test when the glucose levels are < 50 or 60, or > 450 or 500 mg/dl. It varies with manufacturer.

The use of reagent strips for urine testing, for example, Clinistix, Diastix, Testape, and Clinitest tablets) are less desirable for glucose accuracy than the self-monitoring metered devices. Clients who are unable to perform a finger stick and use the meter machine should use the urine testing method to evaluate blood glucose levels.

Purpose

- To check the blood glucose level.

Clinical Problems

Decreased Level: Insulin overdose.

Elevated Level: Diabetes mellitus, hyperalimentation, excessive stress.

Drugs That May Increase Glucose Value: Steroids, thiazide diuretics.

Procedure

- NPO prior to the test unless otherwise instructed.

Blood: *Finger-Stick Capillary Method*
- Check procedure on the specific glucose monitoring device.
- Cleanse the finger site with alcohol; wipe dry.
- Puncture the lateral side of the finger. Wipe off first drop of blood. Do not "milk" the finger.
- Let a large drop of blood drop onto the reagent strip. The blood should cover the pad of the strip.
- Place the reagent strip into the meter for reading. Follow directions on the meter.
- Apply pressure to the site until bleeding has stopped.

Heelstick: Use the same method for obtaining a finger stick; however, hold the heel in a dependent position to allow the blood drop to accumulate. The use of a capillary tube to obtain the blood specimen may be necessary for blood glucose testing.

Urine

Clinitest: Dip the reagent strip into the urine specimen, remove the strip, wait 10 seconds, read by comparing strip to the color blocks.

Diastix: Dip the reagent strip into the urine specimen, remove the strip, wait 30 seconds, read by comparing strip to the color chart.

Tes-tape: Tear off 1½ inches of reagent tape, dip into the urine specimen, remove tape, wait 60 seconds, read tape by comparing the dark part of tape to color chart.

Factors Affecting Laboratory Results

Blood

- Insufficient blood drop for the test.
- Milking the finger can cause false-low results.

Urine

- Stale urine interferes with test results.
- Drugs that may cause a false-negative result include levodopa, aspirin, ascorbic acid, tetracycline, and methyldopa.

NURSING IMPLICATIONS WITH RATIONALE

- Obtain a history regarding the client's glucose testing method, including the past glucose testing results.
- Answer the client's questions.

Client Teaching

- Discuss the procedure (blood and/or urine) with the client. Have the client demonstrate the procedure.
- Discuss the course of action the client should take if the test result is abnormal.
- Instruct the client to take insulin or the oral hypoglycemic agent at the prescribed time.
- Tell the client to report immediately signs and symptoms of hypoglycemia or hyperglycemia.
- Instruct the client to keep accurate records of the glucose tests.
- Encourage the client to keep all medical appointments.

Glucose tolerance—oral (OGTT) (serum) and IV (IV-GTT)

Reference Values

Adult:

ORAL GTT

Time	Serum (mg/dl)	Blood (mg/dl)
Fasting	70–110	60–100
½ hour	<160	<150
1 hour	<170	<160
2 hours	<125	<115
3 hours	Fasting level	Fasting level
Urine: negative		

IV GLUCOSE TOLERANCE TEST

Time	Serum (mg/dl)
Fasting	70–110
5 minutes	<250
½ hour	<155
1 hour	<125
2 hours	Fasting level
Urine: negative at fasting and at ½, 1, and 2 hours.	

Child: Depends on the child's age. Infants normally have lower blood sugar levels *(see Glucose—Fasting Blood Sugar).* A child aged 6 or older has results similar to those of the adult.

Description

A glucose tolerance test (GTT) is done to diagnose diabetes mellitus in persons having high-normal or slightly elevated blood sugar values. The test may be indicated when there is a familial history of diabetes, in women having babies weighing 10 lb or more, in persons having extensive surgery or injury, and in persons with obesity problems. The test should *not* be performed if the fasting blood sugar (FBS) is >200 mg/dl. After the age of 60 years, the blood glucose level is usually 10 to 30 mg/dl higher than the "normal range."

The peak glucose level for the oral GTT (OGTT) is ½ to 1 hour after the ingestion of 100 g of glucose, and the blood sugar should return to normal range in 3 hours. Blood samples will be collected at specified times.

The *intravenous glucose tolerance test (IV-GTT)* is considered by many to be more sensitive than the oral GTT, because absorption through the gastrointestinal tract is not involved. The IV-GTT is usually done if the person cannot eat or tolerate the oral glucose. The blood glucose returns to the normal range in 2 hours. However, the values for the OGTT and IV-GTT slightly differ, because IV glucose is absorbed faster.

Hyperinsulinism can be detected with the OGTT. After 1 hour the blood glucose level is usually lower than in the FBS test. The person might develop severe hypoglycemic reactions—there is more insulin being secreted in response to the blood glucose.

Purpose

- To confirm the diagnosis of diabetes mellitus.

Clinical Problems

Decreased Level: Hyperinsulinism, adrenal gland insufficiency, malabsorption, protein malnutrition.

Elevated Level: Diabetes mellitus, latent diabetes, adrenal gland hyperfunction (Cushing's syndrome), hyperlipoproteinemia, stress, infections, extensive surgery or injury, alcoholism, acute myocardial infarction, cancer of the pancreas, insulin resistance conditions (eclampsia, cancer metastases, acidotic conditions), duodenal ulcers. *Drug Influence:* Corticosteroids (cortisone), oral contraceptives, estrogens, diuretics, thiazides, salicylates, ascorbic acid.

Procedure

OGTT

- A diet adequate in carbohydrate should be consumed for 2 to 3 days prior to testing.
- The client remains NPO for 12 hours before the test, except for water.
- No coffee, tea, or smoking is allowed during the test. No food should be eaten.
- Drugs that affect test results should not be taken for 3 days prior to the GTT, if possible.
- Collect 5 ml of venous blood in a red- or gray-top tube for FBS. Collect a fasting urine specimen.
- Give 100 g of glucose, either lemon-flavored solution or glucola. Some physicians will give glucose according to body weight (1.75 g/kg), as in pediatrics.
- Obtain blood and urine specimens ½, 1, 2, and 3 hours after glucose intake.

IV-GTT

- NPO 12 hours before test.
- Administer infusion of 50% glucose over 3 to 4 minutes.
- Obtain blood specimens at fasting, 5 minutes (blood only), ½, 1, and 2 hours.

Factors Affecting Laboratory Results

- Drugs *(see Drug Influence)*.
- Age—older adults have higher blood sugar levels. Insulin secretion is decreased because of the aging process.
- Emotional stress, fever, infections, trauma, being bedridden, and obesity can increase the blood sugar level.
- Strenuous exercise and vomiting might decrease the blood sugar level. Hypoglycemic agents will decrease the blood sugar level.

NURSING IMPLICATIONS WITH RATIONALE

- Notify the laboratory of when (the exact time) the client drank the glucose solution. Laboratory personnel will collect the blood samples at specified times.

Client Teaching

- Explain to the client the procedure for the test. Explain that food, alcohol, and medications are restricted for 12 hours prior to the test. Water is permitted.
- Explain to the client that coffee, tea, and smoking are restricted during the test. Water is allowed and encouraged; however, in some institutions, only 240 ml is permitted.
- Explain to the client that he or she may perspire or feel weak and giddy during the 2 to 3 hours of the test. This is frequently transitory; however, the nurse should be notified, and these symptoms should be recorded. They could be signs of hyperinsulinism.
- Inform the client to minimize his or her activities during the test. Increased activities could affect the glucose results.

Decreased Level

- Observe for signs and symptoms of hypoglycemia, especially when hyperinsulinism is suspected. Symptoms include nervousness; irritability; confusion; weakness; pale, cold, clammy skin; diaphoresis (excessive perspiration); and tachycardia.
- Obtain a history from the client as to when hypoglycemic symptoms occur (e.g., before meals). There may be periods of nervousness, "shakiness," and weakness.
- Explain that eating candy to correct nervousness and weakness should be avoided with hyperinsulinism, because it will temporarily correct the problem (the need for glucose) but will stimulate insulin secretion. Sugar will temporarily correct an insulin reaction in a diabetic.

Elevated Level

- Identify factors affecting glucose results (i.e., emotional stress, infection, vomiting, fever, exercise, inactivity, age, drugs, and body weight). Most of these should be reported to the health care provider.
- Check previous FBS results before the test. A known diabetic normally does not, and in some cases should not, have this test performed because diabetic coma may ensue.

Glucose-6-phosphate dehydrogenase (G6PD or G-6-PD) (blood)

Reference Values

Adult: *Screen Test:* Negative. *Quantitative Test:* 8–18 IU/g Hb, 125–281 U/dl packed RBCs, 251–511 U/10^6 cells, 1211–2111 mIU/ml packed RBCs (varies with methods used).

Child: Similar to adult.

Description

Glucose-6-phosphate dehydrogenase (G6PD) is an enzyme in the red blood cells (RBCs), or erythrocytes. It normally assists in glucose use in the RBCs, uses oxidative substances, and protects the integrity of the RBCs from injury.

A G6PD deficit is a sex-linked genetic defect carried by the female (X) chromosome, which will, in conjunction with infection, disease, and drugs, make a person susceptible to developing hemolytic anemia. With a moderate deficiency of G6PD enzyme, there is no apparent detectable RBC abnormality except for a decrease in the life span of the RBCs. Metabolites from certain drugs possessing an oxidizing action in the RBCs will cause an increased need for G6PD for glucose metabolism. A lack of this enzyme results in hemolysis (destruction of the RBCs) and hemolytic anemia when augmented by an oxidative drug.

Purpose

- To screen for hemolytic anemia.

Clinical Problems

Decreased Level: Hemolytic anemia, diabetes acidosis, infections (bacterial and viral), septicemia. *Drug Influence:* Acetanilid (acetylaniline), aspirin, ascorbic acid, nitrofurantoin (Furadantin), phenecetin, primaquine, thiazide diuretics, probenecid (Benemid), quinidine, quinine, chloramphenicol (Chloromycetin), sulfonamides, vitamin K, tolbutamide (Orinase). *Food:* Fava beans.

Procedure

- The laboratory methods used will vary. Screening tests for G6PD deficiency are methemoglobin reduction (Brewer's test), glutathione stability, dye reduction, and ascorbate and fluorescent spot tests. Check with the laboratory on whether capillary or venous blood is needed.
- Collect 5 ml of venous blood in a lavender-top tube.
- There is no food or fluid restriction.

Factors Affecting Laboratory Results

- Drugs can decrease the level *(see Drug Influence)*.

NURSING IMPLICATIONS WITH RATIONALE

Decreased Level

- Obtain a familial history of RBC enzyme deficiency. Blacks are more prone to G6PD deficiency than whites; however, the degree of anemia is not as severe in blacks as it is in whites.
- Observe for symptoms of hemolysis, such as jaundice of the eyes and skin.
- Check for decreased urinary output. Urine should be voided at a rate of at least 25 ml/hour or 600 ml/day. Prolonged hemolysis (destruction of RBCs) can be toxic to the kidney cells, causing kidney impairment.
- Check the hemology results.
- Record oxidative drugs the client is taking on the laboratory slip. *(See Drug Influence.)* Report your findings to the health care provider. Hemolysis usually occurs 3 days after the susceptible person has taken an oxidative drug. Hemolytic symptoms will disappear 2 to 3 days after the drug has been stopped.

Client Teaching

- Instruct the susceptible person to read labels on patent medicines and not to take drugs that contain phenacetin and aspirin. Most of these drugs, if taken continuously, can cause hemolytic anemia.

Glycosylated hemoglobin

See Hemoglobin A$_1$c (Blood)

Growth hormone (GH), human growth hormone (hGH) (serum)

Somatotrophic Hormone (STH)

Reference Values

Adult: *Male:* <5 ng/ml. *Female:* <10 ng/ml.

Child: <10 ng/ml.

Description

Human growth hormone (hGH), hormone from the anterior pituitary gland, regulates growth of bone and tissue. Growth hormone levels are elevated by protein food, fasting, stress, exercise, and deep sleep.

A low serum hGH level might be the cause of dwarfism. Elevated hGH levels cause gigantism in children and acromegaly in adults. From a random growth hormone level, a positive diagnosis cannot be made; therefore *a growth hormone stimulation or suppression challenge test* would be suggested. A glucose loading GH suppression test should suppress hGH secretion. Failure to suppress hGH levels confirms gigantism (children) or acromegaly (adult).

Purposes

- To determine the presence of human growth hormone deficit or excess.
- To aid in the diagnosis of dwarfism, gigantism, or acromegaly.

Clinical Problems

Decreased Level: Dwarfism in children, hypopituitarism. *Drug Influence:* Cortisone preparations, phenothiazines, glucose.

Elevated Level: Gigantism (children), acromegaly (adult), major surgery, premature and newborn infants. *Drug Influence:* Insulin, estrogens, amphetamines, beta-blockers, levodopa, methyldopa (Aldomet).

Procedure

- Collect 3 to 5 ml of venous blood in a red-top tube, preferably in the early morning. Avoid hemolysis. Deliver the blood specimen immediately to the laboratory, because hGH has a short half-life.
- The client is NPO for 8 to 10 hours except for water.
- Have the client rest for 30 minutes to 1 hour before taking a blood sample.

Factors Affecting Laboratory Results

- Stress, exercise, food (protein), and deep sleep could cause an elevated hGH level.
- Drugs listed in *Drug Influence* could decrease or elevate hGH levels.
- Hemolysis of the blood sample affects test results.

NURSING IMPLICATIONS WITH RATIONALE

- Maintain a quiet environment so that stress will not affect test results.
- Notify the health care provider and/or laboratory if the client is anxious, has eaten, or has exercised before the test.

Client Teaching

- Instruct the client not to eat 8 to 10 hours before the test. Encourage the client to rest and not to exercise prior to the test.
- Inform the client that if the serum hGH is elevated, follow-up testing may be necessary.

Haloperidol (Haldol) (serum)

Reference Values

Adult: *Therapeutic Range:* 3–20 ng/ml. *Peak Time:* PO: 2–6 hours. *Toxic Level:* >50 ng/ml.

Description

Haloperidol is used in the treatment of acute and chronic psychosis, in the manic phase of manic-depressive psychosis, and in some cases of schizophrenia. It is a drug frequently used in psychiatry.

Purposes

- To determine if the therapeutic haloperidol dose is within therapeutic range.
- To check for haloperidol toxicity.

Clinical Problems

Decreased Level: *Drug Influence:* Anticholinergics (used for parkinsonism).
Elevated Level: Overdose of haloperidol.

Procedure

- Collect 3 to 5 ml of venous blood in a red-top tube.
- There is no food or fluid restriction.

Factors Affecting Laboratory Results

- Anticholinergics used for the pseudoparkinsonism effect can decrease the effect of haloperidol.
- Phenothiazines, benzodiazepines, or alcohol taken with haloperidol cause an additive central nervous system depressive effect.

NURSING IMPLICATIONS WITH RATIONALE

- Observe for side effects of haloperidol (i.e., dizziness, syncope, drowsiness, hypotension, pseudoparkinsonism, dry mouth, jaundice [due to large doses over a period of time]).
- Check vital signs.

Client Teaching

- Instruct the client to avoid driving and activities that require alertness when taking haloperidol.
- Instruct the client to avoid alcohol and other depressants that might cause side effects of haloperidol.
- Explain to the client the importance of checking with the health care provider about taking over-the-counter (OTC) drugs. Some OTC drugs might cause side effects.

Haptoglobin (Hp) (serum)

Reference Values

Adult: 60–270 mg/dl; 0.6–2.7 g/l (SI units).

Child: *Newborn:* 0–10 mg/dl (absent in 90%). *Infant (1 to 6 months):* 0–30 mg/dl, then gradual increase.

Description

Haptoglobins are alpha$_2$ globulins in the plasma. These globulin molecules combine with free (released) hemoglobin during red blood cell destruction (hemolysis). A decreased level of serum haptoglobin indicates hemolysis. Haptoglobins are decreased in severe liver disease, hemolytic anemia, and infectious mononucleosis and are elevated in inflammatory diseases, steroid therapy, acute infections, and malignancies. A hemolytic process may be masked in persons taking steroids.

Purposes

- To identify the occurrence of hemolysis.
- To assist in the diagnosis of selected health problems *(see Clinical Problems)*.

Clinical Problems

Decreased Level: Hemolysis, anemias (pernicious, Vitamin B_6 deficiency, hemolytic, sickle cell), severe liver disease (hepatic failure, chronic hepatitis), thrombotic thrombocytopenic purpura, disseminated intravascular coagulation (DIC), malaria.

Elevated Level: Inflammation, acute infections, cancer (lung, large intestine, stomach, breast, liver), Hodgkin's disease, ulcerative colitis, chronic pyelonephritis (active stage), rheumatic fever, acute myocardial infarction. *Drug Influence:* Steroids (cortisone).

Procedure

- Collect 3 to 5 ml of venous blood in a red-top tube. Avoid hemolysis.
- There is no food or fluid restriction.
- Haptoglobin levels can be measured by electrophoresis, radioimmunodiffusion, or spectrophotometry.

Factors Affecting Laboratory Results

- Steroids and inflammation may cause false results. Hemolysis could occur but the serum haptoglobin level may not indicate this.

NURSING IMPLICATIONS WITH RATIONALE

Decreased Level

- Associate a decreased serum haptoglobin level with conditions causing hemolysis, such as hemolytic anemias, severe liver disease, and others.
- Assess the client's vital signs. Report abnormal vital signs, especially if the client is having breathing problems. The oxygen capacity of hemoglobin may be reduced, causing a change in breathing pattern.
- Assess the client's urinary output. Excessive amounts of free hemoglobin may cause renal damage.

Elevated Level

- Associate an elevated serum haptoglobin level with clinical problems, such as infections, inflammation, cancer, steroid therapy, and others.
- Check the serum haptoglobin level. The haptoglobin level may be masked by steroid therapy and inflammation. If hemolysis is suspected, the serum level may be normal instead of low because of steroid therapy or inflammation. Notify the health care provider of the findings.

Heinz bodies (blood)

Reference Values

Negative: Absence of Heinz Bodies; <30% Heinz Bodies present.

Description

Heinz bodies are small, irregular, decomposed particles of hemoglobin that accumulate on the red blood cells' (RBCs) membrane. Normally these bodies are removed by the spleen; however, they can be a cause of hemolytic anemia (hemolysis of RBCs) or hemoglobinopathy (hematologic disorder). After a splenectomy, the Heinz bodies increase in the blood, and the reference value can be >30%.

Purpose

- To aid in the cause of hemolytic anemia.

Clinical Problems

Elevated Levels: Hemolytic anemia, hemoglobinopathies, glucose-6-phosphate dehydrogenase (G-6-PD) deficiency, post-splenectomy. *Drug Influence:* Analgesics including acetaminophen, antimalarials, certain sulfonamides, phenothiazines, phenacetin, procarbazine, nitrofurantoin, chlorates.

Procedure

- Collect 7 ml of venous blood in a lavender-top tube. Avoid hemolysis; gently invert tube.
- There is no food or fluid restriction.

Factors Affecting Laboratory Results

- Hemolysis because of rough handling of blood specimen.
- Drugs that could induce hemolysis. *See Clinical Problems.*
- Blood transfusion(s) within the last week before the test.

NURSING IMPLICATIONS WITH RATIONALE

- Obtain a history from client with regard to past and present health problems, drugs the client is taking, and any recent blood transfusions.
- Assess vital signs; report abnormal findings.
- Report jaundice that could result from red blood cell hemolysis. Bilirubin may be elevated.

Helicobacter pylori (*serum, culture, breath analysis*)

Reference Values

Negative findings. A positive or elevated titer level using enzyme-linked immunosorbent assay (ELISA) serology testing or the urea breath test indicates the presence of *Helicobacter pylori*.

Description

The gram-negative bacillus *Helicobacter pylori* is found in the gastric mucus layer of the epithelium in about 50% of the population by age 55. The majority of persons with the infection remain asymptomatic. *H. pylori* was first identified in 1983 as a cause of peptic ulcer disease. It is recognized as a primary cause of chronic gastritis, and it may progress over years to gastric cancer or gastric lymphoma. *H. pylori* is associated with 70% to 85% of clients with gastric ulcers and with 90% to 95% of duodenal ulcers. Duodenal ulcers due to Zollinger-Ellison syndrome are not associated with *H. pylori*.

The incidence of *H. pylori* increases with age. Between the ages of 45 to 55 the incidence of *H. pylori* antibodies is approximately 20%. The incidence of *H. pylori* grows to 50% over the next 10 years and for persons over 65 years of age, the incidence increases to 75%. This organism is common in blacks.

Eradication of *H. pylori* for asymptomatic clients usually is not suggested or prescribed but is definitely indicated for perforated, bleeding, or refractory ulcers. Treatment to eradicate the infection involves a dual, triple, or quadruple drug therapy program using a variety of drug combinations. Dual-drug therapy (omeprazole and amoxicillin) for 14 days has fewer side effects but is not as effective in eradicating *H. pylori* as the use of triple or quadruple therapy. Quadruple therapy has a 7-day treatment course which eliminates some of the side effects. After the drug therapy program, a 6-week standard acid suppression drug (histamine-2 blocker) usually is recommended.

Purposes

- To detect the cause of gastrointestinal disorder.
- To determine the presence of *H. pylori*.

Clinical Problems

Elevated Level or Positive Culture: Presence of *H. pylori* causing acute or chronic gastritis, peptic ulcer disease, gastric carcinoma, gastric lymphoma.

Procedure

Serum (ELISA)

- No food or fluid restriction is required.
- Collect 7 ml of venous blood in a red-top tube.
- Use of a variety of commercial diagnostic kits.

Culture or Biopsy (Endoscopy)

- Obtain a culture or biopsy using endoscopy for detection of urease produced by *H. pylori*.

Urea Breath Test

- Use the urea breath test to diagnose urease which is given off by *H. pylori*. It has a sensitivity of 92% to 94%.
- The urea test dose is accompanied by radioactive carbon 13 or 14. The expired air is tested for radioactivity.

Factors Affecting Laboratory Results

- None known.

NURSING IMPLICATIONS

- Obtain a familial history of gastrointestinal disorders, such as gastritis or peptic ulcer disease.
- Record symptoms client has related to gastritis or peptic ulcer disease, such as pain, abdominal cramping, gastroesophageal reflux disease, dyspepsia (heartburn), anorexia, nausea, vomiting, gastrointestinal (GI) bleeding, and tarry stools.
- Encourage the client to avoid smoking (if the client smokes) because smoking reduces bicarbonate content in the GI tract, allows reflux of the duodenum into the stomach, and slows the healing process.
- Listen to the client's concerns. Answer the client's questions or refer unknown answers to other health care providers.

Hematocrit (Hct) (blood)

Reference Values

Adult: *Male:* 40–54%, 0.40–0.54 (SI units). *Female:* 36–46%, 0.36–0.46 (SI units). *Panic Value:* <15% and >60%.

Child: *Newborn:* 44–65%. *1 to 3 Years Old:* 29–40%. *4 to 10 Years Old:* 31–43%.

Description

The hematocrit (Hct) is the volume (in milliliters) of packed red blood cells (RBCs) found in 100 ml (1 dl) of blood, expressed as a percentage. For example, a 36% hematocrit would indicate that 36 ml of RBCs were found in 100 ml of blood, or 36 vol/dl. The purpose of the test is to measure the concentration of RBCs (erythrocytes) in the blood.

Low hematocrits are found frequently in anemias and leukemias, and elevated levels are found in dehydration (a relative increase) and polycythemia vera. The hematocrit can be an indicator of the hydration status of the client. As with hemoglobin, an elevated hematocrit could indicate hemoconcentration because of a decrease in fluid volume and an increase in RBCs.

Purposes

- To check the volume of RBCs in the blood.
- To monitor the volume of RBCs in blood during a debilitating illness.

Clinical Problems

Decreased Level: Acute blood loss, anemias (aplastic, hemolytic, folic acid deficiency, pernicious, sideroblastic, sickle cell), leukemias (lymphocytic, myelocytic, monocytic), Hodgkin's disease, lymphosarcoma, malignancy of organs, multiple myeloma, cirrhosis of the liver, protein malnutrition, vitamin deficiencies (thiamine, vitamin C), fistula of the stomach or duodenum, peptic ulcer, chronic renal failure, pregnancy, systemic lupus erythematosus, rheumatoid arthritis (especially juvenile). *Drug Influence:* Antineoplastic agents, antibiotics (chloramphenicol, penicillin), radioactive agents.

Elevated Level: Dehydration/hypovolemia, severe diarrhea, polycythemia vera, erythrocytosis, diabetic acidosis, pulmonary emphysema (later stage), transient cerebral ischemia, eclampsia, surgery, burns.

Procedure

- No food or fluid is restricted.

Venous Blood

- Collect 3 to 5 ml of venous blood in a lavender-top tube. Mix well. The tourniquet should be on for less than 2 minutes.
- Do not take the blood specimen from an arm in which there is an IV line.

Capillary Blood

- Collect capillary blood using the microhematocrit method. Blood is obtained from a finger prick, using a heparinized capillary tube.

Factors Affecting Laboratory Results

- If blood is collected from an extremity that has an IV line, the hematocrit will most likely be low. Avoid using such an extremity.
- If blood is taken to check the hematocrit immediately after moderate to severe blood loss and transfusions, the hematocrit could be normal.
- Age of the client—newborns normally have higher hematocrits because of hemoconcentration.

NURSING IMPLICATIONS WITH RATIONALE

- Explain the procedure to the client. If the microhematocrit method is used, explain that the finger will be cleansed with an alcohol sponge and pricked with a lancet or needle to obtain capillary blood.

Decreased Level

- Relate a decreased hematocrit to clinical problems and drugs. Blood loss and anemias are the most common causes of a low hematocrit. A hematocrit of 30% or less with no known bleeding frequently indicates a moderate to severe anemic condition.
- Assess for signs and symptoms of anemia (fatigue, paleness, and tachycardia).
- Assess changes in vital signs to determine whether shock is present because of blood loss. Symptoms could include rapid pulse, rapid respirations, and normal or decreased blood pressure.
- Recommend a repeat hematocrit several days after moderate/severe bleeding or transfusions. A hematocrit taken immediately after blood loss and after transfusions may appear normal.

Elevated Level

- Relate an elevated hematocrit to clinical problems. Dehydration and hypovolemia are common causes of hematocrit elevation because they result in hemoconcentration.
- Assess for signs and symptoms of dehydration/hypovolemia. A history of vomiting, diarrhea, marked thirst, lack of skin turgor, and shocklike symptoms (rapid pulse and respiration rates) could be indicative of a body fluid deficit.
- Administer IV or oral fluids according to the health care provider's order to reestablish body fluid volume.
- Avoid rapid administration of IV fluids to the older adult, child, or debilitated person so as to prevent overhydration and pulmonary edema. Signs and symptoms of overhydration are constant, irritated cough; dyspnea; hand and/or neck vein engorgement; and chest rales.
- Check the hematocrit daily, if ordered, when reestablishing body fluid volume. If the elevated hematocrit returns to normal, the elevation was due to hemoconcentration.

■ Assess changes in urinary output. A urine output of <25 ml/hour or 600 ml daily could be due to dehydration/hypovolemia. Once body fluids are restored, urine output should be normal.

Hemoglobin (Hb or Hgb) (blood)

Reference Values

Adult: *Male:* 13.5–17 g/dl. *Female:* 12–15 g/dl.
Child: *Newborn:* 14–24 g/dl. *Infant:* 10–17 g/dl. *Child:* 11–16 g/dl.

Description

Hemoglobin (Hb or Hgb), a protein substance found in red blood cells (RBCs), gives blood its red color. Hemoglobin is composed of iron, which is an oxygen carrier. Abnormally high hemoglobin levels may be due to hemoconcentration resulting from dehydration (fluid loss). Low hemoglobin values are related to various clinical problems.

The RBC count and hemoglobin level do not always increase or decrease equally. For instance, a decreased RBC count and a normal or slightly decreased hemoglobin level occur in pernicious anemia, and a normal or slightly decreased RBC and a decreased hemoglobin level occur in iron deficiency (microcytic) anemia.

Purposes

■ To monitor the hemoglobin value in RBCs.
■ To assist in diagnosing anemia.
■ To suggest the presence of body fluid deficit due to an elevated hemoglobin level.

Clinical Problems

Decreased Level: Anemias (iron deficiency, aplastic, hemocytic), severe hemorrhage, cirrhosis of the liver, leukemias, Hodgkin's disease, sarcoidosis, excess IV fluids, cancer (large and small intestine, rectum, liver, bone), thalassemia major, pregnancy, kidney diseases. *Drug Influence:* Antibiotics (chloramphenicol [Chloromycetin], penicillin, tetracycline), aspirin, antineoplastic drugs, doxapram (Dopram), hydantoin derivatives, hydralazine (Apresoline), indomethacin (Indocin), MAO inhibitors, primaquine, rifampin, sulfonamides, trimethadione (Tridione), Vitamin A (large doses).

Elevated Level: Dehydration/hemoconcentration, polycythemia, high altitudes, chronic obstructive lung disease, congestive heart failure, severe burns. *Drug Influence:* Gentamicin, methyldopa (Aldomet).

Procedure

- There is no food or fluid restriction.
- Do not take the blood sample from a hand or arm receiving IV fluid. The tourniquet should be on less than a minute.

Venous Blood: Collect 3 to 5 ml of venous blood in a lavender top tube. Avoid hemolysis.

Capillary Blood: Puncture the cleansed earlobe, finger, or heel with a sterile lancet. Do not squeeze the puncture site tightly, for serous fluid and blood would thus be obtained. Wipe away the first drop of blood. Collect drops of blood quickly in micropipettes with small rubber tops or microhematocrit tubes. Expel blood into the tubes with diluents.

Factors Affecting Laboratory Results

- Drugs could increase or decrease hemoglobin *(see Drug Influence above)*.
- Taking blood from an arm or hand receiving IV fluids could dilute blood sample.
- Leaving the tourniquet on for more than a minute will cause hemostasis, which will result in a falsely elevated hemoglobin level.
- Living in high altitudes will increase hemoglobin levels.
- Decreased fluid intake or fluid loss will increase hemoglobin levels due to hemoconcentration, and excessive fluid intake will decrease hemoglobin levels due to hemodilution.

NURSING IMPLICATIONS WITH RATIONALE

- Explain the procedure to the client.

Decreased Level

- Recognize clinical problems and drugs that could cause a decreased hemoglobin level *(see Clinical Problems)*. Anemia is a common cause, but usually the client is not considered anemic until the hemoglobin level is <10.5 g/dl. Hemorrhage could cause a low hemoglobin level if the blood is not replaced; however, the hemoglobin level does not decrease immediately. It may remain normal for hours or even several days.
- Observe the client for signs and symptoms of anemia (i.e., dizziness, tachycardia, weakness, dyspnea at rest). Symptoms depend on how low the hemoglobin level is (severe anemia).
- Check the hematocrit level if the hemoglobin level is low.

Elevated Level

- Recognize clinical problems and drugs that can cause an increased hemoglobin level *(see Clinical Problems)*. Dehydration is a major transient cause of an elevated level. Once the client is hydrated, the hemoglobin should return to the normal range.

- Observe for signs and symptoms of dehydration (i.e., marked thirst, poor skin turgor, dry mucous membranes, and shocklike symptoms [tachycardia, tachypnea, and, later, decreased blood pressure]).

Client Teaching

- Instruct the client to maintain an adequate fluid intake. Frequently, older adults tend to drink less fluid.

Hemoglobin A_1c (Hgb A_1c or Hb A_1c) (blood)

Glycosylated Hemoglobin (Hgb A_1a, Hgb A_1b, Hgb A_1c, Glycohemoglobin)

Reference Values

Total Glycosylated Hemoglobin: 5.5–9% of total Hgb (Hb).

Adult: *Hgb (Hb)* A_1c: Nondiabetic: 2–5%; Diabetic Control: 2.5–6%; high average: 6.1–7.5%; Diabetic Uncontrolled: >8%.

Child: *Hgb (Hb)* A_1c: Nondiabetic: 1.5–4%.

Description

Hemoglobin A (Hgb or Hb A) comprises of 91 to 95% of total hemoglobin. Glucose molecule is attached to Hb A_1, which is a portion of hemoglobin A. This process of attachment is called *glycosylation* or *glycosylated hemoglobin* or *hemoglobin A_1*. There is a bond between glucose and hemoglobin. Formation of Hb A_1 occurs slowly over 120 days, the life span of red blood cells (RBCs). Hb A_1 is composed of three hemoglobin molecules, Hb A_1a, Hb A_1b, and Hb A_1c of which 70% Hb A_1c is 70% glycosylated (absorbs glucose). The amount of glycosylated hemoglobin depends on the amount of blood glucose available. When the blood glucose level is elevated over a prolonged period of time, the red blood cells (RBCs) become saturated with glucose; glycohemoglobin results.

A glycosylated hemoglobin represents an average blood glucose level during a 1- to 4-month period. This test is used mainly as a measurement of the effectiveness of diabetic therapy. Fasting blood sugar reflects the blood glucose level at a 1-time fasting state; whereas, the Hgb or Hb A_1c is a better indicator of diabetes mellitus control. However, a false decreased Hb A_1c level can be caused by a decrease in red blood cells.

An elevated Hb A_1c >8% indicates uncontrolled diabetes mellitus, and the client is at a high risk of developing long-term complications, such as nephropathy, retinopathy, neuropathy, and/or cardiopathy. Total glycohemoglobin may be a better indicator of diabetes control for clients with anemias or blood loss.

Purposes

- To monitor the effectiveness of diabetic therapy.
- To manage diabetic therapy.
- To provide information regarding the presence of diabetes mellitus.
- To determine the client's compliance with diabetic therapy.

Clinical Problems

Decreased Level: Anemias (pernicious, hemolytic, sickle cell), thalassemia, long-term blood loss, chronic renal failure.

Elevated Level: Uncontrolled diabetes mellitus, hyperglycemia, recently diagnosed diabetes mellitus, alcohol ingestion, pregnancy, hemodialysis. *Drug Influence:* Prolonged cortisone intake, ACTH.

Procedure

- Schedule client 6 to 12 weeks from the lab Hb A$_1$c test.
- Food restriction prior to the test is not required but is suggested.
- Collect 5 ml of venous blood in a lavender- or green-top tube. Avoid hemolysis; send specimen immediately to the laboratory.

Factors Affecting Laboratory Results

- Anemias may cause a low value result.
- Hemolysis of the blood specimen can cause an inaccurate test result.
- Heparin therapy may cause false test result.

NURSING IMPLICATIONS WITH RATIONALE

- Monitor blood and/or urine glucose levels. Compare monthly fasting blood sugar with glycosylated hemoglobin (Hb A$_1$c) test result.
- Check previous fasting blood sugar (FBS) results.
- Determine client's compliance to diabetic treatment regimen.
- Check the dose of daily insulin or oral hypoglycemic agent.
- Recognize clinical problems that can cause a false glycosylated hemoglobin result *(see Clinical Problems)*.
- Observe for signs and symptoms of hyperglycemia.
- Report any complications client has due to diabetes mellitus.

Client Teaching

- Inform the client that fasting prior to the test may or may not be prescribed. Tell the laboratory person if you have not fasted prior to the test.

- Explain the purpose of the test, that is, it measures the effectiveness of the prescribed diabetic therapy.
- Instruct the client to comply with the diabetic treatment regimen, such as prescribed insulin, diet, and glucose monitoring.

Hemoglobin electrophoresis (blood)

Hemoglobins A_1, A_2, F, C, S

Reference Values

Adult: *Hemoglobin (Hb or Hgb) Electrophoresis:* A_1, 95–98% total Hb; A_2, 1.5%; F, <2%; C, 0%; D, 0%; S, 0%.

Child: *Newborn:* Hb, F, 50–80% total Hb. *Infant:* Hb F, 8% total Hb. *Child:* Hb F, 1–2% total Hb after 6 months.

Description

The normal types of hemoglobin are Hb A_1, comprising 95% to 98% of the total hemoglobin, Hb A_2, and Hb F (fetal). If Hb F makes up 5% or more of the total hemoglobin after the age of 6 months, thalassemia (Mediterranean anemia) could be a factor. There are three clinical types of thalassemia; thalassemia major (Hb F >50%), thalassemia minor (increased Hb A_2 value), and thalassemia gene (combination of abnormal hemoglobins).

To identify normal hemoglobin types (A_1, A_2, and F) and abnormal hemoglobin types (Hb C, Hb M, Hb S, and others), a hemoglobin electrophoresis is usually ordered. It is not a routine test, but it is useful for identifying 150 or more types of hemoglobin. Many abnormal hemoglobin types do not produce harmful diseases; the common hemoglobinopathies are identified through electrophoresis.

Hemoglobin S: Hb S is the most common hemoglobin variant. If both genes have Hb S, sickle cell anemia will occur; but if only one gene has Hb S, then the person simply carries the sickle trait. Approximately 1% of the black population in the United States has sickle cell anemia, and 8% to 10% carry the sickle cell trait.

Sickle cell anemia symptoms are usually not present until after the age of 6 months. In some cases Hb S is combined with another abnormal hemoglobin type, Hb C or Hb D. Hb S/C or Hb S/D produces red blood cells (RBCs, erythrocytes) that sickle as with Hb S/S. Those with sickle cell anemia have low oxygen tension (*also see Sickle Cell Test*).

Hemoglobin C: Hb C in the homozygous state (C/C) usually produces mild hemolytic anemia; in the heterozygous state (A/C), it produces the Hb C trait. This occurs more frequently in blacks.

Purpose

- To detect abnormal hemoglobin type in the RBCs (e.g., sickle cell anemia, which is characterized by the S-shaped hemoglobin).

Clinical Problems

HEMOGLOBIN TYPE	ELEVATED LEVEL
Hemoglobin F	Thalassemia (after 6 months)
Hemoglobin C	Hemolytic anemia
Hemoglobin S	Sickle cell anemia

Procedure

- Collect 3 to 5 ml of venous blood in a lavender-top tube. Send immediately to the laboratory. Abnormal hemoglobin is unstable.
- There is no food or fluid restriction.

Factors Affecting Laboratory Results

- Blood transfusions given 4 months before hemoglobin electrophoresis may cause inaccurate results.
- Collection of the blood sample in the wrong color tube can affect results.

NURSING IMPLICATIONS WITH RATIONALE

- Observe for signs and symptoms of sickle cell anemia. Early symptoms are fatigue and weakness. Chronic symptoms are fatigue, dyspnea on exertion, swollen joints, bones that ache, and chest pains. Afflicted persons are susceptible to infection. Sickle cell crisis is usually due to small infarcts to various organs. The crisis usually lasts 5 to 7 days, and immediate care is needed for the symptoms. Normally the hemoglobin level does not change.

Client Teaching

- Encourage the client to seek genetic counseling if he or she has sickle cell anemia or is a carrier of the sickle cell trait.
- Instruct the client with sickle cell anemia to minimize strenuous activity and to avoid high altitudes and extreme cold. Encourage the client to take rest periods.
- Encourage the client to stay away from persons with infections.
- Suggest that the client carry a medical alert bracelet and/or card.

Hepatitis (profile)

Hepatitis A, B, C, D, E

Five major types of hepatitis virus can be identified through laboratory testing: hepatitis A virus (HAV), hepatitis B virus (HBV), hepatitis C virus (HCV), hepatitis D virus (HDV), and hepatitis E virus (HEV). These hepatitis viruses can be detected by testing serum antigens, antibodies, DNA, RNA, and/or the immunoglobins IgG and IgM. The following table differentiates between the hepatitis viruses according to method of transmission, incubation time, jaundice, acute and chronic phases of the disease, carrier status, immunity, and mortality rate.

COMPARISON OF THE TYPES OF VIRAL HEPATITIS

Types of Hepatitis				
Factors Associated With Hepatitis	HAV	HBV	HCV	HDV	HEV
Method of transmission	Enteral (oral–fecal) Water and food	Parenteral Intravenous Sexual Perinatal	Parenteral Sexual (possible) Perinatal	Parenteral Sexual (possible) Perinatal	Enteral (oral–fecal) Water and food
Incubation time	Abrupt onset; 2–12 weeks	Insidious onset; 6–24 weeks	Insidious onset; 2–26 weeks	Abrupt onset; 3–15 weeks	Abrupt onset; 2–8 weeks
Jaundice	Adult: 70%–80% Child: 10%	20%–40%	10%–25%	Varies	25%–60%
Hepatocellular carcinoma	None	Possible	Possible	Possible	None
Acute disease: serum markers	Anti-HAV-IgM	HBsAg, HBeAg, Anti-HBc-IgM	Anti-HCV	HDAg	Anti-HEV
Chronic disease: serum markers	None	HBsAg	Anti-HCV (50% of cases)	Anti-HDV	None
Infective state: serum markers	None (HAV-RNA)	HBsAg, HBeAg, HBV-DNA	Anti-HCV HCV-RNA	Anti-HDV HDV-RNA	None (HEV-RNA)
Fulminant hepatitis	Very low	Very low	Very low	High	Low

COMPARISON OF THE TYPES OF VIRAL HEPATITIS

Factors Associated With Hepatitis	Types of Hepatitis				
	HAV	HBV	HCV	HDV	HEV
Chronic carrier	None	HbsAg (low incidence in adults; high incidence in children)	High incidence	Anti-HDV, HDAg low incidence (10%–15%)	None
Immunity; serum markers	Anti-HAV total, Anti-HAV-IgG	Anti-HBs, Anti-HBc total	None	None	Anti-HEV
Mortality rate	<2%	<2%	<2%	≤30%	<2%

Hepatitis A Virus (HAV): Hepatitis A virus is transmitted primarily by oral–fecal contact. Jaundice is an early sign of HAV which can occur a few days after the viral infection and may last up to 12 weeks. The antibodies to hepatitis A, anti-HAV-IgM and anti-HAV-IgG, are used to confirm the phase of the hepatitis A infection. Anti-HAV-IgM denotes an acute phase of the infection, while anti-HAV-IgG indicates recovery, past infection, or immunity. Approximately 45 to 50% of clients having HAV may have a positive anti-HAV-IgG for life.

Hepatitis B Virus (HBV): The hepatitis B virus was once called serum hepatitis. There are numerous laboratory tests for diagnosing the acute or chronic phase of HBV. These include hepatitis B surface antigen (HBsAg), antibody to HBsAg (anti-HBs), hepatitis B e antigen (HBeAg), antibody to HBeAg (anti-HBe), and antibody to core antigen (anti-HBc-total).

HBsAg: The earliest indicator for diagnosing hepatitis B viral infection is the hepatitis B surface antigen. This serum marker can be present as early as 2 weeks after being infected, and it persists during the acute phase of the infection. If it persists after 6 months, the client could have chronic hepatitis and be a carrier. The hepatitis B vaccine will not cause a positive HBsAg. Clients who have a positive HBsAg should NEVER donate blood.

Antibody to Hepatitis B Surface Antigen (Anti-HBs): With HBV, the acute phase of viral hepatitis B usually lasts for 12 weeks; therefore, HBsAg is absent and anti-HBs (antibodies to HBsAg) develop. This serum marker indicates recovery and immunity to the hepatitis B virus. An anti-HBs-IgM would determine if the client is still infectious. An anti-HBs titer of >10 mIU/ml and without HBsAg presence confirms that the client has recovered from HBV.

Hepatitis B e antigen (HBeAg): This serum marker occurs only with HBsAg. It usually appears one week after HBsAg and disappears before anti-HBs. If HBeAg is still present after 10 weeks, the client could be developing a chronic carrier state.

Antibody to HBeAg (Anti-HBe): The presence of anti-HBe indicates the recovery phase.

Antibody to Core Antigen (Anti-HBc): The anti-HBc occurs with a positive HBsAg approximately 4 to 10 weeks of acute HBV. An elevated anti-HBc-IgM titer indicates the acute infection process. Anti-HBc can detect clients who have been infected with HBV. This serum marker may persist for years, and clients with a positive anti-HBc should not give blood.

Hepatitis C Virus (HCV): HCV is formerly non-A, non-B hepatitis. It is transmitted parenterally. It occurs more frequently with posttransfusion hepatitis, but also should be considered with drug addiction, needle sticks, hemodialysis, and hemophilias. Approximately half of the acute cases of HCV become chronic carriers.

Antibody to Hepatitis C Virus (Anti-HCV): HCV is confirmed by the anti-HCV test. Anti-HCV does not indicate immunity as it can with anti-HBs and anti-HBe.

Hepatitis D Virus (HDV): Hepatitis D (delta) virus is transmitted parenterally. HDV can be present only with HBV. It is coated by the HBsAg and depends on the HBV for replication. HDV is severe and usually occurs 7 to 14 days after an acute, severe HBV infection. It has a low occurrence rate except in IV drug abusers and clients receiving multiple transfusions. Its presence is in the acute phase of HBV or as a chronic carrier of HBV. Of all the types of hepatitis, it has the greatest incidence of fulminant hepatitis and death.

Hepatitis D Antigen (HDAg): Detection of HDAg and HDV-RNA indicates the acute phase of HBV and HDV infection. When HBsAg diminishes, so does HDAg, Anti-HDV appears later and may suggest chronic hepatitis D.

Hepatitis E Virus (HEV): HEV is transmitted by oral–fecal contact and not parenterally. It can result from drinking unsafe water as well as traveling in Mexico, Russia, India, or Africa. It is rare in the United States. Antibodies to hepatitis E (Anti-HEV) detect hepatitis E infection.

Hepatitis A virus (HAV) antibody (HAV ab, anti-HAV) (serum)

Reference Value

None detected.

Description

Hepatitis A virus (HAV), previously called infectious hepatitis, usually is transmitted by oral–fecal contact. The incubation period for HAV is 2 to 6 weeks, not like the 7 to 25 weeks for hepatitis B virus. HAV is not associated with chronic liver disease.

Antibodies to hepatitis A virus (IgM and IgG) indicate the presence or past infection and possible immunity. Anti-HAV IgM (HAV ab IgM) appears early after exposure and is detectable for 4 to 12 weeks. Anti-HAV IgG appears postinfection (>4 weeks), and usually remains present for life. Approximately 50% of the population in the United States have a positive anti-HAV IgG.

Purpose

- To determine the presence or past infection of HAV.

Clinical Problems

Positive: Hepatitis A virus (HAV).

Procedure

- There is no food or fluid restriction.
- Collect 3 to 5 ml of venous blood in a red-top tube.

Factors Affecting Laboratory Results

- None known.

NURSING IMPLICATIONS WITH RATIONALE

- Obtain a history from the client of a possible contact with a person having HAV. Record if the client has eaten shellfish that may have been obtained from contaminated water.

Client Teaching

- Explain to the client that HAV is normally transmitted by oral or fecal contact. A food handler with HAV could transmit the virus if the handler had poor personal hygiene (not washing hands after toileting).
- Alert the client that HAV can spread in institutions such as day-care centers, prisons, and state mental institutions.

Positive Test

- Rest and nutritional dietary intake for several weeks according to the severity of the HAV are indicated. Fatigue is common. Rest periods are necessary as long as jaundice is present.
- Instruct the client that effective personal hygiene is very important.

Hepatitis B surface antigen (HB$_s$Ag) (serum)

Hepatitis-Associated Antigen (HAA)

Reference Values

Adult: Negative.

Child: Negative.

Description

The hepatitis B surface antigen (HG$_s$Ag) test was originally called the Australia antigen test and later the hepatitis-associated antigen (HAA) test. This test is done to determine the presence of hepatitis B virus in the blood in either an active or a carrier state (as in a hepatitis B carrier). Approximately 5% of persons with diseases other than hepatitis B (serum hepatitis) will have a positive HB$_s$Ag test.

The HB$_s$Ag test is routinely performed on the donor's blood to identify the hepatitis B antigen. Transmission of hepatitis B in blood transfusions has greatly diminished through HB$_s$Ag screening of the donor's blood and excluding donors with a history of hepatitis. Though transfusion-related hepatitis B has decreased, the occurrence of hepatitis B is still on the increase.

In hepatitis B, the antigen in the serum can be detected 2 to 24 weeks (average 4 to 8 weeks) after exposure to the virus. The positive HB$_s$Ag may be present 2 to 6 weeks after onset of the clinical disease. Approximately 10% of the clients with positive HB$_s$Ag are carriers, and their tests may remain positive for years.

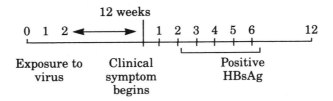

In 75% to 90% of the clients, antibody to hepatitis B surface antigen (called anti-HB$_s$Ag or HB$_s$Ab) is found 2 to 12 weeks after HB$_s$Ag occurs. Anti-HB$_s$Ag can be detected for years after the acute viral infection, but it does not guarantee immunity against future hepatitis infection.

HB$_s$Ag test does not diagnose hepatitis A virus. Two tests for hepatitis A are anti-HAV-IgM (indicates an acute infection) and anti-HAV-IgG (indicates a past exposure).

Purposes

- To screen for the presence of hepatitis B in the client's blood.
- To detect the presence of hepatitis B in the donor's blood.

Clinical Problems

Elevated Level (Positive): Hepatitis B, chronic hepatitis B. *Less Common:* Hemophilia, Down syndrome, Hodgkin's disease, leukemia. *Drug Influence:* Drug addiction.

Procedure

- Collect 5 to 7 ml of venous blood in a red-top tube. Careful handling of the blood sample and washing the hands are most important to keep from contacting the viral hepatitis B.
- There is no food or fluid restriction.

Factors Affecting Laboratory Results

- None known.

NURSING IMPLICATIONS WITH RATIONALE

- Explain to the client the purpose of the test. If the person is a blood donor, the test is automatically done after the unit of blood is taken. Most of these persons do not know that the HB$_S$Ag test and other blood tests are done on donor blood.
- Obtain a history of any previous hepatitis infection and report it to the health care provider.

Elevated Level (Positive Test)

- Handle blood obtained from the client with care, avoiding blood contact with your skin (especially if skin and nail cuts are present). If you accidentally stick yourself with the used needle, you should, in most cases, receive gamma globulin as a preventive measure to avoid the disease.
- Discard all needles and syringes used on clients having hepatitis B. Follow the hospital's isolation procedure.
- Observe for signs and symptoms of hepatitis, such as lethargy, anorexia, nausea and vomiting, fever, dark-colored urine, and jaundice.

Client Teaching

- Instruct the client to get plenty of rest; follow a nutritional diet, if tolerated; and drink fluids (juice and carbonated drinks).

Herpes simplex virus (HSV) antibody test (serum)

HSV-1 and HSV-2

Reference Values

Negative: <1:10.

Positive: *Early Primary Herpes Simplex Infection:* 1:10 to 1:100. *Late Primary Herpes Simplex Infection:* 1:100 to 1:500. *Latent Herpes Simplex Infection:* >1:500. Fourfold titer increase between the acute and convalescent period.

Description

Herpes simplex is an infectious virus that can produce antibody titers. There are two types of herpes simplex; herpes simplex virus type 1 (HSV-1) and herpes simplex virus type 2 (HSV-2). HSV-1 infects the mouth, mostly the mucous membrane around the lip (cold sores), eyes, or upper respiratory tract. HSV-2 is frequently referred to as genital herpes infecting the genitourinary tract. HSV-2 is transmitted primarily through sexual contact and can infect the newborn during vaginal delivery. Neonatal herpes may be mild, resulting in eye infection or skin rash, or it may result in a fatal systemic infection. Congenital herpes is not as common but may be acquired during early pregnancy, resulting in central nervous system disorders causing brain damage.

In addition to the serology blood test, a culture may be obtained to isolate the HSV. HERPCHEK from E.I. duPont de Nemours, Wilmington, Delaware, detects the herpes antigen from scrapings of suspected HSV genital vesicular lesions.

Antibodies for HSV-1 and HSV-2 begin to rise in 7 days and reach peak titers in 4 to 6 weeks after infection. Usually recurrence or reinfection of HSV does not greatly change the titer level. Those infected may have an increased titer level for 6 months after infection or it may persist throughout their life. Genital herpes, HSV-2, tends to be more severe and needs appropriate medical care such as the topical antiviral drug, acyclovir (Zorvirax).

Purposes

- ■ To detect the presence of HSV.
- ■ To diagnose the convalescent phase of HSV.

Clinical Problems

Positive Titer: HSV-1, HSV-2, HSV-1 encephalitis, cervicitis, congenital herpes.

Procedure

- There is no food or fluid restriction.
- Collect 3 to 5 ml of venous blood in a red-top tube. Avoid hemolysis. Deliver the blood sample to the laboratory within 1 hour. Gloves should be worn when obtaining the blood specimen.
- The laboratory slip should indicate whether the test is for HSV-1 or HSV-2, or both.
- Cerebral spinal fluid (CSF) may be obtained to determine the presence of HSV if HSV-1 encephalitis is suspected.

Factors Affecting Laboratory Results

- Hemolysis of the blood sample.
- Not delivering the blood sample to the laboratory within an hour.

NURSING IMPLICATIONS WITH RATIONALE

- Obtain a history from the client of a possible herpes infection of the mouth (HSV-1) or the genital area (HSV-2). Ascertain when the symptoms first occurred.
- Use gloves when inspecting the area because herpes simplex can be infectious.
- Listen to the client's concerns. If the herpes simplex is HSV-2, the client should be encouraged to have her or his sexual partner tested for HSV-2.

Client Teaching

- Inform the pregnant woman that it may be necessary for a cesarean section if the virus is still present at the time of delivery. The health care provider will most likely culture the genital area near the time of birthing.
- Encourage the pregnant client to speak with appropriate health professionals. This helps in alleviating client's fears and making client well-informed.

Heterophile antibody (serum, Mono-Spot)

Reference Values

Adult: Normal, <1.28 titer; abnormal, >1:56 titer.

Child: Same as adult.

Elderly: Normal, slightly higher titer than adult.

Description

This is a test, primarily to check for infectious mononucleosis. Infectious mononucleosis is thought to be caused by the Epstein-Barr virus (EBV).

Heterophiles are a group of antibodies that react to sheep and horse red blood cells; if positive (titer), an agglutination occurs. Titers of 1:56 to 1:224 are highly suspicious of infectious mononucleosis; those of 1:224 or greater are positive for infectious mononucleosis. Elevated heterophile titers occur during the first 2 weeks, peak in 3 weeks, and remain elevated for 6 weeks. Sixty to 80% of persons with infectious mononucleosis have a positive heterophile antibody test.

There are several commercially prepared tests: Monospot by Ortho Diagnostics; Monoscreen by Smith, Kline and Beecham; and Monotest by Wapole. A Mono-Spot test is usually done first; if positive, then the titer test is performed.

Purposes

- To check for an elevated heterophile titer.
- To aid in the diagnosis of infectious mononucleosis.

Clinical Problems

Elevated Level: Infectious mononucleosis, serum sickness, viral infections.

Procedure

Heterophile Antibody
- Collect 3 to 5 ml of venous blood in a red-top tube.
- There is no food or fluid restriction.

Mono-Spot Screening Test: Collect 2 ml of venous blood in a red-top tube. Use a monokit and follow directions. The client's serum is mixed with the guinea pig tissue on one spot of a glass slide, and at another spot on the slide it is mixed with beef red-cell stromata. Unwashed horse red cells are added to both spots. Observe for 1 minute for agglutination. Results of the Mono-Spot test are as follows:

1. If agglutination is stronger at the guinea-pig–kidney-tissue spot, the test is positive for infectious mononucleosis.
2. If agglutination is stronger at the beef red cells, the test is negative for infectious mononucleosis.
3. If agglutination is present at both spots, the test is negative for infectious mononucleosis.
4. If no agglutination is present at either spot, the test is negative.

There is no food or fluid restriction. Usually in infectious mononucleosis the white blood cell differential may show 10% to 25% atypical lymphocytes.

Factors Affecting Laboratory Results

- Serum sickness and Forssman antibodies can cause positive titers.

NURSING IMPLICATIONS WITH RATIONALE

- Explain to the client the procedure for the heterophile antibody test and the Mono-Spot test.
- Obtain a history of the client's contact with any person or persons recently diagnosed as having infectious mononucleosis.
- Observe for signs and symptoms of infectious mononucleosis, such as fever, sore throat, fatigue, swollen glands.
- Determine when the symptoms (fever, fatigue, sore throat) first occurred. A repeat heterophile antibody or Mono-Spot test may be needed if the first was done too early. Elevated titers take 4 to 8 weeks to return to normal.

Client Teaching

- Encourage the client to rest, drink fluids, and follow the health care provider's orders.

Hexosaminidase (total, A, and A and B) (serum, amniotic fluid)

Reference Values

Adult: *Total:* 5–20 U/l. Hexosaminidase A: 55–80%.

Description

Hexosaminidase is a group of enzymes (isoenzymes A and B) responsible for the metabolism of gangliosides. It is found in brain tissue. Lack of the hexosaminidase A causes accumulation of gangliosides in the brain, a condition known as Tay-Sachs disease. The total hexosaminidase may be normal or decreased. This test is used to confirm Tay-Sachs disease or to identify Tay-Sachs carriers.

Tay-Sachs disease is an autosomal-recessive disorder resulting in progressive destruction of the cells of the central nervous system. It is characterized by mental retardation, muscular weakness, and blindness. It affects primarily the Ashkenazic Jewish population. Death usually occurs before the age of 5 years.

Sandhoff's disease, a variant of Tay-Sachs, progresses more rapidly than Tay-Sachs disease. With this disorder there is a deficiency of hexosaminidase A and B. It is not prevalent in any ethnic group.

Purposes

- To diagnose a deficit of hexosaminidase A (Tay-Sachs disease) or hexosaminidase A and B (Sandhoff's disease).
- To identify carriers of Tay-Sachs disease or Sandhoff's disease.

Clinical Problems

Decreased Level: *Hexosaminidase A:* Tay-Sachs disease. *Hexosaminidase A and B:* Sandhoff's disease.

Procedure

- Collect 5 to 7 ml of venous blood in a red-top tube for serum value. Avoid hemolysis.
- Collect cord blood from newborn.
- There is no food or fluid restriction.

Factors Affecting Laboratory Results

- Hemolysis of the blood sample can cause an inaccurate test result.
- Pregnancy could increase total hexosaminidase values. *Note:* Most laboratories will not perform the test on pregnant women.

NURSING IMPLICATIONS WITH RATIONALE

- Talk with the health care provider and genetic counselor when both partners have a hexosaminidase A deficiency. It is important that correct information and answers be given to the couple.

Client Teaching

- Inform the Ashkenazic Jewish couple that the hexosaminidase screening test is to determine if they are Tay-Sachs carriers. Explain to the couple that it is a recessive trait and that both must carry the gene for their offspring to get Tay-Sachs disease.

Human chorionic gonadotropin (HCG) (serum and urine)

Pregnancy Test

Reference Values

Values may be expressed as IU/ml or ng/ml. Check with your laboratory.

Adult: *Serum:* Nonpregnant female: <0.01 IU/ml.

Pregnant (Weeks)	Values
1	0.01–0.04 IU/ml
2	0.03–0.10 IU/ml
4	0.10–1.0 IU/ml
5–12	10–100 IU/ml
13–25	10–30 IU/ml
26–40	5–15 IU/ml

Urine: Nonpregnant: negative; pregnant: 1–12 weeks: 6000–500,000 IU/24 h. Many OTC pregnancy kits available. The woman is usually tested 3 days after missed menstrual period.

Description

Human chorionic gonadotropin (HCG) is a hormone produced by the placenta. In pregnancy HCG appears in the blood and urine 14 to 26 days after the conception, and the HCG concentration peaks in approximately 8 weeks. After the first trimester of pregnancy, HCG production declines. HCG is not found in nonpregnant women, in death of the fetus, or after 3 to 4 days postpartum.

The immunologic test for pregnancy using anti-HCG serum is more sensitive, more accurate, less costly, and easier to perform than the older pregnancy test, which used live animals. The Aschheim-Zondek test and the Friedman test are no longer used.

Certain tumors (such as the hydatidiform mole, chorionepithelioma of the uterus, and choriocarcinoma of the testicle) can cause a positive HCG test. HCG levels may be requested on males for the determination of testicular tumor.

Purposes

- To determine if the client is pregnant.
- To detect a threatened abortion or dead fetus.

Clinical Problems

Decreased Level (Negative): Nonpregnant, dead fetus, postpartum (3 to 4 days), incomplete abortion, threatened abortion (decreased serum value).

Elevated Level (Positive): Pregnancy, hydatidiform mole, chorionepithelioma, choriocarcinoma. *Drug Influence:* Anticonvulsants, hypnotics, tranquilizers (phenothiazines), antiparkinsonism drugs.

Procedure

- Perform the pregnancy test 2 weeks (no earlier than 5 days) after the first missed menstrual period. There are several commercially prepared kits for the immunologic pregnancy test.
- There is no food restriction.

Serum

- Perform the pregnancy test no earlier than 5 days after the first missed menstrual period.
- Collect 3 to 5 ml of venous blood in a red-top tube. Avoid hemolysis.

Urine

- The client should be NPO of fluid for 8 to 12 hours; no food is restricted.
- Take a morning urine specimen (60 ml) with specific gravity >1.010 to the laboratory immediately. A 24-hour urine collection may be requested.
- Instruct the client to follow directions when using a commercial kit.
- Avoid blood in the urine, as false-positive results could occur.

Note: There are many commercial kits; follow the directions on kit.

Factors Affecting Laboratory Results

- Diluted urine (specific gravity <1.010) could cause a false-negative test result.
- Certain drug groups can cause false-positive test results *(see Drug Influence)*.
- Protein and blood in the urine could cause false-positive test results.
- During menopause, there may be an excess secretion of pituitary gonadotropin hormone, which could cause a false-positive result.

NURSING IMPLICATIONS WITH RATIONALE

- Ask the client when she had her last period. The test should be done 5 or more days after the missed period to avoid a false-negative result. Blood in the urine can cause a false-positive result.
- Listen to the client's concerns.

Client Teaching

- Inform the client who plans to use a commercially prepared pregnancy kit to follow the directions carefully.

■ Inform the client that she will receive the results of the test within minutes. Some tests, such as a serum value, may take 1 to 2 hours.

Human immunodeficiency virus type-1 (HIV-1) (serum)*

HIV

Note: The retrovirus designated human immunodeficiency virus-type 2 (HIV-2) differs in genetic structure from HIV-1, but exhibits a pattern of transmission, and causes clinical disease features similar to those of HIV-1; prevalent in Africa, with equal numbers of infected men and women, HIV-2 is generally spread through heterosexual contact as a classic sexually transmitted disease, often concurrent with other genital lesions. HIV-2 cases in the United States are currently more limited; of long-term concern is that the African pattern may, in the future, be duplicated in North America. Use of the term HIV in this section refers to HIV-1 unless otherwise specified.

Reference Values

Antibody Screening: *HIV-1/2 Antibody Screen (ELISA; EIA)*

Adult: Seronegative for antibodies to HIV-1/2; nonreactive.

Child: Seronegative for antibodies to HIV-1/2; nonreactive.

HIV-1 Western Blot, HIV-2 Western Blot (Confirmatory tests that directly detect HIV viral gene proteins)

Adult: Negative.

Child: Negative.

Antigen Screening: *HIV-1 p24 Antigen*

Adult: Negative for p24 antigen of HIV; nonreactive.

Child: Negative for p24 antigen of HIV; nonreactive.

(*Note:* There is no HIV-2 p24 antigen test. Confirmatory test for the HIV-1 p24 antigen is a neutralization.)

Viral Load Tests: (Sensitive assay that measures levels of HIV's ribonucleic acid [RNA] in plasma [to predict disease course]) (Uses polymerase chain reaction [PCR] to amplify HIV RNA.) (Used as marker for basing treatment decisions and evaluating effectiveness of anti-HIV drug therapy [rechecked 4 to 8 weeks after changes in

---

*This test was prepared by Jane Purnell Taylor, RN, MS.

drug therapy as monitoring techniques].) Expressed as the number of copies of HIV RNA in a 1-mL sample of plasma.

Low Numbers: Represents suppressed replication.

High Numbers: Represents increased replication and disease progression.

Description

The retrovirus HIV-1, identified as the cause of acquired immunodeficiency syndrome (AIDS), was first recognized in 1981. However, it is now believed that HIV has existed in human populations for at least 70 years, based on genetic work comparing the genetic composition of many current HIV strains and extrapolation back to a common origin. The infection is expressed along a progressive continuum extending from clinically asymptomatic (although seropositive for HIV-1 antibodies) to expression of a severely damaged (suppressed) immune system (due to T-helper lymphocyte [T4 lymphocyte] destruction) manifested by clinical signs and symptoms, altered laboratory values, and increased susceptibility to AIDS-defining opportunistic infections (including *Pneumocystis carinii* pneumonia, chronic cryptosporidiosis, toxoplasmosis, cryptococcosis, disseminated hisoplasmosis, mycobacterial infection, disseminated cytomegalovirus infection, chronic mucocutaneous or disseminated herpes simplex virus infection, and esophageal, bronchial or pulmonary candidiasis) that rarely cause disease in an immune-competent person, and rarer forms of cancer (including Kaposi's sarcoma and lymphomas [non-Hodgkin lymphoma and primary brain lymphoma]).

The incubation time between HIV infection and the development of HIV-1-related disease is highly individualized. Until recently, it was thought that an initial dormant phase occurred during the early and middle years of the infection. New research now shows that HIV multiplies rapidly, with high viral blood levels developing in the first few weeks of infection. HIV viral antigen may become detectable approximately 2 weeks after infection and lasts for 3 to 5 months. Two to 6 weeks after exposure to HIV, an influenza-type illness (fever, muscle aches, sweating, rash, sore throat, headache, fatigue, swollen lymph nodes) is demonstrable in up to 70 percent of clients. The client recovers, but over a 12-day to 5-year period (most often 6 to 12 weeks) the immune system develops antibodies to the virus (seroconversion). Depending on individual variables, many clients next enter into a symptomless stage of infection that may last up to 8 to 12 years, during which the infection may be unknowingly transmitted. Prevention of transmission is critically important; the recent addition of the HIV-1 p24 antigen test (approved by the FDA in March 1996) may identify HIV infection in a individual within 2 weeks (approximately a week earlier than the anti-HIV-1/2 test), thus narrowing the vulnerable period when the virus may be passed to others while screening tests cannot detect it.

In 1993, the Centers for Disease Control and Prevention (CDC) revised the system by which HIV infection and the definition of AIDS are classified to include the $CD4^+$ T-lymphocyte count as a marker for the degree of immunosuppression related to HIV. This new definition adds to the previous operational definition of

AIDS that included 23 clinical conditions. Now, the definition includes those individuals with pulmonary tuberculosis, recurrent pneumonia (within a 12-month period), and invasive cervical cancer in addition to laboratory confirmation of HIV infection by a $CD4^+$ T-lymphocyte count of $<200/\mu l$ or a $CD4^+$ T-lymphocyte percentage of total lymphocytes of $<14\%$. It is expected that the new working definition will promote earlier diagnosis of those at risk and that treatment modalities will be instituted with close monitoring. New treatment therapies using protease inhibitors (affecting viral reproduction) in combination, and often also including nucleoside, for example, zidovudine, and nonnucleoside, for example, sustiva, reverse transcriptase inhibitors, in early (rather than later) stages of the infection are leading to the hope that HIV may, in the future, be manageable as a chronic disease. Major hurdles to be overcome include development of viral strains resistant to treatment; overwhelmingly expensive drug therapies involving a complex treatment regimen (important to both individuals and the developing countries most afflicted by the AIDS epidemic); product availability; and the ability of the virus to remain hidden (nondetectable) throughout the body (in the brain, testes, lymph nodes) outside the bloodstream.

Although one nonlive attenuated vaccine is undergoing formal trial with volunteers considered at high risk of contracting the HIV virus, no magic-bullet vaccine is expected in the near future. Major difficulty exists due to the continual mutation of HIV-1 into new strains. A national goal, to find a vaccine within 10 years, was established in May 1997, together with creation of an AIDS vaccine research center at The National Institutes of Health. Today, the infection remains preventable, possibly chronically manageable, but not curable. No prognosis is yet forecast for those persons who now exhibit resistant virus; side effects and long-term effects of protease inhibitors are also not fully known.

It is estimated by the Centers for Disease Control and Prevention that as many as 900,000 people in the United States manifested HIV infection, with about 40,000 new infections per year during the 1990s. Through mid-1998, 665,357 have developed AIDS and over 401,028 have died (not specifically from AIDS). AIDS cases represent a reportable condition in the entire United States, District of Columbia, and U.S. Territories. Data reported by local and state health departments are compiled and tracked through a collaborative effort supported by the CDC. However, at issue is whether there should be a move toward conformity among state laws to also require reporting of HIV infection (not just AIDS cases). Approximately 34 states do HIV reporting, which is encouraged by the CDC but opposed by many interest groups on the basis of fear of stigmatization, concerns about privacy, and potential employment discrimination, even though early intervention and treatment is beneficial. States continue to work to develop useful and acceptable coding systems for case reporting.

In the United States, AIDS has become the second leading cause of death for all people ages 25 to 44 as a group (*note:* for men, AIDS is the leading cause; for women, AIDS is the third leading cause; accidents represent the leading cause of death for the total age group collectively). Overall, AIDS incidence decreased 18%

(1996–1997) and 11% (1997–1998). Despite a continued significant decrease in the total number of reported cases, the 1997–1998 data suggest that the hoped-for continued rate of decline in the incidence of AIDS is slowing. The percentage of deaths decreased 42% (1996–1997), dropping to 20% from 1997–1998, while the percentage increase of those living with AIDS by the end of 1998 was 10%, representing 297,137 persons. Estimates are that 1 in 200 young adults in the United States is infected. Women, minorities (Black Americans, Hispanics), and young adults are among the most rapidly escalating groups of affected individuals. As of June 1999, decreases in the number of children diagnosed with AIDS continue; however, the CDC recognizes that, in children, HIV infection status is generally known by 1 year of age with actual onset of AIDS diagnosis possibly delayed by new therapies or not confirmed for an extended period of time. Overall, of the total number of people with HIV, the largest rate of increase is being observed in the heterosexual community. Sexual intercourse is the major cause of infection for women worldwide, rather than other risk factors, such as personal injectable drug abuse. In the United States, however, IV drug use among pregnant women is an important and common risk factor. Women may, however, be involved in relationships in which cultural issues, a perceived imbalance of decision-making power, and/or financial issues affect ability to discuss and hold fast for safer sex. Infected women remain undiagnosed longer than men; thus, women may die earlier because of a lack of early intervention in the disease process. Frequent, severe, and long-lasting vaginal yeast infections (vaginal candidiases) represent an important early clue that HIV infection may be present; in addition, other sexually transmitted diseases may be present together with other gynecologic symptoms/complications (e.g., abnormal Pap tests; incidence of severe pelvic inflammatory disease). Current evidence suggests male-to-female transmission of HIV is more likely based upon anatomic and social factors, including lack of use of barrier-type birth control methods or barrier method failure. It has been found that, in noncondom users, viral load is the greatest predictor of heterosexual HIV transmission. The finding that, in the United States, 8 million individuals under the age of 25 acquire a sexually transmitted disease every year, with 3 million of these being 13 to 19 years of age, is of great concern. National survey data indicate up to 75% of high school students may have had sexual intercourse by the end of 12th grade; only 50% of sexually active high school seniors reported consistent use of a condom, with female high school students reporting lower condom use than males, a finding that reflects lower use by women overall. In addition, should a nonprotected woman become pregnant, the baby of an **untreated** HIV-positive pregnant woman in the United States has a 25.5% chance of being infected before or during birth, or afterward, if breastfed. Perinatal treatment with Zidovudine (antiretroviral drug), and mandatory bottle-feeding have been found to decrease the risk by two-thirds.

Evidence reveals that health care providers in facilities that serve clients at high risk for HIV-1 infection and/or tuberculosis need to maintain a high index of suspicion for the presence of coinfected persons, because progression from latent tuberculosis infection to full-blown tuberculosis disease is more likely when HIV infection is present. HIV-1-seropositive clients should receive a Mantoux tuberculin skin test. Professionals must recall, however, that false-negative skin test reactions (referred to as *anergy*) may occur in those persons who are coinfected. Anergy testing (skin testing using antigens such as tetanus toxoid, mumps, and candida) may be ordered for clients who initially test negative for tuberculosis to determine whether the client is able to react (anergy is the lack of reaction to antigen even though the subject is actually infected with the organism, and increases in the presence of a decreasing CD4$^+$ lymphocyte count). The CDC has determined that latent tuberculosis infection is indicated by an induration at the skin site 5 or more millimeters in diameter in persons who manifest HIV infection. Additional confirmatory studies are then implemented. The goal is to detect latent tuberculosis infection and institute measures to prevent progression to active disease, in addition to protecting others within the environment.

The incidence of positive HIV antibody responses in previously negative health care workers (nurses, physicians, dentists, and laboratory workers) due to acquiring HIV infection while performing occupational responsibilities is statistically low. CDC statistics indicate that, as of December 1999, only 56 documented cases exist, with another 136 possible cases that also involve other risk factors to be considered. Approximately 800,000 needlesticks occur per year using conventional devices. As an outcome of this finding, a national campaign to motivate health care settings to select newer and safer products (particularly protected or needleless equipment) was initiated in 1996. On the federal level, health care workers' needlestick prevention legislation was recently passed that will require protective equipment for needle systems. Exposure of most health care workers to HIV-1 infection is preventable through use of *standard precautions (see Nursing Implications with Rationale)*.

Child-to-child transmission of HIV-1 infection in school and day care settings is rare as 1985 guidelines established through the CDC in regard to infected children remain effective. School-age children are free to participate in unrestricted environments unless personal risk of newly acquired infection exists. Preschool/handicapped children require supervised environments for protection of self and others, especially if lack of body fluid control, biting problems, and/or open, oozing lesions exist. Within day care settings, routine cleaning with disinfectant, use of disposable towels and tissues, hand-washing and glove use by caretakers having hand lesions is sufficient. The potential for transmission of HIV-1 via saliva appears minimal unless the saliva is blood-contaminated (as is more likely in a dental care setting).

Worldwide, the World Health Organization (WHO) estimated that 40 million may exhibit HIV/AIDS by the year 2000, including 10 million HIV-infected infants and children. Approximately 90% of new cases occur in individuals who live in the developing world, including Southeast Asia and Sub-Saharan Africa, with United Nations estimates of the total number currently infected at 22.6 million, over 7.7 million of whom exhibit symptoms of AIDS. The global death toll due to AIDS was 2.6 million in 1998 (85% of these occurred in Africa). By the end of 2000, the number of orphaned African children under age 15 who will have lost 1 or both parents to AIDS is expected to be over 10 million. The pandemic will be stopped only through a reexamination of culture (including gender and sexual customs) and implementation of major prevention strategies. The United Nations estimates that approximately 700,000 cases of HIV exist in eastern Europe and Central Asia—largely among drug users who inject.

Although the HIV-1 virus has been isolated from blood, semen, saliva, vaginal secretions, breast milk, tears, cerebrospinal fluid, amniotic fluid, and urine, actual transmission occurs via infected lymphocytes carried by blood, semen, vaginal secretions, and breast milk. Those *at risk* for acquiring HIV infection include noninfected persons who have unprotected direct sexual contact (vaginal, oral, or rectal) with an infected person of either sex; those with multiple partners; homosexual and bisexual men; persons with hemophilia or related clotting disorders who have received clotting factor concentrates; other recipients of infected blood or blood products (particularly prior to 1985); persons who have had, or have been treated for, syphilis or gonorrhea during the past 12 months; persons who have had a positive screening test for syphilis in the past 12 months without a negative confirmatory test; persons who have been in jail within the past 12 months; those who share infected needles with others as a component of illicit IV drug use; persons who subsequently have sexual contact with someone included in one or more of these groups; and fetuses or neonates exposed to an infected mother during the perinatal period (possibly secondary to maternal IV drug use or maternal heterosexual contact with an IV drug user).

Prevention: Prevention of HIV-1 infection through control of risk-behavior is the only guaranteed effective intervention known. There is no vaccine, intervention, or treatment known to be curative for HIV infection, including use of antiretroviral drugs in combination to lower virus load. Thus, in adults, individual variations may occur in clinical course once AIDS is diagnosed. HIV-infected children have a clinical course which often progresses faster than adults. Today, children with HIV and AIDS are treated with medication and live longer due to therapy, advances, and more reliable and earlier diagnosis. Rate of disease progression is related to viral load more than to when diagnosis was made. Currently, only a minority of children infected through vertical transmission (perinatal transmission) survive beyond 8. In general, antiretroviral therapy is suggested for those persons whose $CD4^+$ T-lymphocyte count is $<500/mm^3$ and prophylaxis for *Pneumocystis carinii* pneumonia is suggested for those with $CD4^+$ T-lymphocyte counts of <200 mm^3.

In August 1993, the CDC acknowledged, based on two solid European studies, that there is evidence that the best (100%) preventive strategy for HIV-1 infection is to avoid intercourse (i.e., practice abstinence) with an infected or unknown partner; however, if intercourse is elected, use of a latex condom is considered a highly effective mechanical barrier to HIV transmission *provided* the latex condom is *consistently and correctly* used (see *Nursing Implications,* below).

Screening of blood products by blood banks in the United States was instituted in 1985 using the enzyme-linked immunosorbent assay (ELISA). Blood banks are required to test donors for antibodies to HIV-1 and -2. Blood banks have also implemented six additional infectious disease tests to ensure safety of the blood reaching hospitals nationally. In March 1996, the FDA-approved HIV-1 p24 antigen test was added to help identify infection earlier (because a person can be infected and have a negative antibody test). Screening of donors and public education have also been enhanced to assure the public concerning blood safety. All blood that tests positive is destroyed. Donors notified of confirmed positive test results are included on a permanent deferral list and asked not to donate in the future. Nationally, the safety record is positive; over 37 million people have received transfusions since 1985, with 38 documented cases of AIDS from that blood. From 1981 through 1998 (reflecting both pre- and post-1985, when screening requirements were implemented), 8,382 cases have been documented, including those who have received transfusions, organs, and donations of tissue and sperm, collectively.

Purposes

- To detect the presence of antibodies to HIV.
- To identify HIV-infected individuals early in the course of the illness in the hope of allowing these persons to benefit from medical intervention.
- To prompt tested individuals (both negative and positive) to reflect upon behaviors of risk to themselves and others that may be changed as an outcome of the counseling process associated with testing.
- To continue to safeguard the available blood supply.

Clinical Problems and Factors Affecting Laboratory Results

Seropositive Test: Blood shows evidence of infection; blood test detects antibodies to HIV-1/2; or viral antigen is detected (p24 antigen of HIV). Recall that a positive test indicative of HIV infection does not diagnose AIDS (which is defined as a clinical diagnosis with defining characteristics). HIV infection is expressed on a continuum from seropositive asymptomatic infection to disease expression. *Note:* Diagnosing HIV infection in children born to HIV-infected mothers is complicated by maternal antibodies that transplacentally affect the fetus, giving a positive HIV antibody result at birth (although only 15% to 30% are truly infected); the antibody usually becomes undetectable by 9 months of age (occasionally as late as 18 months). Thus, standard antibody tests are not reliable, and polymerase chain reaction (PCR) and virus culture are the most specific and sensitive means for detection of infection in children whose mothers are infected. These additional tests can identify 30% to 50% of infected infants at the time of birth and, by 3 to 6 months of age, close to 100%.

Procedure

- A signed consent form for the HIV-1/2 antibody screen is usually required and should include appropriate pre- and postcounseling.
- Collect 5 to 10 ml of venous blood in a red-top tube.
- No food or fluid restriction is required.

Two tests are most commonly employed for HIV-1/2 antibody screening (not for the virus itself). These include enzyme-linked immunosorbent assay (ELISA) and

EIA (enzyme immunoassay). ELISA testing is reliable, specific, and highly sensitive. When a first positive HIV-1 test result occurs, the test is generally repeated twice on the same sample; if two out of three of these tests are positive, an HIV-1 Western Blot and an HIV-2 antibody screen are performed. If the HIV-2 antibody screen is positive, an HIV-2 Western Blot is performed. A second quickly performed confirmatory test commonly used is the IFA (immunofluorescence assay); it is slightly less reliable than the Western Blot. Collectively, when the ELISA plus Western Blot show a persistently positive outcome, the specificity and sensitivity rates are both 99% and the accuracy rate is 99%. False-positive Western Blot results in low-risk populations are possible but less likely than with ELISA. False positive results may require retesting using an alternate laboratory; false-negative results are usually noted when testing is done prior to seroconversion.

When screening is for the HIV-1 p24 antigen, if the client tests positive (reactive) for the antigen the test is repeated twice more on the same sample. A separate confirmatory test (called a *neutralization*) may be performed. If a client tests positive for the antigen but does not neutralize, both an antibody and an antigen test may be redone in approximately 4 weeks; at 8 weeks, just an antibody test may be done. It must be recalled that the HIV-1 p24 antigen is generally undetectable during the asymptomatic phase.

NURSING IMPLICATIONS WITH RATIONALE

- Observe client affect and listen carefully to the client's communication (pattern and content) in regard to HIV/AIDS.
- Recognize the role of education as a highly effective preventive strategy.
- Ascertain the purpose of being tested for each person screened and assess the risk potential for HIV using information provided.
- Obtain a signed consent form from the client for the HIV antibody test and/or antigen screening test.
- Provide clients being screened for HIV antibody or antigen with comprehensive pretest counseling, protection for confidential information obtained, consistently accurate and comprehensive posttest education, support while waiting for test results, and follow-up support and referral as needed.
- Become knowledgeable about commercially available HIV home blood test kits in order to be able to accurately provide advice for clients who may elect initial self-testing and experience a variety of positive and negative issues as an outcome of this choice.
- Compile an accurate/current list of health professionals and resources (phone numbers/addresses) for referral purposes when needed.
- Develop a full knowledge of HIV infection and AIDS-related diseases in order to adequately address actual and potential client concerns in the role of nurse educator.
- Be prepared to clearly explain and clarify meaning of test results for clients who may be experiencing situational crisis associated with the testing process and/or outcome.

- Implement *standard precautions,* which combine the major features of universal (blood and body fluid) precautions (designed to reduce risk of bloodborne pathogen transmission) and body substance isolation (designed to reduce the risk of transmission of pathogens from moist body substances), and apply them to all clients regardless of diagnosis or presumed infection status; these precautions apply to blood, all body fluids, secretions, and excretions (except sweat) regardless of whether visible blood or nonintact skin or mucous membranes is present. The outcome hoped for is that most clients will feel equally treated.

- Protective measures derived from standard precautions include:

  1. Proper handwashing and use of intact latex gloves (preferred to vinyl gloves) prior to invasive procedures and potential contact with blood, body fluids, secretions, excretions, and contaminated items (directly or indirectly); wash hands after glove removal and between same client tasks.

  2. Use of protective masks, full-face shields, and/or eye protection with side pieces during procedures/client care activities likely to generate splashes or sprays of blood, body fluids, secretions, or excretions.

  3. Impervious gowns or aprons, knee-high boots in conditions where splashes or sprays may occur (e.g., surgical or labor and delivery suite); prompt removal of soiled gowns.

  4. Proper disposal of soiled linens in leak-proof bags to prevent skin and mucous membrane exposure and clothing contamination.

  5. Proper handling of tubes, needles, and sharps (no recapping, bending, or separating of needle from disposable syringes); disposal in puncture-free containers in every room, at bedside if possible (only to fill-line); proper clean-up of spills; temporary abstinence from direct client care if caretaker's skin is not intact.

  6. Carry one pair of nonsterile latex gloves in your pocket in case of sudden need to intervene in a risky situation. Place gloves in a puncture-proof pocket container.

  7. Use mouthpieces, resuscitation bags, or other ventilation devices in lieu of mouth-to-mouth methods.

- In obstetric settings, gloves should be worn whenever handling placentas; also when handling newborns who have not had initial baths; when changing diapers, obtaining urine or fecal samples and during suctioning; also when performing heelsticks for blood glucose determination and during Vitamin K administration.

- Request and use tightly fitting collection containers for all laboratory specimens involving blood and body fluids, and place containers into plastic cover bags for safe handling and transport.

- Encourage clients with HIV/AIDS to identify persons with whom they have had sexual contact. At times, clients will tell the nurse names of partners before they tell the health care provider.

- Be nonjudgmental with HIV/AIDS clients and their families with regard to how the illness may have been acquired.
- Monitor laboratory reports for indication of decreasing CD4$^+$ T-lymphocyte cell counts; inform the health care provider.
- Assess for signs and symptoms related to clinical progression toward a depressed immune system, including profound involuntary weight loss, chronic diarrhea, chronic weakness, and intermittent or constant fever.
- Recognize that infants born to HIV/AIDS-infected mothers will exhibit and maintain a positive HIV antibody response (reflecting maternal antibodies) for up to 18 months of age. However, only 15% to 30% are truly infected. Those who do become infected become symptomatic more quickly than adults and may have a decreased survival period. Many children (both infected and noninfected) may by orphaned, if mothers die, necessitating interdisciplinary planning for the family.
- Screen women clients for the presence of frequent vaginal yeast infections.
- Recognize actual and/or at-risk clients for HIV/AIDS. HIV-infected clients should be screened for the presence of coinfection with tuberculosis. Anergy testing may be necessary. Help the client understand the process involved; interpret findings from the PPD test.
- Review client records for adequate immunization status; recognize that HIV-infected clients are also high-risk for coinfection with hepatitis B virus. Screen client records for documentation of hepatitis B vaccine; inform the health care provider of findings; tetanus booster should be current within 10 years; documentation should show receipt of annual flu shot and a single dose of pneumococcal vaccine.
- Be prepared to address anxiety and fear reactions about HIV/AIDS within the public sector.
- Be prepared to address discussions and concerns related to perceived ethical issues related to HIV/AIDS (e.g., voluntary versus mandatory testing for clients and health care workers, reporting outcomes related to confidentiality issues, sex education in the schools, condom distribution programs, and needle exchange programs, among others).
- Include designated care partner and/or family system when identifying stressors and planning and implementing supportive nursing strategies.
- Plan for and provide stress management for health care personnel who work for extended periods of time with clients who experience HIV/AIDS.
- Become knowledgeable concerning institutional policies in compliance with CDC guidelines and the OSHA Bloodborne Pathogen Standard concerning needlestick/penetrating injuries and blood or secretion splash incidents.

Client Teaching

- Provide clients with an overview about HIV and the testing available for antibodies.

- Explain to the client that, if a first HIV test indicates a positive response, a repeat test and confirmatory tests will need to be made prior to reaching any conclusions.
- Explain to the client that a confirmed positive HIV antibody test indicates exposure to HIV that has stimulated an immune system response; the person is infected and able to transmit the infection. Explain that a negative test is not a guarantee that infection has not occurred; variables include the time frame in relation to exposure and when the test is done. For both outcomes, plan strategies with the client to ensure risk reduction related to HIV for both self and others; include relationship and sexual boundary setting as part of the discussion.
- Discuss the meaning of test results for the client's desired or planned life events (e.g., sexual contact, marriage, childbearing, breastfeeding). Refer the client to other health professionals as necessary. Provide the National AIDS Hotline phone number (1–800–342–AIDS) (1–800–342–2437); if needed, suggest Spanish AIDS Hotline (1–800–342–SIDA); Hearing Impaired AIDS Hotline (TDD Service; 1–800–243–7889). Provide these Internet Web sites: American Social Health Association (*www.ashastd.org*) and Centers for Disease Control (*www.cdc.gov/HIV*).
- Explain that there is no definitive cure for HIV/AIDS; however, well-being and survival is affected through early intervention strategies, including early diagnosis and the use of combination drug therapy.
- Stress elimination of substance abuse and to expose oneself to only low-risk sexual behavior as a preventive strategy; explain that sexual abstinence is 100% effective prevention, particularly in regard to infected or unknown partners. Discuss mechanical barrier (latex condom) use with both male and female clients. Stress that, if intercourse is elected, latex condoms should be consistently and correctly used following these guidelines:

   1. Store latex condoms unopened in a safe place not exposed to heat, pressure, or potential puncture.
   2. Use a new latex condom for each act of intercourse; check the expiration date on the package.
   3. Put the condom on before any sexual contact.
   4. Check the condom to be certain no air is trapped inside.
   5. Use only water-based lubricants (oil-based lubricants will quickly dissolve the condom).
   6. Immediately withdraw the penis after sex, holding the condom to prevent slippage.

- If oral sex is a chosen sexual practice, inform the client that dental dams and female condoms are available (e.g., Reality Female Condom). Explain that barrier protection reduces risk somewhat, especially if menstrual blood is present. Unlubricated condoms are available in assorted colors and flavors to use for fellatio.
- If anal sexual activities are engaged in by clients of either sex with same or opposite sex partners, mention that the polyurethane female condom (Reality) is

stronger than latex condoms and might be considered. Stress that a new Reality condom should be used for sex with multiple partners.

■ Inform women clients to seek gynecologic evaluation if an infection is persistent and/or unresponsive to nonprescription treatment (e.g., Monistat–7 and/or Gyne-Lotrimin). Teach clients to wear cotton underwear and avoid douching. Tell clients to not douche prior to a gynecologic examination because PAP tests and specimen quality may be adversely affected.

■ Counsel clients who are contemplating elective surgery with fears about potential blood transfusions to discuss autologous transfusion with their health care provider.

■ Explain to members of the community that casual contact with a person with HIV/AIDS does not put them at high risk for contracting HIV/AIDS. Intimate sexual contract (oral, genital, rectal) with a person with HIV/AIDS puts the individual at high risk.

■ Address anxiety and fear reactions about HIV/AIDS within the public sector. Stress that HIV/AIDS is not spread by insect bites, coughs, sneezes, talking to, shaking hands with, sharing glasses with, embracing, sharing spoons with, or sharing a household with an HIV/AIDS-infected client. Stress that there is only one documented case that involved deep kissing; however, gum bleeding was a known factor for both of the persons involved; saliva is considered low risk because of its being low in lymphocytes.

■ Encourage childbearing-age women to voluntarily and routinely be tested for their HIV status to assist with childbearing decisions and allow for early intervention with any subsequent offspring.

■ Explain to HIV-positive pregnant clients that the American College of Obstetricians and Gynecologists (ACOG) currently recommends (effective July 1999) that all HIV-positive pregnant women should be offered scheduled C-section deliveries at 38 weeks' gestation to decrease the risk of transmission to the newborn; also that HIV risk to the infant can be further reduced to approximately 2% when a combination of a scheduled C-section plus treatment with ZDV (Zidovudine) is employed (as compared with a 25% risk when untreated vaginal delivery is elected).

■ Inform infected pregnant women that internal fetal monitoring will not be used during labor (to maintain fetal skin integrity and prevent exposure to potentially bloody amniotic fluid).

■ Explain that breastfeeding is permitted if a client is initially negative and remains so at the time of delivery; breastfeeding is not initiated when the mother is untested for HIV or determined to be positive, because breast milk contains HIV-infected lymphocytes, colostrum has high concentrations, and maternal nipples may become sore and crack, with potential HIV exposure for the neonate.

■ Inform families that HIV-infected infants and children will need to receive all routine immunizations *except* oral polio vaccine. Only injectable killed polio vaccine should be given. These babies should also receive flu shots (if 6 months of age or older) in the fall of the year. Non-infected children who live with HIV-positive persons should also receive flu injection, and Hepatitis B vaccine should be given employing standard vaccination guidelines.

- Discuss with client the need to have a tetanus booster that is current within 10 years; also, the client should be instructed to receive an annual flu shot and a single dose of pneumococcal vaccine.
- Encourage low-risk healthy individuals to donate blood because sterile needles are used and are discarded with no risk of infection. The donor does not have contact with other blood.
- Advise clients not to use the toothbrushes or razors of high risk or HIV/AIDS infected clients because of the possibility of blood contamination; women should be taught to safely dispose of menstrual blood-containing products.

Human leukocyte antigen (HLA) (serum)

HLA Typing, Organ-Donor Tissue Typing

Reference Values

Histocompatibility match or nonmatch; no norms.

Description

Nucleated cells, including leukocytes, platelets, and many tissue cells, have antigens of the human leukocyte antigen (HLA) system on their surface membranes. These antigens are classified into five different series: A, B, C, D, and DR (D-related). There are many groups of these five series (20 A antigens, 40 B antigens, 8 C antigens, 12 D antigens, and 10 DR antigens) that can be HLA phenotyped to determine histocompatibility.

Testing for HLA antigens is useful in determining tissue typing for recipients and donors for organ transplants, paternity testing, and genetic counseling associated with susceptibility to certain diseases. A putative father who does not have any antigen pair identical to one of the child's is excluded as the father.

Purposes

- To screen for histocompatibilty in tissue typing.
- To determine paternity of the child.

Clinical Problems

Positive Histocompatibility: Tissue compatibility for grafts and organ transplants, father of child.

Procedure

- Collect 5 to 7 ml of venous blood in a green-top tube. Avoid hemolysis. Blood samples should be tested immediately.
- There is no food or fluid restriction.

Factors Affecting Laboratory Results

- Hemolysis of the blood sample.
- Blood transfusion in the last 3 days could affect test results.

NURSING IMPLICATIONS WITH RATIONALE

- Encourage the client to express concerns related to health problems.

Human placental lactogen (hPL) (serum)

Chorionic Somatomammotropin

Reference Values

Adult: *Nonpregnant Female:* <0.5 µg/ml.

Pregnant Female:

Weeks of Gestation	Reference Values
5–7	1.0 µg/ml
8–27	<4.6 µg/ml
28–31	2.4–6.0 µg/ml
32–35	3.7–7.7 µg/ml
36–term	5.0–10.0 µg/ml

Male: <0.5 µg/ml.

Description

Human placental lactogen (hPL), a hormone produced by the placenta, can be detected in the maternal blood after 5 weeks of gestation. The hPL increases slowly throughout the pregnancy. This test is useful for evaluating placental function and fetal well-being in high-risk pregnancies, especially from the 28th week to term. A marked decrease in the serum hPL level during the third trimester of pregnancy is indicative of fetal distress; however, additional testing is recommended to determine fetal distress. A serum estriol and nonstress test are frequently ordered to verify the hPL test result.

Purposes

- To evaluate placental function.
- To determine fetal well-being after the 28th week to term.

Clinical Problems

Decreased Level: Fetal distress, toxemia of pregnancy, threatened-abortion, trophoblastic neoplastic disease (hydatidiform mole, choriocarcinoma).

Elevated Level: Multiple pregnancy, diabetes mellitus, bronchogenic carcinoma, liver tumor, lymphoma.

Procedure

- Collect 5 to 7 ml of venous blood in a red-top or green-top tube. Avoid hemolysis.
- The hPL level fluctuates; therefore the test might need to be repeated.
- There is no food or fluid restriction.

Factors Affecting Laboratory Results

- Hemolysis of the blood sample.

NURSING IMPLICATIONS WITH RATIONALE

- Record the gestation week on the laboratory slip.
- Correlate the serum hPL result with the serum or urine estriol level. The human placental lactogen levels can fluctuate daily, so the hPL test is usually repeated, and other tests for detecting fetal distress are also ordered.

Client Teaching

- Inform the client that the test may be repeated because of frequent hPL fluctuations. Explain that other tests are usually ordered to monitor the fetal well-being.

Hydroxybutyric dehydrogenase (HBD) (serum)

Hydroxybutyrate Dehydrogenase (HBDH),
Alpha-Hydroxybutyric Dehydrogenase

Reference Values

140–350 IU/l, 114–290 U/l. Ratio LD to HBD: from 1.2 to 1, to 1.5 to 1.

Description

Hydroxybutyric dehydrogenase (HBD) enzyme is similar to the isoenzyme of lactate dehydrogenase, LD_1. HBD is found primarily in the heart muscle but also can be found in the brain and kidneys. This test is conducted to diagnose a myocardial infarction (MI). Frequently it is used as a substitute for LD electrophoresis, which is a more costly test. Also, HBD levels are sustained longer than aspartate aminotransferase, creatine phosphokinase, and LD levels. HBD levels rise 8 to 10 hours following an MI, peak in 2 to 4 days, and can remain elevated up to 18 days. Liver disease can complicate the use of HBD for diagnosing MI because an elevated LD_5 (liver) isoenzyme can cause an elevated HBD level. If there is a history of liver disease, then LD electrophoresis (identifying LD isoenzymes) should be used instead of HBD.

HBD is a useful test for aiding in the diagnosis of MI, mainly because other cardiac enzymes return to baseline sooner than HBD. However, HBD should not be the only test used for diagnosing MI, and it usually is not the first group of laboratory tests used for diagnosing an acute MI.

Purposes

- To aid in the diagnosis of an MI, especially a latent MI, when other cardiac enzymes do not show an increase.
- To monitor cardiac enzyme activity when LD electrophoresis is unavailable or too expensive to monitor.

Clinical Problems

Elevated Level: Myocardial infarction (MI), liver disease, nephrotic syndrome, leukemia, lymphomas, anemias (hemolytic or megaloblastic).

Procedure

- There is no food or fluid restriction.
- Collect 5 to 7 ml of venous blood in a red-top tube. A gray-top tube may also be used. Avoid hemolysis caused by rough handling. Send the specimen immediately to the laboratory.

- Do not freeze blood specimen; enzyme activity is lost during freezing. The specimen could be refrigerated but the temperature should not be below 0°C, or 32°F.

Factors Affecting Laboratory Results

- Hemolysis of the blood specimen could cause a false elevation in the HBD level.
- Frozen blood specimen.
- Delay in taking the blood sample to the laboratory.

NURSING IMPLICATIONS WITH RATIONALE

- Obtain a history of the health problem.
- Monitor vital signs and electrocardiogram. Report abnormal findings to the health care provider.
- Monitor cardiac enzyme levels. Report abnormal levels to the health care provider.
- Provide comfort measures for the client.
- Encourage the client to report immediately chest discomfort/pain or shortness of breath.

17-hydroxycorticosteroids (17-OHCS) (urine)

Corticoids 17-OH, Porter-Silber Chromogens

Reference Values

Adult: *Male:* 3–12 mg/24 h. *Female:* 2–10 mg/24 h. Average 2–12 mg/24 h.

Elderly: Lower than adult.

Child: *Infant to 1 year:* <1 mg/24 h. *2 to 4 years:* 1–2 mg/24 h. *5 to 12 years:* 2–6 mg/24 h.

Description

17-OHCS are metabolites of adrenocortical steroid hormones, mostly of cortisol, and are excreted in the urine. Because the excretion of the metabolites is diurnal, varying in rate of excretion, a 24-hour urine specimen is necessary for accuracy of test results. This test is useful for assessing adrenocortical hormone function. An increased urinary concentration of 17-OHCS may indicate hyperadrenalism, and a decreased urinary concentration may indicate hypoadrenalism.

Purposes

- To assess adrenocortical hormone function.
- To detect disorders caused by deficit or excess of adrenocortical hormone.

Clinical Problems

Decreased Level: Addison's disease, adrogenital syndrome, hypopituitarism, myxedema (hypothroidism). *Drug Influence:* Calcium gluconate, dexamethasone (Decadron), phenytoin (Dilantin), promethazine (Phenergan), reserpine (Serpasil).

Elevated Level: Cushing's syndrome, adrenal cancer, eclampsia, hyperpituitarism, hyperthyroidism, extreme stress. *Drug Influence:* Antibiotics (cloxacillin, erythromycin), acetazolamide (Diamox), ascorbic acid, chloral hydrate, chlordiazepoxide (Librium), chlorothiazide (Diuril), chlorpromazine (Thorazine), colchicine, cortisone, digoxin, digitoxin, estrogen, hydroxyzine (Atarax), iodides, oral contraceptives, meprobamate (Equanil or Miltown), methenamine (Urex), paraldehyde, quinine, quinidine, spironolactone (Aldactone).

Procedure

- Collect urine in a large container/bottle, and add an acid preservative to prevent bacterial degradation of the steroids. The urine collection should be refrigerated if no preservative is added. No toilet paper or feces should be in the urine.
- Label container with client's name, date, and exact time of collection (e.g., 9/23/04, 7:20 AM to 9/24/04, 7:30 AM).
- Withhold drugs (with health care provider's approval) for 3 days before the test to prevent false results. Any drugs given should be listed on the laboratory slip.
- No food or fluid is restricted, except for coffee and tea. Fluid intake should be encouraged.

Factors Affecting Laboratory Results

- Drugs *(see Drug Influence)*. Cortisone can elevate the urinary levels of 17-OHCS, and dexamethasone (Decadron), a potent cortisone derivative, can decrease the 17-OHCS level. The potent cortisone drug inhibits ACTH production, which causes a decrease in adrenocortical hormone secretion.
- If the 24-hour urine sample is not refrigerated or does not contain a preservative, the results of the test could be inaccurate.

NURSING IMPLICATIONS WITH RATIONALE

- Encourage the client to drink six to eight glasses of water or other fluid (except coffee) during the 24-hour test.
- Check the drugs the client is receiving, and withhold drugs (with the health care provider's permission) that may interfere with test results. Many times, medication cannot be withheld; in such cases, the drugs given should be listed on the laboratory slip and reported.

- Explain to the client and family that all urine should be saved during a 24-hour period and that there should be no toilet paper or feces in the urine.
- Label the urine bottle with the client's name and the date and exact time for the urine collection (e.g., 11/3/04, 7:20 AM to 11/4/04, 7:22 AM).
- Post a notice of urine collection on the client's door or bed and in the Kardex.
- Check the results of the plasma cortisol and 17-ketosteroids tests.

Decreased Level

- Observe for signs and symptoms of hypoadrenalism (Addison's disease). These symptoms include fatigue, weakness, weight loss, bronze coloration of the skin, postural hypotension, arrhythmia, craving of salty food, and fasting hypoglycemia. Report your findings to the health care provider.

Elevated Level

- Observe for signs and symptoms of hyperadrenalism (Cushing's syndrome). These symptoms include fluid retention, "moon face," hirsutism, "buffalo hump," hypertension, hyperglycemia, petechiae, and ecchymosis. Report your findings to the health care provider.

5-Hydroxyindoleacetic acid (5-HIAA) (urine)

5-OH-Indoleacetic Acid, Serotonin Metabolite

Reference Values

Adult: *Qualitative Random Samples:* Negative. *Quantitative 24 Hours:* 2–10 mg/24 h.

Child: Not usually done—results would be similar to adult results.

Description

5-Hydroxyindoleacetic acid (5-HIAA), a metabolite of serotonin, is excreted in the urine as the result of carcinoid tumors found in the appendix or in the intestinal wall. Serotonin is a vasoconstricting hormone secreted by the argentaffin cells of the gastrointestinal tract and is responsible for peristalsis. Carcinoid tumor cells, which secrete excess serotonin, are of low-grade malignancy. Early removal of this type of tumor ensures an 80 to 90% chance of cure. There have been reports of some noncarcinoid tumors producing high levels of 5-HIAA.

Certain foods may elevate the 5-HIAA urinary levels, and certain drugs may elevate or decrease the 5-HIAA urinary levels. More than one random sample of urine for the 5-HIAA test may be needed to avoid false-positive or false-negative results. The 24-hour urine test usually follows the random urine screening test.

Purposes

- To confirm carcinoid tumor of the intestine.
- To compare with other laboratory tests for confirmation of carcinoid tumor.

Clinical Problems

Decreased Level: *Drug Influence* (depresses 5-HIAA): ACTH, heparin, imipramine (Tofranil), isoniazid (INH), MAO inhibitors, methyldopa (Aldomet), phenothiazines (chlorpromazine [Thorazine]), promethazine (Phenergan).

Elevated Level: Carcinoid tumors of the appendix and intestine, carcinoid tumor with metastasis (>100 mg/24 h), sciatica pain (severe), skeletal and smooth muscle spasm. *Drug Influence:* Acetophenetidin (Phenacetin), glyceryl guaiacolate, methamphetamine (Methampex or Desoxyn), reserpine (Serpasil). *Foods:* Bananas, pineapple, avocados, plums, eggplant, walnuts.

Procedure

- Eliminate the foods and drugs listed above for 3 days before the test, if possible.

Qualitative Random Urine Sample (for screening purposes): Collect a random urine sample and take it to the laboratory. If the urine sample is not tested immediately, it should be refrigerated. Collection of a random urine sample may need to be repeated to verify the results. The random urine screening test is usually done first, and if the test is positive, a 24-hour urine test for 5-HIAA is ordered.

Quantitative 24-Hour Urine Collection: Collect urine for 24 hours in a large container with a preservative. Some laboratories require no preservative, but the urine should be refrigerated during the 24-hour collection time. Label the bottle and laboratory slip with the client's name and the date and exact times of the urine collection (e.g., 6/24/04, 7:00 AM to 6/25/04, 7:00 AM).

- Foods (except for those listed) and fluids are not restricted.

Factors Affecting Laboratory Results

- Foods *(see Foods)*.
- Drugs *(see Drug Influence)*.
- A 24-hour urine sample that does not have a preservative and/or has not been refrigerated. (Check with the laboratory about the urine preservative and refrigeration.)

NURSING IMPLICATIONS WITH RATIONALE

- Instruct the client not to eat bananas, pineapple, avocados, plums, eggplant, or walnuts for 3 days before the test. Foods and fluid other than those mentioned are permitted before and during the test.

- Instruct the client and family not to throw away any urine during the 24-hour collection time. Instruct the client not to discard toilet paper or feces in the urine.
- Inform the heath care provider (HCP) of any drugs the client is taking that could cause a false-positive or false-negative result. These drugs should not be taken for 3 days before the test, if possible; if they are, the names of the drugs should be listed on the laboratory slip and recorded in the client's chart.
- Check the 5-HIAA result of the random sample urine test and inform the HCP if the result is unknown. A repeat test may be needed if the client has taken drugs that can depress the 5-HIAA or if the test is negative. If the urine test is positive, the HCP may order the 5-HIAA 24-hour urine test.

Hydroxyproline (urine)

Reference Values

Adult >40 Years Old: 15–42 mg/24 h; 115–310 µmol/24 h; 0.4–4.5 mg/2 h; 3–38 µmol/2.

Child 11–18 Years Old: Much higher than adults.

Description

Hydroxyproline, an amino acid found in collagen, is increased during bone growth and bone disease. Collagen is a component of bone, cartilage, and skin. Urine hydroxyproline levels increase when there is collagen breakdown, as in bone destruction. Levels of hydroxyproline are higher during the night, in teenagers, and during the third trimester of pregnancy.

Urine excretion of hydroxyproline is an effective test for monitoring the progress of Paget's disease (bone lesions, mainly of the long bones). Hydroxyproline levels decrease during treatment therapy for bone disorders.

Purposes

- To aid in the detection of bone disorders.
- To monitor the effect of treatment for bone disorders.

Clinical Problems

Decreased Level: Malnutrition, hypopituitarism, hypoparathyroidism. *Drug Influence:* Aspirin, ascorbic acid, glucocorticoids, calcitonin, plicamycin.

Elevated Level: Paget's disease, metastatic bone tumor, osteoporosis, bone growth, acromegaly.

Procedure

- Food and fluids are restricted for 8 to 12 hours before the 2-hour hydroxyproline test.
- The client should avoid meat, poultry, fish, jelly, and gelatin for 24 to 48 hours prior to the test.
- Collect a 2-hour or 24-hour urine specimen. A preservative is usually added to prevent degradation of hydroxyproline.
- Label the specimen with the client's sex and age and the exact time of urine collection.
- Keep the urine container refrigerated, and take it to the laboratory immediately following the specified urine collection time.

Factors Affecting Laboratory Results

- Drug influence *(see Clinical Problems)*, decreased level.
- Meats and gelatin can cause false-positive test results.
- Faulty collection of urine specimen (e.g., not refrigerating the urine container).

NURSING IMPLICATIONS WITH RATIONALE

- Obtain a health and drug history. Record drugs the client is taking. If the client is receiving drugs to control bone disorder (e.g., Paget's disease), the urine hydroxyproline level is expected to be lower.
- Provide comfort (i.e., position changes, pain medication) to alleviate pain.
- Be supportive of the client and family. Answer questions or refer the question to other health care providers.

Client Teaching

- Instruct the client to avoid meats and gelatin products for 24 to 48 hours prior to the test because these foods can increase urine hydroxyproline levels. If the client consumes these foods prior to the test, it should be noted on the laboratory slip and health care providers informed.
- Explain the procedure of urine collection to the client. Inform the client that the urine container should be refrigerated. If any of the urine is discarded accidently, the test should be restarted the next day.

Immunoglobulins (Ig) (serum)

IgG, IgA, IgM, IgD, IgE

Reference Values

	Total Ig (99%; mg/dl)	IgG (80%; mg/dl)	IgA (15%; mg/dl)	IgM (4%; mg/dl)	IgD (0.2%; mg/dl)	IgE (0.0002% U/ml)
Adult	900–2,200	650–1,700	70–400	40–350	0–8	<40
						(IgE 0–120 mg/dl)
6–16 yr	800–1,700	700–1,650	80–230	45–260		<62
4–6 yr	700–1,700	550–1,500	50–175	22–100		<25
1–3 yr	400–1,500	300–1,400	20–150	40–230		<10
6 mo	225–1,200	200–1,100	10–90	10–80		
3 mo	325–750	275–750	5–55	15–70		
Newborn	650–1,450	700–1,480	0–12	5–30		

Description

Immunoglobulins (Ig) are classes (groups) of proteins referred to as antibodies; they can be divided into five groups found in gamma globulin. Immunoglobulin is produced by the action of B lymphocytes and plasma cells, and, as is characteristic of all antibody actions, immunoglobulin responds to invading foreign antigens. As individuals are exposed to antigens, immunoglobulin (antibody) production occurs. With further exposure to the same antigen, immunity results.

The five classes of immunoglobulins—IgG, IgA, IgM, IgD, and IgE—are separated by the process of immunoelectrophoresis. Of these five classes, IgG, IgA, and IgM are the important ones, because they make up most of the total gamma globulin.

The immunologic functions of the immunoglobulins are as follows:

IgG: IgG is the major immunoglobulin. IgG results from secondary exposure to the foreign antigen and is responsible for antiviral and antibacterial activity. This antibody passes through the placental barrier and provides early immunity for the newborn. The IgG response is longer and stronger than that of the other immunoglobulins.

IgA: This immunoglobulin is found in the secretions of the respiratory, gastrointestinal, and genitourinary tracts, tears, and saliva. Its purpose is to protect mucous membranes from invading organisms (viruses, certain bacteria—*Escherichia coli* and *Clostridium tetani*). IgA does not pass the placental barrier. Those having congenital IgA deficiency are prone to autoimmune disease.

IgM: IgM antibodies are produced 48 to 72 hours after an antigen enters the body and are responsible for primary immunity. This immunoglobulin produces antibody activity against rheumatoid factors, gram-negative organisms, and the ABO blood group. IgM activates the complement system by destroying antigenic substances. Because it does not pass the placental barrier, the serum value is low in newborns; however, it is produced early in life and the level increases after 9 months of age.

IgD: Unknown.

IgE: This immunoglobulin increases during allergic reactions and anaphylaxis.

Purposes

- To identify the occurrence of total or a specific elevated immunoglobulin.
- To associate a specific immunoglobulin elevation with a health problem *(see Clinical Problems)*.

Clinical Problems

Ig	Decreased Level	Elevated Level
IgG	Lymphocytic leukemia Agammaglobulinemia Preeclampsia Amyloidosis	Infections—all types Severe malnutrition Chronic granulomatous infection Hyperimmunization Liver disease Rheumatic fever Sarcoidosis
IgA	Lymphocytic leukemia Agammaglobulinemia Malignancies	Autoimmune disorders Rheumatic fever Chronic infections Liver disease
IgM	Lymphocytic leukemia Agammaglobulinemia Amyloidosis	Lymphosarcoma Brucellosis Trypanosomiasis Relapsing fever Infectious mononucleosis Rubella virus in newborns
IgE		Allergic reactions (asthma) Skin sensitivity Drug influence Tetanus toxoid Tetanus antitoxin Gamma globulin

Procedure

- Collect 5 to 7 ml of venous blood in a red-top tube.
- Record on the laboratory slip whether the client has received any vaccination or immunization, including toxoid, within the last 6 months; or any blood transfusion, gamma globulin, or tetanus antitoxin injections in the last 6 weeks.

- There is no food or fluid restriction. Some laboratories request that the client refrain from eating and drinking 12 hours before the test. Check with your laboratory.

Factors Affecting Laboratory Results

- Immunizations and toxoids received in the last 6 months, and blood transfusions, tetanus antitoxin, and gamma globulin received in the last 6 weeks can affect immunoglobulin results.

NURSING IMPLICATIONS WITH RATIONALE

- Obtain a history from the client concerning previous vaccination or immunization, including toxoids (tetanus), received in the last 6 months and blood transfusions or injections of gamma globulin or tetanus antitoxin received in the last 6 weeks.
- Report to the health care provider and record on the client's chart and the laboratory slip if the client has received recent blood transfusions, immunization or injections of toxoids, tetanus antitoxin, and gamma globulins.
- Check the client's temperature periodically.

Client Teaching

- Instruct the client to avoid infections by using preventive measures (i.e., to avoid being around persons with colds, to get adequate rest, to eat balanced meals, and to maintain an adequate fluid intake).

Insulin (serum), insulin antibody

Reference Values

Adult: *Serum Insulin:* 5–25 μU/ml, 10–250 μIU/ml. *Panic Value:* 7 μU/ml.
Insulin Antibody Test: <4% serum binding of pork and beef insulin.

Description

Insulin, a hormone from the beta cells of the pancreas, is essential in transporting glucose to the cells for metabolism. Increased glucose levels stimulate insulin secretion.

Serum insulin and blood glucose levels are compared to determine the glucose disorder. Serum insulin is valuable in diagnosing insulinoma (islet cell tumor) and islet cell hyperplasia and in evaluating insulin production in diabetes mellitus. In insulinoma the serum insulin is high, and blood glucose is <30 mg/dl. Hyperinsulinemia can occur in obesity as well as in insulinoma.

The *insulin antibody test* is ordered when a diabetic, taking pork or beef insulin, requires larger and larger insulin dosages. Insulin antibodies develop as the result of impurities in animal insulins. These antibodies are of immunoglobulin types (i.e., IgG [most], IgM, IgE). The IgG antibodies neutralize the insulin, thus preventing glucose metabolism. IgM antibodies can cause insulin resistance, and IgE could be responsible for allergic effects.

Purposes

- To assist in the detection of an early pre-hyperglycemic diabetes mellitus state.
- To check for the presence of insulin antibody that can affect insulin absorption and dosage.

Clinical Problems

Decreased Level: Diabetes mellitus. *Drug Influence:* Insulin.

Elevated Level: Insulinoma, insulin-resistant diabetic state, Cushing's syndrome, obesity. *Drug Influence:* Cortisone preparations, oral contraceptives, thyroid hormones, epinephrine, levodopa.

Procedure

- Collect 3 to 5 ml of venous blood in a red-top tube. Avoid hemolysis. The blood sample should be chilled. Serum must be separated within 30 minutes of collection. If blood glucose is needed, collect 3 to 5 ml in a gray-top or red-top tube.
- Food and fluids are restricted for 10 to 12 hours prior to the test. Insulin secretion reaches its peak in 30 minutes to 2 hours after meals.
- Withhold medications that could affect test results, such as insulin and cortisone, until after the test.

Factors Affecting Laboratory Tests

- Drugs such as insulin, cortisone, oral contraceptives, and hormones could increase serum insulin levels.
- Hemolysis of the blood sample and not chilling the specimen could affect results.

NURSING IMPLICATIONS WITH RATIONALE

- Obtain a history of glucose disorders from the client or family. Report the client's complaints.
- Report if the client's insulin dosage has increased over a period of time in response to an increase in blood sugar.
- Be alert for signs and symptoms of hypoglycemia. If insulinoma is highly suspected, keep IV dextrose 50% available.

Client Teaching

- Explain to the client the importance of remaining NPO and resting (not exercising) before the test. Food and exercising increase blood glucose, thus increasing serum insulin level. Incorrect test results would occur.
- Teach client to report signs and symptoms of insulin reaction (i.e., nervousness, sweating, weakness, rapid pulse rate, confusion).

International normalized ratio (INR) (plasma)

Reference Values

Oral Anticoagulant Therapy: 2.0–3.0 INR.

Higher Value for Mechanical Heart Value: 2.5–3.5 INR.

Description

The international normalized ratio (INR) was devised to monitor more correctly anticoagulant therapy for clients receiving warfarin (Coumadin) therapy. The World Health Organization (WHO) recommends the use of INR for a more consistent reporting of prothrombin time results. The INR is calculated by the use of a nomogram demonstrating the relationship between the INR and the prothrombin time (PT) ratio. Usually both PT and INR values are reported for monitoring Coumadin therapy.

Refer to PT for the purposes, clinical problems, procedure, and factors effecting laboratory results, nursing implications, and client teaching.

Inulin clearance

Reference Values

Adult: *Average Range for 21–69 Years:* 90–130 ml/min. 21–39 *Years: Male:* 90–168 ml/min. *Female:* 84–150 ml/min. 40–49 *Years: Male:* 78–162 ml/min. *Female:* 82–146 ml/min. 50–69 *Years: Male:* 68–137 ml/min. *Female:* 66–130 ml/min. 70–79 *Years: Male:* 42–122 ml/min. *Female:* 45–121 ml/min.

Child: <11 *Years:* 82–122 ml/min. 11–20 *Years:* 85–125 ml/min.

Description

The inulin clearance test is a reliable test used to assess the glomerular filtration rate (GFR) in relation to renal function. The substance given for the test is inulin, an inert sugar that is not metabolized nor absorbed from the renal tubules but is rapidly filtered through the glomeruli. If glomerular filtration is normal, the inulin clearance should be equivalent to the GFR. Decreased levels occur when >50% of renal cells are nonfunctioning, thus indicating impaired glomerular filtration. Normal decreased glomerular filtration can occur during the aging process. Inulin clearance test is not suggested for a client who has a history of congestive heart failure (CHF).

Inulin clearance test is very time consuming and is not frequently performed. Blood urea nitrogen, serum creatinine, and creatinine clearance test are normally ordered to determine renal function.

Purpose

- To assess renal function.

Clinical Problems

Decreased Level: Acute and chronic glomerulonephritis, acute tubular necrosis, nephrosclerosis, advanced chronic bilateral pyelonephritis, renal atherosclerosis, CHF, renal malignancy, polycystic kidney disease, shock. *Drug Influence:* Aminoglycosides, penicillin preparations, amphotericin B, and phenacetin.

Procedure

Check your laboratory policy for consistency with this procedure.

- The client should not eat food for 4 hours prior to the test. Exercise should be avoided.
- Collect 7 ml of venous blood in a green-top tube for use as a control blood sample.
- The client is to drink a quart of water (4 water glassesful) in 30 to 60 minutes prior to the test.
- Insert a Foley catheter (indwelling urinary catheter) and save the urine for a baseline urine specimen.
- Start an IV line using 500 ml of 5% dextrose in water (D_5W) using a Y tubing set.
- Prepare 25 ml of 10% inulin for IV bolus. Inulin may be difficult to dilute; therefore, warming the vial may be necessary.
- Inject intravenously 25 ml of 10% inulin over 4 minutes.
- Wait 30 minutes and begin the infusion of 500 ml of 1.5% inulin solution using an IV pump at the rate of 4 ml/min or 240 ml/h.
- Obtain 4 urine samples: 30, 50, 70, and 90 minutes after the 1.5% inulin solution was started. Clamp the catheter between each collected urine specimen. Some institutions require three urine specimens, 20 minutes apart. Urine specimens should be refrigerated if not sent immediately to the laboratory.

- Collect four blood samples of 10 ml each in a green-top tube at 40, 60, 80, and 95 minutes after the 1.5% inulin solution was started. Some institutions require two blood samples, 20 minutes apart. Blood samples should be sent immediately to the laboratory.
- Label each specimen with the time of collection and the amount of inulin used.
- Remove the Foley catheter.

Factors Affecting Laboratory Results

- Hemolysis of the blood samples from rough handling can cause a false-negative result.
- Failure to infuse the inulin solution at the constant rate, prescribed rate of flow.
- Failure to collect the blood and urine specimens at the prescribed times and/or not labeling specimen correctly.
- Inadequate urine output due to inadequate water intake.

NURSING IMPLICATIONS WITH RATIONALE

- Assess vital signs. Auscultate the lungs to check for chest rales and check for peripheral edema. Excess fluid intake may increase the already overloaded vascular system. Report findings.
- Assess the urine output and fluid intake. Urine output of <600 ml/day can indicate renal dysfunction or inadequate fluid intake.
- Use the 25 ml of 10% inulin for IV bolus within 1 hour of preparation.
- One nurse should be assigned to monitor the test to maintain the correct procedure.

Client Teaching

- Explain the procedure for the inulin clearance test to the client (see Procedure). This may be written for the client so that he or she can follow the procedure.
- Inform the client that a catheter will be inserted in the bladder for the duration of the test. It will be removed following the test.
- Instruct the client not to eat for 4 hours before the test and not to exercise.
- Tell the client that the test usually takes about 2 hours. Explain that there will be four to five blood samples drawn and four to five urine samples collected according to the prescribed policy.
- Listen to the client's concerns. Answer questions.

Iron (Fe), total iron-binding capacity (TIBC), transferrin, percent (transferrin) saturation (serum)

Iron-Binding Capacity (IBC), Transferrin Saturation

Reference Values

	Serum Iron	TIBC	Serum Transferrin	Saturation
Adult	50–150 µg/dl 10–27 µmol/l (SI units) Males slightly higher	250–450 µg/dl	200–430 mg/dl	30–50% (male) 20–35% (female)
Elderly	60–80 µg/dl	<250 µg/dl		
Child				
Newborn	100–270 µg/dl	60–175 µg/dl	125–275 mg/dl	
Infant		100–400 µg/dl		
6 months–2 years:	40–100 µg/dl	100–135 µg/dl		
>2 years:		40–100 µg/dl		

Description

Iron is absorbed from the duodenum and upper jejunum; the amount absorbed usually covers the amount of iron that has been lost. The average daily iron intake is 10–20 mg. With severe iron deficiency, the amount of iron absorbed will be greatly increased.

Iron is coupled with the iron-transporting protein transferrin. Transferrin is responsible for transporting iron to the bone marrow for the purpose of hemoglobin synthesis (see Transferrin). The storage compound for iron is ferritin (see Ferritin).

Total iron-binding capacity (TIBC) measures the maximum amount of iron that can bind to the protein transferrin. The level of TIBC decreases with age. Normally, TIBC is two to three times greater than serum iron level.

Transferrin can be measured as serum and as percent of saturation (transferrin saturation). The transferrin saturation is the ratio between serum iron and TIBC relating to the availability of transferrin in binding with iron. Transferrin saturation is given in percent and the percentage is determined by using the following formula:

$$\text{Transferrin saturation \%} = \frac{\text{serum iron level}}{\text{TIBC}} \times 100$$

Serum iron, TIBC, transferrin, and percent (transferrin) saturation values are needed to adequately diagnose iron deficiency anemia and other disorders. The table below gives the various tests used for diagnosing health problems related to iron and transferrin imbalances.

SERUM IRON, TIBC, TRANSFERRIN, AND TRANSFERRIN SATURATION

Serum Iron	TIBC	Transferrin	Transferrin Saturation	Health Problems
Low	High	High	Low	Iron deficiency anemia
Low	Low	Low	Normal	Chronic illness: cancer, infection, cirrhosis
High	Normal or low	Low	Very high	Iron therapy overload

Purposes

- To determine a probable cause of iron excess (e.g., hemolysis) or deficit (e.g., iron deficiency anemia).
- To compare serum iron and TIBC for diagnosing iron deficiency anemia.

Clinical Problems

Decreased Levels: *Serum Iron:* Iron deficiency anemia; cancer of the stomach, intestine, rectum, breast; rheumatoid arthritis; bleeding peptic ulcer; protein malnutrition; low-birth-weight infants, blood loss, burns. *TIBC:* Hemochromatosis, anemias (hemolytic, pernicious, sickle cell), hypoproteinemia, renal failure, cirrhosis of the liver, infections, cancer of the gastrointestinal tract. *Drug Influence:* Cortisone preparations, dextran, testosterone. *Transferrin:* Anemia of chronic disease, hepatic damage, renal disease, cancer, acute or chronic infection. *Percent Saturation:* Chronic iron deficiency anemia, anemia of chronic disease.

Elevated Levels: *Serum Iron:* Hemochromatosis (excessive iron deposits), anemias (hemolytic, pernicious, folic acid deficiency), liver damage, thalassemia, lead toxicity. *TIBC:* Microcytic anemia, acute and chronic blood loss, polycythemia. *Drug Influence:* Oral contraceptives. *Transferrin:* Iron deficiency. *Percent Saturation:* Anemias (hemolytic, sideroblastic) hemochromatosis, iron overload. *Drug Influence:* Oral contraceptives, iron preparations.

Procedure

- Collect 5 to 7 ml of venous blood in a red-top tube. Avoid hemolysis because it can cause false-positive readings.

269

■ The client should refrain from eating or drinking for 8 hours before the test. Serum iron levels are usually higher in the morning and following food intake.

Factors Affecting Laboratory Results

■ Hemolysis of the blood sample.
■ Oral iron medications and recent blood transfusion.

NURSING IMPLICATIONS WITH RATIONALE

Decreased Level (Serum Iron)

■ Observe for signs and symptoms of iron deficiency anemia (i.e., pallor, fatigue, headache, tachycardia, dyspnea on exertion).
■ Check with the laboratory about whether the client should refrain from eating and drinking prior to the test.

Client Teaching

■ Instruct the client to eat foods rich in iron (i.e., liver, shellfish, lean meat, egg yolks, dried fruits, whole grain, wines, and cereals). Milk has little or no iron. Nutritional instruction is particularly important for preschool and adolescent children and for pregnant women.
■ Recommend rest and avoidance of strenuous activity before test.
■ Instruct the client on how to take iron supplements. Iron should be given following meals or snacks because it irritates the gastric mucosa. Orange juice and ascorbic acid promote iron absorption.
■ Explain to the client that iron supplements can cause constipation and that the stools will have a tarry appearance.

Elevated Level

■ Observe for signs and symptoms of hemochromatosis (i.e., bronze pigmentation of the skin, dysrhythmias, and heart failure).

Ketone bodies, acetone (urine)

Reference Values

Adult: Negative test.
Child: Negative test.

Description

(See Acetone, Ketone Bodies [Serum].)

Ketone bodies are produced to provide energy when carbohydrates (CHO) cannot be used, as in diabetic acidosis and starvation/malnutrition. When these excess ketones are produced, ketosis (in the blood) results, thus exhausting the alkaline reserve (e.g., bicarbonates) of the body, causing an acidotic state. Ketonuria (ketone bodies in the urine) occurs as a result of ketosis.

In testing for ketonuria, Acetest tablets are used to detect the two principal ketones (acetone and acetoacetic acid) in the urine. Ketostix can also be used, but this test method is more specific for acetoacetic acid.

Purpose

- To detect the presence of an acidotic state.

Clinical Problems

Positive Result: Diabetic acidosis (ketoacidosis), starvation/malnutrition, reducing diet (↓ CHO), fasting, severe vomiting, heat stroke, fetal death. *Drug Influence:* Ascorbic acid, levodopa compounds, insulin, isopropyl alcohol, paraldehyde, pyridium, dyes used for the tests—bromsulfophthalein (BSP) and phenolsulfonphthalein (PSP).

Procedure

Collect a random urine specimen. Two tests are usually performed, as follows.

Acetest: Place an Acetest tablet on a clean surface (preferably a white paper towel), and put a drop of fresh urine on the tablet. Wait 30 seconds, and if the tablet changes color (lavender, medium purple, or dark purple), the result is positive for ketones.

The test is usually done on the same urine used for testing for glycosuria. The Clinitest is used for determining glycosuria, and the Acetest, for ketonuria.

Ketostix: Dip a reagent stick in fresh urine. Wait 15 seconds and compare it to the color chart. This test is more sensitive to acetoacetic acid than it is to acetone.

The urine should be fresh or refrigerated in a closed container. Waiting may cause false-negative results because of the instability of acetone.

There is no food or fluid restriction.

Factors Affecting Laboratory Results

- A low-carbohydrate diet or a high-fat diet can cause false-positive results.
- Certain drugs can cause false-positive results *(see Drug Influence)*.
- Urine kept at room temperature for 1 hour or more before testing may cause a false-negative result.
- Urinary tract infection—bacteria in the urine—will cause a loss of acetoacetic acid.

■ Juvenile diabetics are more prone to ketonuria (ketosis) than adults.

NURSING IMPLICATIONS WITH RATIONALE

Positive Result

■ Relate ketonuria to diabetic acidosis (ketoacidosis), starvation, fasting, or a low-carbohydrate diet. In severe diabetic acidosis, both ketonuria and glycosuria may be present. This would not be true in severe vomiting, starvation, reducing diets, and heat stroke, because in such cases only ketonuria would be present.

■ Explain to the client that the urine should be freshly voided. Only 1 ml is needed. Acetone is lost in the urine if it stands at room temperature because it is volatile.

■ Test and record the results of the Acetest and Clinitest on the client's chart. Notify the health care provider if results are abnormal.

■ Assess for signs and symptoms of diabetic acidosis, such as rapid, vigorous breathing; restlessness; confusion; sweet-smelling breath; and a positive Clinitest and Acetest.

Client Teaching

■ Instruct client how to use the Acetest and Clinitest.

■ Answer the client's questions concerning urine testing and diabetes mellitus.

17-Ketosteroids (17-KS) (urine)

Reference Values

Adult: *Male:* 5–25 mg/24 h. *Female:* 5–15 mg/24 h.

Elderly: 4–8 mg/24 h.

Child: *Infant:* <1 mg/24 h. *1–3 Years Old:* <2 mg/24 h. *3–6 Years Old:* <3 mg/24 h. *7–10 Years Old:* <4 mg/24 h. *10–12 Years Old: Male:* <6 mg/24 h; *Female:* <5 mg/24 h.

Adolescent: *Male:* 3–15 mg/24 h. *Female:* 3–12 mg/24 h.

Description

17-Ketosteroids (17-KS) are metabolites of male hormones that are secreted from the testes and adrenal cortex. 17-KS are excreted in the urine. In men, approximately one-third of the hormone metabolites come from the testes, and two-thirds come from the adrenal cortex. In women, nearly all of the excreted hormones (androgens) are derived from the adrenal cortex.

Because most of the 17-KS is derived from the adrenal cortex and not from the testes, the 17-KS level is more useful for diagnosing adrenal cortex dysfunction. This test is also useful for determining pituitary and gonadal hormone function. Usually plasma cortisol and 17-OHCS determinations are requested at the same time to further confirm adrenal dysfunctions.

Purpose

- To assist in the diagnosis of adrenal cortex dysfunction.

Clinical Problems

Decreased Level: Adrenal cortical hypofunction (Addison's disease), hypogonadism, hypopituitarism, nephrosis, myxedema, severe debilitating diseases. *Drug Influence:* Thiazide diuretics, chlordiazepoxide (Librium), estrogen, oral contraceptives, paraldehyde, reserpine, probenecid (Benemid), promazine, meprobamate (Miltown),* quinidine, quinine.

Elevated Level: Adrenocorticotropic hormone therapy, adrenal cortical hyperfunction (adrenocortical hyperplasia, Cushing's syndrome, adrenocortical carcinoma), testicular neoplasm, ovarian neoplasm, hyperpituitarism, hirsutism, severe stress (burns, surgery, infectious diseases). *Drug Influence:* Acetazolamide (Diamox); antibiotics (chloramphenicol [Chloromycetin], cloxacillin, erythromycin), chlorpromazine (Thorazine), hydralazine, meprobamate (Miltown),* phenothiazines, spironolactone (Aldactone), phenazopyridine, dexamethasone (Decadron).

Procedure

- There is no food or fluid restriction.
- Drugs that interfere with test results should not be given for 48 hours before the test. Check with the health care provider first.
- Collect a 24-hour urine specimen in a large container, and keep the container on ice or refrigerated. An acid preservative is usually added to keep the urine at a pH <4.5, thus preventing steroid decomposition by bacterial growth.
- List on the laboratory slip the client's sex and age.
- Label container with the client's name, date, and exact time of collection, such as 9/23/03, 7:30 AM to 9/24/03, 7:32 AM.
- Postpone the test if the female has her menstrual period. Blood in the urine can cause false-positive results.

Factors Affecting Laboratory Results

- Drugs *(see Drug Influence above)*.

---

*Meprobamate may increase or decrease the 17-KS value.

NURSING IMPLICATIONS WITH RATIONALE

- List on the laboratory slip the client's sex and age. If the client is a male, the laboratory results should be slightly higher than if the client is a female. In addition, if the client is over 65 years old, the test results should be low or low normal.
- Encourage the client to increase fluid intake.

Client Teaching

- Explain to the client and family that all urine will be collected for 24 hours in the large urine container/bottle, which is on ice or refrigerated. Inform the client that he or she should not put toilet paper or feces in the urine, and not to urinate directly into the collection container. The container could contain an acid preservative which could "splash" while urinating.

Decreased Level

- Observe for the signs and symptoms of adrenal gland insufficiency (Addison's disease), such as weakness, weight loss, polyuria, hypotension, increased pulse rate, and shock (if severe).
- Record fluid intake and output. Report if the client's urine output is greater than normal (>2000 ml/24 h).
- Monitor weight loss. In Addison's disease, sodium is not retained; therefore both sodium and water are lost. Weight loss and dehydration usually occur.

Client Teaching

- Encourage the client to wear an identification bracelet containing emergency information.

Elevated Level

- Observe for signs and symptoms of adrenal gland hyperfunction (Cushing's syndrome), such as moon face, hirsutism, weight gain, a cervicodorsal fat pad (buffalo hump), a bleeding tendency, hyperglycemia, and edema in the extremities.
- Check serum potassium and blood glucose levels. Hypokalemia and hyperglycemia frequently occur; potassium supplements and insulin or a low-carbohydrate diet may be indicated.

Lactic acid (blood)

Reference Values

Adult: *Arterial Blood:* 0.5–2.0 mmol/l, <11.3 mg/dl. *Venous Blood:* 0.5–1.5 mmol/l, 8.1–15.3 mg/dl. *Panic Range:* >5 mEq/l, >45 mg/dl.

Description

Blood lactic acid or lactate is an indicator of the presence of lactic acidosis. Lactic acidosis is suspected if the anion gap is >17 mEq/l and pH is decreased.

Shock and severe dehydration cause cell catabolism (cell breakdown) and an accumulation of acid metabolites, such as lactic acid. Excess lactic acid can decrease pH and cause lactic acidosis.

Purpose

- To detect the presence of acidosis related to shock, trauma, or severe illness *(see Anion Gap).*

Clinical Problems

Decreased Level: High lactic dehydrogenase (LDH) value.

Elevated Level: Shock, severe dehydration, severe trauma, ketoacidosis, severe infections, neoplastic conditions, hepatic failure, renal disease, alcoholism, salicylate toxicity (severe), chronic alcoholism.

Procedure

- Collect 5 to 7 ml of blood in a green-top tube.
- Inform the client to avoid hand clenching, which can lead to a buildup of lactic acid caused by a release of lactic acid from muscle of the clenched hand.
- Avoid using a tourniquet if possible. It could increase the blood lactic acid level.
- Deliver blood specimen on ice to the laboratory immediately.

Factors Affecting Laboratory Results

- Delivery to the laboratory of an arterial blood specimen not on ice could cause an inaccurate result.
- Use of tourniquet could elevate lactic acid value.

NURSING IMPLICATIONS WITH RATIONALE

Elevated Level

- Associate an elevated lactic acid value with shock, severe dehydration, severe trauma, severe infection, and other conditions.
- Observe for signs and symptoms of acidosis, dyspnea, or Kussmaul's breathing, increased pulse rate, decreased pH, decreased serum carbon dioxide value, and decreased arterial bicarbonate value.
- Be supportive of the client and family. If shock is present, anxiety and fear are common.

Lactic (lactate) dehydrogenase (LD or LDH), LDH isoenzymes (serum)

Reference Values

Adult: *Total LDH:* 100–190 IU/l, 70–250 U/l. Values can differ according to the method used.

Isoenzymes: LDH_1, 14–26%; LDH_2, 27–37%; LDH_3, 13–26%; LDH_4, 8–16%; LDH_5, 6–16%. Differences of 2% to 4% are considered normal.

Child: *Newborn:* 300–1500 IU/l. *Child:* 50–150 IU/l; 110–295 U/l.

Description

Lactic dehydrogenase (LDH) is an intracellular enzyme present in nearly all metabolizing cells, with the highest concentrations in the heart, skeletal muscle, liver, kidney, brain, and red blood cells (RBCs). LDH has two distinct subunits—M (muscle) and H (heart). These subunits are combined in different formations to make five isoenzymes.

- LDH_1: cardiac fraction; H, H, H, H; in heart, RBCs, kidneys, brain (some).
- LDH_2: cardiac fraction; H, H, H, M; in heart, RBCs, kidneys, brain (some).
- LDH_3: pulmonary fraction; H, H, M, M; in lungs and other tissues; spleen, pancreas, adrenal, thyroid, lymphatics.
- LDH_4: hepatic fraction; H, M, M, M; liver, skeletal muscle, kidneys and brain (some).
- LDH_5: hepatic fraction; M, M, M, M; liver, skeletal muscle, kidneys (some).

Like other enzymatic tests, such as the creatine phosphokinase (CPK) and aspartate aminotransferase (AST) tests, serum LDH and LDH_1 are used for diagnosing acute myocardial infarction (MI). A high serum LDH (total) level occurs 12 to 24 hours after the infarction, reaches its peak in 2 to 5 days, and remains elevated for 6 to 12 days, making it a useful test for delayed diagnosis of MI. A flipped LDH_1/LDH_2 ratio, with LDH_1 the highest, indicates a myocardial infarction.

LDH_3 is linked to pulmonary diseases, and LDH_5 is linked to liver and skeletal muscle diseases. In acute hepatitis, total LDH rises, and the LDH_5 usually rises before jaundice develops and falls before the bilirubin level does.

Purposes

- To aid in the diagnosis of myocardial or skeletal muscle damage.
- To compare test results with other cardiac enzyme tests (i.e., CPK, AST).
- To check LDH isoenzyme results to determine organ involvement.

Clinical Problems

Elevated Level: Acute MI, cerebrovascular accident, cancer (lung, bone, intestines, liver, breast, cervix, testes, kidney, stomach, melanoma of the skin), acute leukemia, acute pulmonary infarction, infectious mononucleosis, anemias (pernicious, folic acid deficiency, sickle cell, acquired hemolytic), acute hepatitis, shock, skeletal muscular disease, heat stroke. *Drug Influence:* Narcotics (codeine, morphine, meperidine [Demerol]).

Procedure

- Collect 5 to 7 ml of venous blood in a red-top tube. Avoid hemolysis.
- List on the laboratory slip any narcotics or intramuscular (IM) injections the client received within 8 hours before the test.
- There is no food or fluid restriction.

Factors Affecting Laboratory Results

- Narcotic drugs and IM injections can elevate serum LDH levels.
- Hemolysis of the blood sample can cause an elevated serum LDH level; the enzyme is plentiful in the RBCs.

NURSING IMPLICATIONS WITH RATIONALE

Elevated Level

- Obtain a history of the client's discomfort. A complaint of severe indigestion several days before could be indicative of an acute MI. All information should be recorded and reported.
- Assess for signs and symptoms of an acute MI (i.e., pale or gray color, sharp stabbing pain or heavy pressure pain, shortness of breath, diaphoresis, nausea and vomiting, and indigestion).

Client Teaching
■ Instruct the client to notify the nurse of any recurrence of chest discomfort or to seek medical care for indigestion of several days.

Lactose tolerance

Reference Values

Adult: *Normal:* 20–50 mg/dl rise from fasting blood glucose without abdominal symptoms of cramps and diarrhea. *Abnormal:* <20 mg/dl of glucose rise from fasting blood glucose with abdominal cramps and diarrhea.

Description

Lactase, an enzyme from the small intestine, digests lactose, which is a sugar found in milk. The lactose tolerance test identifies clients with a deficiency of the enzyme lactase, which leads to an intolerance of lactose, found in milk. With an absence of lactase, lactose cannot be absorbed from the small intestine and is excreted through the bowel undigested, causing the client to have abdominal cramps and watery diarrhea.

This test is similar to a glucose tolerance test except that lactose is ingested instead of glucose. A flat curve of <20 mg/dl rise of the fasting glucose indicates lactose intolerance.

Purposes

■ To compare serum and urine lactose results for determining lactase deficit.
■ To diagnose lactose intolerance.

Clinical Problems

Decreased Level of Glucose: Lactose intolerance.

Procedure

■ The client should not eat or drink after midnight or at least 8 hours prior to the test.
■ Collect 5 to 7 ml of a fasting venous blood specimen in a gray-top tube.
■ The client drinks 50 g to 100 g of lactose in 200 to 300 ml of water in 5 to 10 minutes. If severe lactase deficiency is suspected, the lactose dosage may be decreased.
■ Collect blood samples following lactose ingestion in 30 minutes and in 1, 2, and 3 hours.
■ If the lactose tolerance test is abnormal, a glucose tolerance test may be ordered.

Factors Affecting Laboratory Results

- In the diabetic, an abnormal lactose tolerance can be due to abnormal carbohydrate metabolism.
- Twenty percent of individuals can have either a false-positive or false-negative test result.

NURSING IMPLICATIONS WITH RATIONALE

- Obtain a history from the client of abdominal cramps and diarrhea that occur following ingestion of milk. Notify the health care provider of finding because this usually indicates lactose intolerance. The test may be canceled.
- Explain the procedure to the client.
- Assess the client during and following the procedure for symptoms of abdominal cramps, pain, nausea, and watery diarrhea. Report findings.

Client Teaching

- Instruct the client with a lactose intolerance to buy lactose-free milk. It can be purchased in most grocery stores.

LDH isoenzymes

See Lactic Dehydrogenase

Lead (blood)

Reference Values

Adult: *Normal:* 10–20 μg/dl. *Acceptable:* 20–40 μg/dl. *Excessive:* 40–80 μg/dl. *Toxic:* 80 μg/dl.

Child: *Normal:* 10–20 μg/dl. *Acceptable:* 20–30 μg/dl. *Excessive:* 30–50 μg/dl. *Toxic:* 50 μg/dl.

Description

Excessive lead exposure due to occupational contact is a hazard to adults; however, most industries will accept a 40-μg/dl blood lead level as a normal value. Lead toxicity can occur in children from eating chipped, lead-based paint found in old houses. Sources of lead include leaded gasoline (fumes), lead-based paint, unglazed pottery, and "moonshine" whiskey prepared in lead containers.

Lead is usually excreted rapidly in the urine, but if excessive lead exposure persists, the lead will accumulate in the bone and soft tissues. Chronic lead poisoning is more common than acute poisoning. Lead colic (crampy abdominal pain) occurs in both acute and chronic lead poisoning.

Purpose

- To check for lead toxicity.

Clinical Problems

Elevated Level: Leaded gasoline, including fumes; lead-based paint; unglazed pottery; batteries; lead containers used for storage; heat stroke (mobilizes lead stored in the body).

Procedure

- Collect 5 to 7 ml of venous blood in a brown- or royal blue-top tube.
- There is no food or fluid restriction.
- Urine may be requested for a 24-hour quantitative test; a lead-free container must be used.

Factors Affecting Laboratory Results

- None reported.

NURSING IMPLICATIONS WITH RATIONALE

Elevated Level

- Obtain a history from the client and/or parent concerning lead exposure. Record this history on the chart, and report the information to the health care provider.
- Observe for signs and symptoms of lead poisoning: lead colic (crampy abdominal pain), constipation, occasional bloody diarrhea, behavioral changes (from lethargy to hyperactivity, aggression, impulsiveness), tremors, and confusion.
- Monitor the urinary output, because lead toxicity can decrease kidney function. A urine output of <25 ml/h should be reported.
- Monitor the medical treatment for removing body lead such as chelation therapy. The principal chelating agent is calcium disodium edetate, which combines metal with calcium substance.
- Provide adequate fluid intake. Adequate hydration prevents hemoconcentration.

Client Teaching

- Instruct clients who are exposed to lead (in their occupations) that blood levels should be monitored. These persons should definitely keep medical appointments.
- Suggest to parents ways of satisfying children's hunger through the attention method of providing psychological satisfaction that will replace that gained by eating lead chips.

LE cell test; lupus erythematosus cell test (blood)

Lupus Test, LE Prep, LE Preparation, LE Slide Cell Test

Reference Values

Adult: Negative, no LE cells.

Child: Negative.

Description

The lupus erythematosus (LE) cell test, a screening test for systemic lupus erythematosus (SLE), is a nonspecific test. Positive results have been reported in those having rheumatoid arthritis, scleroderma, and lupus induced by drugs, such as penicillin, tetracycline, dilantin, oral contraceptives. The test is positive in 60% to 80% of those having SLE. Antinuclear antibodies (ANA) or antideoxyribonucleic acid (anti-DNA) are more sensitive tests for lupus and should be used to confirm SLE. The LE cell test has been replaced by the ANA test.

Purposes

- To aid in the diagnosis of SLE.
- To compare with ANA and/or anti-DNA tests for diagnosing SLE.

Clinical Problems

Elevated Level: Systemic lupus erythematosus (SLE), scleroderma, rheumatoid arthritis, chronic hepatitis. *Drug Influence:* Hydralazine (Apresoline), procainamide (Pronestyl), quinidine, anticonvulsants (phenytoin [Dilantin], Mesantoin, Tridione), oral contraceptives, methysergide, antibiotics (penicillin, tetracycline, streptomycin), sulfonamides, methyldopa (Aldomet), isoniazid (INH), clofibrate, reserpine, phenylbutazone.

Procedure

- Collect 3 to 5 ml of venous blood in a red-top tube.
- There is no food or fluid restriction.
- List on the laboratory slip drugs taken that might affect test result.

Factors Affecting Laboratory Results

- Certain drugs can cause false-positive test results *(see Drug Influence)*.
- Hemolysis of the blood sample could affect test result.

NURSING IMPLICATIONS WITH RATIONALE

- Compare LE cell test results with those of serum ANA or anti-DNA, or both. The LE test should not be the only test used to diagnose SLE.
- Observe for signs and symptoms of SLE (i.e., fatigue, fever, rash [butterfly over the nose], leukopenia, thrombocytopenia).
- Be supportive of the client and family.

Client Teaching

- Instruct the client to have daily rest periods, which help to decrease symptoms.

Lecithin/sphingomyelin (L/S) ratio (amniotic fluid)

Reference Values

Before 35 Weeks of Gestation: 1:1. *Lecithin (L):* 6–9 mg/dl. *Sphingomyelin (S):* 4–6 mg/dl.

After 35 Weeks of Gestation: 4:1. *Lecithin (L):* 15–21 mg/dl. *Sphingomyelin (S):* 4–6 mg/dl.

Description

The lecithin/sphingomyelin (L/S) ratio can be used to predict neonatal respiratory distress syndrome (also called hyaline membrane disease) before delivery. Lecithin (L), a phospholipid, is responsible mostly for the formation of alveolar surfactant. Surfactant lubricates the alveolar lining and inhibits alveolar collapse, thus preventing atelectasis. Sphingomyelin (S) is another phospholipid, the value of which remains the same throughout pregnancy. A marked rise in amniotic lecithin after 35 weeks (to a level three or four times higher than that of sphingomyelin) is considered normal, and so chances for having hyaline membrane disease are small. The L/S ratio is also used to determine fetal maturity in the event that the gestation period is uncertain. In this situation, the L/S ratio is determined at intervals of a period of several weeks.

Purpose

- To check for possible neonatal respiratory distress syndrome (hyaline membrane disease) prior to delivery.

Clinical Problems

Decreased Ratio after 35 Weeks: Respiratory distress syndrome, hyaline membrane disease.

Procedure

- The physician obtains amniotic fluid by the method of amniocentesis. The specimen should be cooled immediately to prevent the destruction of lecithin by certain enzymes in the amniotic fluid. The specimen should be frozen if testing cannot be done at a specified time (check with the laboratory).
- Care should be taken to prevent puncture of the mother's bladder. If urine in the specimen is suspected, then the specimen should be tested for urea and potassium. If these two levels are higher than blood levels, the specimen could be urine and not amniotic fluid. Ultrasound is frequently used when obtaining amniotic fluid.
- There is no food, fluid, or drug restriction.

Factors Affecting Laboratory Results

- Maternal vaginal secretions or a bloody tap into the amniotic fluid may cause a falsely increased reading for lecithin.
- The amniotic fluid specimen should be tested immediately to prevent inaccurate results.

NURSING IMPLICATIONS WITH RATIONALE

- Check the procedures for amniocentesis. Explain the procedure to the client. Assist the health care provider in obtaining amniotic fluid.
- Obtain a fetal history of problems occurring during gestation. Also, ask for and report information on any previous children born with respiratory distress syndrome.
- Be supportive of the mother and her family before, during, and after the test. Remain with the client and answer her questions, if possible, or refer her questions to appropriate professional personnel.
- Assess the newborn at delivery for respiratory complications (substernal retractions, increased respiratory rate, labored breathing, and expiratory grunts).

Legionnaires' antibody (serum)

Reference Value

Negative.

Description

Legionnaires' disease, caused by a gram-negative bacillus, *Legionella pneumophila,* causes acute respiratory infections such as severe, consolidated pneumonia. This organism is in the soil and water (lakes, streams, reservoirs) and is passed by inhalation of the bacillus in water aerosolized through plumbing fixtures (shower heads, whirlpool baths) and air conditioning systems (cooling towers and condensers). The bacteria can be isolated from blood, sputum, pleural fluid, and lung-tissue specimen.

A fourfold rise in antibody titer >1:128 during the acute and convalescent phase or a single titer >1:256 is evidence of the disease. Several blood samples and a tissue specimen are useful in confirming legionnaires' disease.

Purpose

- To diagnose the presence of legionnaires' disease.

Clinical Problems

Elevated Antibody Titer: Legionnaires' disease.

Procedure

- Collect 3 to 5 ml of venous blood in a red-top tube. Tissue specimen from the lung or bronchiole site may be used.
- There is no food or fluid restriction.

Factors Affecting Laboratory Results

- None known.

NURSING IMPLICATIONS WITH RATIONALE

- Obtain a history from the client as to where he or she has been in the last week, such as hotel or other institutional site.
- Assess the client's respiratory status by inspection, palpation, percussion, and auscultation.

- Observe for signs and symptoms of legionnaires' disease, such as malaise, high fever, chills, cough, chest pain, and tachypnea. Fever rises rapidly to 39°C to 41°C or to 102°F to 105°F.

Client Teaching

- Inform the client that legionnaires' disease is not transmitted from person to person but through aerosol means such as exhaust vents and fans.

Leucine aminopeptidase (LAP) (serum)

Reference Values

Adult: 8–22 μU/ml, 12–33 IU/l, 75–200 U/ml, 20–50 U/l at 37°C (SI units). Varies according to laboratory method.

Description

The leucine aminopeptidase (LAP) enzyme is produced by the liver and tends to parallel serum alkaline phosphatase (ALP), except that the LAP level is normal in bone disease or malabsorption syndrome. LAP is not an indicator of pancreatic carcinoma, as was once thought, but it is an indicator for biliary obstruction caused by liver metastases and choledocholithiasis.

This enzyme test is not frequently ordered but is useful as a supplement test in evaluating hepatobiliary disease.

Purpose

- To compare with other liver enzyme tests for diagnosing liver disease.

Clinical Problems

Elevated Level: Cancer of the liver, extrahepatic biliary obstruction (stones), acute necrosis of the liver, viral hepatitis.

Procedure

- Collect 3 to 5 ml of venous blood in a red-top tube.
- There is no food or fluid restriction.

Factors Affecting Laboratory Results

- None reported.

| **NURSING IMPLICATIONS WITH RATIONALE**

Elevated Level

- Compare LAP with other tests for liver dysfunction, such as the alkaline phosphatase (ALP), alanine aminotransferase (ALT, or SGPT), and gamma glutamyl transpeptidase (GGT) tests. The LAP test is frequently used to verify the results of other laboratory tests. It is not considered as sensitive as the other tests, and therefore it it not as commonly used.

Leukoagglutinin test (serum)

Reference Values

Negative: No dye uptake.

Positive: Dye uptake in the lymphoctes.

Description

Leukoagglutinins are antibodies that react with white blood cells (WBCs) and may cause a febrile and/or a transfusion reaction. Usually the leukagglutinin antibodies develop after the client has received WBCs through transfusions or pregnancies. To detect leukoagglutinins, the recipient's serum is tested with the donor's lymphocytes. The lymphocytes are examined under the microscope for cell damage. Agglutinating antibodies may be present in the donor or recipient's plasma.

Purpose

- To detect leukoagglutinin antibodies that may be a contributing factor to transfusion reaction.

Clinical Problems

Positive Test: Pregnancies, numerous transfusions.

Procedure

- Collect 10 ml of venous blood in a red-top tube.
- There is no food or fluid restriction.

Factors Affecting Laboratory Results

- Blood transfusion or dextran that has been previously administered.

NURSING IMPLICATIONS WITH RATIONALE

- Obtain a history of past blood transfusions and ascertain whether adverse effects occurred.
- Record baseline vital signs. Vital signs (VS) can be compared with those taken during a transfusion or if a transfusion reaction occurs. Acetaminophen may be prescribed prior to a transfusion to avoid febrile state if indicated.
- Administer leukocyte-poor blood that has been separated from the donor's blood when necessary to avoid a transfusion reaction.

Client Teaching

- Listen to the client's concerns. Answer questions or contact other health professionals.

Lidocaine hydrochloride (blood, serum, plasma)

Xylocaine

Reference Values

Therapeutic Range: *Adult:* 1.5–5.0 μg/ml; 6.0–22.5 μmol/l (SI units). *Child:* Similar to adult.

Toxic Level: *Adult:* .6 mg/ml. *Child:* Similar to adult.

Description

For treating acute ventricular arrhythmia, IV lidocaine is one of the drugs of choice. It obtains its antiarrhythmic effect by suppressing automaticity and increasing the electrical stimulation threshold of the ventricle. Lidocaine is also used as a local anesthetic.

Lidocaine is metabolized in the liver to active metabolites; about 70% of the metabolites are bound to plasma protein. An initial bolus of parenteral lidocaine (50 to 100 mg) has a half-life of 10 minutes; however, the half-life is lengthened to 2 hours with continuous IV administration. Steady state occurs 6 to 12 hours after IV lidocaine infusion. Ninety percent of the drug is excreted in the urine as metabolites and 10% excreted unchanged.

Monitoring lidocaine levels is necessary to maintain therapeutic level and to avoid lidocaine toxicity. The maximum dose of lidocaine IV and bolus is 300 mg/h.

Purposes

- To monitor lidocaine levels for therapeutic effect.
- To check for lidocaine toxicity.

Clinical Problems

Decreased Level: *Drug Influence:* Barbiturates, phenytoin (Dilantin).

Elevated Level: *Excess Dosage of Lidocaine:* Shock, liver and heart diseases. *Drug Influence:* Cimetidine (Tagamet), propranolol (Inderal).

Procedure

- Collect 3 to 5 ml in a red-top tube. Draw blood specimen 6 to 12 hours after starting lidocaine therapy for dysrhythmia prophylaxis. Then check serum levels daily as ordered.
- Record dose, time, and route (bolus or infusion) of lidocaine administration on the laboratory requisition slip.
- There is no food or fluid restriction.

Factors Affecting Laboratory Results

- Incorrect blood-collecting tube. Check with the laboratory for the type of collecting tube.

NURSING IMPLICATIONS WITH RATIONALE

- Monitor therapeutic drug level every 12 hours, especially when cardiac or liver insufficiency exists. The maximum dose is 300 mg/h.
- Regulate the IV rate using microchamber tubing and an infusion pump. Normally, no more than 4 mg/min should be infused.

Elevated Level

- Observe for signs and symptoms of side effects of lidocaine and of lidocaine toxicity (drowsiness, dizziness, lightheadedness, confusion, disorientation, irritability, apprehension, double vision). High doses (>9 μg/ml, 38.4 μmol/l) may produce convulsions, hypotension, bradycardia, and shock.

Lipase (serum)

Reference Values

Adult: 20–180 IU/l, 114–286 U/l, 14–280 U/l (SI units). Norms vary among laboratories.

Child: *Infant:* 9–105 IU/l at 37°C. *Child:* 20–136 IU/l at 37°C.

Description

Lipase, an enzyme secreted by the pancreas, aids in digesting fats. Lipase, like amylase, appears in the blood stream following damage to the pancreas. Acute pancreatitis is the commonest cause for an elevated serum lipase level. Lipase and amylase levels increase early in the disease, but serum lipase can be elevated for up to 14 days after an acute episode, whereas the serum amylase returns to normal after approximately 3 days. Serum lipase is useful for a late diagnosis of acute pancreatitis.

Purpose

- To suggest acute pancreatitis or other pancreatic disorders *(see Clinical Problems)*.

Clinical Problems

Decreased Level: Late cancer of the pancreas, hepatitis.

Elevated Level: Acute and chronic pancreatitis, cancer of the pancreas (early stage), perforated ulcer, obstruction of the pancreatic duct, acute cholecystitis (some cases), acute renal failure (early stage). *Drug Influence:* Codeine, morphine, meperidine (Demerol), bethanechol (Urecholine) steroids, guanethidine.

Procedure

- Collect 3 to 5 ml of venous blood in a red-top tube. Avoid hemolysis.
- NPO except water for 8 to 12 hours.
- Narcotics should be withheld for 24 hours prior to the test. If narcotics are administered within the 24 hours, the drug and the time administered should be written on the laboratory slip.

Factors Affecting Laboratory Results

- Most narcotic drugs elevate the serum lipase level.
- Food eaten within 8 hours prior to the test may interfere with serum lipase levels.
- The presence of hemoglobin and calcium ions may cause a decreased serum lipase level.

Elevated Level

- Relate elevated serum lipase and amylase levels to acute pancreatitis.
- Notify the health care provider when abdominal pain persists for several days. A serum lipase determination may be ordered because it is an effective test for latent diagnosis of acute pancreatitis. Lipase levels may remain elevated in the blood for 2 weeks.

Lipoproteins, lipoprotein electrophoresis, lipids (serum)

Reference Values

Adult: *Total:* 400–800 mg/dl, 4–8 g/l (SI units). *Cholesterol:* 150–240 mg/dl (see test on cholesterol). *Triglycerides:* 10–190 mg/dl (see test on triglycerides). *Phospholipids:* 150–380 mg/dl.

LDL: 60–160 mg/dl. *Risk for CHD:* High: >160 mg/dl. Moderate: 130–159 mg/dl. Low: <130 mg/dl. Desirable: 100 mg/dl.

HDL: 29–77 mg/dl. *Risk for CHD:* High: <35 mg/dl. Moderate: 35–45 mg/dl. Low: 46–59 mg/dl. Very low: >60 mg/dl.

Child: *See tests on cholesterol and triglycerides.*

Description

Lipoproteins are lipids bound to protein, and the three main lipoproteins are cholesterol, triglycerides, and phospholipids. The two fractions of lipoproteins—alpha (α), high-density lipoproteins (HDL), and beta (β), low-density lipoproteins (chylomicrons, VLDL, LDL)—can be separated by electrophoresis. The beta groups are the largest contributors of atherosclerosis and coronary artery disease. HDL, called "friendly lipids," are composed of 50% protein and do aid in decreasing plaque deposits in blood vessels.

LIPOPROTEIN CLASSIFICATION

Subgroup Classes of Lipoproteins	Protein Composition (%)	Cholesterol (%)	Triglycerides (%)	Phospholipids (%)
Chylomicrons	2	3	90	5
Very low-density (VLDL, pre-beta)	10	10	70	10

LIPOPROTEIN CLASSIFICATION

Subgroup Classes of Lipoproteins	Protein Composition (%)	Cholesterol (%)	Triglycerides (%)	Phospholipids (%)
Low-density (LDL, beta)	25	45	10	20
High-density HDL, alpha	50	20	Trace	30

Adapted from Henry, J. B. *Todd-Sanford-Davidsohn: Clinical diagnosis and management by laboratory methods* (17th ed., p. 183), Philadelphia: Saunders, 1984.

Increased lipoproteins (hyperlipidemia or hyperlipoproteinemia) can be phenotyped into five major types (I, IIA and IIB, III, IV, V). Cholesterol and triglycerides are the two lipids in each type found in varying amounts. With type II, the cholesterol is highly elevated, and the triglycerides are slightly increased. With type IV, the triglycerides are highly elevated, and the cholesterol is slightly increased. Types II and IV are the commonest phenotypes and are the most prevalent in atherosclerosis and coronary artery disease (CAD).

LIPOPROTEIN PHENOTYPE: HYPERLIPIDEMIA

Type	Lipid Composition*
I	Increased chylomicrons, increased triglycerides; rare pattern of hyperlipidemia
IIA	Increased beta (low-density) lipoproteins (LDL); increased cholesterol, slightly increased triglycerides or normal; common pattern of hyperlipidemia
IIB	Increased beta and pre-beta lipoproteins; both cholesterol and triglycerides are elevated; common pattern of hyperlipidemia
III	Moderately increased cholesterol and triglycerides; uncommon pattern of hyperlipidemia
IV	Increase of pre-beta (very low-density) lipoproteins (VLDL); slightly increased cholesterol and markedly increased triglycerides; common pattern of hyperlipidemia
V	Increased chylomicrons, VLDL, and triglycerides, and slightly increased cholesterol; uncommon pattern of hyperlipidemia

*Types II and IV are increased in atherosclerosis and coronary artery diseases.

Purposes

- To identify clients with hyperlipoproteinemia.
- To distinguish between the phenotypes of lipidemias.
- To monitor lipid counts for clients with hyperlipidemia.

Clinical Problems

Decreased Level: Tangier disease, chronic obstructive lung disease. *Drug Influence: See Cholesterol and Triglycerides.*

Elevated Level: Hyperlipoproteinemia, acute myocardial infarction (AMI), hypothyroidism, diabetes mellitus, nephrotic syndrome, eclampsia, Laënnec's cirrhosis, multiple myeloma, diet (high in saturated fats). *Drug Influence: See Cholesterol and Triglycerides.*

Procedure

- NPO except for water for 12 to 14 hours prior to the test. The client should be on a regular diet for 3 days before the test. No alcohol intake for 24 hours.
- Collect 7 to 10 ml of venous blood in a red-top tube.

Factors Affecting Laboratory Results

- A diet high in saturated fats and sugar could elevate test results.
- Certain drugs can increase or decrease serum lipoproteins *(see Clinical Problems, Drug Influence for Cholesterol and Triglycerides).*

NURSING IMPLICATIONS WITH RATIONALE

- Check the client's serum cholesterol, serum triglyceride LDL, and HDL levels. This information is helpful for teaching purposes and in answering the client's questions.

Client Teaching

- Instruct the client with hyperlipoproteinemia to avoid foods high in saturated fats and sugar (i.e., bacon, cream, butter, fatty meats, and candy).
- Answer client's questions concerning risk of CAD related to LDL and HDL.

Lithium (serum)

Eskalith, Lithobid, Esthalith CR, Lithotabs, Cibalith

Reference Values

Adult: *Normal:* Negative. *Therapeutic:* 0.8–1.2 mEq/l. *Toxic:* >1.5 mEq/l. *Lethal:* >4.0 mEq/l.

Child: Not usually given to children.

Description

Lithium, or lithium salt, is used to treat manic-depressive psychosis. This agent is used to correct the mania in manic-depression and to prevent depression. Because therapeutic and toxic lithium levels are narrow, serum lithium should be closely monitored.

Lithium salt was first used in the 1940s as a salt substitute; this practice was abandoned in the late 1940s because of its high toxicity. It was not used in the United States until after 1965 and then was used for treatment of manic depression.

Purposes

- To identify lithium toxicity.
- To monitor lithium levels for therapeutic effect and toxicity.

Clinical Problems

Elevated Level: *Toxicity:* Lithium carbonate (Eskalith, Lithane, Lithonate), lithium bromide.

Procedure

- Collect 5 to 7 ml of venous blood in a red-top tube 8 to 12 hours after the last lithium dose.
- There is no food or fluid restriction.
- The lithium tolerance test may be ordered instead of the conventional blood sample. A base blood specimen is obtained, and then the lithium dose is given. Blood specimens are collected 1, 3, and 6 hours after the lithium dose.

Factors Affecting Laboratory Results

- None reported.

NURSING IMPLICATIONS WITH RATIONALE

- Observe for signs and symptoms of lithium overdose (slurred speech, muscle spasm, confusion, and nystagmus). Lithium dosage should be lower in the older adult (over 65 years) than in the middle-aged adult. Lithium test results should always be reported to the health care provider because of the narrow range of the "therapeutic" dosage.

Client Teaching

- Instruct the client to take the prescribed lithium dosage daily and to keep his or her medical appointments. Periodic blood specimens will need to be drawn to determine lithium levels.

- Suggest to the nursing mother taking lithium that the pediatrician should be notified before she breastfeeds the infant. Breast milk can contain high levels of lithium.
- Encourage adequate fluid and sodium intake while the client is maintained on lithium. Lithium inhibits antidiuretic hormone secretion, causing body water loss. Diuretics should be avoided.

Lupus erythematosus cell

See LE cell

Luteinizing hormone (LH) (serum and urine)

Interstitial Cell-Stimulating Hormone (ICSH)

Reference Values

Ranges vary among laboratories.

Serum: *Adult:* Female: Follicular phase: 5–30 **mIU/ml**. Midcycle: 50–150 **mIU/ml**. Luteal phase: 2–25 mIU/ml. *Postmenopausal:* 40–100 mIU/ml. Male: 5–25 mIU/ml. *Child:* 6–12 years: <10 mIU/ml; 13–18 years: <20 mIU/ml.

Urine: *Adult:* Female: Follicular Phase: 5–25 IU/24 h. Midcycle: 30–90 IU/24 h. Luteal phase: 2–24 IU/24 h. Postmenopausal: >40 IU/24 h. Male: 7–25 IU/mL.

Description

Luteinizing hormone (LH), gonadotropic hormone secreted by the anterior pituitary gland, is needed (with follicle-stimulating hormone [FSH]) for ovulation to occur. After ovulation, LH aids in stimulating the corpus luteum in secreting progesterone. FSH values are frequently evaluated with LH values. In men, LH stimulates testosterone production, and with FSH, they influence the development and maturation of spermatozoa.

LH is usually ordered to evaluate infertility in women and men. High-serum values are related to gonadal dysfunction, and low serum values are related to hypothalamus or pituitary failure. Women taking oral contraceptives have an absence of midcycle LH peak until the contraceptives are discontinued. This test might be used to evaluate hormonal therapy for inducing ovulation.

Purposes

- To evaluate the serum or urine LH level for determining the cause of hormonal dysfunction.
- To identify the gynecologic problem related to excess or deficit of LH.

Clinical Problems

Decreased Level: Hypogonadotropinism (defects in pituitary gland or hypothalamus), anovulation, amenorrhea (pituitary failure), hypophysectomy, testicular failure, hypothalamic dysfunction, adrenal hyperplasia or tumors. *Drug Influence:* Oral contraceptives, estrogen compounds, testosterone administration.

Elevated Level: Amenorrhea (ovarian failure), tumors (pituitary, testicular), precocious puberty, testicular failure, Turner's syndrome, Klinefelter's syndrome, premature menopause, Stein-Leventhal syndrome, polycystic ovary syndrome, liver disease.

Procedure

Serum

- Collect 3 to 5 ml of venous blood in a red-top or lavender-top tube. Avoid hemolysis. Daily blood samples must be taken at the same time each day to determine if ovulation occurs.
- There is no food or fluid restriction.
- Note on the laboratory slip the phase of the menstrual cycle, client's age, and if client is postmenopausal.
- Withhold 24 to 48 hours before the test medications that could interfere with test results (check with health care provider).

Urine

- Collect 24-hour urine specimen in a container with a preservative, or keep refrigerated if no preservative is added.
- Label the specimen with the client's name, date, and time.

Factors Affecting Laboratory Results

- Hormones (estrogen, progesterone, and testosterone) and oral contraceptives could decrease plasma LH value.
- Hemolysis of the blood sample could affect test result.
- Collection of the daily specimen at different times of the day may cause inaccurate result.

NURSING IMPLICATIONS WITH RATIONALE

- Obtain a menstrual history from the client. Record the menstrual phase on the laboratory slip.
- Check with the health care provider (HCP) about withholding medications that could affect test results.
- Encourage the client to express concerns about infertility or other health problems.
- Be supportive of client and family.

Client Teaching

- Instruct client to express concerns to HCP and to keep an accurate account of her menstrual cycle.

Lyme disease (antibody)

Reference Value

Titer: Negative; <1:256.

Description

Borrelia burgdorferi is the spirochete that causes Lyme disease. Several tick vectors, primarily the deer tick, carry the spirochete. Lyme disease is most prevalent in the northeastern states, upper midwestern states, and western states.

A reddish, macular lesion usually occurs about 1 week after the tick bite. It can affect the central nervous system and the peripheral nervous system, causing a neuritis or aseptic meningitis. Also it can affect the heart and joints, causing transient electrocardiographic abnormalities, carditis, and problems in one or more joints, mostly the knees, leading to arthritis (may take from a few weeks to 2 years to become symptomatic).

Purpose

- To detect the occurrence of Lyme disease.

Clinical Problems

Positive Titer: Lyme disease.

Procedure

- Collect 3 to 5 ml of venous blood in a red-top tube.

- There is no food or fluid restriction.

Factors Affecting Laboratory Results

- Persons with a high rheumatoid factor could have a false-positive test result.

NURSING IMPLICATIONS WITH RATIONALE

- Report a history of a tick bite.
- Assess for a macular lesion at the site of the tick bite and elsewhere.
- Check titer level. A fourfold rise in titer is indicative of a recent infection.

Client Teaching

- Instruct the client to wear clothing that covers entirely the extremities when in the woods and areas infested by ticks and deer.
- Instruct the client to see his or her health care provider immediately if bitten by a tick or if a macular lesion results from a tick bite. Antibiotic therapy is frequently started.
- Inform the client that the commonest complication of Lyme disease is arthritis. Others are cardiac dysrhythmias, carditis, and neuritis.

Lymphocytes (T and B) (blood)

T and B Lymphocytes; Lymphocyte Marker Studies;
Lymphocyte Subset Typing

Reference Values

Adult: *T Cells:* 60–80%, 600–2400 cells/µl. *B Cells:* 4–16%, 50–250 cells/µl.

Description

The two categories of lymphocytes are T lymphocytes and B lymphocytes. The T lymphocytes are associated with cell-mediated immune responses (cellular immunity), such as rejection of transplant and graft, tumor immunity, and microorganism (bacterial and viral) death. If the surface of the host's tissue cell is altered, the T cells might perceive that altered cell as foreign and attack it. This might be helpful if the altered surface is of tumor development; however, this T-cell attack might give rise to autoimmune disease.

The B lymphocytes, derived from bone marrow, are responsible for humoral immunity. The B cells synthesize immunoglobulins to react to specific antigens. An interaction between T and B lymphocytes is necessary for a satisfactory immune response.

Measurement of T and B lymphocytes is valuable for diagnosing autoimmune diseases (i.e., immunosuppressive diseases such as acquired immunodeficiency syndrome [AIDS], lymphoma, and lymphocytic leukemia). T and B cells can be used to monitor changes during the treatment of immunosuppressive diseases.

Purposes

- To detect selected autoimmune diseases, such as lymphoma and lymphocytic leukemia.
- To monitor the effects of treatment for immunosuppressive diseases, such as AIDS.

Clinical Problems

Decreased Level: *T Lymphocytes:* Lymphoma, systemic lupus erythematosus (SLE), thymic hypoplasia (DiGeorge's syndrome), acute viral infections. *Drug Influence:* Immunosuppressive agents. *B Lymphocytes:* IgG, IgA, IgM deficiency, lymphomas, nephrotic syndrome, sex-linked agammaglobulinemia. *T and B Lymphocytes:* Immunodeficiency diseases.

Elevated Level: *T Lymphocytes:* Autoimmune disorders such as Graves' disease. *B Lymphocytes:* Acute and chronic lymphocytic leukemias, multiple myeloma, Waldenström's macroglobulinemia.

Procedure

- Collect two 10-ml samples of venous blood in two lavender-top tubes. Refrigerate blood samples. *Check the laboratory procedures in your institution.*
- There is no food or fluid restriction.

Factors Affecting Laboratory Result

- An insufficient amount of blood drawn for the test could affect test result.

NURSING IMPLICATIONS WITH RATIONALE

- Keep the client free from exposure to infection.
- Observe for signs and symptoms of lymphocytic leukemias (i.e., fatigue, pallor, vesicular skin lesions, increased white blood cell count).

Client Teaching

- Teach the client to stay away from persons with colds or communicable diseases.

Magnesium (Mg) (serum)

Reference Values

Adult: 1.5–2.5 mEq/l, 1.8–3.0 mg/dl.

Child: *Newborn:* 1.4–2.9 mEq/l. *Child:* 1.6–2.6 mEq/l.

Description

Magnesium is most plentiful in the cells (intracellular fluid). One third of the magnesium ingested is absorbed through the small intestine, and the remaining unabsorbed magnesium is excreted in the stools. The absorbed magnesium is eventually excreted through the kidneys.

As with potassium, sodium, and calcium, magnesium is needed for neuromuscular activity. Magnesium influences use of potassium, calcium, and protein, and when there is a magnesium deficit, there is frequently a potassium and calcium deficit. Magnesium is also responsible for the transport of sodium and potassium across the cell membranes. Another function of magnesium is its activation of enzymes for carbohydrate and protein metabolism.

Magnesium is found in most foods, so it would be difficult for a person who maintains a normal diet to have a magnesium deficiency. The daily required magnesium intake for an adult is 200 to 300 mg, or 0.2 to 0.3 g.

A serum magnesium deficit is known as hypomagnesemia, and a serum magnesium excess is called hypermagnesemia.

Purposes

- To detect hypomagnesemia or hypermagnesemia.
- To monitor magnesium levels when there is a probable magnesium loss.

Clinical Problems

Decreased Level: Protein malnutrition, malabsorption, cirrhosis of the liver, alcoholism, hypoparathyroidism, hyperaldosteronism, hypokalemia (decreased potassium), IV solutions without magnesium, chronic diarrhea, bowel resection complications, dehydration. *Drug Influence:* Diuretics (mercurial, ethacrynic acid [Edecrin]), calcium gluconate, amphotericin B, neomycin, insulin.

Elevated Level: Severe dehydration, renal failure, leukemia (lymphocytic and myelocytic), diabetes mellitus (early phase). *Drug Influence:* Antacids (Maalox, Mylanta, Aludrox, DiGel), laxatives (epsom salts [$MgSO_4$], milk of magnesia, magnesium citrate).

Procedure

- Collect 3 to 5 ml of venous blood in a red-top tube. Avoid hemolysis.
- There is no food or fluid restriction.

Factors Affecting Laboratory Results

- Hypokalemia and hypocalcemia will decrease the magnesium level.
- Drugs: Laxatives and antacids containing magnesium can cause hypermagnesemia, and diuretics, calcium gluconate, and insulin can cause hypomagnesemia. Insulin moves magnesium back into the cells, causing a serum magnesium deficit.

NURSING IMPLICATIONS WITH RATIONALE

Decreased Level

- Observe for signs and symptoms of hypomagnesemia, such as tetany symptoms (twitching and tremors, carpopedal spasm, generalized spasticity), restlessness, confusion, and arrhythmia. Neuromuscular irritability can be mistakenly attributed to hypocalcemia.
- Check serum potassium, sodium, calcium, and magnesium levels. Electrolyte deficits may accompany a magnesium deficit. If hypokalemia and hypomagnesemia are present, potassium supplements will not completely correct the potassium deficit until the magnesium deficit is corrected.
- Check for a positive Chvostek's sign by tapping the facial nerve in front of the ear and observing for spasm of the cheek and twitching at the corner of the lip.
- Report to the health care provider if the client has been NPO and receiving IV fluids without magnesium salts for weeks. Hyperalimentation solutions should contain magnesium.
- Check clients receiving digitalis preparations for digitalis intoxication (anorexia, nausea, vomiting, bradycardia). A magnesium deficit enhances the action of digitalis, causing digitalis toxicity.
- Assess renal function when the client is receiving magnesium supplements. Excess magnesium is excreted by the kidneys.
- Assess eletrocardiographic changes. A flat or inverted T wave can be indicative of hypomagnesemia. It can also indicate hypokalemia.
- Administer IV magnesium sulfate in solution slowly to prevent a hot or flushed feeling.
- Have IV calcium gluconate available to reverse hypermagnesemia due to overcorrection. Calcium antagonizes the sedative effect of magnesium.

Client Teaching

- Instruct the client to eat foods rich in magnesium (fish, seafood, meats, green vegetables, whole grains, and nuts).

Elevated Level

- Observe for signs and symptoms of hypermagnesemia, such as flushing, a feeling of warmth, increased perspiration (with the magnesium level at 3 to 4 mEq/l), muscular weakness, diminished reflex, respiratory distress, hypotension, a sedative effect (with the magnesium level at 9 to 10 mEq/l).
- Monitor urinary output. Effective urinary output (>750 ml daily) will decrease the serum magnesium level.
- Assess the client's level of sensorium and muscle activity.
- Assess ECG changes. A peaked T-wave and wide QRS complex can indicate hyperkalemia (increased potassium) and hypermagnesemia, so the serum potassium and magnesium levels should be checked.
- Provide adequate fluids to improve kidney function and to restore body fluids. Dehydration can cause hemoconcentration and, as a result, magnesium excess.
- Check for digitalis intoxication if the client is receiving calcium gluconate for hypermagnesemia. Calcium excess enhances the action of digitalis.

Client Teaching

- Instruct clients to avoid constant use of laxatives and antacids containing magnesium. Suggest to clients that they check drug labels.

Malaria (blood)

Reference Values

Adult: Negative.

Child: Negative.

Description

Malaria is caused by malarial parasites transmitted by mosquitoes. The parasites rupture the red blood cells (hemolysis), causing the client to have chills and fever.

Malarial parasites can be detected by blood smears (venous or capillary blood). Blood samples are usually taken in the presence of chills and fever daily for 3 days or at specified times—every 6 or 12 hours.

Purpose

- To identify the presence of malarial parasites.

Clinical Problems

Positive: Malaria (*Plasmodium* species).

Procedure

- Venous or capillary blood can be used for the malarial smear.
- Collect 5 ml in a lavender-top tube.
- There is no food or fluid restriction.

Factors Affecting Laboratory Results

- None known.

NURSING IMPLICATIONS WITH RATIONALE

- Explain the procedure to the client. The client should inform the nurse when he or she is having chills and fever, because a blood sample is usually requested at that time. The blood sample may also be requested daily for 3 days or at specified times during the day.
- Monitor the client's temperature every 4 hours or as ordered. Record temperature changes.
- Report chills and fever to the health care provider.

Melanin (urine)

Reference Values

Negative for melanogen or melanin.

Description

The melanin urine test is prescribed to verify the presence or progression of a melanoma. Melanin, a pigment in the body, is highly elevated in malignant melanoma. With metastatic melanoma, melanin metabolites, melanogens, are usually found in high concentration in the urine. If the urine is exposed to air for many hours, melanogen is converted to melanin and the urine becomes deep brown and later black. Twenty-five percent of clients with malignant melanoma have melanogen in the urine (melanogenuria). Further testing is necessary to determine the extent of disease.

Purposes

- To detect melanogenuria.
- To aid in the detection of malignant melanoma.

Clinical Problems

Elevated Level: Malignant melanoma. *Drug Influence:* Aspirin and aspirin compounds.

Procedure

- There is no food or fluid restriction.
- Collect a random urine specimen and send it immediately to the laboratory.

Factors Affecting Laboratory Results

- Aspirin can give a false-positive test result.
- When urine is left for hours at room temperature, the melanogen will convert to melanin and urine will become dark brown.

NURSING IMPLICATIONS WITH RATIONALE

- Obtain a history of health problems and drugs the client is currently taking. Drugs that contain aspirin can cause a false-positive test result.
- Listen to the client's concerns. Answer questions or refer the questions to other health professionals.

Client Teaching

- Instruct the client concerning urine collection. The urine container should be taken immediately to the laboratory.

Methemoglobin (blood)

Hemoglobin M, Hb M

Reference Values

Normal: <1.5% of the total hemoglobin; 0.06–0.24 g/dl; 9.2–37.0 μmol/l (SI units).

Positive: >20–70%, complaints of headache, dizziness, fatigue, tachycardia; >70%, death.

Description

Methemoglobin (Hb M) occurs when the deoxygenated heme (iron portion of hemoglobin) is oxidized to a ferric state. In the ferric state, the heme cannot combine with oxygen; thus, cyanosis without dyspnea or other cardiovascular problems may result. Methemoglobinemia may be acquired from chemicals, radiation, and such drugs as nitrites, nitrates, certain sulfonamides, antimalarials, local anesthetics, or inherited enzyme deficiency. Poisoning from occupational or environmental contact could cause methemoglobinemia. A deficiency in the glucose-6-phosphate dehydrogenase (G-6-PD) enhances the production of Hb M.

   If newborns are cyanotic after oxygen has been given, the methemoglobin level should be checked. Infants are more prone to develop methemoglobinemia.

Purposes

- To detect methoglobin in the blood caused from an acquired chemical or drug condition.
- To detect congenital methemoglobinemia.

Clinical Problems

Elevated Level

Acquired or hereditiary methemoglobinemia, radiation, carbon monoxide poisoning, smoking. *Drug Influence:* Bromo-Seltzer, nitrates (include silver nitrate topical preparation), nitrites, nitrous oxide, nitroglycerin, antimalarials, analgesics, certain sulfonamides, fluoroquinolones, benzene derivatives such as chlorobenzene, phenacetin, isoniazid, lidocaine, chlorates. *Food Influence:* Sausage and other foods that contain nitrites.

Procedure

- Collect 7 ml of venous blood in a lavender-top or green-top tube. Keep blood specimen on ice. Deliver blood specimen to the laboratory within 1 hour.
- There is no food or fluid restriction.

Factors Affecting Laboratory Results

- Certain drugs and foods can cause false results *(see Clinical Problems)*.
- Not keeping the blood specimen chilled (on ice) and not delivering the specimen to the laboratory within 1 hour.

NURSING IMPLICATIONS WITH RATIONALE

- Obtain a history of the health complaints, drugs and food the client is consuming. Certain drugs can enhance the production of Hb M *(see Clinical Problems)*. Excessive use of Bromo-Seltzer can increase the Hb M level.
- Check vital signs. Continuously monitor heart rate with a pulse oximetry.
- Check O_2 saturation with the pulse oximetry or arterial blood gases (ABGs).

- Administer oxygen. Blood transfusions may be prescribed.

Client Teaching

- Encourage client to rest if dizziness, fatigue, and headaches occur.
- Explain to the client that the health care provider may discontinue a drug that may be causing an increase in Hb M production.

Mumps antibody (serum)

Reference Values

Negative: <1:8 titer.

Positive or Immunization: >1:8 (recent infection or immunization undetermined).

Description

Mumps, infectious parotitis, is an acute, contagious viral infection causing an inflammation of the parotid and salivary glands. The mumps virus can be spread by droplets or by direct contact with the saliva of an infected person. Complications of mumps include (1) in adolescent or adult males, unilateral orchitis in approximately 20% of reported cases, (2) in adult women, oophoritis, and (3) in persons of all ages and genders, meningoencephalitis in 1% to 10% of infected cases.

Diagnosis may be made by blood specimen, culture of saliva, or mumps skin test. With a blood specimen there should be two blood samples taken, one during the acute phase and one during the convalescent phase. For those persons that are at high risk or who have not had mumps, there is a vaccine to provide immunity.

Purpose

- To detect the presence of the mumps antibody in a person who may be at risk.

Clinical Problems

Positive: Mumps virus. *Complications:* Orchitis, oophoritis, meningoencephalitis.

Procedure

- Collect a total of two 3- to 5-ml samples of venous blood in a red-top tube, 1 to 2 weeks apart. The first specimen is drawn during the acute phase and the second is taken 1 to 2 weeks later during the convalescent phase. Avoid hemolysis.

■ There is no food or fluid restriction.

Factors Affecting Laboratory Results

■ Hemolysis of the blood sample.
■ Obtaining one blood specimen only. A total of two blood samples should be obtained to determine not only the acute phase but also when the convalescent phase begins.

NURSING IMPLICATIONS WITH RATIONALE

■ Assess the client for symptoms of mumps, which can include malaise, headache, chills, fever, pain below the ear, and swelling of the parotid glands.
■ Assess if the client has been in contact with a person diagnosed as having mumps. Clients who are suspected of having mumps may be isolated up to 9 days after swelling occurs.
■ Check if the client had received the mumps vaccine. Those who develop mumps normally have a lifetime immunity.

Client Teaching

■ Explain to the client that he or she is to return for a second blood test. This is necessary to determine the convalescent phase of the mumps infection.
■ Explain to the client that mumps is contagious and he or she should be isolated for approximately 9 days from persons who have never had mumps or the vaccine.

Myoglobin (serum)

Reference Values

Adult: 12–90 ng/ml, 12–90 µg/l.
Female: 12–75 ng/ml, 12–75 µg/l.
Male: 20–90 ng/ml, 20–90 µg/l.

Description

Myoglobin is an oxygen-binding protein, similar to hemoglobin, that is found in skeletal and cardiac muscle cells. Myoglobin is released into circulation after an injury. Increased serum myoglobin occurs about 2 to 6 hours following muscle tissue damage. Serum myoglobin level reaches its peak following a myocardial infarction (MI) in approximately 8 to 12 hours. Elevated serum myoglobin (myoglobinemia) is short-lived; in 50% of persons having an MI, the serum level begins to return to normal range in 12 to 18 hours. Urine myoglobin may be detected for 3 to 7 days following muscle injury.

Because serum myoglobin is nonspecific concerning which muscle is damaged, myocardium or skeletal, cardiac enzymes should also be ordered. Creatine phosphokinase (CPK) and CPK isoenzyme, CPK-MB, should be checked because this enzyme rises early after an MI. Assessment of signs and symptoms of an acute MI need to be considered along with the blood tests. This test is not performed following cardioversion or after an angina attack.

Purpose

- To detect myoglobin protein, which is released in high amount during skeletal or cardiac muscle injury.

Clinical Problems

Elevated Level: Acute MI, skeletal muscle injury, severe burns, polymyositis, trauma, surgical procedure, acute alcohol intoxicity with delirium tremens, renal failure, metabolic stress.

Procedure

- There is no food or fluid restriction.
- Collect 3 to 5 ml of venous blood in a red-top tube. Avoid hemolysis. The blood sample should be drawn soon after an acute MI; following acute pain.

Factors Affecting Laboratory Results

- Blood sample taken for serum myoglobin a day or two after an acute injury or myocardial infarction.
- Hemolysis of the blood specimen.

NURSING IMPLICATIONS WITH RATIONALE

- Obtain a history of current discomfort. Differentiate, if possible, between heart and skeletal muscle discomfort. Record and inform the health care provider of your findings.
- Assess the client for signs and symptoms of an MI, such as sharp-penetrating pain, intense chest pressure, diaphoresis, dyspnea, nausea and vomiting, indigestion. Report findings immediately.
- Check vital signs. Compare with baseline vital signs. Report changes immediately.
- Compare serum myoglobin results with cardiac enzyme tests. Serum myoglobin usually increases before CPK; however, serum myoglobin elevation could indicate skeletal muscle injury. Various laboratory tests, history, and symptoms need to be considered.

Client Teaching

- Instruct the client to inform you when pain occurs or recurs. Have client describe the pain (type, intensity, duration).
- Allow client and family member(s) time to express their concerns. As necessary, refer questions to other health care providers.

Myoglobin (urine)

Reference Values

Adult: None detected.

Description

Myoglobin is an oxygen-binding protein, similar to hemoglobin, that is found in skeletal and cardiac muscle cells. Myoglobin is released into circulation soon after a muscle tissue injury (skeletal or cardiac) occurs *(see Myboglobin [serum])*. Myoglobin passes rapidly from the blood through the glomeruli in the kidney and is excreted in the urine. Myoglobinuria can appear within 3 hours after a myocardial infarction (MI) and may be present in the urine up to 72 hours or longer. Usually the serum myoglobin level returns to normal range within 18 to 36 hours.

Besides indicating myocardial damage due to a MI, myoglobinuria may occur following a traumatic muscle tissue injury, severe ischemia, diabetic ketoacidosis, delirium tremens, systemic infection with fever, severe burns, and muscular dystropy. Client's symptoms and other tests should be considered to determine cause of urine myoglobin.

Purpose

See myoglobin (Serum).

Clinical Problems

Elevated Level: Acute MI, skeletal muscle tissue injury, crush injuries from trauma, severe burns, surgical procedure, polymyositis, delirium tremens, metabolic stress.

Procedure

- There is no food or fluid restriction.
- Collect 5 to 10 ml of random urine specimen in a sterile plastic container. Deliver the urine specimen to the laboratory.

Factors Affecting the Laboratory Results

- Collecting the urine specimen within 3 hours of an acute injury. A repeat urine specimen should be collected 24 hours after the injury (skeletal or cardiac).

NURSING IMPLICATIONS WITH RATIONALE

- Obtain a history of the current muscle discomfort (skeletal or cardiac). Report your findings.
- Assess the client for signs and symptoms of an MI, such as sharp-penetrating pain in the chest, radiating pain in the left arm, diaphoresis, dyspnea, nausea, and vomiting. Report your findings immediately.
- Check vital signs and report abnormal findings.
- Compare elevated serum myoglobin level with positive urine myoglobin. Cardiac enzymes should also be ordered.

Client Teaching

- Explain the procedure for urine collection to the client. Urine should be collected in a sterile plastic container. The client should clean the urinary orifice before urinating into the container.
- Instruct the client to give the urine specimen to the health provider immediately so that the urine can be delivered to the laboratory. Urine should be tested soon after it is given.
- Answer client's and family's questions. Unknown answers should be referred to the appropriate health professional.

5'Nucleotidase (5'N or 5'NT) (serum)

Reference Values

Adult: <17 U/l.

Pregnancy (Third Trimester): Slightly above normal value.

Child: Values lower than adults.

Description

This is a liver enzyme test that aids in the diagnosis of hepatobiliary disease. 5'Nucleotidase (5'N) is not elevated in bone disorders as is alkaline phosphatase (ALP); therefore it is useful in determining the origin of the problem. Elevated ALP and 5'N indicate liver disorder. Elevated ALP and normal 5'N indicate bone disorder.

Usually several liver enzyme tests (i.e., ALP, leucine aminopeptidase [LAP], gamma-glutamyl transferase [GGT]) are performed to evaluate liver function.

Purpose

- To compare test results with other liver enzyme tests for diagnosing a liver disorder.

Clinical Problems

Elevated Level: Cirrhosis of the liver, biliary obstruction from calculi and tumor, and metastasis to the liver. *Drug Influence:* Phenothiazines, narcotics (codeine, morphine, meperidine [Demerol]).

Procedure

- Collect 3 to 5 ml of venous blood in a red-top tube. Avoid hemolysis.
- There is no food or fluid restriction.

Factors Affecting Laboratory Results

- Hemolysis of the blood specimen.

NURSING IMPLICATIONS WITH RATIONALE

- Check the venipuncture site; clients with liver disorders tend to have prolonged clotting times.

Elevated Level

- Compare 5'N levels with other liver enzyme levels. Elevated ALP, GGT, LAP, and 5'N values indicate that the problem is of liver origin.

Client Teaching

- Instruct the client that there could be a tendency toward bleeding. If bleeding occurs from the mouth, rectum, or elsewhere, the health care provider should be notified.
- Encourage the client to eat well-balanced meals, especially if the condition is cirrhosis of the liver or cancer of the liver.

Occult blood (feces)

Reference Values

Adult: Negative.

Child: Negative.

Note: A diet rich in meats, poultry, fish, and drugs (cortisone, aspirin, potassium) could cause a false-positive occult blood test.

Description

Occult (nonvisible or hidden) blood in the feces usually indicates gastrointestinal bleeding. Bright red blood from the rectum can be indicative of bleeding from the lower large intestine (e.g., hemorrhoids), and tarry black stools indicate blood loss of >50 ml from the upper GI tract.

Occult blood in the feces may be present days or several weeks after a single bleeding episode. False-positive occult blood test results may be due to ingestion of meats, poultry, fish, and certain drugs.

Purpose

- To detect blood in the feces.

Clinical Problems

Negative Results: *Drug Influence:* Ascorbic acid (large amounts of vitamin C).

Positive Results: Bleeding, peptic ulcer, gastritis, gastric carcinoma, bleeding esophageal varices, colitis, intestinal carcinoma, diverticulitis. *Drug Influence:* Aspirin, steroids (cortisone preparations), colchicine, iron preparations, iodine, indomethacin (Indocin), reserpine, potassium preparations, thiazide diuretics, bromides.

Procedure

- There are a variety of blood-test reagents that may be used to test for occult blood. Some are more sensitive than others. Orthotolidine (Occultest) is considered the most sensitive test, more sensitive than the guaiac (least sensitive).
- Meats, poultry, and fish should be avoided for 3 days prior to stool specimen, especially if orthotolidine or benzidine tests are used.
- Obtain a single, random stool specimen and send it to the laboratory. Only a small amount of fecal material is needed. Stool may be obtained from a rectal examination. Many times the stool test is done on the nursing floor using a commercial kit.
- List on the laboratory slip drugs the client is taking that could affect test results.
- The stool specimen does not need to be kept warm or examined immediately.

Factors Affecting Laboratory Results

- Drugs *(see Drug Influence)*.
- Foods: meats; poultry; fish; and green, leafy vegetables can cause a false-positive test result.
- Urine and soap solution in the feces may affect the test result.

NURSING IMPLICATIONS WITH RATIONALE

Client Teaching

- Instruct the client not to eat meats, poultry, or fish for 3 days prior to the test. Green, leafy vegetables, if eaten in abundance, could cause a false-positive test result.
- Instruct the client not to take drugs that could cause false-positive results for 3 days before the test, if possible.

Positive Result for Occult Blood

- Obtain a history of recent or past bleeding episodes. Inform the health care provider of a history of GI bleeding.
- Inform the health care provider if the client is receiving medication that could cause a false-positive test result *(see Drug Influence)*.
- Determine whether the client has had epigastric pain between meals. This type of pain could be indicative of a peptic ulcer.
- Be sure the stool is not contaminated with menstrual discharge.

Client Teaching

- Encourage the client to report abnormal-colored stools (e.g., tarry stools). Oral iron preparations can cause the stools to be black.

Opiates (urine)

Reference Values

Negative.

Toxic Values: *Codeine:* >0.005 mg/dl (0.2 µmol/l). *Hydromorphone:* >0.1 mg/dl (5 µmol/l). *Meperidine:* >0.5 mg/dl (20 µmol/l). *Methadone:* >0.2 mg/dl (10 µmol/l). *Morphone:* >0.005 mg/dl (0.2 µmol/l). *Propoxyphene:* >0.5 mg/dl (20 µmol/l).

Description

Testing for opiates is primarily done to screen for drug abuse or narcotic toxicity, or to check the progress of opiate detoxification. Specific opiates, such as codeine, morphine, methadone, hydromorphone, and meperidine, can be individually tested. Urine is the preferred specimen for checking for opiates; however, gastric secretions could be analyzed.

The liver detoxifies opiates and the urine excretes 90% of the opiates in 24 hours. The peak effect of opiates in the body occurs in approximately 1 hour.

Purposes

- To detect the presence of opiates.
- To check for opiate toxicity.
- To monitor the progress of opiate detoxification.

Clinical Problems

Elevated Level: Specific opiate presence or toxicity: *Drug Influence:* Use of other opiates.

Procedure

- There is no food or fluid restriction.
- Collect a random urine specimen and send the specimen immediately to the laboratory.
- List drugs taken by the client in the last 24 hours on the lab sheet, including over-the-counter drugs.
- Refrigerate the urine specimen if the test can not be done immediately.

Factors Affecting Laboratory Results

- Delay in testing the urine specimen without it being refrigerated.

NURSING IMPLICATIONS WITH RATIONALE

- Have the client sign a consent form if necessary.
- Explain the test procedure to the client.
- Obtain a drug history including over-the-counter drugs. Explain that the drug information will be given to the health care provider.
- Send the random urine specimen immediately to the laboratory. If the opiate test is for methadone, a 24-hour urine specimen is needed. Inform the laboratory that the urine specimen should be tested immediately or refrigerated. Delay in testing could result in false-negative test result.
- Listen to the client's concerns. Be available to discuss drug problems or refer the discussion to an appropriate health care provider.

Osmolality (serum)

Reference Values

Adult: 280–300 mOsm/kg.

Panic Values: <240 mOsm/kg and >320 mOsm/kg.

Child: 270–290 mOsm/kg.

Description

Serum osmolality is an indicator of serum concentration. It measures the number of dissolved particles (electrolytes, urea, sugar) in the serum and is helpful in the diagnosis of fluid and electrolyte imbalances. Sodium contributes 85% to 90% of the serum osmolality; changes in osmolality usually result from changes in the serum sodium concentration. Double the serum sodium can give a rough estimate of the serum osmolality.

The hydration status of the patient is usually determined by the serum osmolality. An increased value (>300 mOsm/kg) indicates hemoconcentration due to dehydration; a decreased value (<280 mOsm/kg) indicates hemodilution due to overhydration, or water excess. An osmometer is used in laboratories to determine serum osmolality; however, if the serum sodium, urea, and sugar levels are known, the serum osmolality can be calculated by the nurse as follows.

$$\text{Serum osmolality} = 2 \times \text{Serum sodium} + \frac{\text{BUN}}{3} + \frac{\text{Sugar}}{18}$$

Purposes

- To monitor body fluid balance.
- To determine the occurrence of body fluid overload or dehydration.

Clinical Problems

Decreased Level: Excessive fluid intake, cancer of the bronchus and lung, adrenal cortical hypofunction, IV 5% dextrose in water (D_5W), syndrome of inappropriate diuretic hormone (SIADH).

Elevated Level: Diabetes insipidus, dehydration, hypernatremia, hyperglycemia, uremia.

Procedure

- Collect 5 to 7 ml of venous blood in a red-top tube. Avoid hemolysis.
- There is no food or fluid restriction.

Factors Affecting Laboratory Results

- Hyperglycemia increases the serum osmolality.

NURSING IMPLICATIONS WITH RATIONALE

Decreased Level

- Observe for signs and symptoms of overhydration, such as a constant, irritated cough; dyspnea; neck- and hand-vein engorgement; and chest rales.
- Observe for signs and symptoms of water intoxication, such as headaches, confusion, and irritability. Excessive amounts of hyposmolar solutions can "superdilute" the intravascular fluid.

Client Teaching

- Instruct the client to decrease fluid intake.

Elevated Level

- Assess for signs and symptoms of dehydration (thirst, dry mucous membranes, poor skin turgor, and shocklike symptoms).
- Check for glycosuria. Increased sugar in the urine could indicate the presence of hyperglycemia.
- Check the serum sodium, urea, and glucose for increased values. Calculate the serum osmolality by either doubling the serum sodium or using the formula given in the description.

Client Teaching

- Encourage the client to increase fluid intake.

Osmolality (urine)

Reference Values

Adult: 50–1200 mOsm/kg/H_2O, average 200–800 mOsm/kg H_2O.

Child: *Newborn:* 100–600 mOsm/kg/H_2O. *Child:* Same as adult.

Description

The urine osmolality test is more accurate than the specific gravity in determining the urine concentration, because its value reflects the number of particles, ions, and molecules and is not unduly influenced by large molecules. Specific gravity measures the quantity and nature of the particles, such as sugar, protein, and IV dyes (these elevate specific gravity but have little effect on osmolality).

The urine osmolality fluctuates in the same way that the urine-specific gravity does, and it can be low or high according to the client's state of hydration. A dehydrated client with normal kidney function could have a urine osmolality of 1000 mOsm/kg H2O or more. When hemoconcentration occurs as a result of acidosis, shock, or hyperglycemia, the serum osmolality is elevated, and so should the urine osmolality be elevated.

If serum hyposmolality and hyponatremia occur with urine hyperosmolality, the problem is most likely the syndrome of inappropriate antiduretic hormone secretion (SIADH). ADH causes water reabsorption from the kidney, thus diluting the serum.

Purposes

See Osmolality (Serum).

Clinical Problems

Decreased Level: Excessive water intake, continuous IV 5% dextrose in water (D₅W), diabetes insipidus, glomerulonephritis, acute renal failure, sickle cell anemia, multiple myeloma. *Drug Influence:* Diuretics.

Elevated Level: High-protein diet, SIADH, Addison's disease (adrenal gland insufficiency), dehydration, hyperglycemia with glycosuria.

Procedure

- Give a high-protein diet for 3 days prior to the urine osmolality test. Check with your laboratory.
- Restrict fluids for 8 to 12 hours before the test.
- Collect a random, morning, urine specimen. The first urine specimen in the morning is discarded, and the second specimen, taken 2 hours later, is sent to the laboratory. Urine osmolality should be high in the morning.
- Send the urine specimen to the laboratory.

Factors Affecting Laboratory Results

- Diuretics can cause urine hyperosmolality.
- A high-protein diet can cause urine hyperosmolality.

NURSING IMPLICATIONS WITH RATIONALE

- Explain to the client that the purpose of the test is to determine the kidney's ability to concentrate urine.
- Explain the procedure of the test if it requires more than a random urine sample for urine osmolality. A high-protein diet is taken for 3 days before the test, and oral fluids are restricted the night before. The first urine specimen of the morn-

ing is discarded, and the second specimen, taken an hour or two later, is sent to the laboratory.

Decreased Level

- Determine whether the decreased urine osmolality could be caused by excessive intake of water (>2 quarts daily) or continuous IV administration of D_5W in water. A urine osmolality that remains <200 mOsm/kg after fluids are restricted could be indicative of early kidney impairment.
- Explain to the client the need to decrease excessive water intake.
- Report to the health care provider when the client is receiving D_5W continuously without any other solutes, such as saline (NaCl). The D_5W not only dilutes the urine, it can decrease the serum osmolality and cause water intoxication.
- Observe for signs and symptoms of water intoxication, such as headaches, confusion, irritability, weight gain, and, later, cerebral edema (if severe).

Elevated Level

- Determine the hydration status of the client. Dehydration will cause an elevated urine osmolality as well as elevated serum osmolality. A urine osmolality of 1000 mOsm/kg is not abnormal if the client has a decreased fluid intake.
- Check the serum osmolality. If the serum is hyposmolar and the urine is hyperosmolar, the problem could be due to SIADH. SIADH frequently occurs after surgery, trauma, or pain and will correct itself in a day or two. The function of ADH is to promote water reabsorption from the kidney tubules. The serum is diluted, and the decreased urine is concentrated.
- Keep an accurate intake and output record. The fluid intake should be comparable to the urine output.

Client Teaching

- Instruct clients on high-protein diets to increase water intake.

Osmotic fragility of erythrocytes (blood)

Erythrocyte Osmotic Fragility, Red Cell Fragility

Reference Values

Adult

	% HEMOLYSIS	
% Saline (NaCl)	Fresh Blood (<3 hours)	Incubated at 37°C (24-hour blood)
0.30	97–100	85–100
0.35	90–98	75–100
0.40	50–95	65–100
0.45	5–45	55–95
0.50	0–5	40–85
0.55	0	15–65
0.60	0	0–40

Child: Similar to adult.

Description

This is an infrequently performed test.

Water is normally exchanged between cells and extracellular fluid according to the osmolality (concentration) of fluid. Erythrocyte (red blood cell, RBC) fluid and plasma have similar ionic concentrations, iso-osmolar or isotonic. When there is an imbalance in one of the fluids, osmosis occurs. Fluid moves from the fluid with the lesser concentration to the fluid with the greater concentration. If erythrocytes are placed in a hypo-osmolar solution, fluid with less than the normal serum/plasma osmolality (<280 mOsm/kg) will move into the erythrocytes, causing them to swell and eventually to rupture.

The erythrocyte osmotic fragility test determines the erythrocytes' ability to resist hemolysis (RBC destruction) in a hypo-osmolar solution. Erythrocytes are placed in various concentrations of saline. If hemolysis occurs at a slightly hypo-osmolar concentration of saline (0.36% to 0.73% solution), there is increased osmotic fragility, and if hemolysis occurs at a severely hypo-osmolar concentration of saline, there is decreased osmotic fragility. With increased fragility, the erythrocytes are usually spherical, and with decreased fragility, the erythrocytes are thin and flat.

Purpose

■ To determine erythrocyte osmotic fragility in a hypo-osmolar solution.

Clinical Problems

Decreased Level: Anemias (iron deficiency, folic acid deficiency, vitamin B_6 deficiency, sickle cell), thalassemia major and minor (Mediterranean anemia or Cooley's anemia), hemoglobin C disease,* polycythemia vera, after splenectomy, acute and subacute necrosis of the liver, obstructive jaundice.

Elevated Level: Hereditary spherocytosis, transfusion (incompatibility—ABO and Rh), acquired hemolytic anemia (autoimmune), hemoglobin C disease,* chemical or drug poisonings, chronic lymphocytic leukemia, burns (thermal).

Procedure

- The test is usually performed on fresh blood less than 3 hours old and/or on 24-hour-old blood incubated at 37°C.
- Collect 7 ml of venous blood in a lavender-top or green-top tube. The tube should be filled to its capacity. A drop of blood is placed in tubes with decreasing saline concentration.
- Hemolysis is frequently determined by a colorimeter.
- There is no food or fluid restriction.

Factors Affecting Laboratory Results

- Plasma pH, temperature, glucose concentration, and oxygen saturation of the blood affect the osmotic fragility.
- Older erythrocytes have increased osmotic fragility.
- A blood sample more than 3 hours old may show an increase in osmotic fragility.

NURSING IMPLICATIONS WITH RATIONALE

Decreased Level

- Identify clinical problems related to a decreased erythrocyte osmotic fragility. Normally, complete hemolysis occurs with 0.30% saline. Thin, flat cells are usually resistant to hemolysis at 0.30%.
- Assess for signs and symptoms of anemias, such as fatigue, weakness, tachycardia, and dyspnea.

Elevated Level

- Identify clinical problems related to an increased erythrocyte osmotic fragility (i.e., transfusion incompatibility, acquired hemolytic anemia, and chemical or drug poisoning [see Clinical Problems]).
- Monitor temperature when the client receives a blood transfusion. A slightly elevated temperature is an early sign of transfusion reaction.
- Observe for signs and symptoms of transfusion reactions other than changes in temperature (i.e., rash, difficulty in breathing, and an increased pulse rate).

---

*Decreased or increased fragility may occur in hemoglobin C disease.

Ova and parasites (O and P) (feces)

Reference Values

Adult: Negative.

Child: Negative.

Description

Parasites may be present in various forms in the intestine, including the ova (eggs), larvae (immature form), cysts (inactive stage), and trophozoites (motile form) of protozoa. It is vitally important to detect parasites so that proper treatment can be ordered. Some of the organisms identified are amoeba, flagellates, tapeworms, hookworms, and roundworms. A history of recent travel outside the United States should be reported to the laboratory, because it may help in identifying the parasite.

Purpose

- To identify specific ova and parasites in fecal matter.

Clinical Problems

Positive Result: Protozoa—*Balantidium coli, Chilomastix mesnili, Entamoeba histolytica, Giardia lamblia, Trichomonas hominis;* helminths (adults)—*Ascaris lumbricoides* (roundworm), *Diphyllobothrium latum* (fish tapeworm), *Enterobius vermicularis* (pinworm), *Necator americanus* (American hookworm), *Strongyloides stercoralis* (threadworm), *Taenia saginata* (beef tapeworm), *Taenia solium* (pork tapeworm).

Procedure

- Collect stool specimens for 3 days or every other day. Stool specimens should be taken immediately to the laboratory.
- Mark on the laboratory slip the countries the client has visited outside the United States in the last 1 to 3 years.
- A loose or liquid stool is more likely to indicate that trophozoites are present. The stool must be kept warm and taken to the laboratory within 30 minutes. If the stool is semiformed or well formed, it does not need to be kept warm but should be taken to the laboratory at once.
- If the stool is tested for tapeworm, the entire stool should be sent to the laboratory so that the head (scolex) of the tapeworm can be identified. The tapeworm will continue to grow as long as the head is lodged in the intestine.
- Anal swabs are used to check for pinworm eggs, and the swabbing should be done in the morning before defecation or the morning bath.
- No tissue paper or urine should be allowed in the fecal collection.

- Avoid taking mineral oil, castor oil, Metamucil, barium, antacids, or tetracycline for 1 week before the test.
- Laboratory results are available in 24 to 48 hours.

Factors Affecting Laboratory Results

- Urine, toilet paper, soap, disinfectants, antibiotics, antacids, barium, harsh laxatives, and hypertonic saline enemas (Fleet) may affect the result of the test.

NURSING IMPLICATIONS WITH RATIONALE

- Administer a mild laxative or normal saline enema, with the health care provider's approval, to obtain the stool specimen, if necessary.
- Take the fresh stool specimen to the laboratory immediately.
- Report if the client is taking antacids and/or antibiotics or has received barium in the last 7 days. These agents can alter the stool examination for parasites and ova.
- Obtain a history of the client's recent travel. Certain parasites are common to certain countries, and the health care provider and laboratory should be notified of this information.
- Handle the stool specimen with care to prevent parasitic contamination of yourself and other clients.
- Check for occult blood in the stool. The worm attaches itself to the bowel's lining.

Client Teaching

- Explain to the client the procedure for collecting the stool specimen. The stool should be collected in the morning, preferably before a bath. Explain to the client that he or she should not use soap or a Fleet enema, for this may destroy the parasite. The stool specimen should be obtained before treatment is initiated.
- Instruct the client not to put urine or toilet paper in the sterile bedpan. Disinfectants should not be used, because they can cause the ova to deteriorate.
- Instruct the client to wash hands thoroughly after urinating and defecating.

Parathyroid hormone (PTH) (serum)

Parathormone

Reference Values

Adult: *Intact PTH:* 11–54 pg/ml; *C-Terminal PTH:* 50–330 pg/ml; *N-Terminal PTH:* 8–24 pg/ml.

Description

Parathyroid hormone (PTH), secreted by the parathyroid glands, regulates the concentration of calcium and phosphorus in the extracellular fluid. The main function of PTH is to promote calcium reabsorption and phosphorus excretion. Serum calcium levels affect the secretion of PTH: low serum calcium levels stimulate the secretion of PTH; high serum calcium levels inhibit PTH secretion.

Two forms of PTH, inactive C-terminal PTH and active N-terminal PTH, are used in diagnosing parathyroid disorders. C-terminal assays (PTH-C) are an effective indicator of chronic hyperparathyroidism. N-terminal assays (PTH-N) detect acute changes in the PTH secretion, can differentiate between hypercalcemia due to malignancy or parathyroid disorder, and are useful for monitoring client's response to PTH therapy. Both assays and serum calcium values are used in diagnosing early and borderline parathyroid disorders.

Purposes

- To identify hypo- or hyperparathyroidism *(see Clinical Problems)*.
- To monitor the client's response to PTH therapy.

Clinical Problems

Decreased Level: *PTH-C Levels:* Hypoparathyroidism, nonparathyroid hypercalcemia. *PTH-N Levels:* Hypoparathyroidism, nonparathyroid hypercalcemia, certain tumors, pseudohyperparathyroidism. *PTH (Serum):* Hypoparathyroidism, nonparathyroid hypercalcemia, Graves disease, sarcoidosis.

Elevated Level: *PTH-C Levels:* Secondary hyperparathyroidism, tumors, hypercalcemia, pseudohypoparathyroidism. *PTH-N Levels:* Primary and secondary hyperparathyroidism, pseudohypoparathyroidism. *PTH (serum):* Primary and secondary hyperparathyroidism, hypercalcemia, chronic renal failure, pseudohyperparathyroidism (defect in renal tubular response).

Procedure

- NPO for 8 hours prior to the test.

- Collect 5 to 7 ml of venous blood in a red-top tube in the morning. Morning PTH is usually at its lowest point. Avoid hemolysis. Two tubes may be required (5 ml each). N-terminal PTH is unstable and needs to be chilled or frozen if test is not immediately run.
- N-terminal PTH levels decrease during hemodialysis; therefore, collect blood specimens prior to dialysis.

Factors Affecting Laboratory Results

- Using a nonchilled tube for N-terminal PTH affects test result.
- Food, especially milk products, might lower the PTH level.
- Hemolysis of the blood sample could cause inaccurate results.

NURSING IMPLICATIONS AND RATIONALE

- Check with the laboratory to verify the procedure for collecting blood sample(s).
- Assess for signs and symptoms of hypocalcemia (tetany; i.e., muscular twitching and tremors, paresthesia [tingling and numbness of fingers], spasmodic contractions).
- Assess for signs and symptoms of hypercalcemia (i.e., lethargy, muscle flaccidity, weakness, headaches, nausea and vomiting).

Client Teaching

- Instruct the client not to eat until after the blood sample is taken. Explain to the client that foods high in calcium can affect test results.

Partial thromboplastin time (PTT), activated partial thromboplastin time (APTT) (plasma)

Reference Values

Adult: Results vary in accordance with equipment and laboratory values. **PTT:** 60–70 seconds. **APTT:** 20–35 seconds.

Child: Increased above adult level.

Anticoagulant Therapy: 1.5–2.5 times the control in seconds.

Note: Most laboratories do APTT only.

Description

The partial thromboplastin time (PTT) is a screening test used to detect deficiencies in all clotting factors except VII and XIII and to detect platelet variations. It is more sensitive than the prothrombin time (PT) in detecting minor deficiencies but is not as sensitive as the activated partial thromboplastin time (APTT).

The PTT is useful for monitoring heparin therapy. Heparin doses are adjusted according to the PTT test.

The APTT is more sensitive in detecting clotting factor defects than the PTT, because the activator added in vitro shortens the clotting time. By shortening the clotting time, minor clotting defects can be detected.

The APTT is similar to the PTT, except that the thromboplastin reagent used in the APTT test contains an activator (kaolin, celite, or ellagic acid) for identification of deficient factors. This test is commonly used to monitor heparin therapy.

Purposes

- To monitor heparin therapy.
- To screen for clotting factor deficiencies.

Clinical Problems

Decreased Level: Extensive cancer.

Increased Level: Factor deficiency (factors V, VIII [hemophilia], IX [Christmas disease], X, XI, XII), cirrhosis of the liver, vitamin K deficiency, hypofibrinogenemia, prothrombin deficiency, von Willebrand's disease (vascular hemophilia), disseminated intravascular coagulation (DIC), leukemias (myelocytic, monocytic), malaria. *Drug Influence:* Heparin, salicylates.

Procedure

- Collect 3 to 5 ml of venous blood in a blue-top tube. The tube should be filled to its capacity.
- An activated thromboplastin mixture (thromboplastin reagent and an activator, such as kaolin) is added to the patient's plasma sample and the control sample. When a small amount of calcium solution is added, the stopwatch is started; it is stopped when fibrin strands are noted. The tests are usually duplicated and should agree to within 1 to 1.5 seconds. The test can also be done using a "fibronmeter."
- There is no food or fluid restriction.

Factors Affecting Laboratory Results

- A clotted blood sample.
- A test (collection) tube without an anticoagulant.

NURSING IMPLICATIONS WITH RATIONALE

- Check the APTT or PTT and report the results to the health care provider. The heparin dosage may need to be adjusted. The APTT range for heparin therapy is 1.5 to 2.5 times the normal value.

- Assess the client for signs and symptoms of bleeding (purpura [skin], hematuria, and nosebleeds).
- Administer heparin subcutaneously or intravenously through a heparin lock. Do not aspirate when giving heparin subcutaneously, because a hematoma (blood tumor) could occur at the injection site.

Parvovirus B 19 antibody (serum)

Reference Values

Negative: No IgG and IgM antibodies to parvovirus B 19.

Description

The parvovirus B 19, a human virus, destroys red blood cells (RBCs) and interferes with RBC production. This virus occurs more frequently in children. Erythema infectiosum causes a low-grade fever and rash, particularly in children; hydrops fetalis and aplastic anemia are associated with the parvovirus B 19.

The presence of IgM antibodies to parvovirus B 19 can indicate an acute infection, and the IgG antibodies can indicate a past infection or immunity. Joint inflammation and purpura are other clinical manifestations of the parvovirus B 19. A positive parvovirus B 19 has been associated with organ transplants; therefore, a serologic assessment should be made on organ donors.

Purposes

- To detect the presence of parvovirus B 19 antibody.
- To aid in the diagnosis of erythema infectiosum.

Clinical Problems

Positive Test: Erythema infectiosum (most common), transient aplastic anemia, joint arthritis, hydrops fetalis, fetal loss, bone marrow failure (aplastic anemia), chronic anemia in immunocompromised clients.

Procedure

- Collect 5 ml of venous blood in a red-top tube. Avoid hemolysis (shaking tube or rough handling of the blood specimen). Keep blood specimen on ice.
- Take precaution with collection and delivery of the blood specimen to avoid spread of infection.
- There is no food or fluid restriction.

Factors Affecting Laboratory Results

- Hemolysis of the blood specimen.
- Blood specimen not kept cold or on ice.

NURSING IMPLICATIONS WITH RATIONALE

- Obtain a history of the health complaint from the child, parent, or family member. List symptoms.
- Record vital signs. Report abnormal findings.

Client Teaching

- Explain to the organ donors that a blood test may be prescribed to rule out the presence of a virus antibody (parvovirus B 19 antibody) that may affect organ donation. It is for preventive purposes.
- Answer the parent or family members' questions concerning the child or client condition or refer the person(s) to other health professionals for correct answers.

Pepsinogen I (serum)

Reference Values

Adult: 124–142 ng/ml; 124–142 µg/l (SI units).

Child: *Premature Infant:* 20–24 ng/ml (SEM) × 1; 20–24 µg/l (SI units). *<1 Year:* 72–82 ng/ml; 72–82 µg/l (SI units). *1–2 Years:* 90–106 ng/ml; 90–106 µg/l (SI units). *3–6 Years:* 80–104 ng/ml; 80–104 µg/l (SI units). *7–10 Years:* 77–103 ng/ml; 77–103 µg/l (SI units). *11–14 Years:* 96–118 ng/ml; 96–118 µg/l (SI units).

Description

There are seven fractions of pepsinogens in the blood; five are classified as pepsinogen I (PG-I), which are secreted from the lumen of the stomach. The secretion of pepsinogen I is controlled by the hormone gastrin. Pepsinogen I is converted to pepsin when the stomach pH is acidic. Pepsin is needed in the process of digestion of proteins. Low gastrin and pepsinogen I levels are specific for atrophic gastritis. An elevated pepsinogen I level frequently occurs with duodenal ulcer. A high PG-I level can be inherited as an autosomal dominant trait.

Purpose

- To determine the cause of the gastric disorder.

Clinical Problems

Decreased Level: Atropic gastritis, gastric cancer, achlorhydria, pernicious anemia, Addison's disease, myxedema, hypopituitarism.

Elevated Level: Duodenal ulcer, acute gastritis, Zollinger-Ellison syndrome, hypergastrinemia.

Procedure

- NPO 8 to 12 hours before the test.
- Collect 5 to 7 ml of venous blood in a red-top tube.

Factors Affecting Laboratory Results

- Poor renal output can cause an elevated serum pepsinogen I level.

NURSING IMPLICATIONS WITH RATIONALE

- Assess the client's renal function, such as adequate urine output and blood urea nitrogen and serum creatinine levels. Poor renal function can cause a false-elevated serum PG-I level.
- Assess the client for complaints of gastric discomfort. Record findings.

Client Teaching

- Instruct the client that the test requires a fasting blood specimen; therefore, the client should take nothing by mouth after midnight.
- Instruct the client to inform you of any abdominal discomfort. The time of gastric or intestinal discomfort should be recorded.

Phenothiazines (serum)

Reference Values

Adult

Drug	Therapeutic Range	Peak Time	Toxic Level
Chlorpromazine (Thorazine)	50–300 ng/ml	2 to 4 hours	>750 ng/ml
Prochlorperazine (Compazine)	50–300 ng/ml	2 to 4 hours	>1000 ng/ml

(continued)

Drug	Therapeutic Range	Peak Time	Toxic Level
Thioridazine (Mellaril)	100–600 ng/ml 0.2–2.6 mg/l	2 to 4 hours	>2000 ng/ml >10 mg/l
Trifluoperazine (Stelazine)	50–300 ng/ml	2 to 4 hours	>1000 ng/ml

Description

Phenothiazines are major tranquilizers (neurolytics) used for the treatment of psychosis and emesis. The phenothiazines have many active metabolites that are excreted in the urine. Thus phenothiazines can be measured in the urine and also in gastric fluids. Because phenothiazines are metabolized to many metabolites, the serum value is difficult to measure.

The phenothiazines have a wide therapeutic index. Consequently large dosage or large overdoses are relatively safe. However, extremely large overdoses can cause drug toxicity.

Purposes

- To monitor a specific phenothiazine level for therapeutic effect.
- To check for specific phenothiazine toxicity.

Clinical Problems

Decreased Level: *Drug Influence:* Antacids, anticholinergics (for pseudoparkinsonism).

Elevated Level: Phenothiazide overdose.

Procedure

- Collect 7 ml of venous blood in a red-top tube.
- There is no food or fluid restriction.

Factors Affecting Laboratory Results

- Barbiturates and other antipsychotic agents enhance the phenothiazine effect.
- Antacids slow down the phenothiazine absorption, and anticholinergics taken for the pseudoparkinsonism effect can decrease the phenothiazine effect.

NURSING IMPLICATIONS WITH RATIONALE

- Obtain a history from the client concerning drug dosage and frequency.
- Determine if the client smokes. Smoking increases metabolism of the drug, and the drug dosage might need to be increased.

- Check liver enzyme laboratory tests, especially if the client is taking chlorpromazine (Thorazine). Taking chlorpromazine for a long period of time could have an effect on the liver.
- Observe for side effects of phenothiazines, especially the common pseudoparkinsonism effect (muscle rigidity, tremors, bent-over position when walking).

Client Teaching

- Explain to the client the importance of taking the prescribed drug dosage. Desired effect from the drug would not be obtained if the client were underdosed.
- Inform the client to use protective suntan lotion, because photosensitivity is common with phenothiazines.
- Advise the client to check with the health care provider before taking over-the-counter drugs to avoid side effects.
- Inform the client that the urine may be pink or red-brown when taking chlorpromazine (Thorazine).

Phenylketonuria (PKU) (urine), Guthrie test for PKU (blood)

Reference Values

Adult: PKU and Guthrie test not usually done.

Child: *Phenylalanine:* 0.5–2.0 mg/dl. *PKU:* Negative, but positive when the serum phenylalanine is 12–15 mg/dl. *Guthrie:* Negative, but positive when the serum phenylalanine is 4 mg/dl.

Description

The urine phenylketonuria (PKU) and Guthrie (blood) tests are two screening tests used for detecting a hepatic enzyme deficiency, phenylalanine hydroxylase, that prevents the conversion of phenylalanine (amino acid) to tyrosine in the infant. Phenylalanine from milk and other protein products accumulates in the blood and tissues and can lead to brain damage and mental retardation.

At birth the newborn's serum phenylalanine level is <2 mg/dl because of the mother's enzyme activity. After the third day of life or after 48 hours of milk ingestion, the serum level increases if phenylalanine is not metabolized.

The Guthrie procedure is the test of choice because a positive test result occurs when the serum phenylalanine reaches 4 mg/dl at 3 to 5 days of life after milk ingestion. A positive Guthrie test does not always indicate PKU, but if it is positive, a specific blood phenylalanine test should be performed. The PKU urine test is done after the infant is 3 to 4 weeks old and should be repeated a week or two later. Significant brain damage usually occurs when the serum level is 15 mg/dl. If either the Guthrie test or the urine PKU is positive, the infant should be maintained on a low phenylalanine diet for 6 to 8 years.

Purposes

- To screen for phenylalanine hydroxylase deficiency.
- To repeat phenylketonuria test as indicated.

Clinical Problems

Elevated Level: PKU, low-birth-weight infants, hepatic encephalopathy, septicemia, galactosemia. *Drug Influence:* Aspirin and salicylate compounds, chlorpromazine (Thorazine), ketone bodies.

Procedure

Guthrie Test (Guthrie Bacterial Inhibition Test): Phenylalanine promotes bacterial growth *(Bacillus subtilis)* when the serum level is >4 mg/dl.

- Cleanse the infant's heel, and prick it with a sterile lancet. Obtain several drops of blood on the filter paper. The surface of the filter paper is streaked with *Bacillus subtilis,* and if the bacillus grows, the test is positive. Check the procedure outlined by your institution.
- The test should not be done before 2 to 4 days of milk intake, either cow's milk or breast milk, and is preferably done on or after the fourth day.
- Note on the laboratory slip the date of birth and the date the first milk was ingested.

*Urine PKU: There are several urine tests for detecting phenylpyruvic acid. All use the reagent ferric chloride, which causes the urine specimen to turn green when positive. The Phenistix is a dipstick with ferric salt in the filter paper; it is dipped in fresh urine or pressed against a wet diaper. The dipstick will turn green if positive.

- The urine PKU test should be done 3 to 6 weeks after birth, preferably at the fourth week. It is usually not positive for PKU until the serum phenylalanine levels are between 10 and 15 mg/dl.
- The infant should be receiving milk for accurate Guthrie and urine PKU test results.

Factors Affecting Laboratory Results

- Urine that is not fresh can cause an inaccurate result.
- Vomiting and/or decreased milk intake may cause a normal serum phenylalanine level in the infant with PKU.
- Aspirins and salicylate compounds can cause a false-positive result.

---

*Most state laws require a repeat blood test instead of a urine test because it is more reliable.

- Early PKU testing before the infant is 3 days old (Guthrie) or 2 weeks old (Phenistix) may cause a false-negative test result.

NURSING IMPLICATIONS WITH RATIONALE

Elevated Level

- Relate positive Guthrie and urine PKU test results to the clinical problem, phenylketonuria.
- Explain to the mother the screening tests used to detect PKU. The Guthrie test is normally done while the mother and infant are in the hospital. Many pediatricians want the urine PKU done at home by the parent or in the doctor's office 3 to 4 weeks after birth as a follow-up test.
- Determine whether the infant has been taking adequate feedings (cow's milk or breast milk) before performing the Guthrie test. Vomiting and/or refusing to eat are common problems of PKU infants. This may cause a normal serum phenylalanine level.
- Obtain history if mother was a "PKU baby." If so, the mother should be on a low-phenylalanine diet before and during pregnancy.

Client Teaching

- Instruct the mother how to perform a urine PKU test accurately. A fresh, wet diaper or a fresh urine specimen should be used.
- Instruct the mother that the baby should not receive aspirin or salicylate compounds for 24 hours before testing the urine. A false-positive test could result. Tylenol should be given instead of aspirin.
- Tell the mother which foods the baby should and should not have. The preferred milk substitute is Lofenalac (Mead Johnson and Co.), an enzymic casein hydrolysate with vitamins and minerals. It provides a balanced nutritional formula. Other low-phenylalanine foods are fruits, fruit juices, vegetables, cereals, and breads. High-protein foods should be avoided (e.g., milk shakes, ice cream, and cheese). It is thought that after the age of 6 to 8 years, 90% of the brain growth has occurred, and the diet does not need to be as restrictive.

Phenytoin sodium (serum)

Diphenylhydantoin (Dilantin)

Reference Values

Therapeutic Range: *Adult:* As an anticonvulsant, 10–20 µg/ml, 39.6–79.3 µmol/l (SI units). As an antiarrhythmic, 10–18 µg/ml, 39.6–71.4 µmol/l (SI units). *In saliva:* 1–2 µg/ml, 4–9 µmol/l.

Toxic Level: *Adult:* >20 µg/ml, >79.3 µmol/l (SI units). *Child:* >15–20 µg/ml, 56–79 µmol/l (SI units).

Description

Phenytoin (Dilantin) reduces voltage, frequency, and spread of electrical discharges within the motor cortex. It is used to prevent and control grand-mal seizures. Phenytoin is also used as an antiarrhythmic drug for decreasing force of myocardial contraction, improving atrioventricular conduction depressed by a digitalis preparation, and prolonging the refractory period of the heart contraction.

Phenytoin sodium is absorbed from the gastrointestinal tract within 3 to 12 hours. Foods and antacids can decrease its absorption rate. Neonates and infants during their first 2 to 3 months of age cannot absorb phenytoin, so other anticonvulsants should be used during that period of time.

Approximately 90% to 95% of phenytoin is bound to plasma proteins, and the remainder is free. About 5% to 10% of the drug is excreted unchanged in the urine. Half-life in adults is an average of 24 hours and in children is an average of 15 hours. Frequent monitoring of serum phenytoin levels is indicated for checking therapeutic level and for avoiding toxic level. It takes about 5 to 10 days to obtain steady state. With a change in phenytoin dosage, resampling is suggested in 48 hours.

General signs and symptoms of phenytoin toxicity include nystagmus (rapid movement of the eyeball), slurred speech, gingival hyperplasia, ataxia, drowsiness, lethargy, and confusion. IM injection might cause a slow and erratic absorption. Oral and IV routes (not to exceed 50 mg/min push) are preferred.

Purpose

■ To monitor phenytoin (Dilantin) levels.

Clinical Problems

Decreased Level: Pregnancy, infectious mononucleosis. *Drug Influence:* Alcohol, carbamazepine (Tegretol), folate.

Elevated Level: Phenytoin overdose, uremia, liver disease. *Drug Influence:* Aspirin, phenylbutazone (Butazolidin), dicumarol, chloramphenicol (Chloromycetin), sulfisoxazole (Gantrisin), chlorothiazide (Diuril), tranquilizers (chlordiazepoxide [Librium], chlorpromazine [Thorazine], prochlorperazine [Compazine], diazepam [Valium]), isoniazid (INH), phenobarbital, propoxyphene (Darvon).

Procedure

- Collect 5 to 7 ml of venous blood in a red-top tube. Avoid hemolysis.
- Record the dose, route, and last dose administered on the laboratory requisition slip. List drugs the client is taking that could affect test results.
- There is no food or fluid restriction.

Factors Affecting Laboratory Results

- Hemolysis of the blood specimen.
- Drugs that increase serum phenytoin level *(see Drug Influence above).*

NURSING IMPLICATIONS WITH RATIONALE

- Check serum phenytoin result and immediately report nontherapeutic levels to the health care provider.
- Record dose, route, and last time the drug was given on the requisition slip.
- Note the method of drug administration. The oral and IV routes are commonly chosen methods for administration. The IM route might cause a slow and erratic absorption.

Elevated Level

- Observe for signs and symptoms of phenytoin toxicity, such as nystagmus, slurred speech, ataxia, drowsiness, lethargy, confusion, and rash.

Phosphorus (P)—inorganic (serum)

Phosphate (PO$_4$)

Reference Values

Adult: 1.7–2.6 mEq/l or 2.5–4.5 mg/dl; 0.78–1.52 mmol/l (SI units).
Child: *Newborn:* 3.5–8.6 mg/dl. *Infant:* 4.5–6.7 mg/dl. *Child:* 4.5–5.5 mg/dl.
Elderly: Slightly lower than adult.

Description

Phosphorus is the principal intracellular anion; however, most of phosphorus exists in the blood as phosphate. From 80% to 85% of the total phosphates in the body are combined with calcium in the teeth and bones.

Phosphorus is the laboratory term used, because phosphates are converted into inorganic phosphorus for the test. Functions of phosphorus include metabolism of carbohydrates and fats, maintenance of the acid-base balance, use of B vitamins, promotion of nerve and muscle activity, and transmission of hereditary traits.

Phosphorus (P) metabolism is associated with calcium (Ca) metabolism. Both ions need Vitamin D for their absorption from the gastrointestinal tract. Phosphorus and calcium concentrations are controlled by the parathyroid hormone. Usually there is a reciprocal relationship between calcium and phosphorus: when serum phosphorus levels increase, serum calcium levels decrease, and when serum phosphorus levels decrease, serum calcium levels increase. In certain neoplastic bone diseases, this relationship is no longer true, because both calcium and phosphorus are increased.

A high serum phosphorus level is called *hyperphosphatemia,* which is usually associated with kidney dysfunction (poor urinary output). *Hypophosphatemia* means a low serum phosphorus level.

Purposes

- To check phosphorus level.
- To monitor phosphorus levels during renal insufficiency or failure.
- To compare the phosphorus level with those of other electrolytes (i.e., potassium, calcium).

Clinical Problems

Decreased Level: Starvation, malabsorption syndrome, hyperparathyroidism, hypercalcemia, hypomagnesemia, chronic alcoholism, Vitamin D deficiency, diabetic acidosis, myxedema, continuous IV fluids with glucose. *Drug Influence:* Antacids such as aluminum hydroxide (Amphojel), epinephrine (adrenalin), insulin, mannitol.

Elevated Level: Renal insufficiency, renal failure, hypoparathyroidism, hypocalcemia, hypervitaminosis D, bone tumors, acromegaly, fractures (healing). *Drug Influence:* Antibiotics (methicillin, tetracyclines), phenytoin (Dilantin), heparin, Lipomul, laxatives with phosphate.

Procedure

- Collect 3 to 5 ml of venous blood in a red-top tube. Avoid hemolysis.
- The client should be NPO except for water for 8 hours before the test. Some laboratories will require NPO for 4 hours. Carbohydrate lowers serum phosphorus levels because phosphate goes into the cells with glucose.

- The blood sample should be taken to the laboratory within 30 minutes. The serum should be separated from the red blood cells (RBCs) quickly.

Factors Affecting Laboratory Results

- A high-carbohydrate diet and IV fluids with glucose can lower the serum phosphorus level; hence a fasting specimen is needed.
- Hemolysis of the blood sample can increase the serum phosphorus level. When RBCs rupture, they release intracellular phosphate into the serum.
- Late delivery of the blood sample (>30 minutes) may cause the release of phosphorus from the blood cells into the serum. The serum should be separated from the blood clot within 30 minutes.
- Drugs (see Drug Influence above). Amphojel can lower the serum phosphorus level.

NURSING IMPLICATIONS WITH RATIONALE

- Hold medications in the morning until the blood sample is taken.
- Hold IV fluid with glucose for 4 to 8 hours before the blood test, if possible. Glucose can lower the serum phosphorus level by promoting the shift of phosphate back into the cells.

Decreased Level

- Check the serum phosphorus, calcium, and magnesium levels, and report changes to the health care provider if the serum levels are unknown. An elevated calcium level causes a decreased phosphorus level.
- Monitor oral and IV phosphorus replacements. Some of the oral phosphate salts (Neutrophos) come in capsules, which are indicated if nausea is present. Administer IV phosphate (KH_2PO_4) slowly to prevent hyperphosphatemia.
- Observe for signs and symptoms of hypophosphatemia, such as anorexia and pain in the muscles and bone.
- Observe for signs and symptoms of hypocalcemia (tetany) while the client is receiving phosphate supplements.

Client Teaching

- Instruct the client to eat foods rich in phosphorus (i.e., meats [beef, pork, turkey], milk, whole grain cereals, and almonds) if the decrease is caused by malnutrition. Most carbonated drinks are high in phosphates.
- Instruct the client not to take antacids that contain aluminum hydroxide (Amphojel). Phosphorus binds with aluminum hydroxide; a low serum phosphorus level results.

Elevated Level

- Check the serum phosphorus, calcium, and magnesium levels. Observe for signs and symptoms of hypocalcemia (tetany); with an increased phosphorus level, calcium is usually low.
- Monitor urinary output. A decreased urine output (<25 ml/h or <600 ml/day) can increase the serum phosphorus level. Notify the health care provider of changes in urinary status.

Client Teaching

- Instruct the client to eat foods that are low in phosphorus (i.e., vegetables). Instruct the client to avoid drinking carbonated sodas that contain phosphates.

Plasminogen (plasma)

Reference Values

Adult: 2.5–5.2 U/ml, 7–16 mg/dl; 3.8–8.4 CTA (Council on Thrombolytic Agents).

Description

Plasminogen, inactive precursor of plasmin, is converted to plasmin, which activates the fibrinolytic process, a breakdown of fibrin clots in prevention of coagulation. Because plasmin cannot be measured in its active form in blood, plasminogen is measured to evaluate fibrinolysis. A decrease in plasminogen concentrate can indicate a tendency for thrombosis and also a serious secondary disease process (disseminated intravascular coagulation [DIC]).

Plasminogen is frequently monitored during administration of thrombolytic agents, such as streptokinase and urokinase, that are used to dissolve blood clots following an acute myocardial infarction (AMI). This test is also helpful in evaluating DIC.

Purposes

- To monitor the effect of thrombolytic therapy.
- To evaluate DIC.

Clinical Problems

Decreased Level: DIC, liver disease (cirrhosis), thrombolytic therapy, tumors, preeclampsia. *Drug Influence:* Streptokinase.

Elevated Level: Acute infection, MI, stress, surgery, trauma, malignant disease. *Drug Influence:* Oral contraceptives.

Procedure

- Collect 5 ml of venous blood in a blue-top tube. Avoid hemolysis. Avoid leaving the tourniquet on too long.
- There is no food or fluid restriction.

Factors Affecting Laboratory Results

- Hemolysis of the blood sample can affect results.
- Prolonged use of tourniquet could decrease plasma plasminogen level.
- Drugs *(see Drug Influence)*.

NURSING IMPLICATIONS WITH RATIONALE

- Assess for bleeding tendencies, apprehension, petechiae, bleeding from orifices, tachycardia, and, later, hypotension.
- Check other laboratory findings (e.g., fibrin degradation products [FDPs]).
- Monitor vital signs.

Platelet aggregation and adhesions (blood)

Reference Values

Adult: Aggregation in 3 to 5 minutes.

Description

Platelet aggregation test measures the ability of platelets adhering to each other when mixed with an aggregating agent such as collagen, ADP, or ristocetin. This test is performed to detect abnormality in platelet function and to aid in diagnosing hereditary and acquired platelet deficiencies such as von Willebrand's disease. Increased bleeding tendencies result from a decrease in platelet aggregation time.

The platelet adhesion test, like platelet aggregation, evaluates platelet function and helps to confirm hereditary diseases such as von Willebrand's disease. This test is also performed on clients taking large doses of aspirin for several weeks and on persons having a prolonged bleeding time. It is not performed in many laboratories because of the difficulty in standardizing the technique.

Clinical Problems

Decreased Platelet Aggregation: von Willebrand's disease, Bernard-Soulier syndrome, Glanzmann's disease (thrombasthenia), leukemia, idiopathic thrombocytopenia purpura, platelet release defects, afibrinogenemia, cirrhosis of the liver, uremia. *Drug Influence:* Aspirin and aspirin compounds, antiinflammatory agents (ibuprofen [Motrin], indomethacin [Indocin], phenylbutazone [Butazolidin]), 5-fluorouracil, phenothiazines, tricyclic antidepressants, diazepam (Valium), antihistamines, dipyridamole (Persantine), cortisone preparations, theophylline, cocaine, marijuana.

Elevated Platelet Aggregation: Diabetes mellitus, hyperlipemia, hypercoagulability.

Procedure

- Collect 5 to 7 ml of venous blood in a blue-top tube. Avoid hemolysis.
- The client should be NPO, including no medications, after midnight, except for water.
- Allow no aspirin or aspirin compounds for 7 to 10 days prior to the test. List drugs the client is taking on the laboratory slip.

Factors Affecting Laboratory Results

- Foods high in fat content eaten before the test: Hyperlipemia increases platelet aggregation.
- Drugs that inhibit platelet aggregation *(see Drug Influence)*.

NURSING IMPLICATIONS WITH RATIONALE

- Obtain a drug history from the client. Record and underline names of drugs the client is taking that could prolong platelet aggregation.
- List names of drugs that the client is taking that could affect test results on the laboratory slip.
- Check for bleeding tendencies, petechiae, purpura.

Client Teaching

- Instruct the client about the importance of not taking aspirin and aspirin compounds 7 to 10 days before the test (check with the health care provider about the time period to avoid aspirin intake). Aspirin inhibits clotting time or prolongs bleeding time; thus the test could be invalidated.
- Inform the client that no medications, food, or fluids, except water, should be taken after midnight before the test (it may be necessary to take some medications before test; check with health care provider).

Platelet antibody test (blood)

Platelet Antibody Detection Test, Antiplatelet Antibody Detection

Reference Values

Negative.

Description

When client become sensitized to platelet antigens of transfused blood, platelet antibodies (autoantibodies) develop and thus cause thrombocytopenia because of destruction to the platelets. The platelet autoantibodies are IgG immunoglobulins of autoimmune origin. With idiopathic thrombocytopenic purpura (ITP), platelet autoantibodies are present.

Drug-induced thrombocytopenia is caused by platelet-associated IgG autoantibodies because of hypersensitivity to certain drugs. Some of the drugs that may cause drug-induced immunologic thrombocytopenia include salicylates, acetaminophen, antibiotics (sulfonamides, penicillin, cephalosporins), quinidine and quinidine-like drugs, gold, cimetidine, oral hypoglycemic agents, heparin, digoxin.

Maternal-fetal platelet antigen incompatibility can occur if the mother has ITP autoantibodies that are passed to the fetus. Neonatal thrombocytopenia may result.

Purpose

- To detect the present of platelet antibodies.

Clinical Problems

Positive Test: Thrombocytopenia because of platelet autoantibodies, idiopathic thrombocytopenic purpura, posttransfusion purpura, drug-induced thrombocytopenia.

Drug that may cause drug-induced thrombocytopenia: See description.

Procedure

- No food or fluid restriction is required.
- Collect two (2) 10 ml of venous blood in a blue-top tube. Deliver to the laboratory immediately with the time of collection written on the requisition form.

NURSING IMPLICATIONS WITH RATIONALE

- Obtain a drug history from the client.
- Check platelet count. If thrombocytopenia is present, a platelet antibody test may be ordered.

- Check for sites of petechiae, purpura. Report findings.

Client Teaching
- Instruct the client to report any abnormal bleeding.
- Listen to client's and family's concerns.

Platelet count (blood—thrombocytes)

Reference Values

Adult: 150,000–400,000 μl (mean, 250,000 μl), 0.15–0.4 × 10^{12}/l (SI units).

Child: *Premature:* 100,000–300,000 μl. *Newborn:* 150,000–300,000 μl. *Infant:* 200,000–475,000 μl (mm³ or K/Ul may be used for ul).

Description

Platelets (thrombocytes) are basic elements in the blood that promote coagulation. Platelets are much smaller than erythrocytes. They clump and stick to rough surfaces and injured sites when blood coagulation is needed. A decrease in circulating platelets of <50% of the normal value will cause bleeding; if the decrease is severe (<50,000 μl), hemorrhaging might occur.

Thrombocytopenia means platelet deficiency or a low platelet count. It is commonly associated with leukemias, aplastic anemia, and idiopathic thrombocytopenic purpura. Increased platelet counts (thrombocytosis) occur in polycythemia, in fractures, and after splenectomy.

Purposes
- To check the platelet count.
- To monitor the platelet count during cancer chemotherapy.

Clinical Problems

Decreased Level: Idiopathic thrombocytopenic purpura, multiple myeloma, cancer (bone, gastrointestinal tract, brain), leukemias (lymphocytic, myelocytic, monocytic), anemias (aplastic, iron deficiency, pernicious, folic acid deficiency, sickle cell), liver disease (cirrhosis, chronic active hepatitis), systemic lupus erythematosus, disseminated intravascular coagulopathy, kidney diseases, eclampsia, acute rheumatic fever. *Drug Influence:* Antibiotics (chloromycetin, streptomycin), sulfonamides, aspirin (salicylates), quinidine, quinine, acetazolamide (Diamox), amidopyrine, thiazide diuretics, meprobamate (Equanil), phenylbutazone (Butazolidin), tolbutamide (Orinase), vaccine injections, chemotherapeutic agents.

Elevated Level: Polycythemia vera, trauma (surgery, fractures), postsplenectomy, acute blood loss (peaks in 7 to 10 days), metastatic carcinoma, pulmonary embolism, high altitudes, tuberculosis, reticulocytosis, severe exercise. *Drug Influence:* Epinephrine (adrenalin).

Procedure

- There is no food or fluid restriction.

Venous Blood: Collect 3 to 5 ml of venous blood in a lavender-top tube.

Capillary Blood: Discard the first few drips. Collect a drop of blood from a finger puncture, and dilute the blood immediately with the appropriate diluting solution.

Factors Affecting Laboratory Results

- Chemotherapy and x-ray therapy can cause a decreased platelet count.
- Drugs *(see Drug Influence)*.

NURSING IMPLICATIONS WITH RATIONALE

- Explain to the client that the purpose of the blood test is to determine the platelet count, or give a similar explanation.
- Check the platelet count, especially with bleeding episodes, and report abnormal levels.

Decreased Level

- Observe for signs and symptoms of bleeding (skin [purpura, petechiae] or gastrointestinal [hematemesis, rectal bleeding]). Record findings on the chart, and report them to the health care provider.
- Monitor the platelet count, especially when the client is receiving chemotherapy or radiation therapy for cancer.

Client Teaching

- Instruct the client to avoid injury, if possible. Mild injury could cause bleeding.

Porphobilinogen (urine)

Reference Values

Adult: *Random (qualitative):* Negative. *24-Hour (quantitative):* 0–2 mg/24 h.
Child: Same as adult.

Description

Porphobilinogen is one of the precursors of porphyrins, and large amounts are excreted during an acute attack of porphyria. Between attacks there may not be an appreciable amount of porphobilinogen present. The test should be conducted during the acute phase.

The urine porphobilinogen test is ordered to detect the presence of prophyrias. Porphyrias are inherent metabolic disorders that affect the synthesis of heme or hemoglobin. Congenital porphyria (erythropoietic porphyria) is characterized by pinkish brown-stained teeth, pinkish yellow to reddish black urine, and skin photosensitivity. Uroporphyrin and coproporphyrin I are excreted.

Hereditary hepatic porphyria can be divided into three types: acute intermittent porphyria, variegate porphyria, and hereditary coproporphyria. During an acute attack of porphyria, the urine becomes deep red and there are mental disturbances and severe abdominal pain. These attacks mimic various diseases such as appendicitis and pancreatitis; the leukocyte (white blood cell) count becomes elevated. Barbiturates, alcohol, and estrogen can precipitate an acute attack of porphyria.

Purpose

- To detect the presence of porphyrias.

Clinical Problems

Elevated Level: Acute intermittent porphyria, variegate porphyria, secondary malignant neoplasm, Hodgkin's disease, cirrhosis of the liver (occasionally). *Drug Influence:* Antibiotics (penicillin, tetracyclines); antiseptics (phenol compounds, phenazopyridine [Pyridium]), barbiturates, hypnotics, phenothiazines (chlorpromazine [Thorazine]), procaine, sulfonamides.

Procedure

Qualitative (Screening Test)

- Collect a random sample of 30 ml or more of fresh urine during or immediately after an acute attack of porphyria. The client has acute abdominal pain.
- Protect the specimen from light.

Quantitative (24 Hour)

- Collect the urine in a dark container. If it is collected in a clear container, protect it from light and refrigerate. The container should have an acidic preservative. Delta amino levulinic acid (ALA), which forms porphobilinogen, is not stable unless the urine is acidic. Urine should be collected immediately after the client has an acute attack.
- Have the client void, discard the urine, and then save all urine for 24 hours.
- Label the specimen with the date and the exact time the test started and ended.
- Encourage the client to take fluids. There is no food restriction.

Factors Affecting Laboratory Results

- Exposure of the urine sample to light.
- Drugs (*see Drug Influence above*).
- Contamination of the urine with toilet paper or feces.

NURSING IMPLICATIONS WITH RATIONALE

Patient Teaching

- Explain the procedure to the client and family and tell them not to throw away any urine. Tell them that urine should not be exposed to light and should be refrigerated.
- Inform the client that he or she should not contaminate the urine with toilet paper or stools.

Elevated Level

- Recognize that this test is usually done during an acute attack (acute abdominal pain) to detect porphyria.
- Observe and report urine color prior to an acute attack. The urine color should be amber to burgundy.
- Observe for signs and symptoms of an acute porphyria attack, such as severe abdominal pain (colicky), mental disturbances, and neuropathy. Respiratory distress could occur.

Client Teaching

- Instruct the client with porphyria to stay away from bright sunlight. Skin photosensitivity is a common problem, and skin lesions could result. Suggest that the client use sun screen on exposed skin areas and wear protective clothing.
- Instruct the client not to take barbiturates, alcohol, or estrogens without permission. These agents can precipitate an acute attack of porphyria.

Porphyrins—coproporphyrins, uroporphyrins (urine)

Reference Values

Coproporphyrins: *Adult:* Random: 3–20 μg/dl. Quantitative: 50–160 μg/24 h. *Child:* 0–80 μg/24 h.

Uroporphyrins: *Adult:* Random: Negative. Quantitative: <30 μg/24 h. *Child:* 10–30 μg/24 h.

Description

Porphyrins are used in the synthesis of hemoglobin and of any hemoproteins that are carriers of oxygen. The porphyrins are eliminated from the body in feces and urine, mainly as coproporphyrins I and III and as uroporphyrins. Normal excretion of coproporphyrins is minimal, but the amount excreted rises during liver damage, lead poisoning, and congenital porphyria (an inherent error of metabolism).

There is an increase in urine porphobilinogen with disorders of porphyrin metabolism. Porphobilinogen is one of the precursors of porphyrins (formed in the liver).

Purposes

- To monitor porphyrin levels.
- To aid in the diagnosis of selected disease entities *(see Clinical Problems)*.

Clinical Problems

Elevated Level: Lead toxicity, cirrhosis of the liver, acute intermittent porphyria, viral hepatitis, infectious mononucleosis, porphyria variegata, prophyria cutanea tarda, acquired hemolytic anemia (autoimmune). *Drug Influence:* Antibiotics (tetracyclines, penicillin), antiseptics (ethoxazene [Diaphenyl], phenazopyridine [Pyridium]), sulfonamides (sulfamethoxazole [Gantanol], sulfisoxazole [Gantrisin]), barbiturates and hypnotics, phenothiazines such as chlorpromazine (Thorazine), procaine.

Procedure

- Collect urine in a dark container containing the preservative sodium carbonate. If a large, clear container is used, protect it from light and refrigerate it.
- Have the client void, discard the urine, and then save all urine for 24 hours.
- Label the specimen with the exact date and time the test started and ended (e.g., 7/24/03, 7:00 AM to 7/25/03, 7:01 AM).
- There is no food or fluid restriction.

Factors Affecting Laboratory Results

- Exposure of the urine to light.
- Drugs *(see Drug Influence)*.
- Contamination of the urine with toilet paper and feces.

NURSING IMPLICATIONS WITH RATIONALE

Client Teaching

- Explain the procedure to the client. Inform the client and family that all urine must be saved for 24 hours. Emphasize that the urine should *not* be exposed to light.
- Inform the client not to contaminate the urine with toilet paper or feces.

Elevated Level

- Recognize clinical problems and drugs related to elevated porphyrin levels. Liver disease and lead poisoning cause an excessive amount of coproporphyrin III to be excreted.
- Observe the color of a urine specimen exposed to light. A pinkish or red color should be reported.

Potassium (K) (serum)

Reference Values

Adult: 3.5–5.3 mEq/l; 3.5–5.3 mmol/l (SI units).

Panic Values: <2.5 mEq/l and >7.0 mEq/l.

Child: *Infant:* 3.6–5.8 mEq/l. *Child:* 3.5–5.5 mEq/l.

Description

Potassium is the electrolyte found most abundantly in intracellular fluids (cells). The serum potassium level has a narrow range, and cardiac arrest could occur if serum level is <2.5 mEq/l or >7.0 mEq/l.

Eighty to 90% of the body potassium is excreted by the kidneys. When there is tissue breakdown, potassium leaves the cells and enters the extracellular fluid (interstitial and intravascular fluids). With adequate kidney functions, the potassium in the intravascular fluid (plasma/blood vessels) will be excreted, and with excessive potassium excretion, a serum potassium deficit (hypokalemia) occurs. However, if the kidneys are excreting <600 ml of urine daily, potassium will accumulate in the intravascular fluid and serum potassium excess (hyperkalemia) will occur.

The body does not conserve potassium, and the kidneys excrete an average of 40 mEq/l daily (the range is 25 to 120 mEq/l/24 h), even with a low dietary potassium intake. The daily potassium requirement is 3 to 4 g, or 40 to 60 mEq/l.

Purposes

- To check the potassium level.
- To detect the presence of hypo- or hyperkalemia.
- To monitor potassium levels during health problems (i.e., renal insufficiency, debilitating illness, cancer), and with certain drugs (e.g., thiazide diuretics).

Clinical Problems

Decreased Level: Vomiting/diarrhea, dehydration, malnutrition/starvation, crash diet, stress (trauma, injury, or surgery), gastric suction, intestinal fistulas, diabetic acidosis, burns, renal tubular disorders, hyperaldosteronism, excessive ingestion of licorice, excessive ingestion of glucose, alkalosis (metabolic). *Drug Influence:* Potassium-wasting diuretics (furosemide [Lasix], thiazides [Hydrodiuril], ethacrynic acid [Edecrin]), steroids (cortisone, estrogen), antibiotics (gentamicin, amphotericin, polymyxin B), bicarbonate, insulin, laxatives, lithium carbonate, sodium polystyrene sulfonate-(Kayexalate), salicylates (aspirin).

Increased Level: Oliguria and anuria, acute renal failure, IV potassium in fluids, Addison's disease (adrenocortical hormone), crushed injury and burns (with kidney shutdown), acidosis (metabolic or lactic). *Drug Influence:* Potassium-sparing diuretics, spironolactone (Aldactone), triamterene (Dyrenium), antibiotics (penicillin G potassium), cephaloridine (Loridin), heparin, epinephrine, histamine, isoniazid.

Procedure

- Collect 3 to 5 ml of venous blood in a red-top tube. Avoid hemolysis.
- Avoid leaving the tourniquet on for >2 minutes if possible.
- Food, fluid, and drug restrictions are not necessary.

Factors Affecting Laboratory Results

- The hydration status of the client can cause false potassium test values. Overhydration can cause a false serum-potassium deficit through hemodilution. Dehydration can cause a serum potassium excess through hemoconcentration. After the client is hydrated, his or her serum potassium level may be normal or slightly low.
- The use of a tourniquet can cause an increase in the serum potassium level.
- Hemolysis of the specimen (blood) can result in a high serum-potassium level.
- Drugs *(see Drug Influence).*

NURSING IMPLICATIONS WITH RATIONALE

- Compare serum potassium levels with urine potassium levels. When the serum potassium level is decreased, the urine potassium level is frequently increased, and vice versa.

Decreased Level

- Observe for signs and symptoms of hypokalemia, such as vertigo (dizziness), hypotension, cardiac dysrhythmias, nausea, vomiting, diarrhea, abdominal distention, decreased peristalsis, muscle weakness, and leg cramps.
- Record intake and output. Polyuria can cause an excessive loss of potassium. Potassium is not conserved well in the body, and the kidney excretes potassium regardless of potassium intake.
- Report serum potassium levels <3.5 mEq/l. If the potassium level is 3.0 to 3.5 mEq/l, it will take 100 to 200 mEq/l of potassium chloride (KCl) to raise the potassium level 1 mEq/l. If the potassium level is 2.9 mEq/l or less, it will take 200 to 400 mEq/l of KCl to raise the level 1 mEq/l.
- Determine the client's hydration status when hypokalemia is present. Over-hydration can dilute the serum potassium level.
- Recognize behavioral changes as a sign of hypokalemia. Low potassium levels can cause confusion, irritability, and mental depression. The serum potassium level should be checked in the presence of any behavioral changes.
- Report electrocardiographic changes. A prolonged and depressed ST segment and a flat or inverted T-wave is indicative of hypokalemia.
- Dilute oral potassium supplements in at least 4 oz of water or juice. Potassium is a corrosive agent and is most irritating to the gastric mucosa.
- Monitor the serum potassium level in clients receiving potassium-wasting diuretics and steroids. Examples of potassium-wasting diuretics are Hydrodiuril, Lasix, and Edecrin. Cortisone steroids (such as prednisone) cause sodium retention and potassium excretion.
- Assess for signs and symptoms of digitalis toxicity when the client is receiving a digitalis preparation and a potassium-wasting diuretic or steroid. A lower serum-potassium level enhances the action of digitalis. Signs and symptoms of digitalis toxicity are nausea and vomiting, anorexia, bradycardia, cardiac dysrhythmia, and visual disturbances.
- Monitor serum chloride, serum magnesium, and serum protein test results when hypokalemia is present. Correcting a potassium deficit with potassium only is not effective if chloride, magnesium, and protein levels are also low.
- Administer IV KCl in a liter of parenteral fluids. Never give an IV or bolus push of KCl, because cardiac arrest can occur. Parenteral KCl can only be administered intravenously when it is diluted (20 to 40 mEq per liter) and should never be given subcutaneously or intramuscularly. Concentrated IV KCl is irritating to the heart muscle and to the veins, causing phlebitis.
- Check the IV site when the client is receiving KCl in IV fluids. Infiltrated potassium is most irritating to the subcutaneous tissues (fatty tissues) and can cause tissue sloughing.
- Measure gastrointestinal fluid loss from suctioning, vomiting, or diarrhea for appropriate potassium and other electrolyte replacement. Potassium, sodium, hydrogen, and chloride are most plentiful in the gastrointestinal tract.
- Irrigate gastrointestinal tubes with normal saline solution to prevent electrolyte loss.

Client Teaching

■ Instruct the client and family to eat foods high in potassium (fruits, dry fruits, vegetables, meats, nuts, coffee, tea, cocoa, and colas). The daily potassium requirement is 3 to 4 g, or 40 to 60 mEq/l.

■ Teach clients to eat foods rich in potassium when they are taking drugs and foods that decrease body potassium (i.e., cortisone, potassium-wasting diuretics, laxatives, lithium carbonate, salicylates, insulin, glucose, and licorice).

Increased Level

■ Observe for signs and symptoms of hyperkalemia, or serum potassium excess (slow pulse rate [bradycardia], abdominal cramps, oliguria or anuria, tingling, and twitching or numbness of the extremities).

■ Assess urine output to determine renal function. Urine output should be at least 25 ml/h, or 600 ml daily, and a urine output of <600 ml/day could cause hyperkalemia.

■ Report serum potassium levels >5.3 mEq/l. High serum-potassium levels can cause cardiac arrest.

■ Regulate the rate of IV fluids so that no more than 10 mEq KCl are administered per hour. Rapid administration of KCl intravenously can result in hyperkalemia.

■ Check the age of whole blood before administering it to a client with hyperkalemia. Blood 2 weeks old or older has an elevated serum potassium level.

■ Assess the client's serum potassium level every 6 to 8 hours when it is elevated (>6.5 mEq/l) and during treatment for hyperkalemia. The serum potassium level can change frequently during treatment.

■ Monitor the electrocardiogram for QRS spread and peaked T-waves (signs of hyperkalemia). The pulse rate may be rapid, but if hyperkalemia persists, bradycardia or slow pulse can occur.

■ Restrict potassium intake when the serum potassium level is >6.0 mEq/l.

■ Monitor clients receiving various medical treatments for hyperkalemia for signs and symptoms of continuous hyperkalemia or developing hypokalemia. The various medical treatments are as follows: (1) IV sodium bicarbonate increases the pH, causing potassium to shift back into the cells; (2) IV glucose and insulin can also cause potassium to shift back into the cells and are usually effective for 6 hours; (3) calcium gluconate decreases the myocardial irritability resulting from hyperkalemia but does not decrease the serum potassium level; (4) sodium polystyrene sulfonate (Kayexalate) is a drug used as ion (resin) exchange, sodium for potassium. It can be administered orally or rectally and is considered the most effective method for treating hyperkalemia.

■ Notify the health care provider if the client is receiving a digitalis preparation when calcium gluconate is given. An elevated serum calcium level enhances the action of digitalis, causing digitalis toxicity.

■ Observe for signs and symptoms of hypokalemia when administering Kayexalate for a prolonged period of time (2 or more days).

Potassium (K) (urine)

Reference Values

Adult: *Broad Range:* 25–100 mEq/24 h. *Average Range:* 40–80 mEq/24 h, 40–80 mmoL/24 h (SI units).

Child: 17–57 mEq/24 h.

Description

Eighty to 90% of the body's potassium is excreted in the urine. A 24-hour urine potassium level is a valuable indicator of serum potassium status. A decrease in urinary potassium can indicate hyperkalemia (elevated serum potassium), and an increase in urinary potassium can indicate hypokalemia (low serum potassium) or may result from an increased potassium intake. If the kidneys are not functioning properly and there is decreased urine output (oliguria), the potassium excreted in the urine will be decreased and the serum potassium level will be elevated.

Purposes

See Potassium (Serum).

Clinical Problems

Decreased Level: Elevated serum potassium level, acute renal failure, diarrhea. *Drug Influence:* Potassium-sparing diuretics (e.g., Aldactone).

Elevated Level: Decreases serum potassium level, dehydration/starvation, chronic renal failure, diabetic acidosis, vomiting and gastric suction, increased adrenal cortical hormone or Cushing's disease, salicylate toxicity. *Drug Influence:* Potassium-wasting diuretics (e.g., Hydrodiuril, Lasix), prednisone.

Procedure

- The 24-hour urine specimen should be kept on ice or refrigerated.
- There is no food or fluid restriction.
- Potassium supplements given as salt replacement should be eliminated for 48 hours.

Factors Affecting Laboratory Results

- Failure to refrigerate the urine container affects test results.
- Fecal material and toilet paper contaminate urine specimen.
- Vomiting or gastric suctioning can cause hypokalemia due to potassium loss from the gastrointestinal tract, and the accompanying metabolic alkalosis can

cause an increase in urinary potassium loss. With a high urinary potassium excretion, the hypokalemic state could become more severe.

NURSING IMPLICATIONS WITH RATIONALE

Decreased Level

- Explain to the client that the purpose of the test is to determine whether the kidneys are excreting an adequate amount of potassium or whether the body is retaining it.
- Instruct the client to save all of his or her urine for 24 hours and to place it in the container, which should be on ice or refrigerated.
- Observe for signs and symptoms of hyperkalemia. When urinary potassium excretion is decreased, the serum potassium level may be increased. Signs and symptoms of hyperkalemia are oliguria, abdominal cramps, bradycardia, and tingling, twitching, or numbness in the extremities. Check the arterial pH or the serum carbon dioxide (CO_2) levels. If metabolic acidosis is present (decreased pH and serum CO_2), the serum potassium may be elevated and the urinary potassium may be decreased. Potassium is frequently retained in the body during metabolic acidosis.

Metabolic acidosis: $\downarrow$ pH, $\downarrow$ serum $CO_2 \rightarrow \uparrow$ serum K, $\downarrow$ urinary K.

Elevated Level

- Explain to the client that an increase in potassium intake or the use of diuretics (potassium wasting) will result in an excess urinary potassium excretion.
- Observe for signs and symptoms of hypokalemia. When urinary potassium excretion is increased, the serum potassium level is frequently decreased. Signs and symptoms of hypokalemia are vertigo (dizziness), hypotension, cardiac dysrhythmia, muscle weakness, and decreased peristalsis.
- Determine arterial pH or serum CO_2 levels. If metabolic alkalosis is present (elevated pH and serum CO_2), the serum potassium level may be low and the urine potassium may be increased. Hydrogen and potassium are excreted together in the urine and alkalosis results. Vomiting and gastric suction can cause metabolic alkalosis.

Metabolic alkalosis: $\uparrow$ pH, $\uparrow$ serum $CO_2 \rightarrow \downarrow$ serum K, $\uparrow$ urinary K.

Prealbumin (PA) antibody assay (serum)

Transthyretin (TTR)

Reference Value

17–40 mg/dl.

Description

Prealbumin, also known as thyroxin-binding protein or transthyretin, is a test used primarily for nutritional assessment. Transthyretin, a transport protein, is a precursor of albumin. Prealbumin has a shorter half-life (2 to 4 days) than albumin (20 to 24 days). This test is more sensitive for determining nutritional status and liver dysfunction than an albumin test.

Purposes

- To assess the client's nutritional status.
- To evaluate the client's nutritional needs postsurgery, and for the critically ill.

Clinical Problems

Decreased Level: Protein-wasting diseases, malnutrition, inflammation, malignancy, cirrhosis of the liver, zinc deficiency. *Drug Influence:* Estrogen, oral contraceptives.

Elevated Level: Hodgkin's disease. *Drug Influence:* Steroids, nonsteroidal anti-inflammatory drugs (NSAIDs).

Procedure

- Collect 2 to 5 ml of venous blood in a red-top tube.
- Avoid hemolysis.
- There is no food or fluid restriction.

Factors Affecting Laboratory Results

- Hemolysis can cause a false test result.

NURSING IMPLICATIONS WITH RATIONALE

- Obtain a history of the client's nutritional intake. Record findings; relate findings to the health care providers (i.e., the physician or dietitian).
- Check vital signs and weight.
- Listen to the client's concerns; answer questions or refer them to other health care providers.

Client Teaching
- Inform the client of ways in which nutritional status can be improved.

Pregnanediol (urine)

Reference Values

Adult: *Male:* 0.1–1.5 mg/24 h. *Female:* 0.5–1.5 mg/24 h (proliferative phase), 2–7 mg/24 h (luteal phase), 0.1–1.0 mg/24 h (postmenopausal).

PREGNANCY	
Gestation weeks	**mg/24 h**
10–19	5–25
20–28	15–42
28–32	25–49

Child: 0.4–1.0 mg/24 h.

Description

Pregnanediol is the major metabolite of progesterone produced by the ovary during the secretory phase of the menstrual cycle (second half) and by the placenta. Progesterone is responsible for uterine changes after ovulation and for maintaining pregnancy after fertilization. A steady rise in urinary pregnanediol levels occurs during pregnancy, and a decrease in these levels indicates placental (not fetal) dysfunction and the possibility of an abortion. Progesterone therapy would be indicated when urine pregnanediol is decreased.

Urinary pregnanediol levels may be used to determine menstrual disturbances and are used to verify ovulation in those who have not been able to become pregnant. The pregnanediol levels rise rapidly after ovulation, and they can be used as an indicator of ovulation time. This test should not be mistaken for the pregnanetriol test.

Purposes

- To determine the occurrence of placental dysfunction.
- To compare test results with those of other laboratory tests for determining the cause of a menstrual disorder.

Clinical Problems

Decreased Level: Amenorrhea (menstrual disorder), ovarian hypofunction, threatened abortion, pregnancy complicated by intrauterine death, benign neoplasms of the ovary and breast, lutein cell tumor of the ovary, preeclampsia.

Elevated Level: Pregnancy, ovarian cyst, choriocarcinoma of the ovary, adrenal cortex hyperplasia.

Procedure

- Collect urine over a 24-hour period in a large container or bottle with preservative, and keep it refrigerated.
- Label the bottle with the client's name and the dates and exact times of collection (e.g., 4/10/04, 8:00 AM to 4/11/04, 8:00 AM).
- Record on the laboratory slip the date of the last menstrual period.
- Take the urine bottle to the laboratory immediately after the urine collection has been completed.
- There is no food or fluid restriction.
- The urine may also be used to determine estradiol (E_3) levels in conjunction with the pregnanediol levels.

Factors Affecting Laboratory Results

- Toilet paper and feces in the urine.
- An unrefrigerated urine collection that has not been analyzed for several days.

NURSING IMPLICATIONS WITH RATIONALE

- Ask when the client had her last period; this should be recorded on the laboratory slip.

Client Teaching

- Explain to the client the procedure for collecting urine. Explain that all urine should be saved and placed in the labeled container in the refrigerator.
- Instruct the client not to put toilet paper or feces in the urine.

Decreased Level

- Recognize clinical problems that may cause a decreased pregnanediol level, such as menstrual disorder (amenorrhea), threatened abortion, and complicated pregnancy.
- Obtain a history of menstrual changes (menstruation patterns—frequency, length of period, flow, and discomfort).
- Obtain a history of pregnancy complications or problems. Record when the client had her last menstrual period and whether bleeding is present (how long has it occurred, how much bleeding, and is it continuous?).
- Give support to the client and family by listening, spending time with them, and answering questions, if possible. Supportive care can reduce anxiety.

- Monitor the urine pregnanediol levels if several tests have been ordered over a period of days or weeks. The levels can indicate progesterone production and whether progesterone therapy is needed.

Elevated Level

- Recognize clinical problems that can cause an elevated pregnanediol level, such as pregnancy and an ovarian cyst. The pregnanediol level should increase during pregnancy. After 18 to 24 weeks, the level should be 13 to 22 mg/24 h, and after 28 to 32 weeks, the level should be 27 to 47 mg/24 h. In the last 2 weeks of pregnancy, the urine pregnanediol level decreases.

Pregnanetriol (urine)

Reference Values

Adult: *Male:* 0.4–2.4 mg/24 h. *Female:* 0.5–2.0 mg/24 h.
Child: *Infant:* 0–0.2 mg/24 h. *Child:* 0–1.0 mg/24 h.

Description

Pregnanetriol (17-hydroxyprogesterone) comes from adrenal corticoid synthesis. It should not be mistaken for pregnanediol because it is not a derivative of progesterone. The pregnanetriol test is useful in diagnosing congenital adrenocortical hyperplasia.

Purpose

- To detect anterior pituitary hypofunction or adrenocortical hyperfunction.

Clinical Problems

Decreased Level: Anterior pituitary hypofunction.

Elevated Level: Adrenogenital syndrome, congenital adrenocortical hyperplasia, adrenocortical hyperfunction, malignant neoplasm of the adrenal gland.

Procedure

- Collect urine for 24 hours in a large, refrigerated container. No preservative is needed.
- Label the bottle with the client's name, dates, and exact times of collection (e.g., 2/3/04, 8:00 AM to 2/4/04, 8:02 AM).
- There is no food or fluid restriction.

Factors Affecting Laboratory Results

- None known.

NURSING IMPLICATIONS WITH RATIONALE

- Monitor urine pregnanetriol levels with cortisone replacement.

Client Teaching

- Instruct the client and family to save all urine for 24 hours, to keep the urine refrigerated, and not to put toilet paper or feces in the urine.

Procainamide hydrochloride (serum)

Pronestyl, Procan, Procamide

Reference Values

Therapeutic Range: *Adult:* 4–10 µg/ml, 5–30 µg/ml for sum of procainamide + NAPA. *Child:* Not done.

Toxic Level: *Adults:* >10 µg/ml, >30 µg/ml sum of procainamide + NAPA.

Description

Procainamide (Pronestyl, Procan), an antiarrhythmic agent, is used to treat cardiac arrhythmias. It acts by prolonging refractory period of the heart, reducing conduction velocity, and decreasing myocardial excitability. This drug is absorbed readily from the gastrointestinal tract and is metabolized by the liver to active metabolites.

Procainamide can be administered orally, intramuscularly, and intravenously; the commonest method is oral administration. The peak level occurs 1½ hours after oral administration. The steady state is about 24 hours after ingestion with good renal function. The half-life for procainamide is about 3 to 4 hours and for the metabolite *N*-acetylprocainamide (NAPA) about 6 to 8 hours. Approximately 50% of the drug is excreted unchanged in the urine.

Common side effects of this drug are nausea, vomiting, bitter taste, hypotension, bradycardia. Lupus erythematosus-like syndrome occurs in about 30% to 40% of clients on long-term procainamide therapy (1 year or more).

Purposes

- To monitor procainamide levels for therapeutic effect.
- To check for procainamide toxicity.

Clinical Problems

Elevated Level: Overdose of procainamide, renal disease, liver disease. *Drug Influence:* Acetazolamide (Diamox), cimetidine (Tagamet), sodium bicarbonate. Increased hypotensive effect with methyldopa (Aldomet), reserpine (Serpasil).

Procedure

- Collect 3 to 5 ml of venous blood in a red-top tube.
- Record the dose, route, and last time the drug was administered on the laboratory requisition slip.
- Obtain blood samples during the peak level, 1 to 2 hours after oral administration, or 1/2 hour after IV administration.
- A trough level (before next dose) may be requested.
- There is no food or fluid restriction.

Factors Affecting Laboratory Results

- Drugs *(see Drug Influence)* could elevate the serum procainamide level.

NURSING IMPLICATIONS WITH RATIONALE

- Report the client with a history of renal disease to the health care provider. The procainamide dose might need to be adjusted.
- Monitor the serum procainamide level frequently, because one serum sample is not enough for evaluating therapy.
- Monitor IV procainamide; it should not exceed 25 to 50 mg/min.
- Administer oral dosage 1 hour before or 2 hours after meals with a glass of water to increase absorption.
- Assess vital signs frequently during oral and parenteral drug therapy. Report if the pulse rate and blood pressure decrease substantially from baseline levels. Fever may occur during the first few days of therapy. Report temperature elevation.

Elevated Level

- Observe for signs and symptoms of side effects and procainamide overdose, such as anorexia, nausea, vomiting, bitter taste, dizziness, mental changes, muscle and joint pain, rash, hypotension, and bradycardia.
- Observe for signs and symptoms of lupus erythematosus-like syndrome (skin rash, erythema, fever, polyarthralgias, pleuritic pain). These symptoms are reversible.

Progesterone (serum)

Reference Values

Adult: *Female:* Follicular Phase: 0.1–1.5 ng/ml, 20–150 ng/dl. Luteal Phase: 2–28 ng/ml, 250–2800 ng/dl. Postmenopausal: <1.0 ng/ml, <100 ng/dl. *Pregnancy:* First Trimester: 9–50 ng/ml. Second Trimester: 18–150 ng/ml. Third Trimester: 60–260 ng/ml. *Male:* <1.0 ng/ml, <100 ng/dl.

Description

Progesterone, a hormone produced primarily by the corpus luteum of the ovaries and in a small amount by the adrenal cortex, peaks during the luteal phase of the menstrual cycle for 4 to 5 days and during pregnancy. It prepares the endometrium for implantation of the fertilized egg. Only a small amount of progesterone is detected in the blood, because most is metabolized in the liver to pregnanediol, a progesterone metabolite.

Serum progesterone is useful in evaluating infertility problems, in confirming ovulation, and in assessing placental functions in pregnancy. A urine pregnanediol might be ordered to verify serum progesterone results.

Purposes

- To aid in the diagnosis of an ovarian or adrenal tumor.
- To assist in the diagnosis of placental failure.
- To evaluate infertility problems resulting from a decreased progesterone level.

Clinical Problems

Decreased Levels: Gonadal dysfunction, luteum deficiency, threatened abortion, toxemia of pregnancy, placental failure, fetal death. *Drug Influence:* Oral contraceptives.

Elevated Levels: Ovulation, pregnancy, ovarian cysts, tumors of the ovary or adrenal gland. *Drug Influence:* ACTH, progesterone preparations.

Procedure

- Collect 5 to 7 ml of venous blood in a red-top (preferred) or green-top tube. Avoid hemolysis. Invert the green-top tube several times to mix with the anticoagulant in the tube.
- There is no food or fluid restriction.
- Note on the laboratory slip the phase of the client's menstrual cycle or weeks of gestation if pregnant.

Factors Affecting Laboratory Results

- Hemolysis from rough handling of the blood sample.
- Progesterone and estrogen therapy.

NURSING IMPLICATIONS WITH RATIONALE

- Obtain a history from the client of her menstrual phase or weeks or months of gestation. Record findings.

Client Teaching

- Inform the client that the blood test may be repeated or that a urine test may be ordered. Repeated tests at different times are usually for information concerning progesterone secretion.
- Listen to the client's concerns and fears. If unable to answer client's questions, direct to appropriate health professionals.

Prolactin (PRL) serum

Lactogenic Hormone, Lactogen

Reference Value

Female: *Nonpregnant:* Follicular Phase: 0–23 ng/ml. Luteal Phase: 0–40 ng/ml. Postmenopausal: <12 ng/ml. **Pregnant:** First Trimester: <80 ng/ml. Second Trimester: <160 ng/ml. Third Trimester: <400 ng/ml.

Male: 0.1–20 ng/ml.

Pituitary Adenoma: >100–300 ng/ml.

Description

Prolactin, a hormone secreted by the anterior pituitary gland, is necessary in the development of the mammary glands for lactation and for stimulating and maintaining lactation postpartum. If the mother does not breastfeed, serum prolactin falls to normal range.

Serum prolactin levels .100–300 ng/ml in nonpregnant females and in males may indicate a pituitary adenoma (tumor). Bromocriptine (Parlodel) decreases the serum prolactin level and slows tumor growth until the pituitary tumor can be removed.

Prolactin levels may be monitored to determine the effects of surgery, chemotherapy, and/or radiation for treating prolactin-secreting tumors.

Purposes

- To detect various health problems related to an increased prolactin level *(see Clinical Problems)*.
- To check drugs that the client is taking which influence increased prolactin levels.

Clinical Problems

Decreased Levels: Postpartum pituitary infarction. *Drug Influence:* Bromocriptine, levodopa, ergot derivatives, apomorphine.

Elevated Levels: Pregnancy, breastfeeding, pituitary tumor, amenorrhea, ectopic prolactin-secreting tumors (such as of the lung), galactorrhea, hypothalamic disorder, primary hypothyroidism, endometriosis, chronic renal failure, polycystic ovary, Addison's disease, stress, sleep, coitus, exercise. *Drug Influence:* Amphetamine, estrogens, antihistamines, oral contraceptives, phenothiazines, tricyclic antidepressants, monoamine oxidase inhibitors (MAO inhibitors), methyldopa (Aldomet), haloperidol (Haldol), cimetidine (Tagamet), procainamide derivatives, reserpine (Serpasil), isoniazid (INH), verapamil.

Procedure

- Collect 3 to 5 ml of venous blood in a red- or lavender-top tube. Avoid hemolysis. The client should be awake for 1 to 2 hours before blood test; sleep elevates the serum prolactin level.
- Withhold food, fluid, and medications for 12 hours prior to the test. If a medication needs to be taken within the 12 hours, the drug should be noted on the laboratory slip and recorded on the client's chart.

Factors Affecting Laboratory Results

- Drugs can cause false-positive or -negative laboratory test results *(see Drug Influences)*.
- Exercise, stress, pain, surgical trauma, sleep.

NURSING IMPLICATIONS WITH RATIONALE

- Check with the health care provider to determine if drugs that could affect test results should be withheld for 12 hours before the test. Medication(s) that must be taken before the test should be recorded on the laboratory slip.

Client Teaching

- Inform the client that the blood sample will be drawn after the client is awake for at least 1 hour, preferably 2 hours. Sleep might cause false-positive results.
- Inform the client that test results might not be known for several days.

- Instruct the client to avoid stress and exercise before the test. If the client is experiencing stress or is in pain, report this to the health care provider and record on laboratory slip, because a false-positive test could result.
- Listen to the client's concerns.

Propranolol hydrochloride (blood, serum, or plasma)

Inderal, Detensol, Novopranol

Reference Values

Therapeutic Range: *Adult:* 50–100 ng/ml, 193–386 nmol/l (SI units). *Child:* Not done.

Toxic Level: *Adult:* >150 ng/ml.

Description

Propranolol (Inderal) is a β-adrenergic blocking agent used in the treatment of angina pectoris, cardiac dysrhythmias, hypertension, and, in some cases, migraine headaches (prophylactically only). This drug blocks the cardiac effects of β_1-adrenergic stimulation, causing a decreased heart rate and force of heart contraction. Propranolol also blocks the bronchodilator effect of catecholamines, causing bronchoconstriction. In hypertensive clients it will lower both supine and standing blood pressure by blocking sympathetic flow and suppressing renin activity.

Almost all of oral propranolol is absorbed through the gastrointestinal tract and is metabolized in the liver to a large number of metabolites. Ninety to 95% is bound to plasma protein and is excreted in urine as free and conjugated propranolol and as active metabolites. The half-life of plasma propranolol is 3 to 4 hours. Peak plasma level for the oral dosage form is 1 to 1$\frac{1}{2}$ hours and for an IV dose in 15 minutes. Propranolol crosses the placental and blood-brain barriers.

Careful monitoring for signs and symptoms of side effects of propranolol is necessary to prevent the three commonest symptoms: bradycardia, hypotension, and bronchoconstriction. This drug is contraindicated for clients with asthma and low blood pressure.

Purposes

- To decrease blood pressure and irregular heart rate.
- To monitor propranolol levels for therapeutic effect.

Clinical Problems

Elevated Level: Overdose of propranolol (Inderal), liver and renal diseases. *Drug Influence:* Quinidine, cimetidine (Tagamet).

Procedure

- Collect 5 to 7 ml of venous blood in a red-top tube.
- Record the dose, route, and last-administered dose on the laboratory requisition slip.
- There is no food or fluid restriction.

Factors Affecting Laboratory Results

- Spuriously low values have been reported with the use of certain blood collection tubes.

NURSING IMPLICATIONS WITH RATIONALE

- Record the dose, route, and last time the drug was given on the requisition slip.
- Check serum propranolol level, and report any nontherapeutic level to the health care provider.
- Take the apical pulse and blood pressure before administering propranolol. If the pulse rate and blood pressure are lower than the baseline levels, notify the health care provider before administering the drug.
- Check the daily intake and output and the client's weight. Propranolol can cause sodium retention.
- Recognize that digitalis glycoside (e.g., digoxin) taken with propranolol could cause bradycardia.

Elevated Level

- Observe for signs and symptoms of drug side effects (i.e., decreased pulse rate or bradycardia, decreased blood pressure or hypotension, vertigo, syncope, dyspnea, bronchospasm, nausea, diarrhea, dry eyes, and dry skin).

Client Teaching

- Instruct the client on how to take a radial pulse. Inform the client to notify the health care provider if the pulse rate is lower than the baseline level or if the pulse becomes irregular.
- Explain to the client that propranolol should never be abruptly discontinued. Propranolol is tapered to lower doses over 1 to 2 weeks to prevent withdrawal syndrome (i.e., severe headaches, palpitation, and rebound hypertension).
- Inform the client that before general anesthesia for planned surgery is considered or given, the surgeon and anesthetist should be notified if the client is taking propranolol.

Prostate-specific antigen (PSA) (serum)

Reference Values

Male: *No Prostatic Disorder:* 0–4 ng/ml. *Benign Prostatic Hypertrophy (BPH):* 4–19 ng/ml. *Prostate Cancer:* 10–120 ng/ml (depends on the stage of prostatic cancer).

Description

Prostate-specific antigen (PSA), a glycoprotein from the prostatic tissues, is increased in both benign prostatic hypertrophy (BPH) and prostatic cancer; however, it is markedly increased in prostatic cancer. The PSA value may also be increased after a rectal examination and prostate surgery. PSA is more sensitive than prostatic acid phosphatase (PAP), also known as acid phosphatase (ACP), in early detection of prostatic cancer. The use of PSA and PAP, along with rectal examination, assists with making an accurate diagnosis.

PSA may be used to diagnose or monitor the effect of prostatic cancer treatment with chemotherapy or radiation, determine disease process and prognosis, and detect a recurrence of the tumor. Repeating the PSA test may be necessary.

Purpose

- To aid in the diagnosis of prostatic cancer.

Clinical Problems

Elevated Level: Prostatic cancer, benign prostatic hypertrophy (BPH), prostatitis, prostatic tissue biopsy, prostatic surgery.

Procedure

- Collect blood specimen before rectal and prostate examination.
- Collect 5 ml of venous blood in a red-top tube.
- There is no food or fluid restriction.

Factors Affecting Laboratory Results

- Rectal and prostate examinations can increase serum PSA levels.

NURSING IMPLICATIONS WITH RATIONALE

- Obtain a history regarding changes in urinary pattern, such as interrupted urine flow, frequent urination, especially at night, difficulty in starting and stopping the urine flow, hematuria, and/or pain in the back or during urination.

- Explain to the client that a blood sample will be obtained and test results should be available within 24 hours.
- Be supportive of the client. Provide an atmosphere in which the client feels comfortable expressing his concerns.

Client Teaching

- Instruct the client that a manual rectal examination is usually part of the test regimen to determine prostatic changes. The prostatic palpation should be done *after* the blood sample is drawn.

Protein (total) (serum)

Reference Values

Adult: 6.0–8.0 g/dl.

Child: *Premature:* 4.2–7.6 g/dl. *Newborn:* 4.6–7.4 g/dl. *Infant:* 6.0–6.7 g/dl. *Child:* 6.2–8.0 g/dl.

Description

The total protein is composed mostly of albumin and globulins *(see Protein Electrophoresis)*. The use of the total serum protein test is limited unless the serum albumin, A/G ratio, or protein electrophoresis test is also performed.

The protein level needs to be known to determine the significance of its components. With certain disease entities (i.e., collagen diseases, cancer, and infections), the total serum protein levels may be normal when the protein fractions are either decreased or elevated.

Purposes

- To differentiate between albumin and globulin.
- To monitor protein levels.
- To identify selected health problems associated with protein deficit.

Clinical Problems

Decreased Level: Prolonged malnutrition, starvation, low-protein diet, malabsorption syndrome, cancer of the gastrointestinal tract, ulcerative colitis, Hodgkin's disease, severe liver disease, chronic renal failure, severe burns, water intoxication.

Elevated Level: Dehydration (hemoconcentration), vomiting, diarrhea, multiple myeloma, respiratory distress syndrome, sarcoidosis.

Procedure

- Collect 5 to 7 ml of venous blood in a red-top tube. Avoid hemolysis.
- There is no food or fluid restriction. High-fat foods should be avoided for 24 hours before the test. Check with your laboratory.

Factors Affecting Laboratory Results

- A high-fat diet before the test.

NURSING IMPLICATIONS WITH RATIONALE

Client Teaching

- Instruct the client to avoid eating foods high in fat for 24 hours before the test.

Decreased Level

- Assess the client's dietary intake. If the deficit is due to poor nutrition, encourage the client to increase protein intake (eggs, cheese, meats, beans).
- Plan a well-balanced diet with the client. Collaborate with the dietitian and/or have the dietitian see the client.

Elevated Level

- Recognize clinical problems associated with a serum protein excess. Hemoconcentration caused by dehydration is a frequent cause of total serum protein excess.
- Assess the client for signs and symptoms of dehydration, such as extreme thirst, poor skin turgor, dry mucous membranes, tachycardia, and increased respirations.
- Check urinary output. The serum protein level may be increased (it also could be decreased) with kidney dysfunction. If kidney dysfunction is due to dehydration, vomiting, or diarrhea, the serum protein level will most likely be elevated.
- Monitor fluid replacement (intravenously or orally). The serum protein level should return to normal when the client is adequately hydrated. Care should be taken to prevent overhydration when forcing fluids.

Protein (urine)

Reference Values

Random Specimen: *Negative:* 0–5 mg/dl. *Positive:* 6–2000 mg/dl (trace to +2).
24-Hour Specimen: 25–150 mg/24 h.

Description

Proteinuria is usually caused by renal disease due to glomerular damage and/or impaired renal tubular reabsorption. With a random urine specimen, protein can be detected using a reagent strip or dipstick, such as Combistix. Normally albumin is measured with the dipstick, because it is sensitive to reagent strip. A positive urine specimen (proteinuria) suggests that a 24-hour urine specimen be obtained for quantitative analysis of protein.

The amount of proteinuria in 24 hours is an indicator of the severity of renal involvement. Minimal proteinuria (<500 mg or 0.5 g/24 h) may be associated with chronic pyelonephritis; moderate proteinuria (500 to 4000 mg or 0.5 to 4 g/24 h) may be associated with acute or chronic glomerulonephritis or toxic nephropathies (i.e., use of aminoglycosides [gentamicin]; and marked proteinuria (>4000 mg or >4 g/24 h) may be associated with nephrotic syndrome.

Emotions and physiologic stress may cause transient proteinura. Newborns may have an increased proteinuria during the first 3 days of life.

Purposes

- To compare urine protein level with serum protein level in relation to health problems *(see Clinical Problems)*.
- To identify renal dysfunction with increased protein level in the urine.

Clinical Problems

Decreased Level: Diluted urine. *Drug Influence:* Sulfosalicylic acid.

Elevated Level: *Heavy Proteinuria:* Acute or chronic glomerulonephritis, nephrotic syndrome, lupus nephritis, amyloid disease. *Moderate Proteinuria:* Drug toxicities (aminoglycosides), cardiac disease, acute infectious disease, multiple myeloma, chemical toxicities. *Mild Proteinuria:* Chronic pyelonephritis, polycystic kidney disease, renal tubular disease. *Drug Influence:* Penicillin, gentamicin, sulfonamides, cephalosporins, contrast media, tolbutamide (Orinase), acetazolamide (Diamox), sodium bicarbonate.

Procedure

- There is no food or fluid restriction.
- List drugs client is taking that could affect test results.

Random Urine Specimen

- Collect clean-caught or midstream urine specimen.
- Place the reagent strip/dipstick (e.g., Combistix) in the urine specimen.
- Match the results from the dipstick with the color chart on the bottle.

24-Hour Specimen (Quantitative Analysis Test)

- Have client void prior to test and discard urine. Then save all urine for 24 hours in a urine collection container.

- Keep urine specimen bottle refrigerated or on ice.
- Label the urine bottle with the client's name, date, exact time of collection (e.g., 7/12/04, 8:01 AM to 7/13/04, 8:02 AM).

Factors Affecting Laboratory Results

- Drugs *(see Drug Influence)*.
- Diluted urine.
- Toilet paper or stool in the urine.

NURSING IMPLICATIONS WITH RATIONALE

- Explain the test procedure to the client *(see Procedure)*. Emphasize the importance of following the test procedure for accurate results.
- Record on the laboratory slip all drugs that the client is taking and the date and time of last dose. The health care provider may withhold drugs for 24 hours prior to test.
- Assess for signs and symptoms of renal dysfunction, such as fatigue, decreased urine output, peripheral edema, increased serum creatinine.
- Answer the client's questions or refer the questions to the appropriate health professionals.

Protein electrophoresis (serum)

Reference Values

Adult

	Weight (g/dl)	Percentage of Total Protein
Albumin	3.5–5.0	52–68
Globulin	1.5–3.5	32–48
Alpha-1 (α_1)	0.1–0.4	2–5
Alpha-2 (α_2)	0.4–1.0	7–13
Beta (β)	0.5–1.1	8–14
Gamma (γ)	0.5–1.7	12–22

Child

	Albumin (g/dl)	Globulins (g/dl)			
		α_1	α_2	β	γ
Premature	3.0–4.2	0.1–0.5	0.3–0.7	0.3–1.2	0.3–1.4
Newborn	3.5–5.4	0.1–0.3	0.3–0.5	0.2–0.6	0.2–1.2
Infant	4.4–5.4	0.2–0.4	0.5–0.8	0.5–0.9	0.3–0.8
Child	4.0–5.8	0.1–0.4	0.4–1.0	0.5–1.0	0.3–1.0

Description

Serum proteins are made up of albumin and globulins. Albumin is the smallest of the protein molecules, but it makes up the largest percentage of the total protein value. Changes in the albumin level will affect the total protein value. Albumin plays an important role in maintaining serum colloid osmotic pressure. The globulin molecules are about 2.5 times as large as albumin molecules, but they are not as effective in maintaining osmotic pressure as albumin molecules are.

Serum protein electrophoresis is a process that separates various protein fractions into albumin, alpha-1 (α_1) globulin, alpha-2 (α_2) globulin, beta (β) globulin, and gamma (γ) globulin. The gamma globulins are the body's antibodies, which contribute to immunity.

Purposes

- To differentiate between the protein fractions.
- To determine disease entities among the protein fractions.

Clinical Problems

Protein Fraction	Decreased Level	Elevated Level
Albumin	Chronic liver disease	Dehydration
	Malnutrition	Exercise
	Starvation	
	Malabsorption syndrome	
	Advanced malignancy	
	Leukemia	
	Congestive heart failure	
	Toxemia of pregnancy	
	Nephrotic syndrome	
	Chronic renal failure	
	Burns (severe)	
	Systemic lupus erythematosus (SLE)	

(*continued*)

Protein Fraction	Decreased Level	Elevated Level
Globulin		
α_1	Emphysema due to α_1-antitrypsin deficiency	Pregnancy
		Neoplasm
		Acute and chronic infection
		Tissue necrosis
α_2	Hemolytic anemia	Acute infection
	Severe liver disease	Injury, trauma
		Burns (severe)
		Extensive neoplasms
		Obstructive jaundice
		Rheumatic fever
		Rheumatoid arthritis
		Acute myocardial infarction
		Nephrotic syndrome
β	Hypocholesterolemia	Hypothyroidism
		Biliary cirrhosis
		Kidney nephrosis
		Diabetes mellitus
		Cushing's disease
		Malignant hypertension
γ	Nephrotic syndrome	Collagen disease
	Lymphocytic leukemia	Rheumatoid arthritis
	Lymphosarcoma	Lupus erythematosus
	Hypogammaglobulinemia or agammaglobulinemia	Hodgkin's disease
		Malignant lymphoma
		Chronic lymphocytic leukemia
		Multiple myeloma
		Liver disease

Electrophoretic Patterns		
Pattern I	↓ albumin	Acute stressful situation
	↑ α_2-globulin	Acute infections
		Myocardial infarction
		Severe burns
		Surgery
Pattern II	↓ (slightly) albumin	Chronic infection and inflammation
	↑ (slightly) α_2-globulin	Cirrhosis
	↑ (slightly) γ globulin	Collagen disease (rheumatoid)
Pattern III	↓ (moderately) albumin	Collagen disease (lupus)
	↑ γ globulin	Subacute bacterial endocarditis
	↑ or normal β	Sarcoidosis

Procedure

- Collect 5 to 7 ml of venous blood in a red-top tube. Avoid hemolysis.
- There is no food or fluid restriction.

Factors Affecting Laboratory Results

■ Hemolysis of the blood sample.

NURSING IMPLICATIONS WITH RATIONALE

■ Check the albumin level from the protein electrophoresis results. Many clinical problems are the result of a serum albumin deficit.

■ Assess for peripheral edema in the lower extremities when the albumin level is decreased. Albumin is the major protein compound responsible for plasma colloid osmotic pressure. With a decreased albumin level, fluid seeps out of the blood vessels into the tissue spaces. Cirrhosis of the liver and congestive heart failure are clinical problems that can cause an albumin deficit and edema.

■ Encourage the client to increase protein intake. Malnutrition and cirrhosis of the liver are associated with a poor-protein diet. Suggest foods high in protein (i.e., beans, eggs, meats, and milk).

■ Assess urinary output. Renal and collagen (lupus) diseases occur with abnormal protein fractions. Urine output should be 25 ml/h or 600 ml/24 h.

■ Check for albumin/protein in the urine.

Prothrombin time (PT) (plasma)

Pro-Time, International Normalized Ratio (INR)

Reference Values

Adult: 10–13 seconds (depending on the method and reagents used) or 70–100%. *For Anticoagulant Therapy:* 1.5–2.0 times the control in seconds or 20–30%. INR: 2.0–3.0.

Child: Same as adult.

Description

Prothrombin (factor II of the coagulation factors) is synthesized by the liver and is an inactive precursor in the clotting process *(see Factor Assay).* Prothrombin is converted to thrombin by the action of thromboplastin, which is needed to form a blood clot.

The prothrombin time (PT) measures the clotting ability of factors I (fibrinogen), II (prothrombin), V, VII, and X. Alterations of factors V and VII will prolong the PT for about 2 seconds, or 10% of normal. In liver disease the PT is usually prolonged, because the liver cells cannot synthesize prothrombin.

The major use of the PT is to monitor oral anticoagulant therapy (i.e., with bishydroxycoumarin [dicumarol] and warfarin sodium [Coumadin]).

International Normalized Ratio (INR): It has been recommended that the PT be reported as an International Normalized Ratio (INR). The INR was devised to improve the monitoring process for warfarin anticoagulant therapy. A client's response to the same dose of warfarin varies thus, the INR is used because of it being an international standardized test for PT. The INR is designed for long-term warfarin therapy, and should only be used after the client has been stabilized on warfarin. Stabilization takes at least one week. The INR should not be used when the client is beginning warfarin therapy in order to avoid misleading test results. The target INR range for a client having heart valve replacement is 2.5 to 3.5.

Purposes

- To monitor warfarin anticoagulant therapy.
- To decrease the clotting process.

Clinical Problems

Decreased Level: Thrombophlebitis, myocardial infarction, pulmonary embolism.
Drug Influence: Barbiturates, digitalis preparations, diuretics, diphenhydramine (Benadryl), oral contraceptives, rifampin, metaproterenol (Alupent, Metaprel), Vitamin K.

Increased Level: Liver diseases (cirrhosis of the liver, hepatitis, liver abscess, cancer of the liver), afibrinogenemia, factor II deficiency, factor V deficiency, factor VII deficiency, factor X deficiency, fibrin degradation products (FDP), leukemias, congestive heart failure, erythroblastosis fetalis (hemolytic disease of the newborn).
Drug Influence: Antibiotics (penicillin, streptomycin, carbenicillin, chloramphenicol [Chloromycetin], kanamycin [Kantrex], neomycin, tetracyclines), anticoagulants, oral (dicumarol, warfarin), chlorpromazine (Thorazine), chlordiazepoxide (Librium), diphenylhydantoin (Dilantin), heparin, methyldopa (Aldomet), mithramycin, reserpine (Serpasil), phenylbutazone (Butazolidin), quinidine, salicylates (aspirin), sulfonamides.

Procedure

- The test (collection) tube should contain an anticoagulant, either sodium oxalate or sodium citrate.
- Collect 3 to 5 ml of venous blood in a black-top tube (sodium oxalate). The blood must be tested within 1 hour after it has been drawn. The tube should be filled to its capacity. Some black-top tubes contain sodium citrate, so check with the laboratory.

OR

- Collect 3 to 5 ml of venous blood in a blue-top tube (sodium citrate). The blood should be tested within 2 hours to prevent inactivation of some of the factors. The tube should be filled to its capacity.

- Deliver the blood sample to the laboratory packed in ice. If the blood clots before testing, a new blood sample should be taken.
- Control values are given with the client's PT and/or INR. Control values may change from day to day; this is an indication of the minor variables in the testing conditions.
- There is no food or fluid restriction.
- List on the laboratory slip drugs the client is taking that could affect test results.

Factors Affecting Laboratory Results

- A clotted blood sample will cause an inaccurate result.
- A high-fat diet (decreased PT) and alcohol use (increased PT) may cause an endogenous change of PT production.
- Leaving a blood sample at room temperature for several hours (1 to 4 hours) may affect results.

NURSING IMPLICATIONS WITH RATIONALE

- Explain to the client that the purpose of the test is to determine how fast the blood clots. If the purpose of the test is to monitor anticoagulant therapy, inform the client that blood will be drawn daily or at specified times.
- Hold medications (if possible) that may affect the PT and/or INR until after the test. If such medications *are* given, list the names of the drugs on the laboratory slip and when the last dose was given.
- Take the blood sample immediately to the laboratory for testing. There should be an anticoagulant in the tube, and the blood should fill the tube.

Increased Level

- Monitor the PT and/or INR when the client is receiving anticoagulant therapy. The desired PT with anticoagulant therapy is 1.5 to 2.0 times the control PT in seconds. The PT may be slightly lower when treating cardiac clients—18 to 24 seconds. In clients with a thrombus, the desired PT range is 26 to 40 seconds. When the PT is above 40 seconds, bleeding may occur.
- Inform the health care provider of the client's PT and/or INR daily or as ordered. The health care provider may want the anticoagulant held (drug adjustment) until the current PT has been received. The results are usually called to the floor by the laboratory personnel.
- Observe the client for signs and symptoms of bleeding (purpura [skin] hematuria [Hemastix test], hematemesis, nosebleeds). Report observations to the health care provider and record them in the client's chart.
- Administer Vitamin K intramuscularly as ordered when the PT is over 40 seconds or when there is bleeding. IM injections can cause hematomas at the injection site when anticoagulants are used.

Client Teaching

- Instruct the client not to self-medicate when receiving anticoagulant therapy. Over-the-counter drugs may either increase or decrease the effects of the antico-agulants (drug interaction) and the results of the PT.
- Instruct the client to take the prescribed anticoagulants as ordered by the health care provider or other health care providers. Missed doses could affect the PT.
- Inform the client not to consume alcohol, over a period of time, because it can affect liver function and cause a prolonged PT. A high-fat diet may decrease the PT and INR.
- *(See Partial Thromboplastin Time, Activated Partial Thromboplastin Time.)*

Quinidine (serum)

Reference Values

Therapeutic Range: *Adult:* 2–5 µg/ml, 6.2–15.4 µmol/l (SI units). *Child:* Not done.

Toxic Level: *Adult:* >6 µg/ml, >18.5 µmol/l (SI units).

Description

Quinidine, one of the first antiarrhythmic agents, is used for treating supraventricu-lar and ventricular cardiac arrhythmias. It acts by decreasing the excitability of the heart and increasing the refractory period. Today quinidine is not the drug of choice, because it causes many side effects (i.e., gastrointestinal upset, severe car-diac problems [bradycardia, congestive heart failure, heart block, circulatory col-lapse], hypersensitivity reactions [urticaria, rash], and central nervous system disturbances). The daily dosage of quinidine should be regulated according to the serum therapeutic range.

The half-life of quinidine is 6 to 8 hours. Quinidine is metabolized by the liver, and 20% is excreted unchanged through the kidneys. Sixty to 80% is bound to plasma protein.

Care should be taken when digoxin and quinidine are coadministered. Quini-dine can increase serum digoxin level 2½ times its expected level. As a result of taking the two drugs, digitalis toxicity could appear 3 to 7 days after quinidine ther-apy was started. Both serum digoxin and quinidine levels should be monitored.

Purposes

- To treat an irregular heart rate.

- To monitor quinidine levels for therapeutic effect.
- To check for quinidine toxicity.

Clinical Problems

Decreased Level: *Drug Influence:* Barbiturates, phenytoin (Dilantin), rifampin.

Elevated Level: Overdose of quinidine, renal disease, severe heart failure, and liver disease. *Drug Influence:* Acetazolamide (Diamox), antacids, thiazides.

Procedure

- Collect 3 to 5 ml of venous blood in a red-top tube. Some laboratories may request that a heparinized plasma specimen be collected (i.e., green-top tube).
- Collect the specimen during the peak (2 hours after dose) and/or trough (before the next dose) levels to determine the therapeutic range for the client.
- Record the dose, route, and last-administered dose on the laboratory requisition slip.
- There is no food or fluid restriction.

Factors Affecting Laboratory Results

- Certain drugs might elevate or decrease quinidine concentration in the body *(see Drug Influence)*.
- Certain blood collection tubes may cause small decreases in serum levels.

NURSING IMPLICATIONS WITH RATIONALE

- Record the dose, route, and last-administered dose on the requisition slip. Record drugs the client is taking that might affect the test result.
- Take apical pulse and blood pressure before administering dose. Report pulse and blood pressure changes from base-line levels to the health care provider.

Client Teaching

- Instruct the client on how to take a radial pulse before discharge. Tell client to report significant change of pulse rate from base-line level to the health care provider.
- Inform the client to take quinidine with food to avoid or to decrease gastrointestinal effects.

Elevated Level

- Observe for side effects of quinidine (bradycardia, hypotension, dizziness, nausea, vomiting, diarrhea, skin eruptions).
- Observe for signs and symptoms of digitalis toxicity in clients taking a digitalis preparation concurrently with quinidine.

Rabies antibody test (serum)

Fluorescent Rabies Antibody (FRA)

Reference Values

Indirect fluorescent antibody (IFA) <1:16.

Description

The rabies rhabdovirus affecting the central nervous system may be present in the saliva, brain, spinal cord, urine, and feces of rabid animals. This virus can be transmitted to the human by an infected dog, bat, skunk, squirrel, or other animal and is nearly 100% fatal if the person does not receive treatment before the symptoms occur.

The rabies antibody test is performed to diagnose rabies in animals, and in humans that have been bitten by a rabid animal, to test the effects of rabies immunization on employees working in animal shelters. Brain tissue examined from the rabid animal can confirm the presence of the rabies virus. Both the rabies antibody test and the animal's brain tissue are preferred to positively diagnose rabies that was transmitted to the human. If the animal suspected of having rabies survives longer than 10 days, it is unlikely that the animal is rabid.

Purpose

■ To aid in the diagnosis of rabies in animals and humans.

Clinical Problems

Elevated Titer Count: Rabies transmission.

Procedure

■ Collect 5 to 7 ml of venous blood in a red-top tube. The animal brain should be sent along with the blood sample to the laboratory if possible.
■ There is no food or fluid restriction.

Factors Affecting Laboratory Results

■ None known.

NURSING IMPLICATIONS WITH RATIONALE

■ Obtain a history of the animal bite. Rabies immunoglobulin (RIG) may be given soon after the exposure to neutralize the virus.

- The animal responsible for the animal bite should be captured. If the animal's rabies vaccination is not current, the animal is usually destroyed in order to test the brain tissue. A wait of 10 days to determine the survival of a "wild" animal is not suggested.

Client Teaching

- Suggest to persons working with animals, such as those working in veterinary practices, in kennels, in wildlife areas, and research laboratories, that they receive a preexposure rabies vaccine such as HDVC (human diploid cell rabies vaccine) to protect them from rabies exposure.
- Instruct the person who was bitten or the family to seek medical care immediately. Encourage the family to notify the humane society concerning the animal bite. The animal should be captured.
- Inform the client and/or family that if the animal is not located, then a series of rabies vaccines is necessary and should be taken.
- Answer the client's questions. Refer questions to appropriate health professionals as needed.

Rapid plasma reagin (RPR) (serum)

Reference Values

Adult: Nonreactive.

Child: Nonreactive.

Description

(See Description for VDRL).

The rapid plasma reagin (RPR) test is a rapid screening test for syphilis. A nontreponemal antibody test like the Venereal Disease Research Laboratory test (VDRL), the RPR test detects reagin antibodies in the serum and is more sensitive but less specific than the VDRL. Frequently it is used on donor blood as a syphilis detection test. As with other nonspecific reagin tests, false positives can occur as the result of acute and chronic diseases. A positive RPR test should be verified by the VDRL and/or fluorescent treponemal antibody absorption (FTA-ABS) tests.

Purpose

- To compare test results with other laboratory tests for diagnosing syphilis.

Clinical Problems

Reactive (positive): Syphilis. *False Positive:* Tuberculosis, pneumonia, infectious mononucleosis, chickenpox, smallpox vaccination (recent), rheumatoid arthritis, lupus erythematosus, hepatitis, pregnancy.

Procedure

- Follow the directions on the RPR kit.

OR

- Collect 3 to 5 ml of venous blood in a red-top tube.
- There is no food or fluid restriction.

Factors Affecting Laboratory Results

- False-positive results caused by acute and chronic diseases *(see Clinical Problems for VDRL).*

NURSING IMPLICATIONS WITH RATIONALE

Reactive (Positive)

- Explain to the client that further testing will be done to verify test results.
- If the repeat result is positive, sexual contacts need to be notified to seek treatment.

Red blood cell indices (MCV, MCH, MCHC, RDW) (blood)

Erythrocyte Indices

Reference Values

	Adult	Newborn	Child
RBC count (million/μL × 10^{12}/l [SI units])	Male: 4.6–6.0 Female: 4.0–5.0 4.6–6.0 × 10^{12}L	4.8–7.2 4.8–7.2 × 10^{12}L	3.8–5.5 3.8–5.5 × 10^{12}L
MCV (μm^3 [conventional]) or fl [SI units])	80–98	96–108	82–92
MCH (pg [conventional and SI units])	27–31	32–34	27–31

	Adult	**Newborn**	**Child**
MCHC (% or g/dl [conventional] or SI units)	32%–36% 0.32–0.36	32%–33% 0.32–0.33	32%–36% 0.32–0.36
RDW (coulter S)	11.5–14.5		

Description

Red blood cell (RBC) indices include the RBC count, RBC size (MCV: mean corpuscular volume), weight (MCH: mean corpuscular hemoglobin), hemoglobin concentration (MCHC: mean corpuscular hemoglobin concentration), and size differences (RDW: RBC distribution width). Other names for RBC indices are *erythrocyte indices* and *corpuscular indices*. To identify the types of anemias, the health care provider depends on the following RBC indices:

- *MCV:* MCV indicates the size of RBC: microcytic (small size), normocytic (normal size), and macrocytic (large size). A decreased MCV, or microcyte, might be indicative of iron-deficiency anemia and thalassemia. An example of an increased MCV, or macrocytosis, is pernicious anemia and folic acid anemia. MCV value can be calculated if the RBC count and hematocrit (Hct) are known.

$$MCV = \frac{Hct \times 10}{RBC \ count}$$

- *MCH:* MCH indicates the weight of hemoglobin in the RBC regardless of the size. In macrocytic anemias, the MCH is elevated, and it is decreased in hypochromic anemia. The MCH is derived by dividing the RBC count into 10 times the hemoglobin (Hb) value.

$$MCH = \frac{Hb \times 10}{RBC \ count}$$

- *MCHC:* MCHC indicates the hemoglobin concentration per unit volume of RBCs. A decreased MCHC can indicate a hypochromic anemia. The MCHC can be calculated from MCH and MCV or from hemoglobin and hematocrit.

$$MCH = \frac{MCH \times 100}{MCV} \qquad OR \qquad MCHC = \frac{Hb \times 100}{Hct}$$

- *RDW:* The RBC distribution width (RDW) is the size (width) differences of RBCs. RDW is the measurement of the width of the size distribution curve on a histogram. It is useful in predicting anemias early, before MCV changes and before signs and symptoms occur. An elevated RDW indicates iron deficiency, folic acid deficiency, and Vitamin B_{12} deficiency anemias. RDW and MCV are used to differentiate among various RBC disorders (*see Anemias: RDW and MCV Values*).

ANEMIAS: RDW AND MCV VALUES

RBC Disorder	RDW	MCV
Early factor deficiency (iron, folate, vitamin B_{12})	High	Normal
Iron-deficiency anemia	High	Low
Folic-acid-deficiency anemia	High	High
Vitamin B_{12} deficiency (pernicious anemia)	High	High
Hemolysis (RBC fragmentation)	High	Low
Hemolysis (autoimmune) anemia	High	High
Sickle cell anemia	High	Normal
Sickle cell trait	High	Normal

Purposes

- To monitor RBC count.
- To differentiate between the components of RBC indices to determine a health problem (see Clinical Problems).

Clinical Problems

Indices	Decreased Level	Elevated Level
RBC count	Hemorrhage (blood loss)	Polycythemia vera
	Anemias	Hemoconcentration/dehydration
	Chronic infections	High altitude
	Leukemias	Cor pulmonale
	Multiple myeloma	Cardiovascular disease
	Excessive intravenous fluids	
	Chronic renal failure	
	Pregnancy	
	Overhydration	
MCV	Microcytic anemia: iron deficiency	Macrocytic anemia: aplastic,
	Malignancy	hemolytic, pernicious
	Rheumatoid arthritis	Chronic liver disease
	Hemoglobinopathies	Hypothyroidism (myxedema)
	Thalassemia	Drug influence
	Sickle cell anemia	Vitamin B_{12} deficiency
	Hemoglobin C	Anticonvulsants
	Lead poisoning	Antimetabolics
	Radiation	
MCH	Microcytic, hypochromic anemia	Macrocytic anemias
MCHC	Hypochromic anemia	
	Iron deficiency anemia	
	Thalassemia	
RDW		Iron-deficiency anemia
		Folic-acid-deficiency anemia
		Pernicious anemia
		Homozygous
		hemoglobinopathies
		(S, C, H)

Procedure

- Collect 3 to 5 ml of venous blood in a lavender-top tube. Avoid hemolysis. Avoid leaving the tourniquet on too long.
- There is no food or fluid restriction.
- Usually a particle counter is used that will provide all complete blood cell count (CBC) results along with all the indices.

Factors Affecting Laboratory Results

- Drugs *(see Clinical Problems)*.

NURSING IMPLICATIONS WITH RATIONALE

Decreased Level

- Relate a decreased RBC count, MCV, MCH, and MCHC to clinical problems.
- Assess for the cause(s) of a decreased RBC count. Check for blood loss, and obtain a history of anemias, renal insufficiency, chronic infection, or leukemia. Determine whether the client is overhydrated.
- Observe for signs and symptoms of advanced iron-deficiency anemia (fatigue, pallor, dyspnea on exertion, tachycardia, and headache). Chronic symptoms include cracked corners of the mouth, smooth tongue, dysphagia, and numbness and tingling of the extremities. With mild iron deficiency the client is usually asymptomatic.

Client Teaching

- Instruct the client to follow the medical regimen, such as iron-supplement therapy and a diet rich in iron.
- Instruct the client to eat foods rich in iron (i.e., liver, red meats, green vegetables, and iron-fortified bread).
- Explain to the client who is taking iron supplements that the stools usually appear dark in color (tarry appearance). Tell the client to take an iron medication with meals. Milk and antacids can interfere with iron absorption.

Elevated Level

- Relate an elevated RBC count, MCV, MCH, MCHC, and RDW to clinical problems and drugs.
- Assess for signs and symptoms of hemoconcentration. Dehydration, shock, and severe diarrhea are some of the causes of hemoconcentration that can elevate the RBC count.

Renin (plasma)

Reference Values

Adult: *Normal-Sodium Diet: Supine:* 0.2–2.3 ng/ml. *Upright:* 1.6–4.3 ng/ml. *Restricted-Sodium Diet: Upright:* 4.1–10.8 ng/ml.

Child: *1–3 Years:* 1.7–11.0 ng/ml; *3–5 Years:* 1.0–6.5 ng/ml; *5–10 Years:* 0.5–6.0 ng/ml.

Description

Renin is an enzyme secreted by the kidneys. This enzyme activates the renin-angiotensin system, which causes vasoconstriction and the release of aldosterone (a hormone from the adrenal medulla that causes sodium and water retention). Vasoconstriction and aldosterone can cause hypertension.

Increased plasma renin levels can occur as a result of hypovolemia and kidney disorders. In addition, postural change (from a recumbent to an upright position) and a decreased sodium (salt) intake will stimulate renin secretion. Plasma renin levels are usually higher from 8:00 AM to noon and lower from noon to 6:00 PM.

Purpose

- To identify a possible cause of hypertension.

Clinical Problems

Decreased Level: Essential hypertension, Cushing's syndrome, diabetes mellitus, hypothyroidism, high-sodium diet. *Drug Influence:* Antihypertensives (methyldopa [Aldomet], guanethidine [Ismelin]), propranolol (Inderal); levodopa.

Elevated Level: Hypertension (malignant, renovascular), hyperaldosteronism, cancer of the kidney, acute renal failure, Addison's disease, cirrhosis, chronic obstructive lung disease, manic-depressive disorder, pregnancy (first trimester), preeclampsia and eclampsia, hyperthyroidism, hypokalemia, low-sodium diet. *Drug Influence:* Estrogens, diuretics, anithypertensives (hydralazine [Apresoline], diazoxide [Hyperstat], nitroprusside), oral contraceptives.

Procedure

- Check with the laboratory and health care provider to determine whether the plasma renin test is to include urine aldosterone and/or urine sodium tests.

Plasma Renin
- Keep the tube and/or syringe cold in an ice bath before collection.

- The tourniquet should be released before the blood is drawn.
- Note on the laboratory slip if the client is in a supine or upright position.
- A normal or low-sodium diet may be indicated.
- Collect 5 to 7 ml of venous blood in a lavender-top tube.
- The blood sample should be placed in an ice bath; after centrifugation, the plasma is separated, frozen immediately to preserve renin activity, and sent to a special laboratory.

Factors Affecting Laboratory Results

- Drugs *(see Drug Influence)*.

NURSING IMPLICATIONS WITH RATIONALE

- Check with the laboratory on procedural changes or modifications.

Elevated Level

- Monitor the client's blood pressure every 4 to 6 hours or as ordered.
- Assess kidney function by recording urinary output. If urinary output is <25 ml/h or 600 ml/day, renal insufficiency should be suspected.

Reticulocyte count (blood)

Reference Values

Adult: 0.5%–1.5% of all RBCs, 25,000–75,000 µl.

$$\text{Reticulocyte count} = \text{reticulocytes (\%)} \times \text{RBC count}$$

Child: *Newborn:* 2.5%–6.5% of all RBCs. *Infant:* 0.5%–3.5% of all RBCs. *Child:* 0.5–2.0% of all RBCs.

Description

The reticulocyte count is an indicator of bone marrow activity and is used for diagnosing anemias. Reticulocytes are immature, nonnucleated red blood cells (RBCs) that are formed in the bone marrow and passed into circulation. Normally there are a small number of reticulocytes in circulation; however, an increased number (count) indicates RBC production acceleration. An increased count could be due to hemorrhage or hemolysis or to treatment of iron deficiency, Vitamin B_{12} deficiency, or folic acid deficiency anemia. This test is also done to check on persons working with radioactive material or receiving radiotherapy. A persistently low count could be suggestive of bone marrow hypofunction or aplastic anemia.

Giving a percentage is not always the most accurate way of reporting the reticulocyte count, especially when the total RBC (erythrocyte) count is *not* within normal range. Both the RBC count and the reticulocyte count should be reported.

Purpose

- To aid in the diagnosis of anemias (pernicious, folic acid deficiency, hemolytic, sickle cell) *(see Clinical Problems)*.

Clinical Problems

Decreased Level: Anemias (pernicious, folic acid deficiency, aplastic), radiation therapy, effects of x-ray irradiation, adrenocortical hypofunction, anterior pituitary hypofunction, cirrhosis of the liver (alcohol suppresses reticulocytes).

Elevated Level: Anemias (hemolytic, sickle cell), thalassemia major, chronic hemorrhage, posthemorrhage (3 to 4 days), treatment for anemias (iron deficiency, Vitamin B_{12}, folic acid), leukemias, erythroblastosis fetalis (hemolytic disease of the newborn), hemoglobin C and D diseases, pregnancy.

Procedure

- Venous or capillary blood could be used for the reticulocyte count test.

Venous Blood

- Collect 3 to 5 ml of venous blood in a lavender-top tube.
- There is no food or fluid restriction.

Capillary Blood

- Cleanse the finger and puncture the skin with a sterile lancet.
- Wipe the first drop of blood away. Collect the blood by using a micropipette. The blood is mixed in equal proportions with methylene blue solution. The reticulocytes stain blue.
- There is no food or fluid restriction.

Factors Affecting Laboratory Results

- The use of the wrong colored-top tube for venous blood. The tube should contain anticoagulant (EDTA).

NURSING IMPLICATIONS WITH RATIONALE

Decreased Level

- Recognize clinical problems related to a decreased reticulocyte count, such as pernicious and aplastic anemias.
- Obtain a history regarding radiation exposure—x-ray and others.

Elevated Level
- Monitor the reticulocyte count when the client is being treated for pernicious anemia or folic acid anemia. There is usually an increase in reticulocytes.

Rheumatoid factor (RF), rheumatoid arthritis (RA) factor, RA latex fixation (serum)

Reference Values

Adult: <1:20 titer; <1:40 chronic inflammatory disease; 1:20–1:80 positive for rheumatoid arthritis and other conditions; >1:80 positive for rheumatoid arthritis.

Child: Not usually done.

Elderly: Slightly increased.

Description

The rheumatoid factor (RF) or rheumatoid arthritis (RA) factor test is a screening test used to detect antibodies (IgM, IgG, or IgA) found in the serum of clients with rheumatoid arthritis. RF occurs in 53% to 94% (average 76%) of clients with rheumatoid arthritis, and if the test is negative, it should be repeated.

The RF tests can be positive in many of the collagen diseases. The RF tests should not be used for monitoring follow-up or treatment stages of RA, because RF tests often remain positive when clinical remissions have been achieved. It also takes approximately 6 months for a significant elevation of titer. For diagnosing and evaluating RA, the ANA and the C-reactive protein agglutination tests are frequently used.

Purposes

- To screen for IgM, IgG, or IgA antibodies present in clients with possible RA.
- To aid in the diagnosis of RA.
- To compare test results in relation to other laboratory tests for diagnosing RA.

Clinical Problems

Elevated Level: Rheumatoid arthritis, lupus erythematosus, dermatomyositis, scleroderma, infectious mononucleosis, tuberculosis, leukemia, sarcoidosis, cirrhosis of the liver, hepatitis, syphilis, chronic infections, old age.

Procedure

- Collect 3 to 5 ml of venous blood in a red-top tube.

■ There is no food or fluid restriction.

Factors Affecting Laboratory Results

■ A positive RF test result frequently remains positive regardless of clinical improvement.

■ The RF test result can be positive in various clinical problems (i.e., collagen diseases, cancer, and liver cirrhosis).

■ The older adult may have an increased RF titer without the disease.

■ Due to the variability in the sensitivity and specificity of these screening tests, positive results must be interpreted in corroboration with the client's clinical status.

NURSING IMPLICATIONS WITH RATIONALE

Elevated Level

■ Relate an increased RF titer to clinical problems. A titer greater than 1:80 is most likely due to RA. Titers between 1:20 and 1:80 could be due to lupus, scleroderma, or liver cirrhosis.

■ Consider the age of the client when the RF is slightly increased. There can be a slight titer increase in the older adult without clinical symptoms of RA. With juvenile rheumatoid arthritis, only 10% of the children have a positive RF titer.

■ Assess for pain in the small joints of the hands and feet (especially the proximal interphalangeal joints), which could be indicative of an early stage of RA.

Rh typing (blood)

Reference Values

Adult: Rh + (positive), Rh − (negative).

Child: Same as adult.

Description

Rh typing is performed when typing donors'/recipients' blood and for cross-matching blood for transfusion. Rh factor (also known as Rh antigen) was first discovered by Landsteiner and Weiner in 1941; it was named Rh because of the use of rhesus monkeys in the research. Rh positive (most common Rh factor) indicates the presence of antigen on red blood cells (RBCs); Rh negative indicates an absence of the antigen.

An Rh-negative woman carrying a fetus with an Rh-positive blood group can cause Rh-positive antigens from the fetus to seep into the mother's blood, causing Rh antibody formation. If the mother develops a high anti-Rh antibody titer, the child can be born with a condition called *erythroblastosis fetalis* (hemolysis of the RBCs). To prevent Rh antibodies, the Rh-negative woman is given Rho(D) immune globulin, such as RhoGAM, within 3 days after delivery with the first child or after a miscarriage to neutralize any anti-Rh antibodies.

Purpose

- To identify the client's Rh factor for pregnancy or for blood transfusion.

Clinical Problems

Elevated Anti-Rh Antibodies: *Infant:* Erythroblastosis fetalis.

Procedure

- Collect 5 ml of venous blood in a red-top tube. Do not use a serum separator tube.
- There is no food or fluid restriction.
- Blood testing for Rh factor (antigen) should be done with care to avoid false-positive and false-negative results.

Factors Affecting Laboratory Results

- None known.

NURSING IMPLICATIONS WITH RATIONALE

- Obtain a history of previous blood transfusions the client has received. If the client is a pregnant woman, determine whether she has been pregnant before and whether the child (children) was (were) born jaundiced.
- Ask the clients if they know their Rh factor. Compare the tested Rh factor with the client's stated Rh factor. This could prevent administering incorrect blood.
- Inform the pregnant woman with Rh-negative factor that her blood will be tested at intervals during her pregnancy to find out whether antibodies are produced. The Rh-negative woman usually receives RhoGAM (Rh immune globulin) after delivery to prevent anti-Rh antibody production.

Rotavirus antigen (feces)

Reference Values

Negative.

Description

Rotavirus is an RNA virus that frequently causes infectious diarrhea in infants and young children, usually between 2 months and 2 years. Forty to 50% of children hospitalized are diagnosed with severe gastroenteritis caused by the rotavirus infection. It is more prevalent in the winter months in the United States; it is year round in the tropical areas. Adults can also become infected with this virus. Clinical symptoms include vomiting (usually precedes diarrhea), diarrhea, fever, and abdominal pain. Symptoms in adults are normally mild.

The rotavirus is mainly transmitted by the fecal-oral route. It can be detected in the stool using electron microscopy or preferably ELISA screening. Kits are available for testing the stool specimen.

Purpose

- To identify the rotavirus that is causing gastroenteritis in infants and young children.

Clinical Problems

Positive Test Result: Gastroenteritis caused by the rotavirus.

Procedure

- There is no food or fluid restriction.
- Obtain liquid stool and place the specimen in a closed container. The container should be placed on ice. A freshly soiled diaper may be used. Take immediately to the laboratory.
- A cotton-tip swab may be used to swab the rectum in a rotating motion. Leave the swab in the rectum for a few seconds for absorption. Place the swab in a tube or container, pack in ice, and send it immediately to the laboratory.
- No preservatives or metal container should be used. It interferes with ELISA testing.

Factors Affecting Laboratory Results

- Not packing the stool specimen in ice can affect test results.
- Insufficient amount of stool specimen.

NURSING IMPLICATIONS WITH RATIONALE

- Obtain a history of diarrhea, vomiting, and fever occurring in the child. Record frequency of the symptoms, and color of the stool and vomitus.
- Take vital signs. Keep a chart of body temperatures.
- Collect stool according to the procedure. Have the specimen container iced and taken immediately to the laboratory.
- Answer the family's questions. Be supportive of the child and family members.

Client Teaching

- Demonstrate to the parent collection of the stool specimen. The stool specimen should be collected during the acute stage.
- Instruct the family member that the stool can be infectious and that the rotavirus could be transmitted to others if precautions are not taken. Hands should be thoroughly washed after changing soiled diapers. Diapers should be carefully placed in plastic bag and properly discarded.
- Instruct the parent to check the child's body temperature at specified intervals.
- Encourage the parent to increase the child's fluid intake, particularly electrolyte-based fluids.
- Inform the parent that the rotavirus is easily transmitted, and there is a higher risk of transmission in nurseries, daycare centers, group homes, and nursing homes.

Rubella antibody detection (serum)

Hemagglutination Inhibition Test (HI or HAI) for Rubella (German Measles)

Reference Values

Adult: *Susceptibility to Rubella:* <1:8 titer. *Past Rubella Exposure:* 1:10–1:32 titer. *Immunity:* 1:32–1:64 titer. *Definite Immunity:* 1:64 titer and higher.

Description

Rubella (German measles) is a mild viral disease of short duration causing a fever and a transient rash. If it occurs in a woman in early pregnancy who is not immune from previous rubella infection and has not received rubella vaccination, the disease can produce serious deformities in her unborn child, especially if exposed during the first 2 months of gestation. Women should be immune to rubella (vaccinated) before marriage and definitely before pregnancy.

The rubella virus produces antibodies (natural immunity) against future rubella infections, but the exact antibody titer in the blood is unknown. Hemagglutination inhibition (HI or HAI) measures rubella antibody titers and is considered sensitive and reliable. If the antibody titer is 1:64 or higher, protection against rubella infection is assured.

Clinical indications for the HAI antibody (screening) test are as follows.

1. To determine the rubella antibody titer of a woman of child-bearing age if she has previously had the rubella infection. She will need the rubella vaccine if her titer is <1:8 (some state <1:20, others 1:32 or less).
2. To determine the rubella antibody titer at the first antepartum visit.
3. To check pregnant women (during their first trimester of pregnancy) at the time of rubella exposure and again in 3 to 4 weeks.
4. To check personnel who work in obstetrics in the hospital, clinic, or physician's office.
5. To diagnose a recent rubella infection in pregnant women (first trimester of pregnancy). The HAI test is done 3 days following the onset of the rash and is repeated 2 to 3 weeks later. A fourfold increase with the second HAI test usually indicates that the rash was due to rubella. A therapeutic abortion might be considered.

Purpose

- To identify clients who are susceptible to rubella or have immunity to the rubella virus.

Clinical Problems

Decreased Level (<1:8): Susceptible to rubella (German measles).

Elevated Level (>1:64): Definite immunity (resistance) to rubella.

Procedure

- Collect 3 to 5 ml of venous blood in a red-top tube.
- There is no food or fluid restriction.

Factors Affecting Laboratory Results

- None known.

NURSING IMPLICATIONS WITH RATIONALE

Patient Teaching

- Explain to the client the HAI antibody titer for rubella susceptibility is <1:8 and for rubella immunity is 1:64 and greater. The antibody titer sufficient to protect the unborn child differs among experts. Some of them feel 1:20 gives adequate immunity, while others think it should be >1:32. All agree that a 1:64 or higher dilution is a definite immunity titer.
- Teach young female adults and families about the need to have their blood checked for rubella immunity (against German measles). This test should be done

before pregnancy, and if the titer is <1:8, they should receive the rubella vaccine. Some states require a rubella test before a marriage license is issued.

- Instruct pregnant women who are susceptible to German measles to avoid exposure to the disease if at all possible. If they have been exposed to German measles or develop a rash, they should notify the obstetrician immediately so that HAI antibody titer testing can be done. Exposure to German measles does not mean that the person will develop the disease, but it does mean that the antibody titer must be monitored. Emphasize the importance of calling the health care provider when exposed to German measles.
- Explain to interested persons some of the fetal abnormalities (congenital heart disease, deafness, mental retardation) that can occur if a woman develops German measles during the first 3 months of pregnancy.

Salicylate (serum)

Reference Values

Adult: *Normal:* Negative. *Therapeutic:* 5 mg (headache); 10–30 mg/dl (rheumatoid arthritis). *Mildly Toxic:* >30 mg/dl. *Severely Toxic:* >50 mg/dl. *Lethal:* >60 mg/dl.

Elderly: *Mildly Toxic:* >25 mg/dl.

Child: *Toxic:* >25 mg/dl.

Description

Salicylate levels are measured to check the therapeutic level, as in the treatment of rheumatic fever, and to check the levels caused by an accidental or deliberate overdose. Blood salicylate reaches its peak in 2 to 3 hours, and the blood level can be elevated for as long as 18 hours.

An overdose of aspirin will cause respiratory alkalosis, and if not corrected, metabolic acidosis will occur in response to cellular breakdown and the increase in organic acids. Prolonged use of salicylates (aspirins) can cause bleeding tendencies, because it inhibits platelet aggregation. It may be toxic in children because it increases the risk of Reye's syndrome.

Purposes

- To monitor salicylate for daily therapeutic range.
- To check for salicylate toxicity.

Clinical Problems

Elevated Level: Overdose or large, continuous doses of acetylsalicyclic acid (aspirin, acetyl salicylic acid), drugs containing aspirin.

Procedure

- Collect 5 to 7 ml of venous blood in a red-top or a green-top tube.
- There is no food or fluid restriction.
- A urine test may also be done as a screening test.

Factors Affecting Laboratory Results

- None reported.

NURSING IMPLICATIONS WITH RATIONALE

- Observe for signs and symptoms of early aspirin overdose (i.e., hyperventilation, flushed skin, and ringing in the ears).
- Obtain a history from the child or parent concerning the approximate number of aspirins taken. A toxic dose for a small child is 3.33 grains/kg, or 200 mg/kg. For a child weighing 15 kg (33 lb), the toxic dose would be 10 adult aspirins (5 grains each). Salicylates are not the choice agent for children with virus because of the possibility of developing Reye's syndrome.
- Recognize that acid-base imbalance is common with salicylate toxicity. Respiratory alkalosis usually occurs first, followed by metabolic acidosis. Symptoms of toxicity usually occur 6 hours following aspirin ingestion. Most of the aspirin has already been absorbed by that time.

Client Teaching

- Instruct the client who takes aspirins constantly that before any surgery the surgeon should be informed of the number of aspirins taken daily. Explain that aspirins will prolong bleeding time.

Schilling test

See Diagnostic Tests

Sedimentation rate

See Erythrocyte Sedimentation Rate—ESR

Semen examination

Reference Values

Semen Examination: *Volume:* 1.5–5.0 ml. *Count:* 60–150 million/ml. *Mobility:* 3 hours >60%. *Normal Forms:* >70%. *Appearance:* Translucent, turbid, viscous. *Viscosity:* Liquid after 30 minutes.

Antisperm Antibody Test: *Adult:* Negative to 1:32.

Description

Semen examination is used as one of the tests to determine the cause of infertility. The sperm count; volume of fluid; percentage of normal, mature spermatozoa (sperms); and percentage of actively mobile spermatozoa are studied when analyzing the semen content. Conception has been reported even when the sperm count has been as low as 10 million/ml.

Sperm count is frequently used to monitor the effectiveness of sterilization after a vasectomy (severing of the vas deferens). The sperm count is checked periodically. In cases of rape, a forensic or medicolegal analysis is done to detect semen in vaginal secretions or on clothes.

The three methods used to collect semen are masturbation, coitus interruptus, and intercourse using a condom. Sexual abstinence is usually required for 3 days before the test. Masturbation is the usual method for obtaining a semen specimen; however, for religious reasons intercourse with a condom is sometimes preferred. With coitus interruptus, only a partial semen specimen may be obtained. A semen specimen may be collected at home or in the health care provider's office.

The *antisperm antibody test* could be ordered to identify a possible cause of infertility. Autoantibodies to sperm might result from a blocking of the efferent ducts in the testes.

Purposes

- To check the sperm count.
- To determine if the decreased sperm count could be the cause of infertility.

Clinical Problems

Decreased Level: Vasectomy; infertility (0–2 million/ml). *Drug Influence:* Antineoplastic agents, estrogen.

Procedure

- Abstinence from intercourse for 3 days before collecting semen.
- Collect semen by:

   1. Masturbation—collect in a clean container.
   2. Coitus interruptus—collect in a clean glass container.
   3. Intercourse with a clean, washed condom—place the condom in a clean container.

- Keep the semen specimen from chilling, and take it immediately to the laboratory. It should be tested within 2 hours after collection—the sooner, the better.
- Alcoholic beverages should be avoided for several days (at least 24 hours) before the test. There is no other fluid or food restriction.

Factors Affecting Laboratory Results

- Recent intercourse (within 3 days) could have an effect on the sperm count.

NURSING IMPLICATIONS WITH RATIONALE

- Explain to the client the purpose of the test. He will most likely know the reason for semen collection and examination, which is either to determine the cause of infertility or to determine the effectiveness of sterilization following vasectomy.
- Be available to discuss methods of semen collection with the client and his spouse/partner (i.e., masturbation, coitus interruptus, and intercourse with a condom). This can be most embarrassing for the man and woman. Some persons prefer to discuss the test in detail with the nurse rather than with the health care provider. Religious beliefs need to be considered.
- Be supportive of the client and his spouse. Be a good listener and give them time to express their concerns.
- Answer their questions. If you are unable to respond, refer the question to the appropriate person (i.e., the health care provider, a clergyman).
- Avoid giving your moral convictions about the test or the surgical procedure (vasectomy).

Serotonin (plasma)

5-Hydroxytryptamine

Reference Values

Adult: 50–175 ng/ml; 10–30 µg/dl, 0.29–1.15 µmol/l (SI units).

Description

Serotonin is produced by the argentaffin cells of the intestinal mucosa. It is transmitted in the body by platelets and acts as a vasoconstrictor to small arterioles after tissue injury. It can also be found in the tissues of the central nervous system and has been classified as one of the neurotransmitters. Other functions of serotonin include contraction of smooth muscle such as in peristalsis, release of the growth hormone, and release of prolactin; it can cause hemocoagulation.

The primary purpose of this test is to confirm the diagnosis of carcinoid tumors of the argentaffin cells in the gastrointestinal tract. Most of serotonin is excreted as the metabolite 5-hydroxyindole-acetic acid (5-HIAA) in the urine. The 5-HIAA urine test should be ordered with the plasma serotonin test. Ectopic production of serotonin can result from oat cell carcinoma of the lung, pancreatic tumors, and thyroid cancer.

Purpose

- To aid in the diagnosis of carcinoid tumors.

Clinical Problems

Decreased Level: Parkinson's disease, Down syndrome, depression, renal insufficiency, phenylketonuria.

Elevated Level: *Carcinoid Tumors:* Ectopic production due to oat cell carcinoma of the lung, pancreatic tumor, thyroid medullary cancer; myocardial infarction, endocarditis, chronic pain, cystic fibrosis. *Drug Influence:* Monoamine oxidase (MAO inhibitors), methyldopa, imipramine, reserpine.

Procedure

- There is no food or fluid restriction.
- Collect 7 to 10 ml of venous blood in a lavender-top tube. The blood specimen should be placed on ice immediately and sent promptly to the laboratory.
- Withhold MAO inhibitors for a week prior to the test with the health care provider's approval. MAO inhibitors taken prior to the test should be noted on the laboratory slip.

Factors Affecting Laboratory Results

- Blood specimen that has not been cooled and not taken immediately to the laboratory. Blood serotonin samples are unstable.
- Certain drugs can increase the plasma serotonin level especially MAO inhibitors *(see Drug Influence)*.
- The drug lithium may decrease or elevate the serotonin in the brain.
- A radioactive scan performed on the client 7 days before the serotonin blood sample is taken.

NURSING IMPLICATIONS WITH RATIONALE

- Obtain a list of drugs the client is taking. Notify the health care provider if the client is taking a drug that could elevate the plasma serotonin level, especially MAO inhibitors.
- Check if a urine 5-HIAA has been ordered. This urine test is usually ordered if a carcinoid tumor is suspected.
- Note if the client has chronic pain, which may increase the plasma serotonin level, or depression, which could decrease the plasma level.

Serum glutamic oxaloacetic transaminase (SGOT)

See Aspartate Aminotransferase

Serum glutamic pyruvic transaminase (SGPT)

See Alanine Aminotransferase

Sickle cell (screening) test (blood)

Reference Values

Adult: 0.

Child: 0.

Description

(See Hemoglobin Electrophoresis.)

Hemoglobin S (sickle cell), an abnormal hemoglobin, causes red blood cells (RBCs; erythrocytes) to form a crescent shape when deprived of oxygen. With adequate oxygen, the RBCs with hemoglobin S will maintain a normal shape.

If a sickle cell screening test is positive for hemoglobin S, hemoglobin electrophoresis should be ordered to differentiate between sickle cell anemia caused by hemoglobin S/S and sickle cell trait caused by hemoglobin A/S. If the patient's hemoglobin level is <10 g/dl or the hematocrit is <30%, test results could be falsely negative.

Purpose

- To screen for sickle cell anemia.

Clinical Problems

Positive Results: Sickle cell anemia, sickle cell trait.

Procedure

- Collect 3 to 7 ml of venous blood in a lavender-top tube.
- If a commercial-test kit (Sickledex) is used, follow the directions given on the kit.
- There is no food or fluid restriction.
- Note on the laboratory slip if blood transfusion was given 3 to 4 months before the screening test. If so, inaccurate results could result.

Factors Affecting Laboratory Results

- A blood transfusion given within 3 to 4 months could cause inaccurate results.
- Hemoglobin <10 g/dl or hematocrit <30% could cause false-negative test results.
- Reagents from the test kit may deteriorate and may no longer be active test agents.
- The test result could be falsely negative in an infant <6 months old.

NURSING IMPLICATIONS WITH RATIONALE

- Explain to the client and/or family that the purpose of the test is to determine the presence of sickle cells (hemoglobin S).

Positive Test Results

- Observe for signs and symptoms of sickle cell anemia. Early symptoms are fatigue and weakness. Chronic symptoms are dyspnea on exertion, swollen joints, "aching bones," and chest pains.

Client Teaching

- Instruct the client to avoid people with infections and colds. Persons with sickle cell anemia are susceptible to infections.
- Encourage the client to seek genetic counseling if he or she has sickle cell anemia or the sickle cell trait.
- Instruct the client with sickle cell anemia to minimize strenuous activity and to avoid high altitudes and extreme cold. Encourage the client to take rest periods.

Sodium (Na) (serum)

Reference Values

Adult: 135–145 mEq/l, 135–145 mmol/l (SI units).

Child: *Infant:* 134–150 mEq/l. *Child:* 135–145 mEq/l.

Description

Sodium (Na) is the major cation in the extracellular fluid (ECF), and it has a water-retaining effect. When there is excess sodium in the ECF, more water will be reabsorbed from the kidneys.

Sodium has many functions. It helps to maintain body fluids, is responsible for conduction of neuromuscular impulses via the sodium pump (sodium shifts into cells as potassium shifts out for cellular activity), it is involved in enzyme activity, and it regulates acid–base balance by combining with chloride or bicarbonate ions.

The body needs approximately 2 to 4 g of sodium daily. The American people daily consume approximately 6 to 12 g (90 to 240 mEq/l) of sodium in the form of salt (NaCl). A teaspoon of salt contains 2.3 g of sodium.

The names for sodium imbalances are *hyponatremia* (serum sodium deficit) and *hypernatremia* (serum sodium excess). When the serum sodium level is 125 mEq/l, sodium replacement with normal saline (0.9% NaCl) should be considered, and if the serum sodium level is 115 mEq/l or lower, concentrated saline solutions (3% or 5% NaCl) might be ordered. When rapidly replacing sodium loss, assessment for overhydration is important.

Purposes

- To monitor the sodium level.
- To detect sodium imbalance (hypo- or hypernatremia).
- To compare the sodium level with that of other electrolytes (i.e., calcium, potassium, chloride).

Clinical Problems

Decreased Level: Vomiting, diarrhea, gastric suction, excessive perspiration, continuous intravenous 5% dextrose in water (D_5W), syndrome of inappropriate antidiuretic hormone (SIADH, due to surgery, trauma, pain, narcotics), low-sodium diet, burns, inflammatory reactions, tissue injury (fluid and sodium shift to the third space); psychogenic polydipsia, salt-wasting renal disease. *Drug Influence:* Potent diuretics (furosemide [Lasix], ethacrynic acid [Edecrin], thiazides, mannitol).

Elevated Level: Dehydration, severe vomiting and diarrhea (water loss is greater than sodium loss), congestive heart failure, Cushing's disease, hepatic failure, high-sodium diet. *Drug Influence:* Cough medicines, cortisone preparations, antibiotics, laxatives, methyldopa (Aldomet), hydralazine (Apresoline), reserpine (Serpasil).

Procedure

- Collect 3 to 5 ml of venous blood in a red- or green-top tube.
- There are no restrictions on food and fluid. If the client has eaten large quantities of foods high in salt content in the last 24 to 48 hours, this should be noted on the laboratory slip and the health care provider should be notified. Sodium is rarely requested alone but is rather given as part of the serum electrolytes (i.e., sodium, potassium, chloride, carbon dioxide).

Factors Affecting Laboratory Results

- A diet high in sodium.
- Drugs—potent diuretics, cortisone preparations, various antihypertensive agents, cough medicines.

NURSING IMPLICATIONS WITH RATIONALE

Decreased Level

- Assess for signs and symptoms of hyponatremia (i.e., apprehension, anxiety, muscular twitching, muscular weakness, headaches, tachycardia, and hypotension).
- Recognize that hyponatremia after surgery is the result of SIADH. There is usually

an excess secretion of antidiuretic hormone for a day or two after surgery, which causes water reabsorption from the kidney and sodium dilution.

- Report if the client has received D₅W infusions for more than 2 days. Hyponatremia and water intoxication could occur. IV fluids with dextrose and one third or one half normal saline solution (0.33% to 0.45%) are frequently ordered.

- Monitor the medical regimen for correcting hyponatremia (i.e., water restriction, normal saline [0.9% percent] solution to correct a serum sodium level of 120 to 130 mEq/l, and 3% or 5% saline to correct a serum sodium level of <115 mEq/l).

- Observe for signs and symptoms of overhydration when the client is receiving 3% or 5% percent saline intravenously. Symptoms of overhydration are a constant, irritated cough; dyspnea; neck- and hand-vein engorgement; and chest rales.

- Check the specific gravity of urine. A specific gravity of <1.010 could indicate hyponatremia.

- Check serum sodium and other laboratory results and report serum electrolyte changes. An extremely low serum sodium level requires that the test be repeated.

- Irrigate nasogastric tubes and wound sites with normal saline instead of sterile water.

- Take vital signs to determine cardiac status during hyponatremia.

- Compare the serum sodium level with the urine sodium level. A low or normal serum sodium and a low urine sodium could indicate sodium retention or a decrease in sodium intake.

Client Teaching

- Encourage the client to avoid drinking only plain water. Suggest fluids with solutes (i.e., broth and juices).

Elevated Level

- Observe for signs and symptoms of hypernatremia (i.e., restlessness; thirst; flushed skin; dry, sticky mucous membranes; a rough, dry tongue; and tachycardia).

- Check for body fluid loss by keeping an accurate intake and output record and weighing the client daily. A liter of fluid will add on approximately 2.5 lb of body weight.

- Check the specific gravity of the urine. A specific gravity >1.030 could indicate hypernatremia.

- Report if the client is receiving IV fluids containing normal saline (0.9% NaCl). A liter of normal saline contains 155 mEq of sodium. The body needs 40 to 70 mEq/l of sodium daily, though the average daily intake for adults is 90 to 240 mEq/l. The maximum daily tolerance of sodium is 400 mEq/l, and if the client receives 3 L of normal saline, he or she will receive 465 mEq/l.

- Observe for edema and overhydration resulting from an elevated serum-sodium level. Signs and symptoms of overhydration are a constant, irritated cough; dyspnea; neck- and hand-vein engorgement; and chest rales.

Client Teaching

- Encourage the client to drink 8 to 10 glasses of water, unless this is contraindicated (for instance, with a history of congestive heart failure).
- Instruct the client to avoid foods that are high in sodium (i.e., corned beef, bacon, ham, tuna fish, cheese, celery, catsup, pickles, olives, and potato chips). Avoid using salt when cooking or at mealtime.

Sodium (Na) (urine)

Reference Values

Adult: 40–220 mEq/l/24 h.

Child: Similar to adult.

Description

Sodium excretion varies according to the sodium intake, aldosterone secretion, urine volume, and disease entities, such as chronic renal failure, adrenal gland dysfunction (Addision's disease and Cushing's syndrome), cirrhosis of the liver, and congestive heart failure.

When the urine sodium level is <40 mEq/24 h, the decreased sodium excretion could be due to sodium retention or decreased sodium intake. The body could be retaining sodium even with a low serum sodium level.

The urine sodium level should be monitored when edema is present and the serum sodium level is low or normal.

Purposes

See Sodium (Serum).

Clinical Problems

Decreased Level: Cushing's syndrome, congestive heart failure, hepatic failure, renal failure, chronic obstructive lung disease (COLD), low sodium (salt) intake. *Drug Influence:* Cortisone preparations.

Elevated Level: Addison's disease, dehydration, essential hypertension, diabetes mellitus, anterior pituitary hypofunction, high sodium intake. *Drug Influence:* Potent diuretics (furosemide [Lasix], ethacrynic acid [Edecrin]).

Procedure

- Collect a 24-hour urine sample and place it in a large specimen container. Label the container with the exact times the urine collection started and ended. First-voided specimen should be discarded.

- The urine specimen should be refrigerated or placed in a container of ice.
- There is no food or fluid restriction.

Factors Affecting Laboratory Results

- A diet high or low in sodium content.
- Drugs such as cortisone and potent diuretics.
- Renal dysfunction.
- Discarded urine.

NURSING IMPLICATIONS WITH RATIONALE

Client Teaching

- Explain the procedure for collecting the 24-hour urine. Inform the client that all voidings (urine) should be placed in the large container. Have clients inform their families of the procedure. Tell the client not to put toilet paper or feces in the urine.

Decreased Level

- Compare the serum sodium level with the urine sodium level. A low or normal serum sodium and a low urine sodium could indicate sodium retention or a decrease in sodium intake.

Elevated Level

- Report if the client is receiving several liters of normal saline solution intravenously (see Sodium [Serum]).

Client Teaching

- Instruct the client to avoid eating foods high in sodium if the cause is due to high-sodium intake.

Testosterone (serum or plasma)

Reference Values

Adult: *Male:* 0.3–1.0 µg/dl, 300–1000 ng/dl. *Female:* 0.03–0.1 µg/dl, 30–100 ng/dl.

Child: *Male:* 12 to 14 Years Old: >0.1 µg/dl, >100 ng/dl.

Description

Testosterone, a male sex hormone, is produced by the testes and adrenal glands in the male and by the ovaries and adrenal glands in the female. It is useful in diagnosing male sexual precocity before the age of 10 years and male infertility.

In males, the highest serum testosterone levels occur in the morning. Serum testosterone is low in both primary and secondary hypogonadism.

Purposes

- To assess testosterone value.
- To detect testicular hypofunction.
- To aid in the diagnosis of male sexual precocity.

Clinical Problems

Decreased Level: Testicular hypofunction. Klinefelter's syndrome (primary hypogonadism), alcoholism, anterior pituitary hypofunction, estrogen therapy, hypopituitarism.

Elevated Level: Male sexual precocity, adrenal hyperplasia or tumor, neoplasm or hyperplasia of ovaries, adrenogenital syndrome in women, polycystic ovaries in females.

Procedure

- Collect 5 to 7 ml of venous blood in a red- or green-top tube. Avoid hemolysis.
- There is no food or fluid restriction.

Factors Affecting Laboratory Results

- None known.

NURSING IMPLICATIONS WITH RATIONALE

Decreased Level

- Determine whether the client is complying with medical treatment for testicular hypofunction or hypogonadism. Discuss the side effects of testosterone.
- Be supportive of the male client and his family concerning physical changes caused by hormonal deficiency.

Elevated Level

- Observe for signs and symptoms of excess testosterone secretion (i.e., hirsutism, masculine voice, and increased muscle mass [especially in women]). Report abnormal findings.

Theophylline (serum)

Aminophylline, Theo-Dur, Theolaire, Slo-Phyllin, Elixophyllin, Sustaire

Reference Values

Therapeutic Range: *Adult:* 5–20 μg/ml, 28–112 μmol/l (SI units). *Elderly:* 5–18 μg/ml. *Premature Infant:* 7–14 μg/ml. *Neonate:* 3–12 μg/ml. *Child:* Same as adult.

Toxic Level: *Adult:* >20 μg/ml, >112 μmol/l (SI units). *Elderly:* Same as adult. *Premature Infant:* >14 μg/ml. *Neonate:* >13 μg/ml. *Child:* Same as adult.

Description

Theophylline, a xanthine derivative, relaxes smooth muscle of the bronchi and pulmonary blood vessels; reduces pulmonary hypertension; stimulates the central nervous system; stimulates myocardium, resulting in an increase in the force of contraction and cardiac output; increases renal blood flow, causing diuresis; and relaxes smooth muscles of the gastrointestinal tract. Usually theophylline products are given to control asthmatic attacks and to treat acute attack. Oral theophylline preparations are well absorbed from the gastrointestinal tract.

Ninety percent of theophylline is metabolized in the liver, with about 60% bound to plasma protein and 40% free. Ten percent of the drug is excreted unchanged in the urine. The half-life of theophylline is 5 to 10 hours in a non-smoker, 3½ to 5 hours in a smoker, and 3½ in children. Peak blood levels after an orally administered dose of theophylline occurs in 1 to 2 hours.

Persons with heart failure or liver disease or who are either very young or elderly could develop theophylline toxicity quickly. Serum theophylline levels in these persons should be monitored frequently.

Early signs and symptoms of theophylline toxicity are anorexia, nausea, vomiting, abdominal discomfort, nervousness, jitters, tachycardia, and cardiac arrhythmias. If severe theophylline toxicity occurs (>30 μg/ml), cardiac dysrhythmias, seizures, respiratory arrest, and/or cardiac arrest might result.

Purpose

■ To monitor theophylline levels.

Clinical Problems

Decreased Level: Smoking. *Drug Influence:* Phenytoin (Dilantin).

Elevated Level: Theophylline overdose, congestive heart failure, liver disease, lung disease, renal disease. *Drug Influence:* Antibiotics (erythromycin, lincomycin), allupurinol, barbiturates, caffeine, cimetidine (Tagamet), furosemide

(Lasix), ephedrine, propranolol (Inderal), sulfonamides, theobromine, other xanthines, flu vaccine.

Procedure

- Collect 3 to 5 ml of venous blood in a red-top tube. Avoid hemolysis.
- Record the name of the drug, dose, route, and last dose administered on the laboratory requisition slip. Test might be ordered for peak levels or for trough levels (before next dose).
- The client should not drink coffee, tea, or colas, or eat chocolates 8 hours prior to the test.
- Note on the laboratory requisition slip drugs the client is taking that could affect test results.
- Do not shake the collecting tube of blood specimen. This could decrease the serum theophylline level.

Factors Affecting Laboratory Results

- Drugs *(see Drug Influence)*; food and fluids, such as chocolate, coffee, tea, and colas, could increase serum theophylline level.
- Shaking the collecting tube vigorously could cause a false-negative test result.

NURSING IMPLICATIONS WITH RATIONALE

- Explain to the client that the purpose of the test is to monitor the therapeutic theophylline level.
- Check the theophylline level and report nontherapeutic levels to the health care provider immediately.
- Record name of the drug, dose, route, and last time drug was given on the requisition slip.
- Record the time the blood sample was drawn on the requisition slip. This informs the laboratory personnel and the health care provider of the theophylline level time (peak or trough before the next dose).

Decreased Level

- Recognize that smoking causes a short half-life and promotes a faster theophylline clearance. The drug phenytoin (Dilantin) has been reported to decrease the theophylline half-life.
- Report if the client is a smoker because a larger dose of theophylline might be needed.

Elevated Level

- Recognize that liver, lung, and renal diseases and certain drugs might cause an elevated serum theophylline level *(see Drug Influence above)*.
- Observe for signs and symptoms of theophylline toxicity (i.e., anorexia, nausea,

vomiting, abdominal discomfort, nervousness, irritability, tachycardia, and cardiac dysrhythmias).

- Monitor pulse rate and report signs of tachycardia and skipped beats.
- Monitor intake and output. Report if client's output has greatly increased because of diuresis.

Client Teaching

- Instruct the client not to drink coffee, teas, or colas, or eat chocolate within 8 hours of the test.

Thyroglobulin antibodies

See Thyroid Antibodies

Thyroid antibodies (TA) (serum)

Thyroglobulin Antibodies or Thyroid Hemagglutination Test

Reference Values

Adult: Negative to 1:20, tanned red cell (TRC) results under 100.

Child: Similar to adult but usually not done.

Description

A thyroid autoimmune disease usually produces thyroid antibodies (antithyroglobulin antibodies and antimicrosomal antibodies). These autoantibodies (against the body's own tissue) combine with thyroglobulin from the thyroid gland and cause inflammatory lesions of the gland.

A serum titer evaluation is ordered to detect the presence of thyroid antibodies. With Hashimoto's thyroiditis, the titer is high, 1:5000. The titer can also be elevated with carcinoma of the thyroid, rheumatoid-collagen diseases, and thyrotoxicosis. A positive thyroid antibodies (TA) test does not always confirm the diagnosis of Hashimoto's thyroiditis, unless the titer is extremely high.

Purposes

- To aid in the diagnosis of Graves' disease.
- To detect the presence of thyroid antibodies, which may cause a thyroid auto-immune disease.

Clinical Problems

Elevated Titer: Hashimoto's thyroiditis, carcinoma of the thyroid gland, pernicious anemia, lupus erythematosus, rheumatoid arthritis, thyrotoxicosis (Graves' disease).

Procedure

- Collect 5 ml of venous blood in a red-top tube. Avoid hemolysis.
- There is no food or fluid restriction.

Factors Affecting Laboratory Results

- Sex (thyroid disease is commoner in women than in men).

NURSING IMPLICATIONS WITH RATIONALE

Elevated Titer Level

- Check serum antithyroglobin antibody titer results and relate them to clinical problems. The test is usually ordered to diagnose Hashimoto's thyroiditis; however, the titer level can be elevated in other clinical conditions (*see Clinical Problems*).
- Obtain a family history of thyroid disease. Determine whether the client has had a viral infection in the last few weeks or months. It is believed that viral infections can trigger autoimmune disease.

Thyroid-stimulating hormone (TSH) (serum)

Reference Values

Adult: 0.35–5.5 µIU/ml, <3 ng/ml.

Newborn: <25 µIU/ml by the third day.

Description

The anterior pituitary gland (anterior hypophysis) secretes thyroid-stimulating hormone (TSH) in response to thyroid-releasing hormone (TRH) from the hypothalamus. TSH stimulates the secretion of thyroxine (T_4) produced in the thyroid gland.

The secretion of TSH is dependent on the negative-feedback system—a decreased T_4 level promotes the release of TRH, which stimulates TSH secretion. An elevated T_4 level suppresses TRH release, which suppresses TSH secretion.

TSH and T_4 levels are frequently measured to differentiate pituitary from thyroid dysfunctions. A decreased T_4 level and a normal or elevated TSH level can indicate a thyroid disorder. A decreased T_4 level with a decreased TSH level can indicate a pituitary disorder.

Purposes

- To suggest secondary hypothyroidism due to pituitary involvement.
- To compare test results with T_4 level to differentiate between pituitary and thyroid dysfunction.

Clinical Problems

Decreased Level: Secondary hypothyroidism (pituitary gland involvement), anterior pituitary hypofunction, Klinefelter's syndrome. *Drug Influence:* Aspirin, steroid, dopamine, heparin.

Elevated Level: Primary hypothyroidism (thyroid gland involvement with a decreased T_4); thyroiditis (Hashimoto's disease, autoimmune disease); cirrhosis of the liver. *Drug Influence:* Antithyroid therapy.

Procedure

- Collect 5 ml of venous blood in a red-top or green-top tube. Avoid hemolysis.
- There is no food or fluid restriction. Shellfish should be avoided for several days prior to the test.

Factors Affecting Laboratory Results

- None known.

NURSING IMPLICATIONS WITH RATIONALE

- Recognize the cause of hypothyroidism by comparing the TSH level with the T_4 level. Decreased TSH and T_4 levels could be due to anterior pituitary dysfunction causing secondary hypothyroidism. A normal or elevated TSH level and a decreased T_4 level could be due to thyroid dysfunction.
- Observe for signs and symptoms of myxedema (hypothyroidism; i.e., anorexia; fatigue; weight gain; dry and flaky skin; puffy face, hands, and feet; abdominal distention; bradycardia; infertility, and ataxia).
- Monitor vital signs before and during treatment for hypothyroidism. Report immediately if tachycardia occurs.
- Refer to the client's triiodothyronine (T_3), T_4, and thyroglobulin results to observe correlations with the TSH result.

Thyroxine (T$_4$) (serum)

Reference Values

Adult: *Reported as Serum Thyroxine:* T$_4$ by column: 4.5–11.5 µg/dl. T$_4$ (RIA): 5–12 µg/dl. Free T$_4$: 1.0–2.3 ng/dl. *Reported as Thyroxine Iodine:* T$_4$ by column: 3.2–7.2 µg/dl.

Child: *Newborn:* 11–23 µg/dl. *1 to 4 Months Old:* 7.5–16.5 µg/dl. *4 to 12 Months Old:* 5.5–14.5 µg/dl. *1 to 6 Years Old:* 5.5–13.5 µg/dl. *6 to 10 Years Old:* 5–12.5 µg/dl.

Description

Thyroxine (T$_4$) is the major hormone secreted by the thyroid gland and is at least 25 times more concentrated than triiodothyronine (T$_3$). The serum T$_4$ levels are commonly used to measure thyroid hormone concentration and the function of the thyroid gland. The use of protein-bound iodine (PBI) is considered obsolete, and this test is seldom performed.

In some institutions the T$_4$ test is required for all newborns (as is the phenyl-ketonuria [PKU] test) to detect a decreased thyroxine secretion, which could lead to irreversible mental retardation.

Purposes

- To determine thyroid function.
- To aid in the diagnosis of hypo- or hyperthyroidism.
- To compare test results with other laboratory thyroid tests.

Clinical Problems

Decreased Level: Hypothyroidism (cretinism, myxedema), protein malnutrition, anterior pituitary hypofunction, strenuous exercise. *Drug Influence:* Cortisone, chlorpromazine (Thorazine), phenytoin (Dilantin), heparin, lithium, sulfonamides, reserpine (Serpasil), testosterone, tolbutamide (Orinase).

Elevated Level: Hyperthyroidism, acute thyroiditis, viral hepatitis, myasthenia gravis, pregnancy, preeclampsia. *Drug Influence:* Oral contraceptives, estrogens, clofibrate.

Procedure

- Various methods are used for measuring T$_4$.
- Thyroid medication will interfere with the T$_4$ by column method. Check with your laboratory for an alternative procedure.
- Collect 5 to 7 ml of venous blood in a red-top tube. Avoid hemolysis.

- There is no food or fluid restriction.
- Note on the laboratory slip drugs the client is taking that could affect test results.

Factors Affecting Laboratory Results

- Drugs *(see Drug Influence)*.

NURSING IMPLICATIONS WITH RATIONALE

Decreased Level

- Observe for signs and symptoms of hypothyroidism (i.e., fatigue, forgetfulness, weight gain, dry skin with poor turgor, dry and thin hair, bradycardia, decreased peripheral circulation, depressed libido, infertility, and constipation).

Elevated Level

- Observe for signs and symptoms of hyperthyroidism (i.e., nervousness, tremors, emotional instability, increased appetite, weight loss, palpitations, tachycardia, diarrhea, decreased fertility, and exophthalmos).
- Monitor the pulse rate. Tachycardia is common and if severe could cause heart failure and cardiac arrest.

Torch screen test

TORCH Battery, TORCH Titer

Reference Values

Maternal: *IgG Titer Antibodies:* Negative. *IgM Titer Antibodies:* Negative.

Infant: Same as maternal; infant should be under 2 months of age.

Description

TORCH stands for toxoplasmosis, rubella, cytomegalovirus (CMV), and herpes simplex. It is a screen test to detect the presence of these organisms in the mother and infant. During pregnancy, TORCH infections can cross the placenta and could result in mild or severe congenital malformation, abortion, or stillbirth. The severe effect from these organisms occurs during the first trimester of pregnancy. Prenatally the TORCH screening test is performed only when a TORCH infection is suspected, such as rubella infection.

TORCH screening test is more frequently performed when congenital infection in the infant is suspected. The IgG titers are compared with both mother's and infant's serum. If the IgG titer level is higher in the infant than mother and the IgM titer is present in the infant, congenital TORCH infection is likely. This test might be repeated in several weeks. Individual testing might be necessary along with clinical information to identify the TORCH infection; rubella and CMV are the commonest.

Purpose

- To detect TORCH infection in newborns and mothers.

Clinical Problems

Positive IgG, IgM Titers: Toxoplasmosis, rubella, CMV, herpes simplex.

Procedure

- Collect 7 ml of venous blood in a red-top tube.
- There is no food or fluid restriction.
- TORCH kits: Follow directions on the kit.

Factors Affecting Laboratory Results

- None known.

NURSING IMPLICATIONS WITH RATIONALE

- Obtain a history from the client about any previous infection.

Client Teaching

- Inform the client that if a positive test result occurs, more testing will be needed.

Toxoplasmosis antibody test (serum)

Reference Values

Titer: <1:4, no previous infection from *T. gondii*.

Titer: 1:4–1:64, past exposure, may persist for life.

Titer: >1:256, recent infection.

Titer: >1:424, acute infection.

Description

Toxoplasma gondii (*T. gondii*) is a protozoan organism that causes the parasitic disease, toxoplasmosis. Twenty-five to 40% of the population in the United States have antibodies to *T. gondii*. Half of these people had been asymptomatic. This organism can remain in body muscle and be dormant for years or life. This organism is transmitted in raw or poorly cooked meat or by ingesting oocysts from feces of infected cats. Transmission from the latter may occur when changing the cat litter.

Congenital form of toxoplasmosis occurs to the fetus when the mother is acutely infected with the *T. gondii* during pregnancy and passed the organism via placenta to the unborn child. Most of these pregnant females having the *T. gondii* are asymptomatic. If the female is infected with *T. gondii* weeks or months before conception, the organism will not affect the fetus. Congenital toxoplasmosis may cause mental retardation, hydrocephalus, microcephalus, and chronic retinitis, and/or lead to fetal death. The Centers for Disease Control recommends a serological test for *T. gondii* antibody titer for all pregnant women before the 20th week (actually earlier is better). There usually is no risk for birth defects; if the titer is low-positive a repeat test may be suggested. However, if the pregnant woman acquires the organism (high titer level) during pregnancy, the fetus is at risk for birth defect. The fetus has been infected with the organism if the antibody titer of the infant persistently increases 2 to 3 months after birth. Toxoplasmosis is not communicable between individuals except for maternal–fetal transfer.

The IGM antibody titer begins to rise 1 week after infection and peaks in 1 to 3 weeks. The IgG antibody titer rises in approximately 4 to 7 days after the IgM antibody, peaks 1 to 3 weeks later, and falls slowly within 6 months. Sulfonamides may be used to treat toxoplasmosis.

Purposes

- To identify the *T. gondii* organism.
- To detect the *T. gondii* organism in pregnant woman before the 20th week.

Clinical Problems

Elevated Titers: Toxoplasmosis. **Low Positive Titer:** Past infection of *T. gondii*. **High Positive Titer:** Current active infection of *T. gondii*.

Procedure

- There is no food or fluid restriction.
- Collect 5 to 7 ml of venous blood in a red-top tube during early weeks of pregnancy or if suggestive symptoms are present. Test may be repeated in 2 weeks to determine if there is a rise in antibody titer.
- For cat owners, meticulous handwashing is essential after changing the cat litter. If possible, pregnant women should not change cat litter.

Factors Affecting Laboratory Results

- None known.

NURSING IMPLICATIONS WITH RATIONALE

- Obtain a history of meat ingested that was raw or poorly cooked or of contact with a cat and cat litter. Ask if the cat roams the street or is completely house bound.
- Check if the client is pregnant and has a cat. Ascertain if the pregnant woman handles the cat litter.
- Check if the client has been or ever had been serologically tested for toxoplasmosis. Chronic toxoplasmosis has a low-positive titer.

Client Teaching

- Instruct the client to cook all meat thoroughly. Raw or poorly cooked meat may have the *T. gondii* organism.
- Instruct the pregnant woman not to handle the cat litter. The feces of the cat could be infected with the *T. gondii* organism and if the pregnant woman is infected, the fetus could also be infected. Not all cats are infected with *T. gondii;* however, cats that roam the streets may have acquired the organism.
- Instruct the pregnant woman with an outdoor cat to inform her obstetrician so that a titer level could be taken and monitored.
- Answer client's questions or refer them to appropriate personnel.

Transferrin (serum)

Siderophilin

Reference Values

Adult: 200–430 mg/dl, 2–4.3 g/l (SI units).

Pregnancy (full-term): 300 mg/dl; 3.0 g/l (SI units).

Newborn: 125–275 mg/dl.

Transferrin Saturation: 20–50%.

Description

Transferrin is a β-globulin protein that is formed in the liver. Iron from the diet is absorbed from the intestinal mucosa and is transported by transferrin to the bone marrow for utilization in hemoglobin (hemoglobin synthesis), and to iron-storage sites such as the muscle. When protein malnutrition is present, serum transferrin levels decrease quickly, even faster than serum albumin levels. Another purpose for transferrin is for stimulation of body growth.

The iron saturation of transferrin, called *transferrin saturation,* is calculated by percent using the following formula.

$$\% \text{ of transferrin saturation} = \frac{\text{serum iron level}}{\text{TIBC}} \times 100\%$$

A transferrin saturation of <15% can indicate chronic iron deficiency anemia and other chronic illnesses.

Additional information concerning iron, total iron-binding capacity (TIBC), and transferrin is discussed on pages 268–270.

Purposes

- To detect a serum transferrin deficit.
- To aid in the diagnosis of chronic iron-deficiency anemia and iron overload.

Clinical Problems

Decreased Level: Chronic iron deficiency anemia (% saturation), protein malnutrition, hepatic damage, renal disease, chronic infection or inflammation, cancer, rheumatoid arthritis, proteinuria, hemolytic states, iron overload.

Elevated Level: Severe iron deficiency, pregnancy, polycythemia, acute hepatitis.
Drug Influence: Oral contraceptives.

Procedure

- NPO for 12 hours before the test. Water is permitted.
- Collect 3 to 5 ml of venous blood in a red-top tube. Avoid hemolysis. The blood specimen should be taken in the morning if the transferrin saturation test is to be performed.

Factors Affecting Laboratory Test

- Hemolysis of the blood sample.
- Pregnancy or use of oral contraceptives may increase the serum transferrin level.

NURSING IMPLICATIONS WITH RATIONALE

- Compare serum transferrin level with serum iron level and the TIBC if these tests were ordered. To determine transferrin saturation (%), serum iron and TIBC values are needed.

Client Teaching

- Instruct the client to eat foods rich in protein, such as meats, beans, and fish.
- Answer questions the client may have or refer the questions to other health professionals.

Transthyretin (TTR)

See Prealbumin Antibody Assay

Tricyclic antidepressants (TCA or TAD) serum

Reference Values

Adult

Drug	Therapeutic Range	Peak Time	Toxic Level
Amitriptyline (Elavil)	125–200 ng/ml	2–12 hours	>500 ng/ml
Desipramine (Norpramin)	125–300 ng/ml	4–6 hours	>500 ng/ml
Doxepin (Sinequan)	150–250 ng/ml	2–4 hours	>500 ng/ml
Imipramine (Tofranil)	150–300 ng/ml	1–2 hours (PO) 30 min (IM)	>500 ng/ml
Nortriptyline (Aventyl)	50–150 ng/ml	8 hours	>200 ng/ml
Protriptyline (Vivactil)	70–170 ng/ml	8–12 hours	>200 ng/ml
Amoxapire (Asendin)	200–400 ng/ml	$1^{1}/_{2}$ hours	>500 ng/ml
Maprotiline (Ludiomil)	200–300 ng/ml	12 hours	>500 ng/ml

Description

Tricyclic antidepressants (TCAs) are useful in treating clinical depression and bipolar disorders. Laboratory measurements for TCAs are used to monitor the therapeutic range, to adjust drug dosages, and to detect toxic levels due to overdose (unintentional or intentional). Peak times should be noted when the client is obtaining maximum effects. The average time at which these drugs reach their steady state varies from days to 1 to 2 weeks. The serious toxic effect of these drugs is cardiotoxicity, which includes depressed myocardial contractility, decreased heart rate, and decreased coronary blood flow.

413

Purposes

- To monitor a specific TCA drug for therapeutic effect.
- To check for a specific TCA toxicity.

Clinical Problems

Decreased Level: *Drug Influence:* Barbiturates, alcohol.

Elevated Level: Overdose of TCAs. *Drug Influence:* Steroids, antipsychotics (neuroleptics).

Procedure

- Collect 3 to 5 ml of venous blood in a red-top tube.
- There is no food or fluid restriction.

Factors Affecting Laboratory Results

- Drugs—barbiturates and alcohol can lower the serum TCAs, and steroids and antipsychotics can elevate serum level.

NURSING IMPLICATIONS WITH RATIONALE

- Obtain a history from the client concerning daily drug dosing, having blood samples taken at regular intervals, and keeping doctor's appointments.
- Record and report noncompliance to drug regimen, if appropriate.

Client Teaching

- Instruct the client to follow the prescribed drug dosage. Explain to the client that if prescribed dose is not taken (undosing), therapeutic effects will not be obtained and depressed feelings might remain. Explain that with overdosing, serious cardiotoxicity might result.
- Encourage the client to express feelings about drug regimen. Listen to the client's concern.
- Explain to the client that when the dose is increased, it may take 7 to 10 days for a clinical change because the half-life is long with most of these agents.
- Explain to the client that when discontinuing the medication, the drug dosage should be tapered to avoid extrapyramidal side effects (EPS).

Triglycerides (serum)

Reference Values

Adult: *12 to 29 Years:* 10–140 mg/dl. *30 to 39 Years:* 20–150 mg/dl. *40 to 49 Years:* 30–160 mg/dl. *>50 Years:* 40–190 mg/dl. 0.44–2.09 mmol/l (SI units).

Child: *Infant:* 5–40 mg/dl. *Child:* 5–11 years: 10–135 mg/dl.

Description

Triglycerides, blood lipids formed by esterification of glycerol and three fatty acids, are carried by the serum lipoproteins. The intestine processes the triglycerides from dietary fatty acids (exogenous), and they are transported in the blood stream as chylomicrons (tiny fat droplets covered by protein), which gives the serum a milky or creamy appearance after a meal rich in fats. The liver is also responsible for manufacturing triglycerides, but these do not travel as chylomicrons. The majority of triglycerides are stored as lipids in the adipose tissue. A function of triglycerides is to provide energy to the heart and skeletal muscles.

Triglycerides are a major contributor to arterial diseases and are frequently compared with cholesterol by the lipoprotein electrophoresis. As the concentration of triglycerides increases, so will the very low-density lipoproteins (VLDL) increase, leading to hyperlipoproteinemia. Alcohol intake can cause a transient elevation of serum triglyceride level.

Purposes

- To monitor triglyceride levels.
- To compare test results with lipoprptein groups (VLDL) that indicate hyperlipemia.

Clinical Problems

Decreased Level: Congenital β-lipoproteinemia, hyperthyroidism, hyperparathyroidism, protein malnutrition, exercise. *Drug Influence:* Ascorbic acid, clofibrate (Atromid-S), phenformin, metformin.

Elevated Level: Hyperlipoproteinemia, acute myocardial infarction, hypertension, cerebral thrombosis, hypothyroidism, nephrotic syndrome, arteriosclerosis, Laënnec's or alcoholic cirrhosis, uncontrolled diabetes mellitus, pancreatitis, Down's syndrome, stress, high-carbohydrate diet, pregnancy. *Drug Influence:* Estrogen, oral contraceptives.

Procedure

- Collect 3 to 5 ml of venous blood in a red-top tube.

- The client should be NPO (food, drink, or medications) after 6 PM the night before the test, except for water. Medications should be held until after blood is drawn. The client should be on a normal diet for several days before the test. No alcohol is allowed for 24 hours prior to the test.
- Note on the laboratory slip if the client's weight has increased or decreased in the last 2 weeks.

Factors Affecting Laboratory Results

- A high-carbohydrate diet and alcohol can elevate the serum triglyceride level.

NURSING IMPLICATIONS WITH RATIONALE

Elevated Level

- Relate clinical problems and drugs to increased serum triglyceride levels. When triglycerides and/or cholesterol are elevated, a lipoprotein electrophoresis is frequently ordered.
- Check the serum cholesterol level. At times only one of the body's lipids will be elevated. If the cholesterol level is elevated, suggest which foods should be avoided (see Cholesterol). Consult with the dietetics department.
- Check to determine if a lipoprotein electrophoresis has been ordered. This is frequently done when the triglycerides are elevated.

Client Teaching

- Instruct the client that he or she is not to eat food or to drink anything except water for 12 to 14 hours before the test. Client should avoid alcoholic intake for 24 hours. Medications may be withheld until after the test. Check with the health care provider and laboratory.
- Instruct the client with a high serum triglyceride level to avoid eating excessive amounts of sugars and carbohydrates as well as dietary fats. The client should be encouraged to eat fruit.

Triiodothyronine (T₃) (serum)

T₃ RIA

Reference Values

Adult: 80–200 ng/dl.

Child: *Newborn:* 40–215 ng/dl. *Age 5 to 10 Years:* 95–240 ng/dl. *10 to 15 Years:* 80–210 ng/dl.

Description

Triiodothyronine (T$_3$), one of the thyroid hormones, is present in small amounts in blood and is more short acting and more potent than thyroxine (T$_4$). Both T$_3$ and T$_4$ have similar actions in the body. Serum T$_3$ is secreted in response to thyroid-stimulating hormone (TSH) from the pituitary gland and thyroid-releasing hormone (TRH) from the hypothalamus and is measured directly by radioimmunoassay (RIA).

Serum T$_3$ RIA measures both bound and free T$_3$. It is effective for diagnosing hyperthyroidism, especially T$_3$ thyrotoxicosis, in which T$_3$ is increased and T$_4$ is in normal range. It is not as reliable for diagnosing hypothyroidism, because T$_3$ remains in normal range. T$_3$ RIA and T$_3$ update are two different tests.

Purposes

- To aid in the diagnosis of hyperthyroidism.
- To compare T$_3$ with T$_4$ for determining a thyroid disorder.

Clinical Problems

Decreased Level: Malnutrition, severe acute illness and trauma. *Drug Influence:* Propylthiouracil, methylthiouracil, methimazole (Tapazole), lithium, phenytoin (Dilantin), propranolol (Inderal), reserpine (Serpasil), salicylates (aspirin), steroids, sulfonamides.

Elevated Level: T$_3$ thyrotoxicosis, Hashimoto's thyroiditis, toxic adenoma. *Drug Influence:* Estrogen, progestins, methadone, liothyronine (T$_3$).

Procedure

- Collect 5 to 7 ml of venous blood in a red-top tube. Avoid hemolysis.
- Send the blood sample to the laboratory as soon as possible.
- Drugs that affect laboratory results should be withheld 24 hours with the health care provider's approval. If the drugs are taken prior to the test, they should be listed on the laboratory slip.

Factors Affecting Laboratory Results

- Drugs *(see Drug Influence)*.
- Hemolysis of the blood specimen from rough handling.

NURSING IMPLICATIONS WITH RATIONALE

- List on the laboratory slip any drugs the client is taking that could cause false-negative or false-positive results.

Elevated Level

- Observe for signs and symptoms of hyperthyroidism (i.e., nervousness, tremors, emotional instability, increased appetite, weight loss, palpitations, tachycardia, diarrrhea, decreased fertility, and exophthalmos [protruding eyeballs]).
- Monitor pulse rate. Tachycardia is common and, if severe, could cause heart failure.

Triiodothyronine resin uptake (T_3 RU) (serum)

T_3 Uptake

Reference Values

Adult: 25–35 relative percentage uptake.

Description

Triiodothyronine (T_3) resin uptake is an indirect measure of free thyronine (T_4), whereas serum T_3 RIA is a direct measurement of T_3. This is an in vitro test in which the client's blood is mixed with radioactive T_3 and synthetic resin material in a test tube. The radioactive T_3 will bind at available thyroid-binding globulin (protein) sites. The unbound radioactive T_3 is added to resin for T_3 uptake. In hyperthyroidism there are few binding sites left, so more T_3 is taken up by the resin, thus causing a high T_3 resin uptake. In hypothyroidism there is less T_3 resin uptake.

This test can be performed when clients receive drugs, diagnostic agents (contrast media), and food containing iodine. Usually this test is not affected by inorganic or organic iodine, but it is affected by radioactive iodine, which interferes with the test reagents.

T_3 RU is one of the thyroid tests but should not be the only test used to determine thyroid dysfunction.

Purposes

- To differentiate between hypo- or hyperthyroidism.
- To compare test result with T_3 for determing thyroid disorder.

Clinical Problems

Decreased Level: Hypothyroidism (cretinism, myxedema), pregnancy, menstruation, thyroiditis (Hashimoto's), acute hepatitis. *Drug Influence:* ACTH,* corticosteroids,*

---

*May cause decreased or elevated T_3, uptake levels.

estrogen, oral contraceptives, antithyroid agents (methimazole, propylthiouracil), thiazides, chlordiazepoxide (Librium), sulfonylureas (e.g., tolbutamide [Orinase]).

Elevated Level: Hyperthyroidism, protein malnutrition, malignancies (breast) and metastatic carcinoma, myasthenia gravis, nephrotic syndrome, uremia, threatened abortion. *Drug Influence:* ACTH,* corticosteroids,* anticoagulants (oral), heparin, phenytoin (Dilantin), phenylbutazone (Butazolidin), salicylates (high doses of aspirin compounds), thyroid agents.

Procedure

- Collect 5 to 7 ml of venous blood in a red-top tube. Avoid hemolysis.
- There is no food or fluid restriction.
- Note on the laboratory slip drugs the client is taking that could affect test results.

Factors Affecting Laboratory Results

- Drugs *(see Drug Influence)*.
- Previous administration of radioactive iodine or other radioactive substances could cause inaccurate results.

NURSING IMPLICATIONS WITH RATIONALE

- List on the laboratory slip any drugs the client is taking that could cause a false-negative or false-positive result. Also note any radioactive substance the client has taken.
- Check results of the T_4 test.

Decreased Level

- Observe for signs and symptoms of hypothyroidism (i.e., fatigue, forgetfulness, weight gain, dry skin with poor turgor, dry and thin hair, bradycardia, decreased peripheral circulation, depressed libido, infertility, and constipation).

Elevated Level

- Observe for signs and symptoms of hyperthyroidism (i.e., nervousness, tremors, emotional instability, increased appetite, weight loss, palpitations, tachycardia, diarrhea, decreased fertility, and exophthalmos [protruding eyeballs]).
- Monitor the pulse rate. Tachycardia is common and, if severe, could cause heart failure and cardiac arrest.

---

*May cause decreased or elevated T_3, uptake levels.

Trypsin (stool)

Reference Values

Adult and Child: Positive in small amounts.

Cystic Fibrosis: Negative at dilutions >1:10.

Description

Trypsin is an enzyme produced in the pancreas. Greater amounts of trypsin is found in stools in young children. Bacteria in the gastrointestinal tract destroys much of the trypsin in stool of older children and adults. With pancreatic insufficiency, the stool trypsin test is usually negative. A sample of stool specimens on three separate days should be sent for testing.

Purposes

- To determine if the stool specimen is negative for trypsin.
- To aid in the diagnosis of a pancreatic disorder or cystic fibrosis.

Clinical Problems

Lack of/Decreased Stool Trypsin: Pancreatic insufficiency, advanced cystic fibrosis, malabsorption (children), chronic pancreatitis.

Procedure

- There is no food or fluid restriction.
- Collect a morning stool specimen, every morning for three consecutive days. Have client defecate in the bedpan. Stool collection from infants may be obtained from the diaper. Use a tongue blade and place the stool specimen in a clean, dry container.
- Deliver the container with the stool specimen immediately to the laboratory. The stool should be tested within 2 hours.

Factors Affecting Laboratory Results

- A stool specimen from a constipated stool could produce a false-negative result, which is due to the extended time the stool is in contact with intestinal bacteria.

NURSING IMPLICATIONS WITH RATIONALE

- Collect the stool specimen and place in a covered container. Send the specimen immediately to the laboratory.
- List on the laboratory slip the age of the client and the time the stool specimen

was collected in addition to the client's name, identification number, and room number, and the date.

- Note on the laboratory slip if the stool specimen was from a constipated stool.

Client Teaching
- Explain the stool collection procedure to the client and/or family member. Inform the client that three stool specimens are needed and that a stool specimen will be collected for the next 3 days.
- Instruct the client to have the bowel movement in a bedpan. The bedpan can be placed on a chair, on a bedside commode, or on the toilet seat area. Stool specimens from infants should be obtained from the diaper.
- Instruct the client not to urinate with the bowel movement and to inform you as soon as the stool is available.

Type and crossmatch

See Rh Typing and Crossmatching

Uric acid (serum)

Reference Values

Adult: *Male:* 3.5–8.0 mg/dl. *Female:* 2.8–6.8 mg/dl (normal range may differ slightly among laboratories). *Panic Values:* >12 mg/dl.

Child: 2.5–5.5 mg/dl.

Elderly: 3.5–8.5 mg/dl.

Description

Uric acid is a by-product of purine metabolism. Elevated urine and serum uric acid levels (hyperuricemia) depend on renal function, purine metabolism rate, and dietary intake of purine foods. Excess quantities of uric acid are excreted in the urine. Uric acid can crystallize in the urinary tract in acidic urine; therefore effective renal function and alkaline urine are necessary with hyperuricemia. The commonest problem associated with hyperuricemia is gout. Uric acid levels frequently change from day to day, thus several uric acid levels may be repeated over several days or weeks.

Clients with elevated serum uric acid should avoid foods high in purine.

Purposes

- To monitor serum uric acid during treatment for gout.
- To aid in the diagnosis of health problems *(see Clinical Problems)*.

Clinical Problems

Decreased Level: Wilson's disease, proximal renal tubular acidosis, folic acid deficiency anemia, burn, pregnancy. *Drug Influence:* Allopurinol, azathioprine (Imuran), coumadin, probenecid (Benemid), sulfinpyrazone (Anturane).

Elevated Level: Gout, alcoholism, leukemias (lymphocytic, myelocytic, monocytic), metastatic cancer, multiple myeloma, severe eclampsia, hyperlipoproteinemia, diabetic mellitus (severe), congestive heart failure, glomerulonephritis, renal failure, stress, lead poisoning, x-ray exposure (excessive), strenuous exercise, high-protein weight-reduction diet, hemolytic anemia, lymphoma. *Drug Influence:* Ascorbic acid, diuretics (acetazolamide [Diamox], thiazides [chlorothiazide], furosemide [Lasix]), levodopa, methyldopa (Aldomet), 6-mercaptopurine, phenothiazines, salicylates (prolonged use), theophylline.

Procedure

- Collect 3 to 5 ml of venous blood in a red-top tube. Avoid hemloysis.
- There is no food or drink restriction; however, in many cases, high-purine foods, such as meats (liver, kidney, brain, heart, and sweetbreads), scallops, and sardines, are restricted for 24 hours before the test.
- List drugs the client is taking that could affect test results on the laboratory slip.

Factors Affecting Laboratory Results

- Excessive stress and fasting could cause an elevated serum uric acid level.
- Foods high in purine *(see Nursing Implications)*.
- Drugs *(see Drug Influence)*.

NURSING IMPLICATIONS WITH RATIONALE

- Check with the health care provider and/or laboratory to determine whether foods high in purine should be restricted.

Elevated Level

- Recognize clinical problems and drugs related to hyperuricemia. Gout is a problem commonly associated with a high serum uric acid.
- Request the dietitian to visit the client to discuss food preference and to plan a low-purine diet.

- Observe for signs and symptoms of gout (i.e., tophi of the ear lobe and joints, joint pain, and edema in the "big" toe). An elevated uric acid level leads to urate deposits in the tissues and in the synovial fluid of joints.
- Monitor the pH of the urine and the amount of the urinary output. The urine pH should be kept alkaline to prevent the formation of uric acid stones in the kidney. A decreased urine output (<600 ml/24 h) with an elevated serum uric acid could indicate kidney disease.
- Check serum urea and serum creatinine levels if the serum uric acid level is elevated and the urinary output is decreased. If the serum urea, creatinine, and uric acid are elevated and the urine output is decreased, kidney dysfunction should definitely be suspected. It could be secondary to another clinical problem.

Client Teaching

- Instruct the client to avoid eating foods that have moderate or high amounts of purines. Examples are as follows.

High (100–1000 mg Purine Nitrogen/100 g Food)	Moderate (9–100 mg Purine Nitrogen/100 g Food)
Brains	Meat
Heart	Poultry
Kidney	Fish
Liver	Shellfish
Sweetbreads	Asparagus
Roe	Beans
Sardines	Mushrooms
Scallops	Peas
Mackerel	Spinach
Anchovies	
Broth	
Consommé	
Mincemeat	

- Instruct the client to decrease alcoholic intake. Ethanol causes renal retention of urate.

Uric acid (urine—24 hour)

Reference Values

Adult: 250–500 mg/24 h (low-purine diet), 250–750 mg/24 h (normal diet).
Child: Similar to adult.

Description

(See Uric Acid [Serum])

Uric acid is the end-product of purine metabolism, which takes place in the bone marrow, muscles, and liver. Excess quantities of uric acid are secreted in the urine, unless there is renal dysfunction caused by obstruction of renal flow.

The main purpose of this 24-hour urine test is to detect and/or to confirm the diagnoses of gout or kidney disease.

Purpose

See Uric Acid (Serum).

Clinical Problems

Decreased Level: Renal diseases (chronic glomerulonephritis, urinary obstruction, uremia), eclampsia (toxemia of pregnancy), lead toxicity. *Drug Influence:* Allopurinol, acetazolamide (Diamox), salicylates (prolonged low doses), triamterene.

Elevated Level: Gout, high-purine diet, leukemias (lymphocytic, myelocytic), polycythemia vera, Fanconi's syndrome, neurologic disorders (cerebral hemorrhage, cerebral thrombosis, brain infarction, cerebral embolism, encephalomyelitis), psychiatric disorders (manic-depressive disease, paranoid states, depressive neurosis), ulcerative colitis, viral hepatitis, x-ray therapy, febrile illnesses. *Drug Influence:* Bishydroxycoumarin, corticosteroids, cytotoxic agents (treatment for cancer), probenecid (Benemid), salicylates (high doses).

Procedure

- Collect a 24-hour sample in a large container and refrigerate. A preservative in the container may be necessary. Check with the laboratory on the need for preservative.
- Label the container with the client's name and the dates and times of urine collection (e.g., 9/23/03, 7:11 AM to 9/24/03, 7:11 AM).
- A diet low or high in purines may be ordered before and/or during the time of urine collection.
- There is no drink restriction.

Factors Affecting Laboratory Results

- Drugs *(see Drug Influence above)*.
- A high- or low-purine diet.
- Excessive x-ray exposure.
- Febrile illnesses.

NURSING IMPLICATIONS WITH RATIONALE

- Monitor urinary output. Poor urine output could indicate inadequate fluid intake or poor kidney function.
- Compare the serum uric acid level with the urine uric acid level. An elevated serum uric acid level (hyperuricemia) and a decreased urine uric acid level can indicate kidney dysfunction. Increased serum and urine uric acid levels are frequently seen in gout, so it is important to obtain both the urine and serum values.
- Check the urine pH, especially if hyperuremia is present. Uric stones can occur when the urine pH is low (acidic). Alkaline urine helps to prevent stones in the urinary tract.

Client Teaching

- Explain to the client the purpose of and procedure for the test. Explain to the client and family that all urine should be saved for 24 hours. Tell the client not to put feces or toilet paper in the urine.
- Instruct the client as to which foods to avoid before and during the test, as ordered by the health care provider.

Urinalysis (routine)

Color, Appearance, Odor, pH, Specific Gravity, Protein, Glucose, Ketones, Blood, Nitrate, and Leukocyte Esterase (WBC)

Reference Values

	Adult	Newborn	Child
Color	Light straw to dark amber		Light straw to dark yellow
Appearance	Clear	Clear	Clear
Odor	Aromatic		Aromatic
pH	4.5–8.0 Average is 6	5–7	4.5–8
Specific gravity (SG)	1.005–1.030 (1.015–1.024, normal fluid intake)	1.001–1.020	1.005–1.030
Protein	(2–8 mg/dl negative reagent strip test)		
Glucose	Negative		Negative
Ketones	Negative		Negative

(continued)

	Adult	Newborn	Child
Blood	Negative		Negative
Microscopic examination			
RBC	1–2 per low power field		Rare
WBC	3–4		0–4
Casts	Occasional hyaline		Rare

Description

Urinalysis is a physical, chemical, and microscopic analysis of the urine. Routine urine tests were performed as early as 1821. Until recently urine was manually tested for individual constituents, but now multiple-reagent strips are used for quick chemical screening.

Urinalysis is useful for diagnosing renal disease or urinary tract infection and for detecting metabolic disease not related to the kidneys. Many routine urinalyses are done in the health care provider's office as well as in the hospital or in a private laboratory. The color, appearance, and odor of the urine are examined, and the pH, protein, glucose ketones, and bilirubin are tested with the reagent strips. Specific gravity is measured with a urinometer, and a microscopic examination of the urinary sediment is performed to detect red and white blood cells (RBCs, WBCs), casts, crystals, and bacteria.

Purposes

- To detect normal versus abnormal urine components.
- To detect glycosuria.
- To aid in the diagnosis of a renal disorder.

Clinical Problems

Property or Constituent	Clinical Conditions/ Problems	Comments
Color		
Colorless (very pale)	Large fluid intake Diabetes insipidus Chronic kidney disease Alcohol ingestion Nervousness	A pale color usually indicates diluted urine, and dark yellow or amber indicates concentrated urine.
Red or red-brown	Hemoglobinuria Porphyrins Menstrual contamination Drug influence Sulfisoxazole with phenazopyridine (Azogantrisin)	Drugs and foods will change the color of the urine.

Property or Constituent	Clinical Conditions/ Problems	Comments
Red or red-brown	Phenytoin (Dilantin)	
	Cascara	
	Chlorpromazine (Thorazine)	
	Docusate Ca (Doxidan)	
	Phenolphthalein (Ex-Lax)	
	Foods	
	Beets	
	Rhubarb	
	Food color	
Orange	Restricted fluid intake	
	Concentrated urine	
	Excess sweating	
	Fever	
	Drug influence	
	Amidopyrine	
	Furazolidone (Furoxone)	
	Nitrofurantoin	
	Phenazopyridine	
	(Pyridium)	
	Sulfonamides	
	Foods and others	
	Carrots (carotene)	
	Rhubarb	
	Food color	
	Bilirubin	
Blue or green	*Pseudomonas* toxemia	
	Drug influence	
	Amitriptyline (Elavil)	
	Methylene blue	
	Methocarbamol (Robaxin)	
	Vitamin B complex	
	Yeast concentrate	
Brown or black	Lysol poisoning	
	Melanin	
	Bilirubin	
	Methemoglobin	
	Porphyrin	
	Drug influence	
	Cascara	
	Chloroquine (Aralen)	
	Iron injectable	
	compounds	
Appearance		
Hazy, cloudy	Bacteria	
	Pus, tissue	
	RBCs	
	WBCs	
	Phosphates	
	Prostatic fluid	

(*continued*)

Property or Constituent	Clinical Conditions/ Problems	Comments
Appearance		
Hazy, cloudy	Spermatozoa	
	Urates, uric acid	
Milky	Fat	
	Pyuria	
Odor		
Ammonia	Urea breakdown by bacteria	
Foul or putrid	Bacteria (UTI)	
Mousey	Phenylketonuria	
Sweet or fruity	Diabetic acidosis (ketoacidosis)	
	Starvation	
Foam		
Yellow—large amounts	Severe cirrhosis of the liver	
	Bilirubin or bile pigment	
pH		
<4.5	Metabolic acidosis	
	Respiratory acidosis	
	Starvation	
	Diarrhea	
	Diet high in meat protein and/ or cranberries	
	Drug influence	
	Ammonium chloride	
	Methenamine mandelate (mandelic acid)	
>8.0	Bacteriuria	
	Urinary tract infection due to *Pseudomonas* or *Proteus*	
	Drug influence	
	Antibiotics	
	Kanamycin	
	Neomycin	
	Streptomycin	
	Sulfonamides	
	Excess salicylates (aspirin)	
	Sodium bicarbonate	
	Acetazolamide (Diamox)	
	Potassium citrate	
	Diet	
	High in citrus fruits	
	High in vegetables	
Specific gravity (SG)		
<1.005	Diabetes insipidus	Low, fixed SG can indicate kidney disease because of inability to concentrate urine.
	Excess fluid intake	
	Overhydration	
	Renal disease	
	Glomerulonephritis	
	Pyelonephritis	
	Polycystic disease	
	Severe potassium deficit	

Property or Constituent	Clinical Conditions/ Problems	Comments
Specific gravity (SG)		
>1.026	Decreased fluid intake	
	Fever	
	Administration of IV dextran, albumin	
	Diabetes mellitus	
	Vomiting, diarrhea	
	Dehydration	
	X-ray contrast media	
Protein		
>8 mg/dl or >80 mg/24 h	Proteinuria	Proteinuria is a sensitive indicator of kidney dysfunction.
	Mild, transitory	
	Protein	
	Exercise	
	Severe stress	
	Cold baths	
	Fever	
	Acute infectious diseases	
	Renal disease	
	Glomerulonephritis	
	Nephrotic syndrome	
	Polycystic kidney	
	Lupus erythematosus	
	Leukemia	
	Multiple myeloma	
	Cardiac disease	
	Toxemia of pregnancy	
	Septicemia	
	Materials	
	Arsenic	
	Mercury	
	Lead	
	Carbon tetrachloride	
	Drug influence	
	Barbiturates	
	Neomycin	
	Massive doses of penicillin	
	Sulfonamides	
<2 mg/dl	Very diluted urine	
Glucose		
>15 mg/dl (random) or +4	Diabetes mellitus	The renal threshold for blood glucose is 160–180 mg/dl.
	CNS disorders	
	Stroke (CVA)	
	Meningitis	Tes-tape should be used in place of Clinitest when the client is receiving drugs.
	Cushing's syndrome	
	Anesthesia	
	Glucose infusions	
	Severe stress	
	Infections	

(continued)

Property or Constituent	Clinical Conditions/ Problems	Comments
Glucose		
>15 mg/dl (random) or +4	Drug influence (false-positive results) Ascorbic acid Aspirin Cephalothin (Keflin) Streptomycin Epinephrine	
Ketones Positive +1 to +3	*See Ketone Bodies, Acetone* Ketoacidosis Starvation A diet high in protein and low in carbohydrates	Acetest or Ketostix should be tested when Clinitest or Tes-tape is tested.
Microscopic Examination of Urinary Sediment		
RBCs: RBCs and RBC casts		
>2 per low power field	Trauma to the kidney Renal disease Pyelonephritis Glomerulonephritis Hydronephrosis Renal calculi Cystitis Lupus nephritis (collagen disease) Aspirins (excess) Anticoagulants Sulfonamides Menstrual contamination	
WBCs: WBC and WBC casts >4 per low power field	Urinary tract infection Fever Strenuous exercise Lupus nephritis Renal diseases	If WBC are present in the urine, a urine culture should be done.
Casts:	Fever Renal disease Heart failure	

Procedure

- Collect a freshly voided urine specimen, approximately 50 ml or more, in a clean, dry container and take it to the laboratory within 30 minutes. An early morning urine specimen collected before breakfast is preferred. The urine specimen could be refrigerated for 6 to 8 hours.
- A clean-caught or midstream urine specimen could be requested if WBCs are in the urine or if bacteria are suspected.

- There is no food or fluid restriction unless the urinalysis is to be done in the early morning.

Factors Affecting Laboratory Results

- A urine specimen that has been sitting for an hour or longer without refrigeration.
- Drugs and foods *(see Clinical Problems)*.
- Feces or toilet paper in the urine.

NURSING IMPLICATIONS WITH RATIONALE

- Assist the client with the urine collection as needed.
- Obtain a history of any drugs the client is currently taking. Such drugs as cascara, Azo gantrisin, nitrofurantoin, Thorazine, sulfonamides, Elavil, Ex-Lax, Pyridium, and others cause a discoloration of the urine. These should be noted on the laboratory slip.
- Assess the fluid status of the client. Urine should be concentrated if the urine specimen is obtained in the morning or if the client has a decreased fluid intake or is dehydrated. An increase in fluid intake will dilute the urine contents.
- Obtain a history of an excess amount of a certain food (e.g., carrots, rhubarb, beets) that can cause a change in the urine color or of foods (e.g., excess amounts of meat, cranberry juice) that could lower the urine pH (acidic).

Client Teaching

- Explain to the client the procedure for collecting the urine. Inform the hospitalized client that an early morning urine specimen taken before breakfast is needed. Instruct the client that approximately one third or one half of a small container of urine is needed. Have the client void in a clean, dry container or a clean urinal or bedpan that can be poured into the container. Inform the client not to put feces or toilet paper in the urine. The urine specimen should be taken to the laboratory within 30 minutes or refrigerated.
- Instruct the client at home to place the fresh morning urine specimen in the refrigerator. The urine specimen, however, should be taken to the laboratory within an hour. Urine is an excellent medium for the growth of bacteria, and the bacterial growth begins approximately one-half hour after collection. Refrigeration may help to retard growth for a short period of time.
- Explain to the client the procedure for a clean-catch or midstream urine collection *(see Cultures)*. This procedure may be requested when culture of the urine is needed as well as for urinalysis.

Urobilinogen (urine)

Reference Values

Adult: *Random:* Negative or <1.0 Ehrlich units. *2-Hour Specimen:* 0.3–1.0 Ehrlich units. *24-Hour Specimen:* 0.5–4.0 mg/24 h, 0.5–4.0 Ehrlich units/24 h, 0.09–4.23 μmol/24 h (SI units).

Child: Similar to adult.

Description

Bile, which is formed mostly from conjugated bilirubin, reaches the duodenum, where the intestinal bacteria change the bilirubin to urobilinogen. Most of the urobilinogen is lost in the feces; a large amount goes back to the liver through the blood stream, where it is reprocessed to bile; and approximately 1% is excreted by the kidneys in the urine.

The urobilinogen test is one of the most sensitive tests for determining liver damage, hemolytic disease, and severe infections. In early hepatitis, mild liver cell damage, or mild toxic injury, the urine urobilinogen level will increase despite an unchanged serum bilirubin level. The urobilinogen level will frequently decrease with severe liver damage, because less bile will be produced. The urobilinogen test might be performed with the urinalysis.

Purpose

■ To aid in determining liver damage.

Clinical Problems

Decreased Level: Biliary obstruction, severe liver disease, cancer of the pancreas, severe inflammatory disease, cholelithiasis, severe diarrhea. *Drug Influence:* Antibiotics (decreasing gut bacteria), ammonium chloride, ascorbic acid (Vitamin C).

Elevated Level: Infectious hepatitis, toxic hepatitis, cirrhosis of the liver (early and recovery stages), hemolytic anemia, pernicious anemia, erythroblastosis fetalis, sickle cell anemia, infectious mononucleosis. *Drug Influence:* Sulfonamides, phenothiazines, acetazolamide (Diamox), cascara, phenazopyridine (Pyridium), methenamine mandelate (Mandelamine), procaine, sodium bicarbonate.

Procedure

■ There is no food or fluid restriction.

Single Specimen

■ The single urine specimen should be fresh and should be tested immediately.

This may be done as part of the routine urinalysis. A reagent color dipstick is dipped in the urine and is compared with a color chart, in Ehrlich units.

2-Hour Urine Specimen

■ Collect 2-hour specimen between 1 and 3 PM or between 2 and 4 PM, because urobilinogen peaks in the afternoon. Urine should be kept refrigerated or in a dark container. Urine should be tested within one-half hour, because urine urobilinogen oxidizes to urobilin (orange substance).
■ Label the container and laboratory slip with the exact time the urine was collected.

24-Hour Urine Specimen

■ Discard the first urine specimen and then start urine collection.
■ Collect 24-hour urine specimen, place in a large container, and keep refrigerated. A preservative may be added to the container. Keep urine collection from the light.
■ Label the container with the client's name, the date, and the time of urine collection.
■ Withhold client's medications that affect test results for 24 hours or until after the test, with the health care provider's permission. If drugs are given, list the drugs on the laboratory slip.

Factors Affecting Laboratory Results

■ Antibiotics decrease the bacterial flora in the intestine.
■ Certain drugs increase the urine urobilinogen level *(see Drug Influence).*
■ pH changes (strongly acidic urine) could cause a decreased urobilinogen level, and strongly alkaline urine could cause an elevated level. Urine sitting for $1/2$ hour or longer may become alkaline.
■ The urobilinogen level is highest in the afternoon and evening. The 2-hour urine specimen is frequently collected in the afternoon.

NURSING IMPLICATIONS WITH RATIONALE

■ Explain to the client the procedure for collecting a 2-hour urine specimen or a 24-hour urine specimen. The bladder should be emptied before starting the 2-hour or 24-hour urine test. Inform the client that all urine must be saved during the specified time.
■ Keep the collected urine from light in a urine container with a preservative. Refrigerate.
■ Label the container and laboratory slip with the exact times urine collection begins and ends (after the last voiding).

Decreased Level

- Relate clinical problems and drugs to decreased urine urobilinogen. Most antibiotics will reduce the bacterial flora in the intestines, thus decreasing the formation of urobilinogen.

Elevated Level

- Check for an elevated urobilinogen level in freshly voided urine with a reagent color dipstick. Record the results of the single test. Note if the client is receiving drugs that could elevate the urobilinogen level.
- Assess for signs and symptoms of jaundice (yellow sclera, skin on the forearm is yellow).

Vancomycin (serum)

Reference Values

Therapeutic Range: *Peak:* 20–40 μg/ml. *Trough:* 5–10 μg/ml.
Toxic Level: >40 μg/ml.

Description

Vancomycin is a potent antibiotic that is prescribed to treat serious gram-positive organisms by inhibiting cell-wall synthesis of the bacteria, thus causing its death. It may be ordered when the bacterium does not respond to penicillins or cephalosporins. Oral vancomycin is poorly absorbed; however, it may be ordered for treating some gastrointestinal infections such as that caused by *Clostridium difficile.* Intravenous vancomycin is the form most likely prescribed. Like aminoglycosides, vancomycin may cause ototoxicity and nephrotoxicity. Peak and trough levels should be closely monitored. The half-life for vancomycin in adults is 4 to 8 hours. In renal insufficiency the half-life can be 4 to 8 days.

Purposes

- To monitor the vancomycin level.
- To check for vancomycin toxicity.

Clinical Problems

Uses: Methicillin-resistant *Staphylococcus aureus,* serious gram-positive organisms, staphylococcal septicemia in cancer.

Procedure

- There is no food or fluid restriction.
- Collect 3 to 5 ml of venous blood in a red-top tube. For peak level, draw a blood sample 30 minutes after administering intravenous vancomycin. For trough level, draw a blood sample prior to administering the next dose of IV vancomycin. Send blood samples immediately to the laboratory.

Factors Affecting Laboratory Results

- Inadequate renal function affects the peak and trough levels. The drug dose needs to be adjusted according to renal function.

NURSING IMPLICATIONS WITH RATIONALE

- Assess renal function. Urine output should be at least 600 ml/day. Vancomycin dose should be adjusted if renal function is inadequate. This drug may cause nephrotoxicity.
- Check hearing. High doses of vancomycin could damage the eighth cranial nerve. This drug may cause ototoxicity.
- Monitor intravenous flow rate for vancomycin. Rapid infusion could cause "red-man's syndrome." The skin becomes red (erythematous) and flushed. Itching may also occur.

Client Teaching

- Inform the client who is ambulatory to save urine so that it can be measured.
- Explain to the client that blood samples will be taken periodically 30 minutes after the drug has been infused and prior to the next drug dose.

Vanillylmandelic acid (VMA) (urine)

Reference Values

Adult: 1.5–7.5 mg/24 h, 7.6–37.9 μ/24 h (SI units).

Child: Adolescent: 1–5 mg/24 h.

Description

Vanillylmandelic (VMA) is the major by-product of catecholamines (epinephrine and norepinephrine). An elevated level of VMA excretion might indicate severe hypertension or tumors of the adrenal medulla (pheochromocytoma in the adult and neuroblastoma and ganglioneuroblastoma in the child). Other methods should be used to verify positive VMA results, such as urine catecholamine.

The VMA test is a simple screening method. However, many foods (bananas, tea, coffee, chocolate, carbonated drinks, etc.) and drugs (aspirin, sulfonamides, some cough medicines, and others) produce false-positive results.

Purpose

- To screen for pheochromocytoma and other health problems, *see Clinical Problems.*

Clinical Problems

Decreased Level: Uremia. *Drug Influence:* clofibrate, antihypertensives (guanethidine [Ismelin], methyldopa [Aldomet], reserpine [Serpasil]), monamine (MAO) inhibitors.

Elevated Level: Pheochromocytoma, neuroblastoma, ganglioblastoma, myasthenia gravis, muscular dystrophy (progressive), physical and mental stress. *Foods:* Fruits (banana), fruit juices, chocolate, tea, coffee, carbonated drinks (except ginger ale), vanilla and vanilla products, candy, mints, jelly, cheese, gelatins, and cough drops. *Drug Influence:* Salicylates (aspirin), sulfonamides, penicillin, chlorpromazine (Thorazine), isoproterenol (Isuprel), levodopa, lithium carbonate, nitroglycerin, glyceryl guaicolate, methenamine (Mandelamine), methocarbamol (Robaxin).

Procedure

- No drugs should be taken for 3 days before the test, *if possible,* especially those listed under *Drug Influence.*
- Insert 10 ml of concentrated hydrochloric acid (HCl) into a large bottle. Some laboratories do not require that a preservative be added to the bottle.
- Label the bottle and laboratory slip with the client's name, dates, and times the urine collection started and ended. Keep the bottle refrigerated during the 24-hour collection time.
- Those foods listed under *Clinical Problems* above should be omitted from the diet for 3 days before the test. Other foods and fluid are not restricted.

Factors Affecting Laboratory Results

- Drugs *(see Drug Influence).*
- Food *(see Clinical Problems).*
- Strenuous exercise will elevate VMA levels.
- Stress will elevate VMA levels.

NURSING IMPLICATIONS WITH RATIONALE

- Monitor vital signs, especially blood pressure. Maintain a blood pressure chart.

Client Teaching

- Explain to the client and family that all urine excreted over the 24-hour period must be saved and kept refrigerated. Inform the client not to put toilet paper or feces in the urine.
- Instruct the client not to eat the foods listed under *Clinical Problems* above for 3 days before the test. Write the restricted foods on a piece of paper for the client's reference.
- Explain to the client that he or she should eat well-balanced meals. Starvation or severe lack of food could increase the VMA levels.
- Encourage the client to avoid emotional stress and physical activity. Stress and activity increase VMA levels. Encourage the client to rest during the test.

VDRL *(venereal disease research laboratory) (serum)*

VDRL Screening Test

Reference Values

Adult: Nonreactive.

Child: Nonreactive.

Description

Syphilis, a venereal disease caused by the spirochete *Treponema pallidum,* is usually transmitted through sexual contact. There are stages of syphilis (primary, secondary, and tertiary) that, left untreated, could lead to death.

Primary Stage: *Duration After Contact:* 3 to 6 weeks. A chancre develops approximately 3 weeks after contact. Spirochetes in the exudate of the chancre lesion (sore) may be visualized with dark-field microscopy. Chancres are generally found in genital areas and in the mouth or on the lips.

Secondary Stage: *Duration After Contact:* 2 weeks to 6 months. Secondary lesions are highly contagious and at times may be visualized on dark-field microscopy. The lesions are usually red papular or "snail track" ulcers and may be seen anywhere on the body, especially in the palms of the hands and the soles of the feet. A relapse may occur in 2 to 4 years; this is called latent syphilis. The client may have a low fever.

Tertiary Stage: *Duration After Contact:* 4 to 20 years. This is referred to as late syphilis. Untreated syphilis (tertiary stage) normally does not have clinical signs;

however, it does affect the person's cardiovascular system and central nervous system. The person may develop cardiac valvular disease, aneurysms, general paresis, blindness, slurred speech, delusions, and "insanity."

Two groups of blood tests are used to identify the spirochete *T. palladum:* the nontreponemal antibody test (VDRL and rapid plasma reagin, RPR) and the fluorescent treponemal antibody absorption test (FTA-ABS, TPI).

The VDRL test is useful for detecting primary syphilis 1 to 3 weeks after the presence of a primary lesion, and for detecting secondary syphilis.

T. pallidum stimulates the development of nonspecific reaginic antibodies in the serum. If these antibodies are present and react with a lipid antigen (cardiolipin), the VDRL test is positive or reactive. A titer about 1:32 can indicate the secondary stage. With tertiary stage syphilis, the VDRL test is not sensitive and may fail to react or may produce variable titers.

The results of the VDRL test may be negative in the early infectious phase of syphilis or could produce biologic false positives (BFP) because of other acute or chronic diseases. If the VDRL test is negative, weekly VDRL tests may be indicated. The RPR test may be used first as a screening test for syphilis.

Purposes

- To detect the presence of *T. pallidum.*
- To screen for primary syphilis 1 to 3 weeks after the appearance of a primary lesion.

Clinical Problems

Nonreactive (negative): *False Negatives:* Early primary stage of syphilis, tertiary stage of syphilis.

Reactive (positive): Syphilis—*T. pallidum* organism. *False Positives (return to nonreactive within 6 months):* Tuberculosis, pneumonia, infectious mononucleosis, chicken pox, smallpox vaccination (recent), subacute bacterial endocarditis, leprosy. *False Positives (chronic; persist longer than 6 months):* Malaria, Hashimoto's thyroiditis, rheumatoid arthritis, progressive systemic sclerosis, systemic lupus erythematosus, hepatitis.

Procedure

- Collect 3 to 5 ml of venous blood in a red-top tube. Avoid hemolysis.
- There is no food or fluid restriction; however, some laboratories require that the client refrain from eating and drinking, so check with the laboratory. Alcohol should not be consumed for 24 hours before the VDRL test.

Factors Affecting Laboratory Results

- Hemolysis of the blood sample could affect test result.
- Alcoholic intake decreases the test reaction.

NURSING IMPLICATIONS WITH RATIONALE

- Instruct the client not to drink alcohol for 24 hours prior to the test. If the client has consumed alcohol, the test may be postponed for 24 hours.
- Obtain a history of any acute or chronic disease. Related BFP may occur with certain diseases (*see Clinical Problems*).
- List present acute and/or chronic diseases in the client's chart and on the laboratory slip and notify the health care provider.
- Interpretation of tests for syphilis requires skill and experience.

Nonreactive (negative)

- Relate a nonreactive VDRL test result to false-negative causes if the history and symptoms are suggestive of syphilis. Test should be repeated weekly for several weeks. Nonreactive (negative) results can occur in the early primary stage of syphilis.

Reactive (positive)

- Relate a reactive VDRL test result to a positive indication of syphilis or a possible false positive due to acute or chronic diseases (*see Clinical Problems*). If the history is suggestive of syphilis but an acute or chronic disease is present, the FTA-ABS or TPI test may be performed.
- Check with the client about receiving treatment for syphilis. If primary syphilis persists for weeks before treatment, the VDRL test could remain positive for up to 6 months after treatment. The test results after treatment for secondary syphilis could remain positive for 12 to 18 months. The history of treatment (where, when, how long, and what drugs) is extremely important. The health department should be notified when there is a positive test result.
- Be supportive of the client. Be willing to listen, and do not make a judgment concerning the client's life-style.
- Elicit from the client his or her sexual contacts so that they can be properly tested and treated. Explain the importance of preventing the transmission of the disease.
- Refer the client to a veneral disease clinic if one is available (with the health care provider's permission). Many clinics have case workers and a good follow-up care program.
- Emphasize the importance of follow-up care. Frequently clients are checked every 3 months for 2 years as a preventive measure for detecting a relapse (syphilis).
- Observe for signs and symptoms of tertiary (late) syphilis (*see Description*). These signs and symptoms should be documented and reported. The VDRL test is usually negative with tertiary syphilis.

Viral culture (blood, biopsy, cerebrospinal fluid, pharynx, rectum, sputum, stool, urine)

Reference Value

Negative culture result.

Description

The virus culture is performed to confirm a suspected viral infection. A blood sample, sputum, and pharyneal swab are the most common specimens obtain for identifying a virus. The specimen is placed on a special viral culture media of growing cells; it will not grow on nonliving media.

Purpose

- To identify a viral infection.

Clinical Problems

Positive: Pneumonia (viral), meningitis (viral), rhinovirus, sinusitus, conjunctivitis, shingles, varicella-zoster virus, herpes simplex, enteroviruses, influenza, cytomegalovirus (CMV).

Procedure

- No food or fluid restriction is required.
- Collect 5 ml of venous blood in a green-top tube. Tube should be chilled. A repeated test is suggested in 14 to 28 days as a convalescent specimen.
- A culturette swab may be used to obtain a specimen from the conjunctiva, lesion, throat, and rectum. The swab should be placed in a chilled viral transport media.
- Obtain 5 ml of cerebrospinal fluid and place in a chilled sterile vial.
- Obtain a midstream, clean caught urine specimen in a sterile container.
- Deliver the specimen immediately to the laboratory.

NURSING IMPLICATIONS WITH RATIONALE

- Obtain a history regarding the possibility of a viral infection. Note the severity of the infection.
- Record symptoms that the client is having in relation to the suspected virus.

Client Teaching

- Explain the procedure for collecting the specimen to the client.

- Inform the client that a second blood sample may be needed in 2 to 4 weeks. Check with the health care provider.
- Listen to the client's concerns.

Vitamin A (serum)

Retinol

Reference Value

Adult: 30–95 μg/dl, 1.05–3.0 μmol/l (SI units), 125–150 IU/dl.

Child: *1 to 6 Years:* 20–43 μg/dl, 0.7–1.5 μmol/l (SI units). *7 to 12 Years:* 26–50 μg/dl, 0.91–1.75 μmol/l (SI units). *13 to 19 Years:* 26–72 μg/dl, 0.91–2.5 μmol/l (SI units).

Description

Vitamin A is a fat-soluble vitamin that is absorbed from the intestine in the presence of lipase and bile. Vitamin A moves to the liver and is stored there as retinyl ester and in the body as retinol. It binds to the serum protein prealbumin.

The functions of Vitamin A include mucous membrane epithelial cell integrity of the eyes, cornea, and the respiratory, gastrointestinal, and genito-urinary tracts; and skin integrity. Vitamin A has played a major role for years in treating acne; however, high doses of Vitamin A can be toxic because it is a fat-soluble vitamin and accumulates in the body tissues. To determine if toxicity is present, a plasma retinyl ester level is obtained. During pregnancy, high doses of Vitamin A may have a teratogenic effect on the fetus. Sufficient intake of Vitamin A maintains cellular integrity, body growth, and night vision.

Purposes

- To detect a Vitamin A deficit.
- To check for Vitamin A toxicity.

Clinical Problems

Decreased Level: Night-blindness; liver, intestinal, or pancreatic diseases; chronic infections; carcinoid syndrome; cystic fibrosis; protein malnutrition; malabsorption; celiac disease. *Drug Influence:* Mineral oil, neomycin, cholestyramine.

Elevated Level: Hypervitaminosis, chronic kidney disease. *Drug Influence:* Glucocorticoids, oral contraceptives.

441

Procedure

- NPO for 8 to 12 hours before the test except for water.
- Collect 5 to 7 ml of venous blood in a red-top tube. Avoid hemolysis and protect the specimen from light. The blood specimen may be placed in a paper bag.

Factors Affecting Laboratory Results

- Selected drugs that can decrease or increase serum level.
- Hemolysis and prolonged exposure of the blood specimen to light.

NURSING IMPLICATIONS WITH RATIONALE

- Explain to the client that food and fluid, except for water, should be avoided until after the test.
- Obtain a history of the client's nutrient intake and supplementary vitamin intake. Note if the client avoids foods that are rich in Vitamin A, such as green leafy and yellow vegetables; yellow fruits such as apricots, canteloupe; eggs, whole milk, liver. Individuals with a well-balanced dietary intake normally do not need vitamin supplements.

Decreased Level—Client Teaching

- Encourage the client to eat foods rich in Vitamin A.
- Inform the client that vitamin supplements can be helpful in preventing vitamin deficiency. The client may wish to contact the health care provider concerning vitamin supplements.

Elevated Level—Client Teaching

- Instruct the client that megadoses of Vitamin A for treating acne can be toxic. Self-treating with Vitamin A may be harmful because it is a fat-soluble vitamin and can have a cumulative effect. The health care provider should be contacted before taking megadoses of Vitamin A.
- Instruct pregnant women that vitamins are usually prescribed during pregnancy; however, megadoses of Vitamin A should be avoided because it may cause a birth defect in the newborn.

Vitamin B₁ (serum and urine)

Thiamine

Reference Values

Serum: 10–60 ng/ml; 5.3–8.0 µg/dl.

Urine: 100–200 µg/24 h.

Description

Vitamin B₁ is a water-soluble vitamin that is absorbed (effectively with the aid of folic acid) in the duodenum and is excreted in the urine. The functions of Vitamin B₁ include the metabolism of carbohydrates, proteins, and fats, and maintaining nerve impulses. Thiamine is one of the B complex vitamins that is given to treat peripheral neuritis caused from alcoholism or beriberi. There are three types of beriberi: (1) wet beriberi, in which the myocardium dilates and becomes flabby, causing heart failure; (2) dry beriberi, characterized by nerve damage, causing peripheral neuritis and atrophy of muscles; and (3) cerebral beriberi (Wernicke-Korsakoff syndrome), which frequently occurs in chronic alcoholics and is characterized by ocular neuropathy and ataxia.

Foods rich in Vitamin B₁ include enriched breads and cereals, yeast, fish, pork, liver, and milk. Asian clients whose diet consists of rice may develop a Vitamin B₁ deficiency. Impaired absorption or utilization of Vitamin B₁ due to intestinal or liver disease contributes to the Vitamin B₁ deficiency.

Purpose

- To detect a Vitamin B₁ deficit.

Clinical Problems

Decreased Level: Chronic alcoholism, beriberi, chronic diarrhea, pregnancy, severe liver disease, malabsorption. *Drug Influence:* Excessive and prolonged use of diuretics.

Procedure

Serum

- NPO for 8 to 12 hours except for water prior to the test.
- Collect 3 to 5 ml of venous blood in a red-top tube (serum) or green-top tube (plasma). Place blood specimen in a paper bag to protect the specimen from light.

Urine

- Discard the first urine specimen.
- Collect a 24-hour urine specimen in a large container (preferably a dark container to avoid light exposure), and keep the container refrigerated.
- Label the container with the client's name, the date, and the exact time of collection, such as 10/30/04, 7 AM to 10/31/04, 7:05 AM.

Factors Affecting Laboratory Results

- Prolonged light exposure to the specimens.
- Toilet paper or feces in the urine collection.
- High consumption of freshwater fish and tea may cause a decrease in Vitamin B_1 levels.

NURSING IMPLICATIONS WITH RATIONALE

- Explain the test procedure to the client.

Client Teaching

- Instruct the client that food and fluids except water are prohibited for 12 hours or overnight (unless otherwise indicated by the health care provider).
- Instruct the client not to place toilet paper or to defecate in the urine specimen.

Decreased Level

- Obtain a history of the client's dietary intake. Note if the client consumes large quantities of alcoholic beverages.
- Note if the client is complaining of tingling and pain in the extremities. This could be an indication of peripheral neuritis.
- Administer oral or injectable thiamine drug (Vitamin B_1) as prescribed.

Client Teaching

- Encourage the client to eat foods rich in Vitamin B_1.
- Encourage the client to avoid alcohol consumption. Refer the client to Alcoholics Anonymous or counseling.

Vitamin B₆ (plasma)

Pyridoxine

Reference Values

Adult: 5–30 ng/ml, 20–120 nmol/l (SI units). Values depend on the method used. *Deficiency:* <5 ng/ml or <20 nmol/l (SI units).

Description

Vitamin B₆, a water-soluble vitamin, is referred to as pyridoxine, pyridoxal, and pyridoxamine. Pyridoxine is converted to pyridoxal and pyridoxamine after absorption. The functions of Vitamin B₆ include heme synthesis and as a coenzyme in amino acid metabolism. Vitamin B₆ may be partially destroyed by heat, so food processing can decrease the availability of Vitamin B₆. Overheating of infant formulas may contribute to Vitamin B₆ deficiency. Certain drugs block Vitamin B₆, such as the long-term use of the antituberculin drug isoniazid (INH). Usually pyridoxine is given with isoniazid.

Foods rich in Vitamin B₆ are whole grains, vegetables, egg, bananas, fish, fowl, and lean meats. Very large doses of Vitamin B₆ can cause peripheral neuropathy; however, this vitamin has a low toxic effect.

Purpose

- To detect a Vitamin B₆ deficit.

Clinical Problems

Decreased Level: Malnutrition, malabsorption, chronic alcoholism, normocytic microcytic anemia, gestational diabetes, pregnancy, lactation, small bowel inflammatory disease, renal failure, asthma, heavy metal intoxication, carpal tunnel syndrome, pellagra. *Drug Influence:* Isoniazid, oral contraceptives, hydralazine, penicillamine, levodopa, anticonvulsants, cycloserine, pyrazinoic acid, tricyclic antidepressants, disulfiram.

Procedure

- NPO for 8 to 12 hours except for water. If the blood specimen was obtained from a nonfasting client, this should be noted on the laboratory slip.
- Collect 3 to 5 ml of venous blood in a lavendar-top tube. Place the blood specimen in a paper bag to avoid light exposure. Time of specimen collection should be noted on the laboratory slip and the specimen should be delivered to the laboratory within 30 minutes.
- 24-hour urine specimen for Vitamin B₆ has limited value.

Factors Affecting Laboratory Results
- Certain drugs can affect test results *(see Drug Influence)*.
- Prolonged exposure of the blood specimen to light.
- Blood specimen not delivered to the laboratory within 30 minutes.

NURSING IMPLICATIONS WITH RATIONALE

- Explain test procedure to the client.

Decreased Level

- Report if the client is taking the antituberculin drug, isoniazid, and is not receiving pyridoxine.
- Observe infant suspected of Vitamin B_6 deficiency for signs and symptoms of irritability, colic, startle reflex, and convulsion.
- Assess children and adults suspected of Vitamin B_6 deficiency for irritability, dermatitis, glossitis, muscle weakness, polyneuritis, and a decrease in lymphocyte count.

Client Teaching

- Instruct the client to eat foods rich in Vitamin B_6, such as whole grains, vegetables, eggs, fish, fowl, lean meats, and bananas. This is particularly necessary for clients with an alcoholic problem, during pregnancy and lactation, and those on strict diets. Vitamin supplements may be necessary.

Vitamin B₁₂ (serum)

Reference Values
Adult: 200–900 pg/ml.

Child: *Newborn:* 160–1200 pg/ml.

Description

Vitamin B_{12} is essential for red blood cell (RBC) maturation and for gastrointestinal and neurologic function. The extrinsic factor of Vitamin B_{12} is obtained from foods and is absorbed in the small intestines when the intrinsic factor is present. The intrinsic factor is produced by the gastric mucosa, and when this factor is missing, pernicious anemia, a megaloblastic anemia, develops.

Purposes

- To detect pernicious anemia as determined by a decreased Vitamin B_{12} level.
- To suggest other health problems *(see Clinical Problems)*.

Clinical Problems

Decreased Level: Pernicious anemia, malabsorption syndrome, liver diseases, hypothyroidism (myxedema), pancreatic insufficiency, sprue, Crohn's disease, gastrectomy. *Drug Influence:* Neomycin, metformin, anticonvulsants, ethanol.

Elevated Level: Acute hepatitis, acute and chronic myelocytic leukemia, polycythemia vera. *Drug Influence:* Oral contraceptives.

Procedure

- Collect 3 to 5 ml of venous blood in a red-top tube. Avoid hemolysis.
- There is no food or fluid restriction.

Factors Affecting Laboratory Results

- Drugs *(see Drug Influences)*.
- Hemolysis of the blood specimen.

NURSING IMPLICATIONS WITH RATIONALE

- Assess for signs and symptoms of pernicious anemia, such as pallor; fatigue; dyspnea; sore mouth; smooth, beefy-red tongue; indigestion; tingling, numbness in the hands and feet; and behavioral changes.

Client Teaching

- Instruct the client to eat foods high in Vitamin B_{12}, such as milk, eggs, meat, and liver. Contact the dietitian to assist the client in meal planning. Intramuscular Vitamin B_{12} may be ordered.

Vitamin C

See Ascorbic Acid

Vitamin D₃ (serum and plasma)

Cholecalciferol

Reference Values

Two Different Vitamin D₃s: Health care provider must specify which ones; 1,25 dihydroxy (kidney) and 25-hydroxy (liver).

1,25 Dihydroxy: 20–76 pg/ml (serum). (Most potent. Stimulates calcium absorption by the small intestine and bone [along with PTH], and increases reabsorption of calcium by kidney.)

25-Hydroxy: 10–55 ng/ml (plasma).

Reference values are usually higher in mid–late summer.

Description

Vitamin D is a fat-soluble vitamin occurring from exposure to the ultraviolet rays of sunlight and is absorbed in the presence of bile and stored in the liver. Most milk and milk products have been fortified with Vitamin D. Vitamin D is needed for calcium absorption from the intestine and reabsorption from the bone.

A decrease in plasma Vitamin D₃ occurs in aging and pregnancy. Rickets in children and osteomalacia in adults are caused by a Vitamin D deficiency. Foods rich in Vitamin D include Vitamin D fortified milk, egg yolk, fish, liver, and butter.

Excess intake of Vitamin D supplements could cause Vitamin D toxicity. Hypercalcemia may occur with megadoses of Vitamin D. Normally the serum calcium levels are checked with Vitamin D₃ levels.

Purposes

- To detect a Vitamin D deficit.
- To check for Vitamin D toxicity when supplements are being taken.

Clinical Problems

Decreased Level: Malabsorption, cirrhosis of the liver, rickets, osteomalacia, steatorrhea, hypoparathyroidism, celiac disease, inflammatory bowel disease. *Drug Influence:* Anticonvulsants, isoniazid, mineral oil, glycocorticoids, aluminum hydroxide, cholestyramine, colestipol.

Elevated Level: Excessive intake of Vitamin D supplements, excessive exposure to sunlight.

Procedure

- NPO for 8 to 12 hours prior to the test. If fasting is not required or if the client did not fast, this should be noted on the laboratory slip.

- Collect 3 to 5 ml of venous blood in a red-top tube (serum) or a green-top tube (plasma).

Factors Affecting Laboratory Results

- Certain drugs can decrease the Vitamin D_3 level *(see Drug Influence)*.
- Insufficient dietary intake of phosphorus can cause a decrease in Vitamin D_3.
- Lack of exposure to sunlight can decrease the Vitamin D_3 level.

NURSING IMPLICATIONS WITH RATIONALE

- Obtain a history from the client of the amount of sunlight exposure. If the client has little to no sunlight exposure, the Vitamin D_3 level will be decreased.
- Determine if the client is taking vitamin supplements and large doses of Vitamin D. Hypervitaminosis D may occur, which can be toxic and could lead to nephrotoxicity.

Client Teaching

- Explain to the client that there should be nothing by mouth overnight prior to the test except for water unless otherwise indicated by the laboratory.

Decreased Level—Client Teaching

- Instruct the client to drink Vitamin D fortified milk and/or take Vitamin D supplements as indicated by the health care provider. Alert the client that massive doses of Vitamin D can be toxic because it is a fat-soluble vitamin and can accumulate in the body.

Vitamin E (serum)

Tocopherol

Reference Values

Adult: 5–20 μg/ml; 0.5–1.8 mg/dl; 12–42 μmol/l (SI units).

Child: 3–15 μg/ml; 0.3–1.0 mg/dl; 7–23 μmol/l (SI units).

Description

Vitamin E is a fat-soluble vitamin that is plentiful in green leafy vegetables, eggs, grains, oils, chicken, and fish. Vitamin E deficiency is not common unless it is due to malnutrition or malabsorption. Megadoses of Vitamin E could impair absorption of vitamins D and K. Vitamin E is needed for muscle growth and development, adequate reproductive function, and neurologic function.

Purposes

- To detect a Vitamin E deficit.
- To improve reproductive and neurologic functions.

Clinical Problems

Decreased Level: Malabsorption, malnutrition, neurologic abnormalities, platelet hyperaggregation, inadequate absorption of lipid, alcoholism, hemolytic anemia, cystic fibrosis. *Drug Influence:* Alcohol, phenytoin, cholestyramine, mineral oil.

Elevated Level: Megadoses of Vitamin E, hyperlipidemia.

Procedure

- There is no food or fluid restriction.
- Collect 3 to 5 ml of venous blood in a red-top tube. Place the blood sample in a paper bag to prevent light exposure. Send the blood specimen to the laboratory within 2 hours.

Factors Affecting Laboratory Results

- Exposure of the blood sample to light.

NURSING IMPLICATIONS WITH RATIONALE

- Obtain a history of dietary intake. Foods rich in Vitamin E include green vegetables, grains, oils, eggs, fish, and chicken.
- Send the blood specimen to the laboratory in a paper bag to avoid light exposure.

Client Teaching

- Encourage the client to eat foods rich in Vitamin E. Explain that Vitamin E aids in muscle development, reproductive function, and neurologic function.
- Answer the client's questions concerning Vitamin E intake. Excessively large doses should not be encouraged.

White blood cells (WBC) total (blood)

Leukocytes

Reference Values

Adult: Total WBC count: 4500–10,000 μl (mm³).

Child: *Newborn:* 9000–30,000 μl; *2 Years:* 6000–17,000 μl; *10 Years:* 4500–13,500 μl.

Description

(See WBC Differential.)

White blood cells (WBCs), or leukocytes, are divided into two groups: the polymorphonuclear leukocytes (neutrophils, eosinophils, and basophils) and the mononuclear leukocytes (monocytes and lymhocytes). Leukocytes are a part of the body's defense system; they respond immediately to foreign invaders by going to the site of involvement. An increase in WBCs is called *leukocytosis,* and a decrease in WBCs is called *leukopenia.*

Purposes

- To assess WBCs as a part of a complete blood count (CBC).
- To determine the presence of an infection.
- To check WBC values for diagnosing health problems *(see Clinical Problems).*

Clinical Problems

Decreased Level: Hematopoietic diseases (aplastic anemia, pernicious anemia, hypersplenism, Gaucher's disease), viral infections, malaria, agranulocytosis, alcoholism, systemic lupus erythematosus (SLE), rheumatoid arthritis. *Drug Influence:* Antibiotics (penicillins, cephalothins, chloramphenicol), acetaminophen (Tylenol), sulfonamides, propylthiouracil, barbiturates, cancer chemotherapy agents, diazepam (Valium), diuretics (furosemide [Lasix], ethacrynic acid [Edecrin]), chlordiazepoxide (Librium), oral hypoglycemic agents, indomethacin (Indocin), methyldopa (Aldomet), rifampin, phenothiazine.

Elevated Level: Acute infection (pneumonia, meningitis, appendicitis, colitis, peritonitis, pancreatitis, pyelonephritis, tuberculosis, tonsillitis, diverticulitis, septicemia, rheumatic fever), tissue necrosis (myocardial infarction, cirrhosis of the liver, burns, cancer of the organs, emphysema, peptic ulcer), leukemias, collagen diseases, hemolytic and sickle cell anemias, parasitic diseases, stress (surgery, fever, long-lasting emotional upset). *Drug Influence:* Aspirin, heparin, digitalis, epinephrine, lithium, histamine, antibiotics (ampicillin, erythromycin, kanamycin, methicillin, tetracyclines, vancomycin, streptomycin), gold compounds, procainamide

(Pronestyl), triamterene (Dyrenium), allopurinol, potassium iodide, hydantoin derivatives, sulfonamides (long acting).

Procedure

Venous Blood

- Collect 3 to 5 ml of venous blood in a lavender-top tube. Avoid hemolysis.
- There is no food or fluid restriction.

Capillary Blood

- Collect blood from a finger puncture with a micropipette.
- Dilute immediately with the proper reagent.

Factors Affecting Laboratory Results

- Drugs that can increase and decrease the WBC count *(see Drug Influence)*.
- The time the blood sample was taken. The WBC count is lower in the morning than in the afternoon.
- The age of the individual. Children can have a high WBC count, especially during the first 5 years of life.

NURSING IMPLICATIONS WITH RATIONALE

- Check the vital signs and note if the temperature and pulse rate are increased. Also check for signs and symptoms of inflammation and infection, such as redness, heat, swelling, drainage at tissue site.
- Notify of changes in the client's condition, such as fever, increased pulse and respiration rate, and leukocytosis.

Client Teaching

- Instruct the client to check the side effects of patent medicines, such as cold medications, which could cause agranulocytosis, severe leukopenia. With agranulocytosis, the major defense system is lost, and the client is susceptible to severe or long-lasting infection.
- Instruct clients with leukopenia to avoid persons with any contagious condition. Their body resistances are reduced, and they are prime candidates for severe colds or infections.

White blood cell differential (blood)

Differential WBC

Reference Values

	DIFFERENTIAL WBC VALUES		
	Adult		**Child**
WBC Type	**%**	**μl (mm³)**	**Same as Adult Except**
Neutrophils (total)	50–70	2500–7000	*Newborn:* 61%. *1-year-old:* 32%
Segments	50–65	2500–6500	
Bands	0–5	0–500	
Eosinophils	1–3	100–300	
Basophils	0.4–1.0	40–100	
Monocytes	4–6	200–600	*1 to 12 years:* 4%–9%
Lymphocytes	25–35	1700–3500	*Newborn:* 34%. *1 year:* 60% *6 years:* 42%. *12 years:* 38%

Description

(See White Blood Cells [WBCs].)

The differential white blood cell (WBC) count, part of the complete blood count (CBC), is composed of five types of WBCs (leukocytes): neutrophils, eosinophils, basophils, monocytes, and lymphocytes. The differential WBC count is expressed as cubic millimeters (mm³, μl) and percent of the total number of WBCs. Neutrophils and lymphocytes make up 80% to 90% of the total WBCs. The differential WBC count provides more specific information related to infections and disease process.

Neutrophils: Neutrophils are the most numerous circulating WBCs, and they respond more rapidly to the inflammatory and tissue injury sites than other types of WBCs. During an *acute* infection, the neutrophils are the body's first line of defense. The segments are mature neutrophils, and the bands are immature ones that multiply quickly during an acute infection.

Eosinophils: Eosinophils increase during allergic and parasitic conditions. With an increase in steroids, either produced by the adrenal glands during stress or administered orally or by injection, eosinophils decrease in number.

Basophils: Basophils increase during the healing process. With an increase in steroids, the basophil count will decrease.

Monocytes: Monocytes are the second line of defense against bacterial infections and foreign substances. They are stronger than neutrophils and can ingest larger particles of debris. Monocytes respond late during the acute phase of infection and inflammatory process, and they continue to function during the chronic phase of phagocytes.

Lymphocytes: Increased lymphocytes (lymphocytosis) occur in chronic and viral infections. Severe lymphocytosis is commonly caused by chronic lymphocytic leukemia. Lymphocytes play a major role in the immune response system as B lymphocytes and T lymphocytes. Like eosinophils, lymphocytes decrease in number during excess adrenocortical hormone secretion or steroid therapy.

Purpose

■ To differentiate between the various types of WBCs for diagnosing health problems *(see Description)*.

Clinical Problems

Decreased Level

Neutrophils: Viral diseases, leukemias (lymphocytic and monocytic), agranulocytosis, aplastic and iron deficiency anemias. *Drug Influence:* Antibiotic therapy, immunosuppressive agents. *Eosinophils:* Stress: burns, shock; adrenocortical hyperfunction. *Drug Influence:* Cortisone, ACTH. *Basophils:* Stress, hypersensitivity reaction, pregnancy, hyperthyroidism. *Monocytes:* Lymphocytic leukemia, aplastic anemia. *Lymphocytes:* Cancer, leukemia, adrenocortical hyperfunction, agranulocytosis, aplastic anemia, multiple sclerosis, renal failure, nephrotic syndrome, systemic lupus erythematosus (SLE).

Elevated Level

Neutrophils: Acute infections (localized and systemic), inflammatory diseases (rheumatoid arthritis, gout, pneumonia), tissue damage (acute myocardial infarction, burns, crushed injury, surgery), Hodgkin's disease, myelocytic leukemia, hemolytic disease of newborns, acute cholecystitis, acute appendicitis, acute pancreatitis. *Drug Influence:* Epinephrine, digitalis, heparin, sulfonamides, lithium, cortisone, ACTH. *Eosinophils:* Allergies, parasitic disease, cancer (bone, ovary, testes, brain), phlebitis, thrombophlebitis, asthma, emphysema, renal disease (renal failure, nephrotic syndrome). *Basophils:* Inflammatory process, leukemia, healing stage of infection or inflammation, acquired hemolytic anemia. *Monocytes:* Viral diseases (infectious mononucleosis, mumps, herpes zoster), parasitic diseases (Rocky Mountain spotted fever, toxoplasmosis, brucellosis), monocytic leukemia, cancer (esophagus, stomach, colon, liver, bone, prostate, uterus, brain, bladder), anemias (sickle cell, hemolytic), collagen diseases (SLE), rheumatoid arthritis, ulcerative colitis. *Lymphocytes:* Lymphocytic leukemia, viral infections (infectious mononucleosis, hepatitis, mumps, rubella, viral pneumonia, pertussis), chronic infections, Hodgkin's disease, multiple myeloma, adrenocortical hypofunction.

Procedure

- Collect 7 ml of venous blood in a lavender-top tube. Avoid hemolysis.
- There is no food or fluid restriction.
- If eosinophils value is needed, record the time that the blood sample was drawn. If drawn in the afternoon or evening, the count could be slightly higher.

Factors Affecting Laboratory Results

- Steroids could decrease eosinophil and lymphocyte values.
- Certain drugs can increase or decrease blood values *(see Drug Influence)*.

NURSING IMPLICATIONS WITH RATIONALE

- Check the WBC count and the differential WBC count. Elevated neutrophils may be indicative of an acute infection. Elevated eosinophils may be a sign of allergy. Increased basophils can be caused by the healing process. Increased monocytes occur during a bacterial infection, and increased lymphocytes occur in chronic or viral infections.
- Assess the client for signs and symptoms of an infection, such as elevated temperature, increased pulse rate, edema, redness, and exudate (wound drainage).
- Assess the client for signs and symptoms of allergies, such as tearing, "runny nose," rash, and more severe reactions.
- Assess for signs and symptoms of healing, such as ability to increase movement at the injured site, and decreased edema and exudate.

Client Teaching

- Instruct the client to report any signs and symptoms of infection, such as the presence of a fever.
- Encourage the client to rest, take medications such as antibiotics as prescribed, increase fluid intake as appropriate, and monitor temperature.

Zinc (plasma)

Reference Values

Plasma: *Adult:* 60–150 μg/dl, 11–23 μmol/l (SI units).

Urine: 150–1250 μg/24 h.

Description

Zinc, a heavy metal, is an element found in the body and required for body growth and metabolism. Approximately 80% of zinc is in the blood cells. About 30% of the zinc ingested is absorbed from the small intestine. Most of the body's excretion of zinc is in the stool and a small amount is excreted in the urine.

Zinc is a component of many enzymes such as carbonic anhydrase, DNA and RNA polymerases, lactic dehydrogenase, and alkaline phosphatase and plays an important role in enzyme catalytic reactions. Plasma zinc levels are requested when a zinc deficiency or toxicity is suspected. Zinc deficiency is not apparent until it becomes severe and is manifested by growth retardation, delayed sexual development, severe dermatitis, alopecia, or poor wound healing. Zinc toxicity is rare, but it can be related to workers inhaling zinc oxide during industry exposure.

Purposes

- To detect a zinc deficiency.
- To determine the cause of diarrhea, growth retardation, delayed sexual development, alopecia, and poor healing.
- To detect zinc toxicity due to industry exposure (inhaling zinc oxide).

Clinical Problems

Decreased Level: Malnutrition, malabsorption, diarrhea, anemia, alcoholism, myocardial infarction, hereditary deficiency, cirrhosis, chronic renal failure, gallbladder disease. *Drug Influence:* Corticosteroids, estrogens, penicillamine, anti-cancer-antimetabolites, cisplatin, diuretics.

Elevated Level: Ingestion of acidic food or beverages from galvanized containers, industrial exposure.

Procedure

- There is no food or fluid restriction.
- Collect 3 to 5 ml of venous blood in a metal-free, navy blue-top tube. Avoid hemolysis.
- Send the blood specimen to the laboratory *immediately.*

Factors Affecting Laboratory Results

- Certain drugs decrease the plasma level *(see Drug Influence).*
- Hemolysis invalidates the test result.
- Use of a tube or needle containing metal.

NURSING IMPLICATIONS WITH RATIONALE

- Obtain a history of the client's nutritional intake. Zinc is present in many foods. Malnutrition, cirrhosis of the liver, alcoholism, or severe diarrhea contributes to a zinc deficit.

- Monitor intravenous therapy including total parenteral nutrition (TPN); continuous use can cause a zinc deficit.
- Check the history for anemia. With sickle cell anemia, the zinc level is decreased because abnormal red blood cells cause excess loss of zinc.

Client Teaching

- Instruct the pregnant client that vitamins prescribed should contain zinc. An increase in zinc requirement is needed during pregnancy and for lactation.
- Instruct client who has poor nutrition to take vitamins. Tell the client to check the label on vitamin container to determine that zinc is one of the elements.

Zinc protoporphyrin (ZPP) (blood)

Free Erythrocyte Protoporphyrin (FEP)

Reference Values

Adult and Child: 15–77 μg/dl, 0.24–1.23 μmol/l (SI units). *Average:* <35 μg/dl; <0.56 μmol/l (SI units).

Description

Zinc protoporphyrin (ZPP) is a screening test to check for lead poisoning and iron deficiency. It can be checked by drawing a blood sample or by use of a hematofluorometer using several drops of blood. With iron deficiency, the ZPP level does not become elevated until after a few weeks. After iron therapy, the ZPP level returns to normal in 2 to 2½ months.

The use of the ZPP test for screening for increased blood lead levels has more than doubled within a year.

Purpose

- To screen for lead poisoning or for iron deficiency.

Clinical Problems

Elevated Level: Lead poisoning, iron deficiency, accelerated erythropoiesis, acute inflammatory processes. *Drug Influence:* Digitalis, riboflavin. *Laboratory Test:* Serum bilirubin can be elevated.

Procedure

- There is no food or fluid restriction.

- Collect 3 to 5 ml in a green- or lavender-top tube. Avoid hemolysis. A hemato-fluorometer with a few drops of blood may be used.

Factors Affecting Laboratory Results

- Hemolysis of the blood sample can increase the ZPP level.

NURSING IMPLICATIONS WITH RATIONALE

- Check with the laboratory concerning the type of blood specimen that should be obtained (drops of blood or use of a hematofluorometer with a few drops of blood).
- Obtain a history from the client or family concerning the child ingesting lead from paint. Older houses may still have lead paint, which could be eaten by a child.
- Obtain a history from the adult client concerning excessive lead exposure due to occupational contact. Other possible contact with lead includes use of unglazed pottery, "moonshine" whiskey prepared in lead containers, lead gasoline fumes (not common today because of unleaded gasoline).
- Compare the blood lead level with the blood ZPP level. Report abnormal findings to the health care provider.
- Observe for signs and symptoms of lead poisoning, such as lead colic (crampy abdominal pain), constipation, occasional bloody diarrhea, behavioral changes (from lethargy to hyperactivity, aggression, impulsiveness), tremors, and confusion.
- Obtain a history of iron deficiency. Check serum iron level, and serum transferrin and ferritin levels. Compare the above levels with the ZPP level.
- Check that blood ZPP levels are repeated after 2 months of iron therapy. ZPP levels should decrease after iron therapy for iron deficiency.

PART TWO

Diagnostic Tests

2

A ■ DIAGNOSTIC TESTS

Acid perfusion

See Esophageal Studies

Amniotic fluid analysis

Amniocentesis, Amnioscopy

Normal Finding

Clear amniotic fluid, no chromosomal or neural tube abnormalities.

Description

Amniotic fluid analysis is useful for detecting chromosomal abnormalities, such as Down's syndrome or mongolism (trisomy 21); neural tube defects (spina bifida); and sex-linked disorders, such as hemophilia; and for determining fetal maturity. The amniotic fluid is obtained by amniocentesis. This procedure involves the insertion of a needle into the suprapubic area after the fetus has been located and manually elevated and the aspiration of 5 to 15 mL of amniotic fluid. Ultrasound may be used to locate the placenta and to determine fetal positions so that needle contact can be avoided. Amniocentesis is performed during the 14th to 16th weeks of pregnancy. It usually is not done before the 14th week because of the insufficient amount of amniotic fluid or after the 16th week if a therapeutic abortion might be suggested.

Analyses of the amniotic fluid may also include color, bilirubin (present in the fluid until the 28th week but absent at full term), meconium (present during stress—e.g., in breech presentation), creatinine, lecithin/sphingomyelin (L/S) ratio (a decreased ratio can indicate respiratory distress syndrome), glucose, lipids, and alpha-fetoprotein (AFP).

Amnioscopy involves insertion of a fiberoptic lighted instrument (amnioscope) into the cervical canal to visualize the amniotic fluid. The color of the amniotic fluid can indicate fetal hypoxia. This test is normally performed close to full term, because it requires cervical dilation. Because there is a risk of rupturing the amniotic membrane and of intrauterine infection, the test is rarely performed.

Purposes

- To detect chromosomal abnormalities, neural tube defects, and sex-linked disorders.

■ To determine fetal maturity.

Clinical Problems

Indications: Chromosomal disorders (e.g., Down syndrome), neural tube defects (e.g., spina bifida), hemolytic disease due to Rh incompatibility; fetal sex (important for sex-linked disorders—e.g., hemophilia), fetal maturity, pulmonary maturity of the fetus (L/S ratio).

Procedure

■ A consent form should be signed.
■ Food and fluids are not restricted.
■ Have the client void before the procedure to prevent puncturing the bladder and aspirating urine.
■ Cleanse the suprapubic area with an antiseptic such as povidone-iodine (Betadine). A local anesthetic is injected at the site for the amniocentesis.
■ The placenta and fetus should be located by ultrasound or manually (fetus only). A 22-gauge spinal needle with stylet is inserted through the skin to the amniotic cavity.
■ 5 to 15 ml of amniotic fluid is aspirated. Apply a small dressing to the needle insertion site.
■ The procedure takes approximately 30 minutes.

Foam Stability Test

This test determines if surfactant from mature fetal lungs is present in the amniotic fluid. When the test tube of amniotic fluid is shaken, bubbles appear around the surface if adequate amounts of surfactant are present.

Factors Affecting Diagnostic Results

■ A traumatic amniocentesis tap may produce blood in the amniotic fluid.

NURSING IMPLICATIONS WITH RATIONALE

■ Recognize when amniocentesis for amniotic fluid analysis is indicated (i.e., with a familial history of sex-linked, genetic, or chromosomal disorders; with a history of previous miscarriages; and in advanced maternal age [>35 years old]). It is not a screening test.
■ Be sure that the client urinates before the test and that the consent form is signed.
■ Be supportive of the woman and her partner. Be a good listener. Allow them time to ask questions and to express any concerns. Refer questions you cannot answer to the appropriate health professionals.

Client Teaching

■ Inform the client that normal results do not guarantee a normal infant, nor do they always predict sex correctly. The health care provider should tell the woman of potential risks, such as premature labor, spontaneous abortion, infection, and fetal or placental bleeding from the needle. These complications rarely occur, but the woman should be told of the risk factors.

■ Instruct the client to notify the health care provider immediately of any of the following: bleeding or leaking fluid from the vagina, abdominal pain or cramping, chills and fever, or lack of fetal movement.

■ Encourage the woman and her partner to seek genetic counseling, especially if a chromosomal abnormality has been determined. Usually the final decision about terminating a pregnancy rests with the pregnant woman and her partner.

Angiography (angiogram)

Arteriography: Cardiac (see Cardiac Catheterization), Cerebral Angiography, Pulmonary Angiography, and Renal Angiography

Normal Finding

Normal structure and potency of the blood vessels.

Description

In vivo angiography was first performed in the 1920s. The terms *angiography* (examination of the blood vessels) and *arteriography* (examination of the arteries) are used interchangeably. A catheter is inserted into the femoral, brachial, subclavian, or carotid artery, and a contrast dye is injected to allow visualization of the blood vessels. Normally the client feels a warm, flushed sensation as the dye is injected. Angiographies are useful for evaluating patency of blood vessels and for identifying abnormal vascularization resulting from neoplasms (tumors). This test may be indicated when computed tomography or radionuclide scanning suggests vascular abnormalities.

The new contrast media have a low osmolality. The older medias were hyperosmolar with a high content of iodine in relation to its solution. Examples of the low-osmolar-contrast media include iopamidol, iohexol, and ioxaglate.

An embolus due to catheter clot formation is the most dangerous complication of angiography. Other complications include puncturing the site causing hematoma and/or hemorrhage, contrast media reactions, and infection.

Cerebral Angiography: Any of the three arteries (femoral, brachial, or carotid) can be used for access. The dye will outline the carotid artery, vertebral artery, large blood vessels of the circle of Willis, and small cerebral arterial branches.

Pulmonary Angiography: The catheter is inserted into the brachial artery (in the arm) or the femoral artery and is threaded to the pulmonary artery. The dye is injected for visualizing pulmonary vessels. During the test the client should be monitored for cardiac dysrhythmias.

Renal Angiography: The catheter is inserted into the femoral artery and is passed upward through the iliac artery and the aorta to the renal artery. This test permits visualization of the renal vessels and the parenchyma. An aortogram is sometimes made with real angiography to detect any vessel abnormality and to show the relationship of the renal arteries to the aorta.

Purposes

- To detect aneurysms, thrombosis, emboli, space-occupying lesions, stenosis, plaques.
- To evaluate cerebral, pulmonary and renal blood flow.

Clinical Problems

Type of Angiography	Indications/Purposes
Cerebral	To detect cerebrovascular aneurysm; cerebral thrombosis; hematomas; tumors from increased vascularization; cerebral plaques or spasm; cerebral fistula
	To determine cerebral blood flow, cause of increased intracranial pressure ($\uparrow$ ICP)
Pulmonary	To detect pulmonary embolism; tumors; aneurysms; congenital defects; vascular changes associated with emphysema, blebs, and bullae; heart abnormality
	To evaluate pulmonary circulation
Renal	To detect renal artery stenosis; renal thrombus or embolus; space-occupying lesions (i.e., tumors, cysts); aneurysms
	To determine the causative factor of hypertension, cause of renal failure
	To evaluate renal circulation

Procedure

All Angiographies

- A consent form should be signed by the client or a designated family member.
- The client should be NPO for 8 to 12 hours before the angiogram. Anticoagulants (heparin) are usually discontinued.
- Record vital signs. Have client void before the test.
- Dentures and metallic objects should be removed before the test.
- The access site should be shaved.
- Premedications (i.e., a sedative or narcotic analgesic), if ordered, are administered an hour before the test. If the client has a history of severe allergic reactions to various substances or drugs, the health care provider may order steroids or antihistamines before and after the procedure as a prophylactic measure.

- Intravenous (IV) fluids may be started before the procedure so that emergency drugs, if needed, may be administered.
- The client lies in a supine position on an x-ray table. A local anesthetic is administered to the injection incisional site.
- The test takes approximately 1 to 2 hours.

Renal: A laxative or cleansing enema is usually ordered the evening before the test.

Pulmonary: Electrocardiography electrodes are attached to the client's chest for cardiac monitoring (tracings of heart activity) during the angiography. Pulmonary pressures are recorded, and blood samples are obtained before the contrast dye is injected.

Factors Affecting Diagnostic Results

- Feces and gas can distort or decrease the visualization of the kidneys.
- Barium sulfate from a recent barium study can interfere with the test results.
- Movement during the filming can distort the x-ray picture.

NURSING IMPLICATIONS WITH RATIONALE

Pretest

- Obtain a client history of hypersensitivity to iodine, seafood, or contrast dye from other x-ray procedures (e.g., intravenous pyelography [IVP]). The health care provider should also know if the client is highly sensitive to other substances. Skin testing could be done before the test, or prophylactic medications (i.e., steroids, antihistamines) may be given prior to and/or following the test.
- Record baseline vital signs.
- Give a laxative or cleansing enema, if ordered. Explain to the client that it will cleanse the lower intestinal tract, allowing better visualization.
- Have the client void, wear a gown, and remove dentures.
- Administer premedications (sedative and narcotic analgesic) as ordered. Check that the consent form has been signed before giving premedications. The client should be in bed with the bed sides up after the premedications are given.
- Encourage the client to ask questions. This test can be frightening to clients, and they will need time to express any concerns.
- Assess for vasovagal reaction (common complication; i.e., decreased pulse rate and blood pressure [BP], cold and clammy skin). Give IV fluids and atropine IV. This reaction lasts about 15 to 20 minutes.

Client Teaching

- Explain the procedure to the client *(see Description and Procedure)*. Inform the client that the radiologist, surgeon, or health care provider will inject a contrast dye into an artery at the groin, elbow, or neck. The area will be numbed, and a catheter will be inserted and threaded with the guidance of fluoroscopy to the appropriate site.

- Inform the client that when the dye is injected he or she will most likely feel a warm, flushed sensation that should last for a minute or two. Explain to the client that the test should not cause pain but can cause some periodic discomfort during the procedure.

Posttest

- Apply pressure on the injection site for 5 to 10 minutes or longer (venous access) or 30 minutes or longer (arterial access) until bleeding has stopped. Check the injection site for bleeding when taking vital signs.
- Monitor vital signs as ordered, such as every 15 minutes for the first hour, every 30 minutes for the next 2 hours, and then every hour for the next 4 hours, or until stable. The temperature should be taken every 4 hours for 24 to 48 hours or as ordered.
- Enforce bed rest for 5 hours for venous access or 6 to 8 hours for arterial access or as ordered. Activities should be restricted for a day.
- Assess the injection site for swelling and for hematoma.
- Check peripheral pulses in the extremities (i.e., dorsalis pedis, femoral, and radial). Absence or weakness in pulse volume should be reported immediately.
- Note the temperature and color of the extremity. Report changes (e.g., color—pale, pain in the extremity, especially distal to access site) to the health care provider immediately. Arterial occlusion to the extremity could occur.
- Apply cold compresses or an ice pack to the injection site for edema or pain, if ordered.
- Monitor electrocardiogram tracings, urine output, and IV fluids. IV fluids and cardiac monitoring may be discontinued after the angiography.
- Inform the client that coughing usually is not abnormal following a pulmonary angiography.
- Assess for dysphagia and for respiratory distress if the carotid artery was used for cerebral angiography.
- Assess for weakness or numbness in an extremity, confusion, slurred speech, or visual changes following a cerebral angiography. These could be symptoms of a transient ischemic attack (TIA), known as a "small stroke."
- Observe for a delayed allergic reaction to the contrast dye (i.e., tachycardia, dyspnea, skin rash, urticaria [hives], decreasing systolic BP, and decreased urine output).
- Be supportive of the client and his or her family. Answer questions, and explain your nursing implications.

Arthrography

Normal Finding

Knee: Normal medial meniscus.

Shoulder: Bicipital tendon sheath, normal joint capsule, and intact subscapular bursa.

Description

Arthrography is an x-ray examination of a joint using air, contrast media, or both in the joint space. The purposes are to detect abnormalities of the cartilage and/or ligaments (e.g., tears) and to visualize structures of the joint capsule.

This procedure is performed when a client complains of persistent knee or shoulder pain or discomfort. Usually it is performed on an outpatient basis.

Arthrography is not indicated if the client is having an acute arthritic attack, has a joint infection, or is pregnant.

Purposes

- To visualize the structures of the joint capsule.
- To detect abnormalities of the cartilage and/or ligaments (tears).

Clinical Problems

Abnormal findings: Osteochondritis dissecans, osteochondral fractures, cartilage abnormalities, synovial abnormalities, tears of the ligaments, and joint capsule abnormalities. *Shoulder:* Adhesive capsulitis, tears of rotator cuff, bicipital tenosynovitis or tears.

Procedure

- Prepare the knee or shoulder area using aseptic technique.
- Local anesthetic is administered to puncture site.
- A needle is inserted into the joint space (e.g., knee), and synovial fluid is aspirated for synovial fluid analysis.
- Air and/or contrast medium is injected into the joint space, and x-rays are taken.
- The knee may be bandaged.
- Food and fluids are not restricted.

Factors Affecting Diagnostic Results

- None known.

NURSING IMPLICATIONS WITH RATIONALE

- Explain the procedure to the client to allay anxiety and fear and to increase the client's cooperation.
- Obtain a client history of allergies to seafood, iodine, and contrast dye. An antihistamine, diphenhydramine (Benadryl), may be given orally or intravenously if there is a history of iodine or seafood hypersensitivity.
- Provide ongoing assessment before, during, and after the procedure, including vital signs, discomfort, and others.

Client Teaching

- Inform the client that changes in body positions may be asked for during the procedure. At other times, the client is to remain still.
- Inform the client that he or she will not be asleep during the arthrography and may ask questions prior, during, and after the test procedure.

Posttest

- Apply an ace bandage to the leg, including the knee, if indicated to decrease swelling and pain.

Client Teaching

- Instruct the client to rest the joint for the time specified, usually 12 hours.
- Inform the client that a crepitant noise may be heard with joint movement. This should stop in a few days; however, if the noise persists, the health care provider should be contacted.
- Instruct the client to apply an ice bag with a cover to the affected joint to decrease swelling if noted. An analgesic for pain and/or discomfort may be ordered or suggested.

Arthroscopy

Normal Finding

Normal lining of the synovial membrane. Cartilage is smooth and white, and ligaments and tendons are intact.

Description

Arthroscopy is an endoscopic examination of the interior aspect of a joint (usually the knee) using a fiberoptic endoscope. Normally an *arthrography* is performed prior to arthroscopy.

Arthroscopy may be used to diagnose meniscal, patellar, extrasynovial, and synovial diseases; to perform joint surgery; and to monitor disease process or the effects of medical or surgical therapeutic regimen. Frequently biopsy or surgery is performed during the test procedure. For a surgical procedure, spinal or general anesthesia is used and for visualization of the interior joint space, a local anesthetic. Arthroscopy is contraindicated if a wound or severe skin infection is present or if the client has severe fibrous ankylosis.

Purposes

- To diagnose meniscal, patellar, extrasynovial, and synovial diseases.
- To perform joint surgery.

Clinical Problems

Abnormal Findings: Meniscal disease with torn lateral or medial meniscus, patellar disease, chondromalacia, patellar fracture, osteochondritis dissecans, osteochondromatosis, torn ligaments, Baker's cysts, synovitis, and rheumatoid and degenerative arthritis.

Procedure

- A consent form should be signed.
- There is no food or fluid restriction for local anesthetic. NPO after midnight for spinal and general anesthesia.
- Local, spinal, or general anesthesia is used, depending on the purpose and procedure for the test.
- Ace bandage and/or tourniquet may be applied to decrease blood volume in the leg.
- The arthroscope is inserted into the interior joint for visualization, for draining fluid from the joint, for biopsy, and/or for surgery.
- A dressing is applied to the incision site of the affected joint.

Factors Affecting Diagnostic Results

- Septic technique used during test procedure could cause pain and discomfort and could further complicate the joint disease.

NURSING IMPLICATIONS WITH RATIONALE

- Check on the type of anesthesia to be used. If general or spinal anesthesia is ordered, inform the client to remain NPO after midnight prior to the test.
- Assess the involved area for possible skin lesion or infection.
- Determine the client's anxiety level, and be available to answer questions. Be prepared to repeat information if the level of anxiety or fear is determined to be high.
- Use aseptic technique throughout the procedure. Sepsis can cause severe complication to the joint and tissues.

Posttest

- Assess the client before, during, and after procedure, including vital signs, bleeding, swelling. Report abnormal findings to the health care provider.
- Apply an ice bag with cover to the area as indicated.
- Administer an analgesic for pain or discomfort as ordered.
- Answer the client's and family members' questions. If unable to, refer the questions to the appropriate health professionals.

Client Teaching

- Instruct the client to avoid excessive use of joint for 2 to 3 days or as ordered. Walking should be minimized.

Barium enema

Lower Gastrointestinal Test, X-Ray Examination of the Colon

Normal Finding

Adult: Normal filling, normal structure of the large colon.

Description

The barium enema test is an x-ray examination of the large intestine (colon) to detect the presence of polyps, an intestinal mass, diverticuli, an intestinal stricture/obstruction, or ulcerations. Barium sulfate (single contrast) or barium sulfate and air (double contrast or air contrast) is administered slowly through a rectal tube into the large colon. The filling process is monitored by fluoroscopy, and then x-rays are taken. The colon must be free of fecal material so that the barium will outline the large intestine to detect any disorders. The double-contrast technique (barium and air) is useful for identifying polyps.

The barium enema test is indicated for clients complaining of lower abdominal pain and cramps; blood, mucus, or pus in the stool; changes in bowel habits; and changes in stool formation. The test can be performed in a hospital, in a clinic, or at a private laboratory.

Purpose

- To detect disorders of the large intestine.

Clinical Problems

Abnormal Findings: Carcinoma (tumor or lesion), inflammatory disease (ulcerative colitis, granulomatous colitis, diverticulitis), diverticulae, fistulas, polyps, intussusception.

Procedure

In most institutions the procedures for the barium enema are similar; however, they usually differ to some degree. Some institutions request that the client maintain a low-residue diet (tender meats, eggs, bread, clear soup, pureed bland vegetables and fruits, potatoes, and boiled milk) for 2 to 3 days before the test. Abdominal x-rays, ultrasound studies, radionuclide scans, and proctosigmoidoscopy should be done *before* the barium enema. It is important that the colon is free of fecal material.

Prepreparation

- Oral medications should not be given for 24 hours before the test, unless indicated by the health care provider. Narcotics and barbiturates could interfere with fecal elimination before and after the test.
- The client should be on a clear-liquid diet for 18 to 24 hours before the test. This would include broth, ginger ale, cola, black coffee or tea with sugar only, gelatin, and syrup from canned fruit. Some institutions permit a white chicken sandwich (*no* butter, lettuce, or mayonnaise) or hard boiled eggs and gelatin for lunch and dinner, then NPO after dinner.
- Encourage the client to increase water and clear liquid intake 24 hours before the test to maintain adequate hydration.
- Prescribe laxatives (castor oil or magnesium citrate) to be taken the day before the test in the late afternoon or early evening (4 PM to 8 PM).
- A cleansing enema or laxative suppository such as bisacodyl (Dulcolax) may be given the evening before the test.
- Saline enemas (maximum three enemas) should be given early in the morning (6 AM) until the returned solution is clear. Some private laboratories have clients use bisacodyl suppositories in the morning instead of the enemas.
- Black coffee or tea is permitted 1 hour before the test. Some institutions permit dry toast.

Postpreparation

- The client should expel the barium in the bathroom or bedpan immediately after the test.
- Fluid intake should be increased for hydration and prevent constipation due to retained barium.
- A laxative, such as milk of magnesia or magnesium citrate, or an oil retention enema should be given to remove the barium from the colon. A laxative may need to be repeated the following day after the test.

Factors Affecting Diagnostic Results

- Inadequate bowel preparation with fecal material remaining in the colon could affect results.
- The use of barium sulfate in upper gastrointestinal and small bowel studies 2 to 3 days before the barium enema test could affect the results.

NURSING IMPLICATIONS WITH RATIONALE

- Review the written procedure for that instituton. Explain the procedure to the client. Procedures do differ from one institution to another. Usually the preparations for a barium enema have similarities (clear liquids, increased fluid intake, laxatives, and cleansing enemas). Fecal material in the large intestine (bowel or colon) should be completely eliminated.
- List the procedure step by step for the client. Most private laboratories and hospitals have written preparation slips. The procedure may be sent to the client at home.
- Emphasize the importance of following dietary restrictions and of bowel preparation. Adequate prepreparation is essential or the test may need to be repeated.
- Notify the health care provider if the client has severe abdominal cramps and pain prior to the test. The barium enema test should not be performed if the client has severe ulcerative colitis, suspected perforation, or tachycardia.

Client Teaching

- Explain to the client that he or she will be lying on a tilting x-ray table for positioning purposes to increase the barium flow into the colon. Explain that a technician will be with him or her and will explain each step of the procedure.
- Inform the client that the test takes approximately $\frac{1}{2}$ to 1 hour to complete. Tell the client to take deep breaths through the mouth, which helps to decrease tension and to promote relaxation.
- Administer a laxative or cleansing enema after the test. Instruct the patient to check the color of the stools for 2 to 3 days. Stools may be light in color because of the barium sulfate. Absence of stool should be reported. Retention of barium sulfate after the test could cause obstruction and/or fecal impaction.

Biopsy (bone marrow, breast, endometrium, kidney, liver)

Normal Finding

Normal cells and tissue from the bone marrow, breast, endometrium of the uterus, kidney, and liver.

Description

Biopsy is the removal and examination of tissue from the body. Usually biopsies are performed to detect malignancy or to identify the presence of a disease process. Biopsies can be obtained by (1) aspiration by applying suction; (2) the brush method, using stiff bristles that scrape fragments of cells and tissue; (3) excision by surgical cutting at tissue site; (4) fine-needle or needle aspiration at tissue site with or without the guidance of ultrasound; (5) insertion of a needle through the skin; and (6) punch biopsy, using a punch-type instrument.

Biopsies are performed on various organs and body structures, such as bone marrow, the breast, endometrium of the uterus, kidney, and liver. The methods used for the biopsy tissues of various organs may differ.

Bone Marrow: The bone marrow is composed of red and yellow marrow. The red marrow produces blood cells and the yellow marrow has fat cells and connective tissue. The sternum and iliac crest are the most common sites for bone marrow aspiration.

Breast: Biopsy of the breast is mainly performed to determine if a breast lesion (nodule or mass) is a cyst or is cancerous. The majority of breast lumps are benign. The site of the breast lesion can be identified with the use of a fixed grid on the mammogram.

Endometrium of the Uterus: Endometrial biopsy can detect polyps, cancer, inflammatory condition and defect in ovulation. The biopsy collection using a probe (blind technique) can be performed in the health care provider's office. Complications include perforation of the uterus, excessive bleeding, and aborting an early pregnancy. This procedure should not be performed if there is purulent discharge from the vagina. An endometrial biopsy differs from a D & C (dilation and curettage) in that dilation of the cervix is not needed. D & C requires general anesthesia because the entire endometrium is curettaged. With an endometrial biopsy, the affected tissue in the uterus could be missed with a sample biopsy; whereas with a D & C the total endometrium is obtained.

Kidney (Renal): A kidney biopsy is usually done with the guidance of ultrasound or fluoroscopy. The biopsy is performed to determine the cause of renal disease, to rule out metastatic malignancy of the kidney, or to determine if rejection of a kidney transplant is occurring. The biopsy can be obtained in three ways: (1) by use of a cystoscope, (2) by excision of the kidney taking a wedge of tissue, and (3) percutaneously using a needle.

Liver: Liver biopsy is not usually done unless the liver enzymes are greatly increased. It is performed to rule out metatastic malignancy or to detect a cyst or the presence of cirrhosis. Ultrasound is used to guide the biopsy needle to the pathologic site. Prior to a liver biopsy, the following laboratory levels should be checked: prothrombin time (PT), partial thromboplastin time (PTT), and platelet count. The liver is vascular and if these laboratory results are abnormal, bleeding could occur following the test procedure.

Purposes

- To identify abnormal tissue from various body sites.
- To detect the presence of a disease process (e.g., cirrhosis).

Clinical Problems

Indications: Blood disorders, malignancies, cysts, polyps, infectious process, progressive disease entities (cirrhosis, nephrosis, lupus nephritis), ovulative defects, rejection of an organ transplant.

Procedure

- A consent form should be signed.
- Baseline vital signs taken.
- Biopsy site is anesthetized.

Bone Marrow

- A local anesthetic is injected at site (sternum or iliac spine).
- A needle with a stylet is inserted through a skin slit into the bone about 3 mm deep.
- The stylet is removed and a 10-ml syringe is attached to the needle. Bone marrow is aspirated; part is used for a blood smear and the remaining amount is placed in a green- or lavender-top tube.

Breast

- Needle aspiration or an excision of breast tissue can be performed.
- The skin is anesthetized; general anesthesia may be used if biopsy tissue is difficult to obtain.
- A mammogram is usually needed to determine the placement of needle or the excision site.
- Tissue obtained from biopsy is placed in formalin and sent immediately to the laboratory. The specimen from a needle aspiration is placed on cytologic slide.

Endometrial of the Uterus

- The client is placed in the lithotomy position.

- A sound (probe) is inserted into the cavity of the uterus to determine its size. This is done as a precaution to prevent perforation of the uterus.
- A suction tube with curette is inserted into the cavity of the uterus, and sample specimens are obtained from the lateral, anterior, and/or posterior uterine wall.
- Specimen(s) is/are placed in formalin solution and sent to the laboratory for histologic testing.

Kidney (Renal)

This test can be performed by use of a cystocope with the brush method, excision of a wedge of renal tissue, or percutaneously with a special needle.

- The client is placed in the prone position.
- With the percutaneous method, the site is determined with the use of ultrasound or fluoroscopy.
- Anesthetic is given according to the procedure chosen.
- With needle insertion, the client is asked to take a breath and hold it. Small tissue specimen is obtained. Pressure is applied to the site to prevent bleeding for approximately 20 minutes, because the kidney tissue is very vascular.

Liver

- NPO for at least 6 hours prior to the test. The liver is less congested without food intake.
- Check that PT, APTT (PTT), and platelet count have been done and documented. Abnormal findings should be reported prior to procedure to decrease/ avoid excessive bleeding following the biopsy.
- A fine needle is inserted, usually with the guidance of ultrasound.
- The client is asked first to take a deep breath, then exhale and hold breath. With expiration the diaphragm is motionless and remains high in the thorax.
- Apply a pressure dressing.
- The tissue specimen is placed in formalin solution or the specimen is swabbed on a slide and fixed in 95% alcohol.
- Place the client on his or her right side to decrease the chance of hemorrhage.

Factors Affecting Diagnostic Results

- Blind biopsy can result in missing the diseased site (tissue).
- Improper care to the tissue specimen.

NURSING IMPLICATIONS WITH RATIONALE

- Check that the consent form has been signed.
- Check that the prescribed laboratory tests have been done.
- Explain the biopsy procedure to the client. Explanation can decrease client anxiety and increase cooperation with the procedure.
- Monitor vital signs as prescribed (i.e., every 15 minutes for the first hour, every 30 minutes for the second hour, and then hourly).

- Observe for bleeding and shortness of breath.

Client Teaching

- Instruct the client to report excessive bleeding immediately to the health care provider.
- Instruct the client to report an elevated temperature.
- Instruct the client to take the prescribed pain medication. If pain intensifies, the health care provider should be notified.
- Advise the client to rest for 24 hours following the test procedure.
- Instruct the client to avoid heavy lifting for at least 24 hours, or longer if indicated (e.g., in liver, renal biopsy).

Kidney

- Increase fluid intake following the biopsy.
- Check bowel sounds for several hours following the test. Abdominal intervention can cause a decrease in bowel sounds (decreased peristalsis).
- Instruct the client to report decreased urination or burning when urinating.

Liver

- Avoid heavy lifting.
- Check bowel sounds for several hours following the test. Report an absence of or decreased bowel sounds.

Bone densitometry

Bone Density (BD), Bone Mineral Density (BMD), Bone Absorptiometry

Normal Finding

Normal bone densitometry scan is determined according to the client's age, sex, and height.

Normal: 1 standard deviation below peak bone mass level.
Osteoporosis: >2.5 standard deviations below peak bone mass level (WHO standard).

Description

Bone density test is to detect early osteoporosis by determining the density of bone mineral content. Clients who have a loss of bone mineral are readily prone to have fractures. The bones that are usually examined are the lumbar spine and the proximal hip (neck of the femur). Other bone site, heel bone, can be evaluated according to the client's symptoms.

The dual energy x-ray absorptiometry (DEXA) measures bone mineral density and only exposes the client to a minimal amount of radiation. Images from the detector/camera are computer analyzed to determine the bone mineral content. The computer can calculate the size and thickness of the bone.

Purposes

- To evaluate the bone mineral density.
- To identify early and progressive osteoporosis.

Clinical Problems

Abnormal Findings: Loss of bone mineral content, early and progressive osteoporosis.

Procedure

- A signed consent form may be required.
- No food or fluid restriction is required.
- Client is to remove all metal objects at the area to be scanned, for example, keys, coins, zippers, belts and others.
- The client lies on an imaging table with a radiation source below and the detector above which measures the bone's radiation absorption.
- The bone density test takes approximately 30 to 60 minutes.

Factors Affecting Diagnostic Results

- Metallic objects in the bone scanning site.
- Previous fractures of the bone may increase the bone density.

NURSING IMPLICATIONS WITH RATIONALE

- Obtain of family history of osteoporosis and client's skeletal problems, such as loss of height, fractures, and others.

Client Teaching

- Explain the procedure for bone density test.
- Inform the client that the test should not cause pain and the radiation is considered minimal.
- Instruct the client to remove all metal objects that would be within the scanning area.
- Tell the client that the test should take approximately 30 to 60 minutes.

Bronchography (bronchogram)

Normal Finding

Normal tracheobronchial structure.

Description

Bronchography is an x-ray test to visualize the trachea, bronchi, and entire bronchial tree after a radiopaque iodine contrast liquid is injected through a catheter into the tracheobronchial space. The bronchi are coated with the contrast dye, and a series of x-rays is then taken. Bronchography may be done in conjunction with bronchoscopy.

Bronchography is contraindicated during pregnancy. This test should also not be done if the client is hypersensitive to anesthetics, iodine, or x-ray dyes.

Purpose

- To detect bronchial obstruction, such as foreign bodies and tumors.

Clinical Problems

Indications: Bronchial obstruction (i.e., foreign bodies, tumors; cysts or cavities; bronchiectasis).

Procedure

- A consent form should be signed.
- The client should be NPO for 6 to 8 hours before the test.
- Oral hygiene should be given the night before the test and in the morning. This will decrease the number of bacteria that could be introduced into the lungs.
- Postural drainage is performed for 3 days before the test. This procedure aids in the removal of bronchial mucus and secretions. An expectorant (i.e., potassium iodide) may be ordered for 1 to 3 days before the test to loosen secretions and could detect an allergy to iodine.
- A sedative and atropine are usually given 1 hour before the test. The sedative/tranquilizer is to promote relaxation; atropine is to reduce secretions during the test.
- A topical anesthetic is sprayed into the pharynx and trachea. A catheter is passed through the nose into the trachea, and a local anesthetic and iodized contrast liquid are injected through the catheter.
- The client is usually asked to change body positions so that the contrast dye can reach most areas of the bronchial tree.

- Following the bronchography procedure, the client may receive nebulization and should perform postural drainage to remove contrast dye. Food and fluids are restricted until the gag (cough) reflex is present.

Factors Affecting Diagnostic Results

- Secretions in the tracheobronchial tree can prevent the contrast dye from coating the bronchial walls.

NURSING IMPLICATIONS WITH RATIONALE

- Obtain a signed consent form. Check that the consent form is signed before premedication is given.
- Explain the procedure of the test. Generally clients are extremely apprehensive about this test and are fearful that they may be unable to breathe. Reassure the client that the airway will not be blocked. Inform the patient that he or she may have a sore throat after the test as the result of catheter irritation.
- Obtain a history of hypersensitivity to anesthetics, iodine, and x-ray dyes. Usually the client will receive an expectorant several days before the test to loosen secretions.
- Record vital signs.

Client Teaching

- Instruct the client how to perform postural drainage (over the side of the bed or in the Trendelenberg position for 15 to 20 minutes 3 times a day). It is important that chest secretions be removed prior to the test to ensure good visualization of the bronchial tree.
- Encourage the client to relax, and teach relaxation techniques.
- Instruct the client to practice good oral hygiene the night before and the morning of the test. Check the oral hygiene procedure. Dentures should be removed before the test.
- Answer the client's questions, and refer questions you cannot answer to other appropriate health professionals. Permit the client time to express his or her concerns.

Posttest

- Assess for signs and symptoms of laryngeal edema (i.e., dyspnea, hoarseness apprehension). This could be caused by a traumatic insertion of the catheter.
- Assess for allergic reaction to the anesthetic and iodized contrast dye (i.e., apprehension, flushing, rash, urticaria [hives], dyspnea, tachycardia, and/or hypotension).
- Check the gag reflex to see that it has returned before offering food and fluids. Have the client swallow and cough, or tickle the posterior pharynx with a

cotton swab; if gag reflex is present, offer ice chips or sips of water before food.

- Monitor vital signs. The temperature may be slightly elevated for 1 or 2 days after the test.
- Check breath signs. If rhonchi and fever are present, notify the health care provider and record on the client's chart.
- Have the client perform postural drainage post-test. This procedure helps with the removal of the contrast dye. Physiologic damage will not occur if some of the dye remains in the lung for a period of time.
- Offer throat lozenges or an ordered medication for sore throat.
- Be supportive of the client and family. Be available to answer their questions.

Bronchoscopy

Normal Finding

Normal structure and lining of the larynx, trachea, and bronchi.

Description

Bronchoscopy is the direct inspection of the larynx, trachea, and bronchi through a standard metal bronchoscope or a flexible fiberoptic bronchoscope called a bronchofibroscope. The flexible fiberoptic bronchoscope has a lens and light at its distal end, and because of its smallness in width and its flexibility, it allows for visualization of the segmental and subsegmental bronchi.

Through the bronchoscope, a catheter brush, biopsy forceps, or biopsy needle can be passed to obtain secretions and tissues for cytologic examination. The two main purposes of bronchoscopy are visualization and specimen collection in the tracheobronchial tree. Other purposes include removal of the secretions and laser of the lesions.

Purposes

- To inspect the larynx, trachea, and bronchus for lesions.
- To remove foreign bodies and secretions from the tracheobronchial area.
- To improve tracheobronchial drainage.

Clinical Problems

Indications: Tracheobronchial lesion (i.e., a tumor), bleeding site, foreign bodies, secretions (liquid and tissue) for cytologic and bacteriologic examinations, mucus plugs, tracheobronchial drainage.

Procedure

- A consent form for bronchoscopy should be signed by the client or an appropriate family member.
- The client should be NPO for 6 hours before the bronchoscopy and preferably for 8 to 12 hours.
- The client should remove dentures, contact lenses, jewelry.
- Obtain a history of hypersensitivity to analgesics, anesthetics, and antibiotics.
- Check vital signs and record.
- Administer premedications.
- Record vital signs, premedications, and when the client voided on the preoperative check list and the client's chart.
- The client will be lying on a table in the supine or semi-Fowler's position with the head hyperextended, or he or she will be seated in a chair. Local anesthetic will be sprayed in the client's throat and nose, and the bronchoscope will be inserted through the client's nose or mouth by the health care provider. It is frequently inserted through the mouth when using the rigid scope and is inserted through the nose when using the fiberoptic scope.
- Specimen containers should be labeled, and specimens should be taken immediately to the laboratory. The procedure takes about 1 hour.

Factors Affecting Diagnostic Results

- Improper labeling of the specimen.
- Failure to take specimens immediately to the laboratory.

NURSING IMPLICATIONS WITH RATIONALE

Pretest

- Explain the procedure to the client. Explanation is important to help allay the client's anxiety.
- Check that the consent form is signed and that the client has voided before administering premedications. One of the drugs usually administered is atropine, which causes dryness of the mouth.
- Check that dentures, contact lenses, and jewelry have been removed.
- Obtain vital signs (VS), and prepare a VS flow chart. Record admission and pretest vital signs, which will serve as baseline VS.
- Advise the client that the procedure takes about 1 hour.

Client Teaching

- Instruct the client to relax before and during the test. The premedications will aid in increasing relaxation and decreasing anxiety. Tell the client the health care provider will inform him or her of how the procedure is progressing. Bronchoscopy usually is performed under local anesthesia but could be performed under general anesthesia. The client should be told whether he or she will receive a local or a general anesthetic.

- Inform the client that the drugs will make him or her feel sleepy and the mouth feel dry. The client should remain in bed, and the bed sides should be up after premedications are given.
- Instruct the client to practice breathing in and out through the nose with the mouth opened. This is important if the bronchoscope is inserted through the mouth.
- Encourage the client to ask questions and give him or her time to express concerns. Inform the client that there may be some discomfort but that the spray will help to decrease it. Inform the client that he or she will receive adequate air exchange. Oxygen can be given through the side arm of the bronchoscope or rigid scope and by mask for fiberoptic scope.
- Inform the client that there may be hoarseness and/or a sore throat after the test.

Posttest

- Recognize the complications that can follow bronchoscopy (i.e., laryngeal edema, bronchospasm, pneumothorax, cardiac dysrhythmias, and bleeding from the biopsy site).
- Check VS until stable and as indicated.
- Elevate the head of the bed (semi-Fowler's position). If the client is unconscious, turn him or her on the side with the head of the bed slightly elevated.
- Assess for signs and symptoms of respiratory difficulty (i.e., dyspnea, wheezing, apprehension, and decreased breath sounds). Notify the health care provider at once.
- Check for hemoptysis (coughing up excessive bloody secretions) and, if found, notify the health care provider. Inform the client that some blood-tinged mucus may be coughed up and that this is not abnormal. It usually occurs following a biopsy or after a traumatic insertion of the bronchoscope.
- Assess the gag (cough) reflex before giving food and liquids. Ask the client to swallow or cough. It normally takes 2 to 8 hours before the gag reflex returns. Offer ice chips and sips of water before offering food.
- Offer the client lozenges or prescribed medication for mild throat irritation after the gag reflex is present.
- Be supportive of the client. Touch the client's hand or arm for reassurance, as necessary.

Client Teaching

- Instruct the client not to smoke for 6 to 8 hours. Smoking may cause the client to cough and start bleeding, especially after a biopsy.
- Inform the client that collection of postbronchoscopic secretions may be required for cytologic testing.

Cardiac catheterization

Cardiac Angiography (Angiocardiography), Coronary Arteriography

Normal Finding

Patency of coronary arteries; normal heart size, structure, valves; normal heart and pulmonary pressures.

Description

The first cardiac catheterization was performed in 1844 on a horse. It was not until 1929 that the first right-cardiac catheterization was performed on a human—the young Dr. Werner Forssmann catheterized himself. During the 1930s and 1940s there were a number of right-cardiac catheterizations done, but the first left-cardiac catheterization was not performed until the early 1950s. In the late 1960s and during the 1970s the procedure and equipment for cardiac catheterization were greatly improved.

Cardiac catheterization is a procedure in which a long catheter is inserted into a vein and artery of the arm or leg. This catheter is threaded to the heart chambers and/or coronary arteries with the guidance of fluoroscopy. Contrast dye is injected for visualizing the heart structures. During injection of the dye, cineangiography is used for filming heart activity. The terms *angiocardiography* and *coronary arteriography* are used interchangeably with the term *cardiac catheterization;* however, with coronary arteriography, dye is injected directly into the coronary arteries, and with angiocardiography, dye is injected into heart, coronary, and/or pulmonary vessels.

With *right-cardiac catheterization,* the catheter is inserted into the femoral vein or an antecubital vein and threaded through the inferior vena cava into the right atrium to the pulmonary artery. Right atrium, right ventricle, and pulmonary artery pressures are measured, and blood samples from the right side of the heart can be obtained. While the dye is being injected, the functions of the tricuspid and pulmonary valves can be observed.

For *left-cardiac catheterization,* the catheter is inserted into the brachial or femoral artery and is advanced retrograde through the aorta to the coronary arteries and/or left ventricle. Dye is injected. The patency of the coronary arteries and/or functions of the aortic and mitral valves and the left ventricle can be observed. This procedure is indicated before heart surgery.

The frequency of complications arising from cardiac catheterizations have decreased to <2%. The complications that can occur, although rare, are myocardial infarction, cardiac dysrhythmias, cardiac tamponade, pulmonary embolism, and cerebral embolism (CVA).

Purposes

- To identify coronary artery disease (CAD).
- To determine cardiac valvular disease.

Clinical Problems

Abnormal Findings: *Right-Sided Cardiac Catheterization:* Tricuspid stenosis, pulmonary stenosis, pulmonary hypertension, septal defects. *Left-Sided Cardiac Catheterization:* Coronary artery disease, partial or complete coronary occlusion, mitral stenosis, mitral regurgitation, aortic regurgitation, aortic stenosis, left ventricular hypertrophy, ventricle aneurysm.

Procedure

- Obtain a signed consent form. Check that the health care provider has discussed possible risk factors before the consent form is signed.
- Food and fluids are restricted for 6 to 8 hours before the test, according to the hospital's policy. Some institutions permit clear liquids until 4 hours before the test.
- Antihistamines (e.g., diphenhydramine [Benadryl]) and steroids may be ordered the evening before and the morning of the test if an allergic reaction is suspected, such as to iodine products.
- Medications are restricted for 6 to 8 hours before the test unless otherwise ordered by the health care provider. Oral anticoagulants are discontinued, or the dosage is reduced to prevent excessive bleeding. Heparin may be ordered to prevent thrombi.
- The injection site of the arm or groin is shaved and cleansed with antiseptics.
- The weight and height of the client should be recorded. These are used to calculate the amount of dye needed (i.e., 1 ml/kg of body weight).
- The client should void before receiving the premedications. Dentures should be removed unless this is not indicated.
- Record baseline VS. Note the volume intensity of pulses. VS should be monitored during the test.
- Premedications may be given $\frac{1}{2}$ to 1 hour before the cardiac catheterization.
- The client is positioned on a padded table. Skin anesthetic is given at the site of catheter insertion. Client lies still during insertion of the catheter and filming.
- A 5% dextrose in water (D_5W) infusion is started at a keep-vein-open (KVO) rate for administering emergency drugs, if needed.
- Eletrocardiography (ECG) leads are applied to the chest skin surface to monitor heart activity.
- A local skin anesthetic is injected at the catheter insertion site. A cutdown to locate the vessel may be needed. The client will feel a hot, flushing sensation for several seconds to a minute as the dye is injected.
- Coughing and deep breathing are frequently requested by the health care provider. Coughing can decrease nausea and dizziness and possible dysrhythmia.
- The procedure takes $1\frac{1}{2}$ to 3 hours.

Factors Affecting Diagnostic Results

- Insufficient amount of contrast dye could affect results.
- Movement by the client could cause complications and interfere with the filming.

NURSING IMPLICATIONS WITH RATIONALE

- Explain to the client that the purpose of the test is to check the coronary arteries for blockage or to check for heart valve defects. This test is almost always done before heart surgery, mostly to determine if heart surgery is necessary.
- Explain the procedure to the client. The cardiologist or cardiac surgeon should explain the risk factors to the client.
- Obtain a client history of allergic reactions to seafood, iodine, or iodine contrast dye used in other x-ray tests (e.g., intravenous pyelography). A skin test may be performed to determine the severity of the allergy. An antihistamine (e.g., diphenhydramine [Benadryl]) may be given the day before and/or the day of the test as a prophylactic measure.
- Record baseline VS, and monitor the VS during the procedure.
- Have the client void and remove dentures before the test. Check that the catheter insertion site has been prepped (shaved and cleansed with an antiseptic).
- Encourage the client to ask questions, and allow the client and family time to express any concerns. Refer questions you cannot answer to the cardiologist or other health professionals.
- Administer premedications $1/2$ to 1 hour before the test. Make sure that the client has voided and that the consent form has been signed before giving the premedications.

Client Teaching

- Inform the client that he or she will be in a special cardiac catheterization room. Give information about the padded table, the ECG leads to monitor heart activity, the IV fluids, which will run slowly, the local skin anesthetic, and instructions that he or she may receive (such as to cough and to breath deeply).
- Inform the client that there should be no pain, except some discomfort at the catheter insertion site and from lying on the back. Instruct the client to ask any questions he or she may have during the test. Tell the client to tell the health care provider of any chest pain or difficulty in breathing during the procedure. The client's ECG and VS are monitored.
- Tell the client that a hot, flushing sensation may be felt for a minute or two because of the dye. The reason for this is a brief vasodilation caused by the dye.
- Tell the client that the test takes approximately $1^1/2$ to 3 hours.

Posttest

- Monitor VS (blood pressure, pulse, respirations) every 15 minutes the first hour, every 30 minutes until stable, or as ordered. Temperatures are monitored for several days.

- Observe the catheter insertion site for bleeding or hematoma. Change dressings as needed.
- Check peripheral pulses below the insertion site; if the femoral artery was used, then check the popliteal and dorsalis pedis pulses; if the brachial artery was used, then check the radial pulse. Note the strength of the pulse beat.
- Assess the client's skin color and temperature.
- Be supportive of the client and family. Answer questions, or refer them to the appropriate health professionals. Communicate with the client about the nursing care being given.
- Administer narcotic analgesics or analgesics as ordered for discomfort. Give antibiotics, if ordered.

Client Teaching

- Instruct the client that he or she is to remain on bed rest for 8 to 12 hours. The client can turn from side to side, and the bed may be elevated 30 degrees. The leg should be extended if the femoral artery was used. If the brachial artery was used, the head of the bed can be slightly elevated; however, the arm should be immobilized for 3 hours. Policy concerning positioning may differ among institutions.
- Encourage fluid intake after the test, unless contraindicated (e.g., in the case of congestive heart failure).

Cervicography (cervigram)

Normal Finding

Normal cervical tissue; no abnormal cells found.

Description

Cervicography is a photographic method to record an image of the cervix. This test may be done in conjunction with a Pap smear, colposcopy, and/or routine gynecologic examination. The Pap smear detects cellular changes; whereas the cervigram is a more sensitive means to detect cervical cancer. It can identify some cancerous lesions that were missed by the Pap smear.

Purpose

- To detect cervical cancer.

Clinical Problems

Abnormal Findings: Cancer of the cervix, invasive cervical cancer.

Procedure

- Food and fluids are not restricted.
- The client is placed in the lithotomy position.
- Acetic acid (5%) is swabbed on the cervical area.
- Pathographs are taken of the cervix.
- Aqueous iodine is then swabbed on the cervix; photos follow.
- An endocervical smear is taken; tissue obtained is applied to a slide(s).

Factors Affecting Diagnostic Results

- Cervical mucus that was not removed from the cervix prior to the application of acetic acid and the photography.

NURSING IMPLICATIONS WITH RATIONALE

- Obtain a signed consent form.
- Obtain a history of any gynecologic health problems (e.g., discharge, abnormal bleeding).
- Explain the procedure to the client. Explain that she may experience some discomfort due to the body position and the procedure; however, the discomfort should be mild and short term.
- Be supportive of the client. Allow the client time to express her fears and concerns.

Client Teaching

- Inform the client that she may experience a brown vaginal discharge following the procedure for a few days. The brown discharge is most likely due to the iodine swabbed on the cervix.
- Instruct the client that if great discomfort or heavy discharge occurs, the health care provider should be informed.

Cholangiography (intravenous, percutaneous, t-tube cholangiography)

Normal Finding

Patent biliary ducts (absence of stones and strictures).

Description

Intravenous (IV) cholangiography examines the biliary ducts (hepatic ducts within the liver, the common hepatic duct, the cystic duct, and the common bile duct) by radiographic and tomographic visualization. Often the gallbladder is not well visualized. The contrast substance, an iodine preparation such as iodipamide meglumine (Cholografin) is injected intravenously. Approximately 15 minutes later x-rays are taken. IV cholangiography is a tedious and time-consuming test, and reactions are commoner with the IV contrast substance than with the oral agents.

Percutaneous cholangiography is indicated when biliary obstruction is suspected. The contrast substance is directly instilled into the biliary tree. The process is visualized by fluoroscopy, and spot films are taken.

T-tube cholangiography, also known as postoperative cholangiography, may be done 7 to 8 hours after a cholecystectomy to explore the common bile duct for patency of the duct and to see if any gallstones are left. During the operation, a T-shaped tube is placed in the common bile duct to promote drainage. The contrast substance is injected into the T-tube. A stone or two could be missed during a cholecystectomy, causing occlusion of the duct.

Clinical Problems

Test	Indications/Purposes
IV cholangiography	To detect stricture, stones, or tumor in the biliary system
Percutaneous cholangiography	To detect obstruction of the biliary system, caused from stones, cancer of the pancreas
T-tube cholangiography	To detect obstruction of the common bile duct from stones or stricture; fistula

Procedure

IV Cholangiography

- A consent form for IV cholangiography should be signed.
- The client should be NPO for 8 hours before the test. Some radiologists encourage fat-free liquids before the test to prevent renal toxicity caused by the injected dye.

- A laxative (i.e., citrate of magnesium or castor oil) may be given the night before the test, and a cleansing enema may be given in the morning. Keeping the gastrointestinal tract clear can prevent shadows in the x-ray films. Check with the radiology department for the exact preparation needed.
- A contrast agent, iodipamide meglumine (Cholografin) is injected intravenously while the client is lying on a tilting x-ray table. X-rays are taken every 15 to 30 minutes until the common bile duct is visualized.

Percutaneous Cholangiography

- A consent form for percutaneous cholangiography should be signed.
- The client should be NPO for 8 hours before the test.
- A laxative the night before and cleansing enema the morning of the test may be ordered.
- Preoperative medications usually include sedatives/tranquilizers. An antibiotic may be ordered for 24 to 72 hours before the test for prophylactic purposes.
- The client is placed on a tilting x-ray table that rotates. The upper right quadrant of the abdomen is cleansed and draped. A local (skin) anesthetic is given.
- The client should exhale and hold his or her breath while a needle is inserted with the guidance of fluoroscopy into the biliary tree. Bile is withdrawn, and the contrast substance is then injected. Spot films are taken.
- A sterile dressing is applied to the puncture site.

T-tube Cholangiography

- A consent form for T-tube cholangiography should be signed.
- The client should be NPO for 8 hours before the test.
- A cleansing enema may be ordered in the morning before the test.
- The client lies on an x-ray table, and a contrast agent such as sodium diatrizoate (Hypaque) is injected into the T-tube and an x-ray is taken. The final x-ray is taken 15 minutes later.
- The T-tube may be removed after the procedure or it may be left in place.

Factors Affecting Diagnostic Results

- Obesity and gas or fecal material in the intestines can affect the clarity of the x-ray.

NURSING IMPLICATIONS WITH RATIONALE

- Explain to the client the purpose and procedure for the IV cholangiography, percutaneous cholangiography, or T-tube cholangiography. Check with your institution to see if procedures differ, and make modifications in your explanation to the client. Explain the procedure step by step for the client, as requested. This can decrease high levels of anxiety.
- Obtain a client history of allergies to seafood, iodine, or x-ray dye. Report a history of allergies to these substances to the health care provider, and record in the client's chart.

- Permit the client to express his or her concerns. Answer questions, if possible. Refer questions you cannot answer to other health professionals.
- Check that the consent form has been signed by the client before giving a sedative and before the test.
- Administer the pre-test orders (i.e., laxatives, sedatives, etc.).
- Inform the client having IV cholangiography that the test may take several hours (up to 4 hours).
- Observe for signs and symptoms of allergic reaction to contrast agents (i.e., nausea; vomiting, flushing; rash; urticaria [hives]; hypotension; slurred, thick speech; and dyspnea).
- Check the infusion site for signs of phlebitis (i.e., pain, redness, swelling). Apply warm compresses to the infusion site if symptoms are present, as ordered.
- Check vital signs as ordered following the percutaneous cholangiography.

Client Teaching

- Instruct the client to remain in bed for 6 hours following percutaneous cholangiography.

Cholecystography (oral)

Gallbladder Radiography, Gallbladder (GB) Series

Normal Finding

Normal size and structure of gallbladder. No gallstones.

Description

Oral cholecystography is an x-ray test used to visualize gallstones in the gallbladder. There are two types of gallstones: radiopaque, usually composed of calcium carbonate, and radiolucent, composed of cholesterol or bile pigment. The radiolucent stones are the commonest ones and can be visualized using contrast material (radiopaque dye) absorbed by the gallbladder. It takes 12 to 14 hours for the dye to be concentrated in the gallbaldder. Nonfunctioning liver cells can hamper the excretion of the radiopaque dye.

Failure to visualize the gallbladder could be due to hypermotility of the bowel (diarrhea), liver disease, obstruction of the cystic duct, and inadequate patient preparation (i.e., a high-fat diet the night before will cause the gallbladder to empty, thus losing the dye). If the gallbladder cannot be visualized using an oral-contrast substance, the IV cholangiography may be ordered.

Immediately after the oral cholecystography test, the client may be given a fat-stimulus meal. Fluoroscopic examination and x-rays are taken to observe the ability of the gallbladder to empty the dye. If x-rays of the gastrointestinal tract are ordered, the gallbladder x-ray should be obtained first, because barium could interfere with the test results.

Purposes

- To detect stones or tumor in the gallbladder.
- To check for obstruction of the cystic duct.

Clinical Problems

Abnormal Findings: Cholelithiasis (gallstones), neoplasms (tumors) of the gallbladder, cholecystitis (inflammation of the gallbladder, with or without stones), obstruction of the cystic duct.

Procedure

- The client should have a fat-free diet 24 hours before the x-ray. Some x-ray departments suggest a high-fat meal at noon to empty the gallbladder and then a low-fat meal in the evening. After the dinner meal the night before the test, the client should be NPO except for sips of water.
- Two hours after the dinner meal, radiopaque tablets are administered according to the directions on the package. There are various commercial contrast agents (i.e., iopanoic acid [Telepaque], calcium or sodium spodate [Oragrafin], iodoalphionic acid [Priodax], and iodipamide meglumine [Cholografin]). The client should take the tablets or capsules (6 tablets of iopanoic acid) 5 minutes apart with a full glass of water (240 ml total).
- No laxatives should be taken until after the x-ray tests. Some x-ray departments request a saline enema the morning of the test to clear the gastrointestinal tract so that fecal material does not interfere with the gallbladder test.
- A high-fat meal (cream, butter, eggs) or synthetic fat-containing substances (Bilevac) may be given in the x-ray department after the fasting x-rays are taken. Post–fatty-meal films will be taken at intervals to determine how fast the gallbladder expels the dye.
- The fasting x-ray tests (stage I) takes from 45 minutes to 1 hour, and the post–fatty-meal tests (stage II) take another hour or two.

Factors Affecting Diagnostic Results

- Inadequate patient preparation (i.e., a high-fat meal the night before, not taking all the tablets).

- Gastrointestinal series, barium enema, thyroid scan, I-131 uptake before the cholecystography test.
- Diarrhea or vomiting, which can inhibit absorption of the contrast substance.
- Liver disease.

NURSING IMPLICATIONS WITH RATIONALE

- Explain the test purpose and procedure to the client. Check your x-ray department's procedure for changes, and modify the procedure if needed. Some institutions send a written procedure to clients who are not hospitalized.
- Obtain a history of allergies the client may have to seafood, iodine, or x-ray dye.
- Observe for signs and symptoms of jaundice (i.e., yellow sclera of the eyes, yellow skin, and a serum bilirubin level >3 mg/dl).
- Administer the radiopaque tablets every 5 minutes with a full glass of water 2 hours after the dinner meal. Clients may take the tablets on their own, but they may need to be reminded.
- Observe for signs and symptoms of allergic reaction to the radiopaque tablets (i.e., elevated temperature, rash, urticaria [hives], hypotension, thick speech, or dyspnea).
- Report vomiting and diarrhea prior to the test to the health care provider. The tablets may not be absorbed because of hypermotility. The test is then canceled.
- Report to the health care provider and/or the x-ray department if the client is scheduled for a barium enema, gastrointestinal series, thyroid scan, or I-131 uptake before the GB series. These tests should be done after the GB series to prevent test interference.

Client Teaching

- Inform the client that the evening meal before the test should be fat free. If there are foods high in fat on the tray (i.e., whole milk, cream, butter, sauces, fatty meats, etc.), the client should not eat them. In some institutions coffee or tea with sugar is given in the morning.
- Explain to the client that it is not uncommon for the test to be repeated and that he or she should not be alarmed. If the test is repeated, the client should remain on a low-fat diet, and the radiopaque tablets should be taken again as directed.
- Inform the client that the test does not hurt. Check to determine if there are two stages of the test; the first stage takes approximately 45 minutes to 1 hour. If the second stage is ordered, the client will receive a high-fat meal or fat-containing agent, and then more x-ray pictures will be taken.

Chorionic villi biopsy (CVB)

Normal Finding

Normal fetal cells.

Description

Chorionic villi sampling can detect early fetal abnormalities. Fetal cells are obtained by suction from fingerlike projections around the embryonic membrane, which eventually becomes the placenta. The test is performed between the eighth and tenth weeks of pregnancy. After the tenth week, maternal cells begin to grow over the villi.

The advantages of CVB over amniocentesis is that CVB may be performed earlier, and results can be obtained in a few days and not weeks. CVB can diagnose many chromosomal and biochemical fetal disorders. The disadvantage is that CVB cannot determine neural-tubal defects and pulmonary maturity.

Purpose

- To detect chromosomal disorders.

Clinical Problems

Indications: Chromosomal disorders, hemoglobinopathies such as sickle cell anemia, lysosomal storage disorders such as Tay-Sachs disease.

Procedure

- A consent form should be signed.
- There is no food or fluid restriction.
- Place the client in the lithotomy position.
- Ultrasound is used to verify the placement of the catheter at the villi. Suction is applied, and tissue is removed from the villi.
- Test takes approximately 30 minutes.

Factors Affecting Diagnostic Results

- Performing test after 10 weeks of gestation.

NURSING IMPLICATIONS WITH RATIONALE

- Obtain a history of last menstrual period (LMP) from the client and a history of family genetic disorders.
- Assess for signs of spontaneous abortion resulting from procedure, such as cramping, bleeding.

- Assess for infection resulting from procedure, such as chills, fever.
- Be supportive of client and family. Be a good listener.

Client Teaching

- Explain to the client that she will be in a lithotomy position and that ultrasound is used during the procedure.
- Instruct the client to report if excessive bleeding or severe cramping occurs after the procedure.

Colonoscopy

Normal Finding

Normal mucosa of the large intestine; absence of pathology.

Description

Colonoscopy is an inspection of the large intestine (colon) using a long, flexible fiberscope (colonoscope). This instrument is inserted anally and is advanced through the rectum, the sigmoid colon, and the large intestine to the cecum. Occasionally fluoroscopy may be used to guide the colonoscope through the intestine and to locate the tip of the colonoscope when it does not advance.

This test is useful for evaluating suspicious lesions in the large colon (i.e., tumor mass, polyps, and inflammatory tissue). Biopsy of the tissue or polyp can be obtained. The biopsy forceps or cytologic brush is passed through the scope to obtain the tissue specimen. Polyps can be removed with the use of an electrocautery snare.

Colonoscopy should not be done on pregnant women near term, following an acute myocardial infarction, after recent abdominal surgery, in acute diverticulitis, in severe (active) ulcerative colitis, or in a confused/uncooperative patient. Occasionally colon perforation is caused by the fiberscope; however, this is rare. Bleeding may be a side effect of the biopsy or polypectomy.

Purposes

- To detect the orgin of lower intestinal bleeding.
- To identify polyps in the large intestine.
- To screen for benign or malignant lesions (tumors) in the colon.

Clinical Problems

Indications: Lower-intestinal bleeding, diverticular disease, or benign or malignant lesions (i.e., polyps or tumors); ulcerative colitis.

Procedure

- A consent form should be signed.
- Specific laboratory tests (hemoglobin, hematocrit, prothrombin time, partial thromboplastin time, and platelet count) should be done within the 2 days before the test.
- Iron medication should be withheld at least 4 days before the procedure. Medications that interfere with coagulation should be withheld for at least 5 days before the procedure.
- A sedative/tranquilizer may be ordered prior to the test to promote relaxation. A narcotic analgesic and a benzodiazepine may be titrated IV during the procedure.
- Glucagon or IV anticholinergics may be given to decrease bowel spasms.
- Barium sulfate from other diagnostic studies can decrease visualization; therefore the study should not be attempted within 10 days to 2 weeks of a barium study.
- Avoid using soapsuds enemas. These can irritate intestine.
- Specimen containers should be labeled with the client's name, date, and the type of tissue.
- Emergency drugs and equipment should be available for hypersensitivity to medications (premedications and anesthetic) and for possible respiratory depression from narcotics and/or tranquilizers.
- Client should be accompanied by someone who can drive him or her home following the test.
- The procedure takes from $\frac{1}{2}$ to $1\frac{1}{2}$ hours.

Preparation A (Use of GoLytely/Colyte Solution)
- Two days prior to test, have client take magnesium citrate at 4 PM.

Day before Test
- Client should prepare GoLytely or Colyte solution according to instructions, and refrigerate solution.
- Client should have a regular lunch.
- Client should have a liquid dinner (i.e., broth, gelatine, etc.).
- Client should drink GoLytely/Colyte as instructed at 7 PM to 10 PM.

Morning of Test
- Client may drink 8 oz of clear liquid (black coffee, tea, water, clear juice) up to 1 hour before test.

Preparation B (72-hour Clear Liquid/Enemas)
- Client should maintain clear liquid diet 3 days before test.
- Client should follow 48-hour Fleet Prep Kit No. 2.

Factors Affecting Diagnostic Results

- A soapsuds enema can cause intestinal irritation.
- Barium sulfate from other diagnostic studies can decrease visualization; therefore the study should not be attempted within 10 days to 2 weeks of a barium study.
- Inadequate bowel preparation with fecal material remaining in the colon will decrease visualization.

NURSING IMPLICATIONS WITH RATIONALE

Pretest

- Explain the procedure of the test. The client lies in the Sims position on left side. A lubricated colonoscope is inserted. Air will be insufflated for better visualization. X-rays may be taken.
- Record baseline vital signs and pertinent laboratory values.
- Report anxiety and fears to the health care provider conducting the procedure.

Client Teaching

- Instruct the client to bring someone to drive him/her home.
- Inform the client that the procedure takes from $\frac{1}{2}$ to $1\frac{1}{2}$ hours.
- Instruct the client to breathe deeply and slowly through the mouth during the insertion of the colonoscope.

Posttest

- Monitor vital signs every $\frac{1}{2}$ hour for at least 1 hour or until stable.
- Assess for anal bleeding, abdominal distention, severe pain, severe abdominal cramps, and fever, and report any of these signs or symptoms to the health care provider *immediately*.

Colposcopy

Normal Finding

Normal appearance of the vagina and cervical structures.

Description

Colposcopy is the examination of the vagina and cervix using a binocular instrument (colposcope) that has a magnifying lens and a light. This test is for identifying precancerous lesions of the cervix and can be performed in the gynecologist's office or in the hospital. After a positive Papanicolaou (Pap) smear or a suspicious cervical lesion, colposcopy is indicated for examining the vagina and cervix more thoroughly. Atypical epithelium, leukoplakia vulvae, and irregular blood vessels can be identified with this procedure, and photographs and a biopsy specimen can be obtained.

Since this test has become more popular, there has been a decreased need for conization (surgical removal of a cone of tissue from the cervical os). Colposcopy is also useful for monitoring women whose mothers received diethylstilbestrol during pregnancy; these women are prone to develop precancerous and cancerous lesions of the vagina and cervix. Colposcopy is used to monitor female patients who have had cervical lesions removed.

Purpose

■ To identify precancerous lesions of the cervix.

Clinical Problems

Indications: Vaginal and cervical lesions, abnormal cervical tissue after a positive Pap smear, irregular blood vessels, leukoplakia vulvae; dysplasia and cervical lesions, vaginal and cervical tissue changes for women whose mothers took diethylstilbestrol during pregnancy.

Procedure

■ A consent form should be signed.
■ Food and fluids are not restricted.
■ The client's clothes should be removed, and the client should wear a gown and be properly draped.
■ The client assumes a lithotomy position (legs in stirrups). A speculum is inserted into the vagina, and a long, dry cotton swab applicator is used to clear away any cervical secretions. Another long cotton-swab applicator with saline may be used to swab the cervix for visualizing vascular patterns.
■ Acetic acid (3%) is applied to the vagina and cervix. This produces color changes in the cervical epithelium and helps in detecting abnormal changes.
■ A biopsy specimen of suspicious tissues and photographs may be taken. Pressure should be applied to control bleeding at the biopsy site, or cautery may be used.
■ A vaginal tampon may be worn after the procedure.
■ The test takes approximately 15 to 20 minutes.

Factors Affecting Diagnostic Results

■ Mucus, cervical secretions, creams, and medications can decrease visualization.

NURSING IMPLICATIONS WITH RATIONALE

■ Explain the purpose and procedure to the client.
■ A consent form should be signed.

- Encourage the client to ask questions and to express any concerns or fears. Reducing anxiety is important for the client and for the test. Remain with the client during the procedure.
- Place the biopsy tissue into a bottle containing a preservative and place the cells, if obtained, on a slide and spray them with a fixative solution.

Client Teaching

- Inform the client that she should not experience pain but that there may be some discomfort with the insertion of the speculum or when the biopsy specimen is taken.
- Tell the client that the test takes 15 to 20 minutes.

Posttest-Client Teaching

- Inform the client that she may have some bleeding for a few hours because of the biopsy. Tell the client that she can use tampons and that if bleeding becomes heavy and it is not her menstrual period, she should call the gynecologist.
- Instruct the client not to have intercourse for a week until the biopsy site is healed or as ordered by the health care provider.
- Inform the client that she should be notified of the results, and tell her to call if she has not heard from the office in a week.

Computed tomography (CT) scan, computed axial tomography (CAT)

CAT Scan, Computed Transaxial Tomography (CTT), EMI Scan

Normal Finding

Normal tissue; no pathologic findings.

Description

The computed tomography (CT) scan was developed in England in 1972 by the Electric Music Industries, Ltd., and was originally called the EMI scan. Other names for the CT scan are computed axial tomography, or CAT scan; computed transaxial (transverse) tomography, or CTT scan; and computer-assisted transaxial tomography, or CATT scan. The preferred term is computed tomography, or CT scan.

The CT scanner produces a narrow x-ray beam that examines body sections from many different angles. The CT scanner can revolve around the client who is lying on a table. It produces a series of cross-sectional images in sequence that build up a three-dimensional picture of the organ or structure. The traditional x-ray takes a flat or frontal picture, which gives a two-dimensional view. The CT scanner is about 100 times more sensitive than the x-ray machine. Although it is a costly diagnostic test, CT scanning is popular because it can diagnose an early stage of disease.

The CT scan can be performed with or without iodine contrast media (dye). It is not an invasive test unless contrast dye is used. The contrast dye causes a greater tissue absorption and is referred to as *contrast enhancement*. This enhancement enables small tumors to be seen.

CT is capable of scanning the head (internal auditory canal, eye orbits, sinuses, neck), abdomen (stomach, small and large intestines, liver, spleen, pancreas, bile duct, kidney, and adrenals), pelvis (bladder, reproductive organs, and small and large bowel within pelvis), chest (lung, heart, mediastinal structure) and bones and joints. Magnetic resonance imaging (MRI), a noninvasive test, has *not* replaced CT scans; see discussion of MRI on pages 559–563.

High-speed and ultrafast electron beam (EBCT) scans are CT terms that are often incorrectly used interchangeably. These terms describe two different CT scanners, high-speed and ultrafast (Electron beam) scanners. Both of these scanners have the ability to perform helical scanning and three-dimensional reconstruction of images. Helical scanning, also known as spiral scanning, is made possible through the use of slip-ring techology. A slip ring has no direct wire connection to the x-ray tube, allowing it to rotate indefinitely in one direction (Bonk). These scanners differ in one very large aspect. The high-speed scanner uses radiographic exposures averaging 1 second, sufficient time to image most anatomy. The EBCT scanner uses radiographic exposures of 100 milliseconds (Wright). This short exposure time is important for it enables the EBCT to accurately image the heart and coronary vessels.

Head and Brain CT: The CT of the brain/head provides three-dimensional views of the brain consisting of cross-sectional images of brain tissue layers. This procedure can differentiate between tumors, aneurysms, cerebral infarction, and intracranial hemorrhage and hematoma. Also this CT scan can detect ventricular displacement or enlargement. Visualization of the pathology can be enhanced with IV iodinated contrast dye. With the availability of brain CT, cerebral angiography and pneumoencephalography are seldom ordered.

Chest (Thoracic) CT: CT of the chest gives a cross-sectional view of the chest at different angles to differentiate between various pathologic conditions: tumors, nodules, cysts, abscesses, hematomas, and aortic aneurysms. It can detect pleural effusion and enlarged lymph nodes in the chest area. The use of IV contrast media aids in highlighting blood vessels, thus identifying abnormalities of the vascular structures. CT of the chest can be useful in evaluating the effects of treatment therapy on the tumor and if metastasis has occurred.

Abdominal CT: CT of the abdomen is useful for diagnosing tumors, obstructions, cysts, hematoma, abscesses, bleeding, perforation, calculi, fibroids, and other pathologic conditions that appear in the liver, biliary tract, pancreas, spleen, GI tract, gallbladder, kidneys, adrenals, uterus and ovaries, and prostate. IV contrast dye may be used to enhance visualization. The kidney and urinary flow is easily seen with the use of contrast dye. Oral contrast media may be used for scanning the GI tract. The CT scan is useful for staging tumors and monitoring the effects of treatment therapy on the tumor.

Spine CT: CT scan of the spine gives cross-sectional images that are displayed as three-dimensional views on a monitor. It is mainly used to view the vertebral area. Contrast dye may be injected into the spinal column via lumbar puncture for clearer visualization. MRI is the preferred study of the spine; however, if MRI is contraindicated or unavailable, then contrast CT would likely be ordered.

Long Bones and Joints CT: Skeletal CT provides cross-sectional images of the bone. This procedure is useful to detect bone and soft tissue tumors and bone metastases. Joint abnormalities can be identified with this CT. Contrast dye may be ordered.

Purposes

- To screen for coronary artery disease; head, liver, and renal lesions; tumors; edema; abscesses; infection; metastatic disease; vascular diseases; stroke; bone destruction.
- To locate foreign objects in soft tissues, such as the eye.

Clinical Problems

CT Type	Abnormal Findings
Head	Cerebral lesions: hematomas, tumors, cysts, abscess, infarction, edema, atrophy, hydrocephalus
Internal auditory canal	Acoustic neuroma, cholesteatoma, bone erosion
Eye orbits	Bone destruction, optic nerve tumors, muscle tumor
Sinus	Bone destruction, sinusitis, polyps, tumors
Neck (soft tissue)	Tumors, abscess, stones in the salivary ducts, enlarged nodes
Abdomen	
Liver	Hepatic lesions: cysts, abscess, tumors, hematomas, cirrhosis with ascites
Biliary	Obstruction due to calculi
Pancreatic	Acute and chronic pancreatitis; pancreatic lesions: tumor, abscess, pseudocysts
Kidney	Renal lesions: tumors, calculi, cysts, congenital anomalies; perirenal hematomas and abscesses
Adrenal	Adrenal tumors
Chest and thoracic	Chest lesions: tumors, cysts, abscesses; aortic aneurysm; enlarged lymph nodes in mediastinum; pleural effusion
Spine	Tumors, paraspinal cysts, vascular malformation, congenital spinal anomalies (e.g., spina bifida, herniated intervertebral disk)
Bony pelvis, long bones, joints	Bone destruction, fractures, tumors
Guided needle biopsy	For lung or liver masses, adrenal mass, kidney

Procedure

General Preparation for All Scans

- A consent form should be signed.
- There is no food or fluid restriction if contrast dye is NOT used.
- For IV contrast injection studies, usually there is NPO (nothing by mouth) 4 hours prior to the CT. Diabetics may be given orange juice instead of water; check with the health care provider or CT supervisor. For PM scheduling: NPO after a liquid breakfast.
- Prescribed medications may be given with a small amount of water prior to the CT scan; check with the health care provider or CT supervisor.
- A mild sedative may be ordered for some clients to alleviate anxiety.
- Client should remain still/motionless during the procedure.
- If contrast media (dye) is ordered and the client is allergic to iodine products, steroids or antihistamines may be given before the scan or may be given IV during the CT scan.

Suggested Prophylactic Premedication for Clients Having Allergy to Contrast Dye

Time Before CT	Drug	Dose
13 hours	Prednisone, PO	50 mg
7 hours	Prednisone, PO	50 mg
1 hour	Prednisone, PO	50 mg
	Benadryl, PO	50 mg
	Zantac, PO	150 mg

Veterans Affairs Medical Center, Wilmington, DE.

- IV infusion or heparin lock insertion may be required prior to test. Use a 19- or 20-gauge needle. Never insert the needle into the antecubital area (anterior bend of the elbow).
- CT scanning usually takes 30 minutes to 1½ hours.

Head CT

- Remove hairpins, braids, clips, and jewelry (earrings) before the test.
- Remove dentures prior to the use of contrast dye.
- A mild sedative or analgesic may be ordered for restless clients or for those who have aches and pains of the neck or back.
- Head is positioned in a cradle, and a wide, rubberized strap is applied snugly around the head to keep it immobilized during test.

Neck CT

- IV contrast media is used. Check general preparation for scan for IV contrast injection studies.

Abdominal and Pelvic CT

- Abdominal x-ray (including the kidneys, ureters, and bladder) may be requested before CT scan.
- The gastrointestinal tract must be free from barium. An enema may be ordered.
- Current laboratory reports of serum creatinine and blood urea nitrogen should be available to determine if there is kidney dysfunction and if so to what degree. These tests should be done 7 days prior to the CT scan with contrast injection.
- For an AM abdominal/pelvic scan, give the oral contrast media (15 oz) between 8 PM and 10 PM the evening before the scan. NPO after 10 PM. One hour prior to the CT, give ½ bottle of the oral contrast. One-half hour prior to the CT, give the remaining ½ bottle of oral contrast.
- For a PM abdominal/pelvic scan, give 1 bottle (15 oz) of oral contrast media at 7 AM the morning of the scan. NPO after 7 AM. One hour prior to the CT, give ½ bottle of the oral contrast. One-half hour prior to the CT, give ½ bottle of the oral contrast.

Chest CT

- A chest x-ray may be requested before a chest scan.
- IV contrast media is frequently given in the left arm.

Spine CT

- NPO is not indicated, because contrast media is usually not ordered.
- Spine x-rays taken prior to scan should be available. Spine CT should be done after myelography.

Bony Pelvis, Long Bone, and Joint CT

- The nuclear medicine study to locate "hot areas" should be done before the CT scan of the bones and joints.

Factors Affecting Diagnostic Results

- Barium sulfate can obscure visualization of the abdominal organs. Barium studies should be performed 4 days before the CT or after the CT.
- Excessive flatus can cause client discomfort and may cause an inaccurate reading.
- Movement can cause artifacts.
- Metal plates in skull and metal bridges.
- Dental fillings.

NURSING IMPLICATIONS WITH RATIONALE

Pretest

- Explain the procedure to the client. The CT scanner is circular, with a doughnut-like opening. The client is strapped to a special table, with the scanner revolving around the body area that is to be examined. Clicking noises will be heard from the scanner. The radiologist or specialized technician is stationed in a control room and can observe and communicate with the client at all times through an intercom system. The test is not painful.

- Inform the client that holding breath may be requested several times during an abdominal scan.
- Inform the client that the CT of the head takes 10 minutes without contrast media and 20 minutes with use of contrast. For body CT, the test takes 30 to 60 minutes.
- Obtain a history of allergies to seafood, iodine, and contrast dye from other x-ray tests. Contrast enhancement is not always done with CT, especially chest and spinal CT scanning.
- Advise the client that if contrast dye is injected IV, a warm, flushed sensation may be felt in the face or body. A salty, "fishy," or metallic taste, and a sensation of urinating (does not occur) may be experienced. Nausea is not uncommon. These sensations usually last for 1 or 2 minutes.
- Observe for signs and symptoms of a severe allergic reaction to the dye (i.e., dyspnea, palpitations, tachycardia, hypotension, itching, and urticaria). Emergency drugs should be available.

Posttest

- Observe for delayed allergic reaction to the contrast dye (i.e., skin rash, urticaria, headache, and vomiting). An oral antihistamine may be ordered for mild reactions.
- If contrast dye has been used, instruct the client to increase fluid intake to enhance the excretion of the dye.
- Be supportive of the client and family. The CT scan can be frightening. The major risk involved is an allergic reaction to the dye.

Client Teaching

- Instruct the client to resume his or her usual level of activity and diet, unless otherwise indicated.

Cordocentesis (see fetoscopy)

Corneal staining

Normal Findings

The cornea is free of injuries.

Description

Corneal staining with fluorescein dye enhances the visualization of corneal injuries, such as scratches and abrasions. The use of slit-lamp examination may be used along with the corneal staining to identify the type of injury to the cornea.

Purpose

- To detect the corneal injury that may have occurred to the cornea of the eye.

Clinical Problems

Abnormal Findings: Corneal abrasions, scratches, and ulcerations.

Procedure

- Signed consent form may be required.
- Flourescein strip deposits the dye by the strip touching the lower conjunctival sac.
- Client closes his/her eyes, opens and closes the eyes again to spread the dye over the cornea.
- With the forehead placed against a bar, the client looks straight ahead, and the eye(s) are examined.
- For several hours after the procedure, blurring may occur.

Factors Affecting Diagnostic Results

- The inability of the client to remain still.

NURSING IMPLICATIONS WITH RATIONALE

- Obtain a history of the eye injury.
- Ask if the client is allergic to dye, particularly fluorescein dye.

Client Teaching

- Inform the client that this procedure should not cause pain, maybe some discomfort.

Cystometry cystometrogram (CMG)

Normal Findings

Adult: Urine stream: Strong and uninterrupted. Normal filling pattern and sensation of fullness. Bladder capacity: 300 to 600 ml; Residual urine: 0 to 30 ml; Urge to void: >150 ml; Fullness felt: >300 ml.

Child: Bladder capacity and urinary flow vary with age.

Description

Cystometry or cystometrogram (CMG) evaluates the neuromuscular function of the bladder. After the instillation of a measured quanity of fluid, this test measures the efficiency of the detrusor muscle, the intravesical pressure and capacity, and the effect of thermal stimulation. CMG is used for evaluating bladder dysfunction caused by neurologic disorder or disease, such as spinal cord injury, stroke, multiple sclerosis, diabetes mellitus, and it also includes stress incontinence, urinary/stress incontinence, and the effects of drugs the client is taking.

Urethral pressure profile (UPP) is frequently performed during the cystometry. A *special* catheter that had been inserted is slowly withdrawn as the urethral pressures are measured. These tests may be conducted in a urologist's office or clinic.

Cystometry is contraindicated for a client with an urinary tract infection (UTI).

Purposes

- To evaluate the detrusor muscle function and tonicity of the bladder.
- To measure the urethral pressures.
- To determine the cause of bladder dysfunction.

Clinical Problems

Abnormal Findings/Causes: Stress incontinence; neurogenic bladder from spinal cord injury, stroke, multiple sclerosis, diabetes mellitus; postoperative urinary dysfuntion, bladder and prostate obstruction.

Procedure

- A signed consent form.
- No food or fluid restriction.
- Have the client urinate into a container attached to a machine that records the force of the urinary flow, amount, and the completion time.
- Insert a retention catheter to measure residual urine volume.
- Test for thermal sensation: Instill 30 to 50 ml of room-temperature normal saline solution (NSS) into the bladder. Client should report the sensation that is felt. The NSS is then withdrawn. Instill 30 ml of 30 to 40° C of NSS. Again the client

reports his/her sensations as, a feeling of warmth, flushing, need to void, and/or discomfort. The bladder is then drained.

- Connect the catheter to a cystometer (a tube to monitor bladder presssures). Normal saline solution, sterile water, OR gas (carbon dioxide) is *slowly* instilled into the bladder. The cystometer graphically records the data. The client tells when he/she can no longer hold the urine without voiding; the liquid instillation is stopped, and the catheter is removed. Client is to void, but not strain when voiding. Again, the voiding pressure is recorded. If gas is used, the gas is withdrawn and the pressures from the urethral wall is obtained.
- The cholinergic drug, bethanechol (Urecholine), an urinary stimulant, may be administered during the cystometric procedure to enhance the bladder tone.
- This test takes approximately 45 minutes to 1 hour.

Factors Affecting Diagnostic Test

- Antihistamines cause relaxation of the bladder muscle and wall, thus, bladder function can be inhibited.

NURSING IMPLICATIONS WITH RATIONALE

- Obtain a history of the client's urinary problem and what drugs the client is taking daily.
- Check vital signs which may be the baseline for the posttest.
- Discuss the procedure with the client.

Client Teaching

- Inform the client that he/she may have a strong urge to urinate during the test and that this is not abnormal. Tell the client to let the urologist know what sensations that he/she may have at various times during the test.

Posttest
Client Teaching

- Inform the client that he/she may have bladder spasms after the test. An analgesic is usually prescribed. After 24 hours, if the bladder spasms continue, the health care provider should be called.
- Notify the health care provider if blood in the urine occurs 4 to 6 hours posttest or after the third voiding.
- Explain to the client who received carbon dioxide gas that it may cause posttest discomfort.
- Instruct the client to report fever, dysuria, or urinary frequency to the health care provider. Urinary tract infection (UTI) may have resulted from this procedure and needs to be reported and treated.
- Encourage the client to increase fluid intake. Measurement of intake and output may be requested.

Cystoscopy, cystography (cystogram)

Normal Finding

Normal structure of the urethra, bladder, prostatic urethra, and ureter orifices.

Description

Cystoscopy is the direct visualization of the bladder wall and urethra with the use of cystoscope (a tubular lighted telescopic lens). Usually this diagnostic test is performed by a urologist. Small renal calculi can be removed from the ureter, bladder, or urethra with this procedure, and a tissue biopsy can be obtained. In addition, *retrograde pyelography* (injection of contrast dye through the catheter into the ureters and renal pelvis) may be performed during the cystoscopy.

Cystoscopy is performed in a cystoscopy room of a hospital or in a urologist's office under general or local anesthesia. Premedications are administered an hour prior to the test.

Cystography is the instillation of a contrast dye into the bladder via a catheter. This procedure can detect a rupture in the bladder, a neurogenic bladder, fistulas, and tumors. The test is useful when x-rays are needed and a cystoscopy or retrograde pyelography is contraindicated.

Purposes

- To detect renal calculi and renal tumor.
- To remove renal stones.
- To determine the cause of hematuria or urinary tract infection (UTI).

Clinical Problems

Abnormal Findings: Hematuria or urinary tract infection; renal calculi (stones), tumors, or prostatic hyperplasia.

Procedure

- A consent form should be signed.
- The client can have a full liquid breakfast the morning of the test if local anesthetic is used. Several glasses of water may be ordered. If general anesthesia is to be administered, the client should be NPO for 8 hours before cystoscopy.
- Record baseline vital signs.
- A narcotic analgesic (meperidine, morphine) may be ordered an hour before the cystoscopy. The procedure is done under local or general anesthesia.

- The client is placed in a lithotomy position (feet or legs in stirrups). A local anesthetic is injected into the urethra. Water may be instilled to enhance better visualization. A urine specimen may be obtained.
- The cystoscopy takes approximately 30 minutes to 1 hour.

Factors Affecting Diagnostic Results

- None reported.

NURSING IMPLICATIONS WITH RATIONALE

Pretest

- Obtain history concerning the presence of cystitis or prostatitis, which could result in sepsis.
- Explain the procedure to the client. Answer, questions or refer questions you cannot answer to the urologist.
- Check with the urologist about the form of anesthesia the client will receive—local or general. Inform the client that a local anesthetic will be injected into the urethra several minutes before the cystoscope is inserted.
- Check that the consent form has been signed before administering the premedications. Normally the drugs are given 1 hour before the test.
- Check with the client concerning hypersensitivity to anesthetics.
- Assess urinary patterns, such as amount, color, odor, specific gravity of the urine.
- Take baseline vital signs.

Client Teaching

- Inform the client that there may be some pressure or burning discomfort during and/or following the test.

Posttest

- Recognize the complications that can occur as a result of the cystoscopy, such as hemorrhaging, perforation of the bladder, urinary retention, and infection.
- Monitor vital signs (VS). Compare with baseline VS. VS may be ordered every half hour until stable.
- Monitor the urinary output for 48 hours following a cystoscopy. If urine output is <200 ml in 8 hours, encourage fluid intake. Anuria could indicate urinary retention due to blood clots or urethral stricture. Report findings to the urologist. An indwelling catheter may be ordered.
- Report and record gross hematuria. Inform the client that blood-tinged urine is not uncommon after a cystoscopic examination.
- Observe for signs and symptoms of an infection (i.e., fever, chills, an increased pulse rate, and pain). Antibiotics may be given before and after the test as a prophylactic measure.
- Apply heat to the lower abdomen to relieve pain and muscle spasm as ordered.

Client Teaching

- Advise the client to avoid alcoholic beverages for 2 days after the test.
- Inform the client that a slight burning sensation when voiding for a day or two is considered normal. Usually the urologist leaves an order for an analgesic.

Echocardiography (echocardiogram)

M-Mode, Two-Dimensional (2D), Spectral Doppler, Color Flow Doppler, Transesphageal, Contrast, and Stress Echocardiography*

Normal Findings

Normal heart size and structure; normal movements of heart valves and heart chambers.

Description

Echocardiography (echocardiogram) is a noninvasive ultrasound test used to identify abnormal heart size, structure, and function, and valvular disease. A hand-held transducer (probe) is moved over the chest in the area of the heart and other specified surrounding areas. The transducer sends and receives high-frequency sound waves. The sound waves that are reflected (echo) from the heart back to the transducer produce pictures. These pictures appear on a television-like screen and are recorded on videotape and moving graph paper.

There are several types of echocardiographic studies, which include M-mode, two-dimensional (2D), spectral doppler, color doppler, transesophageal, contrast, and stress echocardiography. Transesophageal echocardiography (TEE) is gaining popularity for diagnosing and managing a wide range of cardiovascular diseases, such as valvular heart dysfunction and aortic pathology. Stress echocardiography is a valuable tool for assessing myocardial ischemia at half the cost of other cardiac studies.

M-Mode Echocardiography: M-mode echocardiography, the earliest type of echocardiography, is used to record the motion of various heart structures (M is for *motion*). This test assesses the dimension of the left ventricle and its degree of dilatation and contractility related to myocardial disease or volume overload. It is useful for measuring the thickness of the right and left ventricles (hypertrophy). M-mode echocardiography is also used for assessing the cardiac valves and valvular movements for stenosis, regurgitation, or prolapse.

---

*Revised by Frank Di Gregorio, CNMT, RDMS, Director, Community Imaging Center, Wilmington, DE.

Two-Dimensional (2D) Echocardiography: This test employs M-mode echocardiography, which records motion, and provides two-dimensional (cross-sectional) views of the heart structures. It is used to evaluate the size, shape, and movement of the chambers and valves of the heart and it is useful in detecting valvular disease and in assessing congenital heart disease.

Spectral Doppler Echocardiography: Spectral doppler echocardiography measures the amount, speed, and direction of blood passing through the heart valves and heart chambers. A swishing sound is heard as the blood flows throughout the heart. This test can detect tubulent blood flow through the heart valves, which may indicate valvular disease. Septal wall defects may also be detected.

Color Doppler Echocardiography: Color doppler (red and blue) echocardiography shows the direction of blood flowing through the heart. It can identify leaking heart valves (regurgitation) or hardened valves (stenosis), malfunction of prosthetic valves, and the presence of shunts (holes) in the heart. The use of the color doppler compliments 2D echocardiography and the spectral doppler study.

Transesophageal Echocardiography: With transesophageal echocardiography (TEE), a transducer (probe) is attached to an endoscope and is inserted into the esophagus to visualize adjacent cardiac and extracardiac structures with greater acuity than most echocardiography studies, including transthoracic (TTE). TEE can be used in the intensive care unit, emergency department and operating room, as well as in cardiac testing facilities. This type of echocardiography is useful for diagnosing mitral and aortic valvular pathology; determining the presence of a possible intracardiac thrombus in the left atrium; detecting suspected acute dissection of the aorta and endocarditis; monitoring left ventricular function before, during, or after surgery; and evaluating intracardiac repairs during surgery.

This test is contraindicated if esophageal pathology (e.g., strictures, varices, trauma) exists. Also, TEE should not be performed if undiagnosed active gastrointestinal bleeding is occurring or if the client is uncooperative. A light sedative is frequently given prior to testing. TEE can be performed on an unconscious client. TEE is tolerated well, with approximately 1% of clients being intolerant of the esophageal probe. The rate of complications is <0.2%.

Contrast Echocardiography: This test assists in determining intracardiac communications and myocardial ischemia and perfusion defects. Microbubbles are injected into the venous circulation for the purpose of recording showers of echoes by M-mode or 2D tests. The microbubbles pass through the right atrium and ventricle, where they are absorbed in the lung; they do not pass to the left side of the heart. If the microbubbles are detected on the left side of the heart, an intracardiac communication or shunt is present. New contrast agents are under development which may allow visualization of the coronary arteries with echocardiography.

Stress Echocardiography: It may be necessary to evaluate the function of the left ventricle under stress. Physical exercise hampers good imaging, so the ventricle is stressed pharmacologically using the inotropic drugs dobutamine and dipyridamole (Persantine). Dobutamine is a most effective nonexercise stressor. The object of this test is to detect myocardial ischemia caused by coronary artery disease (CAD). To determine perfusion and wall motion abnormalities, dipyridamole and a contrast agent are used. Some facilities use a combination of dipyridamole and dobutamine for stress echocardiographic testing. This combination increases the effectiveness of detecting multivessel coronary artery disease (CAD) from 72% with one pharmacologic agent to 92% using both. Arbutamine is a new inotropic agent in use in Europe and being tested in the United States.

Purposes

- To identify abnormal heart size, structure, and function.
- To detect cardiac valvular disease and septal wall defects.
- To determine the function of prosthetic heart valves.
- To assess the effects of congenital heart disease.
- To monitor left ventricular function before, during, and after surgery.
- To evaluate and rule out CAD.

Clinical Problems

Indications: To detect heart size, structure, and function; heart valvular disease (regurgitation or stenosis of the aortic or mitral valves); congenital heart disease; heart wall damage after a myocardial infarction; cardiomyopathy; mural thrombi; pericardial effusion; aortic pathology; and endocarditis.

Diagnostic Tests	Indications to Determine/Detect
M-mode echocardiography	Dimension of the left ventricle
	Degree of ventricular dilatation and contractility
	Ventricular hypertrophy
	Function of cardiac valves—stenosis or regurgitation
Two-dimensional (2D) echocardiography	Cardiac valvular disease
Spectral doppler echocardiography	Blood flow through heart chambers and valves
	Septal wall defects
Color doppler echocardiography	Direction of blood flow through the heart
	Function of cardiac valves—stenosis or regurgitation
	Function of prosthetic valves
	Presence of shunting in the heart
Transeosphageal echocardiography	Function of left ventricle before, during, or after surgery
	Cardiac valvular disease
	Presence of intracardiac thrombus in left atrium
	Aortic disease (e.g., dissection of aorta)
	Presence of endocarditis
Contrast echocardiography	Perfusion defects
	Presence of shunting in the heart
Stress echocardiography	Function of left ventricle under stress
	Perfusion defects
	Wall motion abnormalities

Procedure

- A consent form should be signed.
- There is no food or fluid restriction.
- No medications should be omitted before the test unless indicated by the institution or health care provider.
- The client undresses from waist up and wears a hospital gown. For the test, the client will be positioned on his or her left side or in the supine position.
- Vital signs are recorded. Three electrode patches are applied to the chest area to monitor heart rate and changes in cardiac rhythm.
- Water-soluble gel is applied to the skin areas that are to be scanned. The transducer (probe), with slight pressure, is moved over different areas of the chest. Some clients may require that pictures be taken under the neck.
- The 2D echo takes about 20 to 30 minutes and the 2D echo with Doppler studies takes approximately 30 to 45 minutes.
- The cardiologist interprets the test result and submits a report to the client's health care provider, who gives the test results to the client.

Transesophageal echocardiography (TEE):

- The client should be NPO for at least 4 hours prior to test.
- A light sedative is given prior to the test.
- An IV sedative (e.g., Versed) is given.
- The endoscopic transducer is inserted into the esophagus.
- The test takes 15 to 30 minutes.
- The client is monitored (Dynamap) during recovery for 1 to 2 hours.

Contrast Echocardiography

- An IV line is inserted for injection of contrast media.

Stress Echocardiography

- The client should be NPO for 4 hours before the test.
- The client may be placed on a treadmill or receive a pharmacologic agent.
- Images are acquired during rest (pretest) and then during stress or immediately following stress (posttest).

Factors Affecting Diagnostic Results

- Large body habitus may cause poor image quality.
- Severe respiratory disease may affect test results.

NURSING IMPLICATIONS WITH RATIONALE

- Obtain a history of the client's physical complaint(s). Complete the pretest form provided by the institution, if available.

- Check that the consent form has been signed.
- Check the client's vital signs and obtain an electrocardiogram (ECG) if indicated by the institution or health care provider. These baseline values are used for comparison purposes.

Client Teaching

- Explain the procedure to the client (see Procedure). Inform the client that the test does not cause pain or discomfort. The test takes approximately 30 minutes, more time if additional testing is done.
- Inform the client that he or she will be positioned on his or her back and/or left side during the test procedure. Changing body position may be asked during testing. If the client is in an uncomfortable position, he or she should tell the technician.
- Instruct the client that a gel will be applied to the skin area that is to be studied. The gel may feel cool. The transducer (probe) is placed on the gel area and moved to different positions. The sound waves are transmitted as a picture, on videotape, and on graph paper.
- Explain to the client that the test results will be submitted to his or her health care provider. If the client does not hear from the health care provider in 1 week, the client should call his or her personal health care provider.
- Answer the client's questions. Refer questions to appropriate health professionals.

Echoencephalography

See Ultrasonography

Electrocardiography (electrocardiogram—ECG or EKG), vectorcardiography (vectorcardiogram—VCG)

Normal Finding

Normal electrocardiogram deflections (P, PR, QRS, ST, and T).

Description

An electrocardiogram (ECG or EKG) records the electrical impulses of the heart by the means of electrodes and a galvanometer (ECG machine). These electrodes are placed on the legs, arms, and chest. Combinations of two electrodes are called bipolar leads (i.e., lead I is the combination of both arm electrodes, lead II is the combination of the right-arm and left-leg electrodes, and lead III is the combination of the left-arm and left-leg electrodes). The unipolar leads are AVF, AVL, and AVR; the A means augmented, V is the voltage, and F is left foot, L is left arm, and R is right arm. There are at least six unipolar chest or precordial leads. A standard ECG consists of 12 leads: six limb leads (I, II, III, AVF, AVL, AVR) and six chest (precordial) leads (V_1, V_2, V_3, V_4, V_5, V_6).

With each cardiac cycle or heartbeat, the sinoatrial node (SA or sinus node) sends an electrical impulse through the atrium, causing atrial contraction or atrial depolarization. The SA node is called the pacemaker, because it controls the heart beat. The impulse is then transmitted to the atrioventricular (AV) node and the bundle of His and travels down the ventricles, causing ventricular contraction or ventricular depolarization. When the atria and the ventricles relax, repolarization and recovery occurs.

The electrical activity that the ECG records is in the form of waves and complexes: P wave (atrial depolarization); QRS complex (ventricular depolarization); and ST segment, T wave, and U wave (ventricular repolarization). An abnormal ECG indicates a disturbance in the electrical activity of the myocardium. A person could have heart disease and have a normal ECG as long as the cardiac problem did not affect the transmission of electrical impulses (Figure 1).

P Wave (Atrial Contraction): The normal time is 0.12 seconds or three small blocks. An enlarged P wave deflection could indicate atrial enlargement, which could be the result of mitral stenosis. An absent or altered P wave could suggest that the electrical impulse did not come from the SA node.

PR Interval (from the P Wave to the Onset of the Q Wave): The normal time interval is 0.2 seconds or five small blocks. An increased interval could imply a conduction delay in the AV node. It could be the result of rheumatic fever or arteriosclerotic heart disease. A short interval could indicate Wolff-Parkinson-White syndrome.

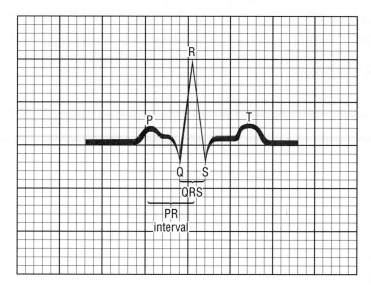

Figure 1.

QRS Complex (Ventricular Contraction): The normal time is <0.12 seconds or three small blocks. An enlarged Q wave may imply an old myocardial infarction. An enlarged R-wave deflection could indicate ventricular hypertrophy (enlargement). An increased time duration may indicate a bundle-branch block.

ST Segment (Beginning Ventricular Repolarization): A depressed ST segment indicates myocardial ischemia (decreased supply of oxygen to the myocardium). An elevated ST segment can indicate acute myocardial infarction or pericarditis. A prolonged ST segment may imply hypocalcemia or hypokalemia. A short ST segment may be due to hypercalcemia.

T Wave (Ventricular Repolarization): A flat or inverted T wave can indicate myocardial ischemia, myocardial infarction, or hypokalemia. A tall, peaked T wave (>10 mm or 10 small blocks in precordial leads, or >5 mm or five small blocks in limb leads) can indicate hyperkalemia.

Vectorcardiogram (VCG): The VCG records electrical impulses from the cardiac cycle, making it similar to the ECG. However, it shows a three-dimensional view (frontal, horizontal, and sagittal planes) of the heart, whereas the ECG shows a two-dimensional view (frontal and horizontal planes). The VCG is considered more sensitive than the ECG for diagnosing a myocardial infarction. It is useful for assessing ventricular hypertrophy in adults and children.

Purposes

- To detect cardiac dysrhythmias.
- To identify eletrolyte imbalance (e.g., hyperkalemia [peaked T wave]).
- To monitor ECG changes during the stress/exercise tests and the recovery phase after a myocardial infarction.

Clinical Problems

Abnormal Findings: Cardiac dysrhythmias, cardiac hypertrophies, myocardial ischemia, electrolyte imbalances (potassium, calcium, and magnesium), myocardial infarction, pericarditis.

Procedure

- Food, fluids, and medications are not restricted, unless otherwise indicated.
- Clothing should be removed to the waist, and the female client should wear a gown.
- Nylon stockings should be removed, and trouser bottoms should be raised.
- The client should lie in a supine position
- The skin surface should be prepared. Excess hair should be shaved from the chest if necessary.
- Electrodes with electropaste or pads are strapped to the four extremities. The color-coded lead wires are inserted into the correct electrodes. Chest electrodes are applied. The lead selector is turned to record the 12 standard leads unless the ECG machine automatically records the lead strips.
- The ECG takes approximately 15 minutes.

Factors Affecting Diagnostic Results

- Body movement and electromagnetic interference during the ECG recording could distort the tracing.
- Poor electrode-to-skin contact will distort tracing.

NURSING IMPLICATIONS WITH RATIONALE

- Record the list of medications the client is taking. The health care provider may want to compare ECG readings to check for improvement and changes; therefore, knowing the drugs the client is taking at the time of the ECG would be helpful.

Client Teaching

- Instruct the client to relax and to breathe normally during the ECG procedure. Tell the client to avoid tightening the muscles, grasping bed rails or other objects, and talking during the ECG tracing.
- Tell the client that the ECG should not cause pain or any great discomfort.
- Inform the client to tell you if he or she is having chest pain during the ECG tracing. Mark the ECG paper at the time the client is having chest pain.
- Allow the client time to ask questions. Refer questions you cannot answer to other health care provider, e.g., physician or cardiologist.
- Inform the client that the ECG takes about 15 minutes.

Posttest

- Remove the electropaste or jelly, if used, from the electrode sites when ECG is completed. Assist the client with dressing, if necessary.

Electroencephalography (electroencephalogram—EEG)

Normal Finding

Adult and Child: Normal tracing, regular short waves.

Description

The electroencephalogram (EEG) measures the electrical impulses produced by brain cells. Electrodes, applied to the scalp surface at predetermined measured positions, record brain-wave activity on moving paper. EEG tracings can detect patterns characteristic of some diseases (i.e., seizure disorders, neoplasms, cerebral vascular accidents, head trauma, and infections of the nervous system). At times, recorded brain waves may be normal when there is pathology.

Another use for the EEG is to determine cerebral death. If the EEG recording gives a flat or straight line for many hours, this usually indicates severe hypoxia and brain death. The cardiovascular functions are usually being maintained through the use of life-support systems (e.g., a respirator, oxygen, and IVs). The neurologist interprets the EEG readings and gives suggestions.

Purposes

- To detect a seizure disorder.
- To identify a brain tumor, abscess, or intracranial hemorrhage.
- To assist in the determination of cerebral death.

Clinical Problems

Abnormal Tracing: Epilepsy, seizures (grand mal, petit mal, psychomotor), brain neoplasms (tumors), brain abscesses, head injury, intracranial hemorrhage, encephalitis, unconsciousness, coma, "brain dead."

Procedure

The procedure may be performed while the client is (1) awake, (2) drowsy, (3) asleep, or (4) undergoing stimuli (hyperventilation or rhythmic flashes of bright light), or (5) a combination of any of these.

Pretest

- The hair should be shampooed the night before the test. Instruct the client not to use oil or hair spray on the hair.
- The decision concerning withdrawal of medications before the EEG is made by the health care provider. Sleeping pills and other sedatives may not be given the night before the test because they can affect the EEG recording.

- Food and fluids are not restricted except *no* coffee, tea, cola, and alcohol before the test.
- The EEG tracing is usually obtained with the client lying down; however, the client could be seated in a reclining chair.
- For a sleep recording, keep the client awake 2 to 3 hours later the night before the test and wake the client up at 6 AM. A sedative such as chloral hydrate may be ordered.
- The EEG test takes approximately 1½ to 2 hours. Flat electrodes will be applied to the scalp.

Posttest

- Remove the collodion or paste from the client's head. Acetone may be used to remove the paste.
- The client should resume normal activity unless he or she has been sedated.

Factors Affecting Diagnostic Results

- Drugs (i.e., sedatives, barbiturates, anticonvulsants, and tranquilizers) can affect test results.
- Alcohol could decrease cerebral impulses.
- Oily hair or the use of hair spray can affect test results.

NURSING IMPLICATIONS WITH RATIONALE

- A consent form should be signed.
- Explain the procedure to the client, step by step. List the important steps on paper for the client if needed.
- Report if the client is taking medications that could change the EEG result.
- Check with the health care provider and/or EEG department in regard to the type or types of recordings ordered (i.e., awake, sleep, stimuli).
- Be supportive of the client. Answer questions and permit the client to express concerns.
- Report to the health care provider and inform the EEG laboratory if the client is extremely anxious, restless, or upset.
- Observe for seizures and describe the seizure activity—the movements and how long they last. Have a tongue blade by the bedside at all times. Chart all seizure activity and the time of its occurrence, because it is very important for the technologist and electroencephalographer to know this.

Client Teaching

- Inform the client that he or she will *not* get an electric shock from the machine (electroencephalograph) and that the machine does not determine the client's intelligence and cannot read the client's mind. Many clients are apprehensive and fearful of this test.

- Encourage the client to eat a meal before the test. Hypoglycemia should be prevented because it can affect normal brain activity. Coffee, tea, cola, and any other stimulants should be avoided. Alcohol is a depressant and can affect the test result.
- Inform the client that the test does not produce pain.
- Advise the client to be calm and to relax during the test. If rest and stimuli (flashing lights) recordings are ordered, inform the client that there will be a brief time when there are flashing lights. Prepare the client, but do not increase the client's apprehension, if possible.
- Inform the client that the test takes 1½ to 2 hours. The room is quiet where the EEG recording is made and is conducive to rest and sleep.
- Instruct the client, after the test that normal activity can be resumed.

Electromyography (electromyogram—EMG)

Normal Finding

At Rest: Minimal electrical activity.

Voluntary Muscle Contraction: Markedly increased electrical activity.

Description

Electromyography (EMG) measures electrical activity of skeletal muscles at rest and during voluntary muscle contraction. A needle electrode is inserted into the skeletal muscle to pick up electrical activity, which can be heard over a loudspeaker, viewed on an oscilloscope, and recorded on graphic paper all at the same time. Normally there is no electrical activity when the muscle is at rest; however, in motor disorders abnormal patterns can occur. With voluntary muscle contraction there is a loud popping sound and increased electrical activity (wave) is recorded.

The test is useful in diagnosing neuromuscular disorders. The EMG can be used to differentiate between myopathy and neuropathy.

Purpose

- To diagnose neuromuscular disorders, such as muscular dystrophy.

Clinical Problems

Abnormal Findings: Muscle disorders (muscular dystrophy), neuromuscular disorders (peripheral neuropathy [i.e., diabetes mellitus, alcoholism], myasthenia gravis, myotonia), central neuronal degeneration (amyotrophic lateral sclerosis [ALS], anterior poliomyelitis).

Procedure

- A consent form should be signed.
- Food and fluids are not restricted, with the exceptions of *no* coffee, tea, colas, or other caffeine drinks, and *no* smoking for at least 3 hours before the EMG.
- Medications such as muscle relaxants, anticholinergics, and cholinergics should be withheld before the test with the approval of the health care provider. If the client needs the specific medication, the time for the test should be rearranged.
- The client lies on a table or stretcher or sits in a chair in a room free of noise. The EMG takes 1 hour but could take longer if a group of muscles is to be tested.
- Needle electrodes are inserted in selected or affected muscles. If the client experiences pain, the needle should be removed and reinserted.
- If serum enzyme tests are ordered (i.e., AST [SGOT], CPK, LDH), the samples should be drawn before the EMG or 5 to 10 days after the test.

Posttest

- If residual pain occurs, analgesic may be given.

Factors Affecting Diagnostic Results

- Pain could cause false reports.
- Age of the client: electrical activity may be decreased in some elderly persons.
- Drugs: muscle relaxants, anticholinergics, and cholinergics could affect the results.
- Fluids that contain caffeine can affect results.

NURSING IMPLICATIONS WITH RATIONALE

- Ask the health care provider (HCP) about withholding client medications that could affect EMG results. If the client takes drugs that could interfere with test results prior to the test, the drugs should be listed on the request slip and recorded in the chart.
- Check the HCP's order for a serum enzyme request. Blood needed for serum enzyme determinants (i.e., AST [SGOT], CPK, LDH) should be drawn before the EMG test.

Client Teaching

- Explain the procedure to the client. Inform the client that the test will not cause electrocution; however, there may be a slight temporary discomfort when the needle electrodes are inserted. If pain persists for several minutes, the client should tell the technician.

- Instruct the client to follow the technician's instructions (i.e., to relax the specified muscle(s) and to contract the muscle(s) when requested). An analgesic may be ordered before and after the test.
- Inform the client that the EMG test usually takes 1 hour, but it could take longer.

Electronystagmography (ENG)

Electronystagmogram

Normal Finding

Normal nystagmus with stimulation; normal vestibular-ocular reflex.

Description

Electromystagmography (ENG) is used to detect physiologic and pathologic nystagmus. This test helps to determine if the problem/abnormality that occurs is in the brain stem, the temporal lobe of the cerebral cortex, auditory nerve, or vestibular-cochlear area. If nystagmus (involuntary rapid eye movement) does not occur with stimulation, the health problem may be due to infection, tumor, ischemia to the surrounding tissues, or degeneration. The pattern of nystagmus helps in differentiating between peripheral and central vertigo.

ENG helps in determining if unilateral hearing loss is caused by the middle ear defect or nerve injury. If nystagmus does not occur with stimulation, the hearing loss is due to auditory nerve damage and not a middle ear problem.

Purposes

- To aid in the diagnosis of lesions in the brain stem or cerebellum
- To identify oculovestibular lesions or abnormalities.

Clinical Problems

Abnormal Findings: Brain stem lesion, cerebellum lesion, 8th cranial nerve injury, vestibular lesion, head trauma, middle ear infection, congenital disorder, peripheral lesions.

Procedure

- A signed consent form is required.
- Avoid applying facial makeup before the test.

- Nothing by mouth (NPO) after midnight. Vomiting frequently occurs with this procedure, thus, NPO for 8 or more hours reduces the chance of vomiting.
- Ear drum should be free of wax.
- Avoid consuming caffeine drinks or alcohol 24 hours prior to the test.
- Avoid sedatives and antivertigo drugs prior to the test.
- The client is seated or is lying while positioned in a darken room.
- Small electrodes are applied around the eyes.
- Test takes about 1 hour.
- Various techniques may be used to stimulate nystagmus, for example, positional, pendulum tracking, gaze position, calibration, and water caloric test.

Positional Technique
- Obtain a baseline recording of eye movement.
- With head erect and eyes looking forward, turn the head quickly to the right and then to the left; repeat the procedure with the eyes closed.
- Various positions are requested, such as sitting up and lying down quickly and lying down and sitting up quickly.

Pendulum Tracking Technique
- Client looks ahead and follows a pendulum.
- With the eyes closed, the client stares straight ahead for 30 seconds.

Gaze Technique
- The client is given a math problem.
- The client closes eyes and solves the math problem in 30 seconds while eye motion is recorded.
- The client looks straight ahead with eyes fixed and head straight; again eye motion is recorded.

Caloric (Water) Test Technique: The test is to evaluate the vesibular part of the 8th cranial nerve.

Note: The client's ear drum should not be perforated.
- The client's head is elevated to 30 degrees and the eyes are to be closed.
- The external auditory canal is irrigated with hot and cold water.
- The client's eyes are opened and the procedure is repeated for 60 seconds. Then the eyes are closed and the procedure is again repeated. The total time is 3 minutes.
- The client may encounter nausea and vomiting during the procedure. Following the test the client should rest until these symptoms have subsided.

Factors Affecting Diagnostic Results
- Sedatives and other CNS depressants.
- Blinking of the eyes.
- Loose electrodes.

NURSING IMPLICATIONS WITH RATIONALE

- Obtain a history of the client's health problems and drugs that are taken daily.
- Explain the procedure(s) to the client. Refer questions with unknown answers to other health professionals.
- Check that the client does not have facial makeup and has not had food in the last 8 hours.

Client Teaching

- Inform the client that he/she may feel nausated or vomit during the procedure. Such feelings should be communicated with the staff.
- Instruct the client to rest following the test procedure. This will decrease feelings of nausea and vomiting.
- Tell the client to follow the staff's instructions and ask questions as needed.

Endoscopic retrograde cholangiopancreatography (ERCP)

Normal Finding

Normal biliary and pancreatic ducts.

Description

Endoscopic retrograde cholangiopancreatography (ERCP) is an imaging technique in which the biliary pancreatic ducts are examined endoscopically after contrast medium is injected into the duodenal papilla. The purpose for this procedure is to identify the cause of a biliary obstruction, which could be stricture, cyst, stones, or tumor. Jaundice is usually present.

ERCP is performed following abdominal ultrasound, computed tomography, liver scanning, and/or biliary tract x-ray studies to confirm or diagnose a hepato-biliary or pancreatic disorder.

Purposes

- To detect biliary stones, stricture, cyst, or tumor.
- To identify biliary obstruction, such as stones or stricture.
- To confirm a biliary or pancreatic disorder.

Clinical Problems

Indications: Biliary stones, stricture, cyst, or tumor; primary cholangitis; cirrhosis;

pancreatic stones, stricture, cysts or pseudocysts, or tumor; chronic pancreatitis; pancreatic fibrosis; or duodenal papilla tumors.

Procedure

- Food and fluids are restricted for at least 8 hours before the test.
- The consent form should be signed prior to premedication.
- Obtain baseline vital signs. Have the client void.
- Premedicate with mild narcotic or sedative. Atropine may be given prior to or after insertion of the endoscope. Atropine relaxes gastrointestinal motility and will cause dryness of mouth.
- Local anesthetic is sprayed in back of throat (pharynx) to decrease the gag reflex prior to the insertion of the fiberoptic endoscope.
- Secretin may be given intravenously to paralyze the duodenum. Contrast medium is injected after the endoscope is at the duodenal papilla and the catheter is in the pancreatic duct.

Factors Affecting Diagnostic Results

- Inability to cannulate biliary and/or pancreatic duct.

NURSING IMPLICATIONS WITH RATIONALE

- Obtain a client history of allergies to seafood, iodine, and contrast dye. Report allergic findings.
- Determine whether the anxiety level may interfere with the client's ability to absorb information concerning the procedure.
- Check that the consent form has been signed prior to premedications.
- Explain to the client that when the contrast medium is injected, there usually is a transient flushing sensation.
- Be supportive of the client prior to and during the test procedure.
- Monitor the vital signs during the test and compare them to baseline vital signs. An increase in the pulse rate could be due to atropine. Rupture within the gastrointestinal tract caused by endoscope perforation could cause shock.

Client Teaching

- Inform the client that the endoscope will not obstruct breathing.
- Inform the client that atropine will make the mouth dry and the tongue feel large or swollen.
- Inform the client that the test takes approximately 1 hour and that lying still on the x-ray table is important.

Posttest

- Monitor vital signs. A rise in temperature might indicate infection (bacteremia or septicemia). Check respirations for respiratory distress resulting from anesthetic spray and/or the endoscope.

- Check skin color. Increased or decreased jaundice is an indicator of a disease process or the result of therapy.
- Check the gag reflex before offering food or drink.
- Check signs and symptoms of urinary retention caused by atropine.

Client Teaching

- Suggest warm saline gargle and/or lozenges to decrease throat discomfort.
- Explain to the client that he or she may have a sore throat for a few days after the test. This is due to the endoscope.

Esophageal acidity

See Esophageal Studies

Esophageal manometry

See Esophageal Studies

Esophageal studies

Esophageal Acidity, Esophageal Manometry, Acid Perfusion (Bernstein Test)

Normal Finding

Esophagus secretions of pH 5 to 6.

Description

Esophageal studies may be performed to determine cause of pyrosis (heartburn) and dysphagia (difficulty in swallowing). Most esophageal problems result from the reflux of gastric juices into the lower part of the esophagus caused by inadequate closure of the cardioesophageal (low esophageal) sphincter.

Gastric secretions are highly acidic, with a pH of 1.0 to 2.5, whereas the pH in the esophagus is 5.0 to 6.0. Backflow of gastric juices causes esophageal irritation or esophagitis.

Esophageal acidity, esophageal manometry, and acid perfusion (Bernstein test) are three common studies performed.

Esophageal Acidity: *One-Time Measurement:* A pH electrode attached to a catheter is passed into the lower esophagus to measure esophageal acidity. Measurement of pH in the esophagus is taken. If there is no acid reflux, hydrochloric acid (HCl) 0.1N is instilled into the stomach. Analysis of esophageal acidity is repeated. A pH <2.0 indicates acid reflux, which is most likely caused by an incompetent lower esophageal sphincter. The one-time measurement of esophageal acidity has largely been replaced by the 24-hour pH monitoring. *24-Hour pH Monitoring:* A pH electrode probe is passed through the nostril into the lower esophagus to measure esophageal acidity. The probe is connected to a recording device, which is worn by the client. The client keeps a diary of all symptoms and activities as they occur and marks them by an indicator on the recorder. After 24 hours the data are analyzed and interpreted.

Esophageal Manometry: This procedure measures esophageal sphincter pressure and records peristaltic contractions (duration and sequence). It detects esophageal motility disorder (e.g., achalasia). The baseline cardioesophageal sphincter pressure is approximately 20 mm Hg. In achalasia, the baseline sphincter pressure could be as high as 50 mm Hg, and the relaxation pressure could be around 24 mm Hg. This indicates that peristalsis is weak and that food and fluid cannot pass into the stomach until the weight of the contents is increased. For spasms of the esophagus, the sphincter is normal and peristalsis has irregular motility and force.

Acid Perfusion (Bernstein Test): This test is useful to distinguish between gastric acid reflux causing "heartburn" or esophagitis, and cardiac involvement (i.e., angina, myocardial infarction). Saline and HCl 0.1N are dripped through tubing, one at a time, into the esophagus. If the client complains of symptoms of esophagitis (i.e., epigastric discomfort, hearburn after ½ hour of IV HCl drip), then the cause is acid reflux. Additional gastrointestinal studies, such as barium swallow and esophagogastroduodenoscopy, are needed to confirm the suspected diagnosis.

Purposes

- To distinguish between gastric acid reflux and cardiac involvement.
- To diagnose gastric acid reflux.
- To determine the cause of heartburn or difficulty in swallowing.

Clinical Problems

Esophageal Acidity: Incompetent lower esophageal sphincter, chronic reflux esophagitis.

Esophageal Manometry: Spasm of esophagus, achalasia, esophageal scleroderma.

Acid Perfusion (Bernstein Test): Esophagitis, epigastric pain or discomfort.

Procedure

- A consent form should be signed.
- Food and fluids are restricted 8 to 12 hours prior to the test. Avoid alcohol intake 24 hours before the test.
- Place client in high Fowler's position.
- Monitor pulse during test procedure to detect arrhythmias from catheter insertion.
- Withhold antacids and autonomic nervous system agents (i.e., anticholinergics, cholinergics, and adrenergic blockers, glucocorticoids, and H_2 blockers [cimetidine, ranitidine]) for 24 hours before the test as indicated, or note on the laboratory slip the last time administered and dosage.

Esophageal Acidity: *One-Time Measurement*

- Catheter with pH electrode is inserted into the esophagus through the client's nostril.
- The client is asked to stimulate acid reflux by performing a Valsalva maneuver or lifting the legs.
- If there is no acid reflux, then 300 ml of HCl 0.1N is administered over 3 minutes, and the Valsalva maneuver or lifting of the legs is repeated.

Esophageal Acidity: *24-Hour pH Monitoring*

- The client should be NPO of solid foods for 8 hours.
- The catheter with the pH probe is inserted into the esophagus through the client's nostril.
- The probe is taped securely at the nose.
- Secure the recorder to the client's belt or provide a shoulder strap.

- The client records symptoms and activities in a diary and on the recorder over a 24-hour period of time.

Esophageal Manometry

- A manometric catheter with a pressure transducer is inserted through the nostril into the esophagus.
- Esophageal sphincter pressure is measured before and after swallowing.
- Peristaltic contractions are recorded.

Acid Perfusion (Bernstein Test)

- A catheter is passed through the nose into the esophagus.
- Saline solution is dripped (6 to 10 ml/min) through the catheter.
- The client is told to indicate when pain occurs.
- HCl 0.1N is dripped through the catheter for $\frac{1}{2}$ hour.
- The client is told to indicate when pain occurs.
- As soon as pain or discomfort is reported, the HCl line is turned off, and saline solution is started until symptoms have subsided.

Factors Affecting Diagnostic Results

- Antacids, anticholinergics, and cimetidine may increase pH, thus reducing acidity and causing false test results.
- Cholinergics, adrenergic blockers, alcohol, or corticosteroids may decrease pH, thus increasing acidity and relaxing the lower esophageal sphincter.

NURSING IMPLICATIONS WITH RATIONALE

- Explain the test procedure(s) to the client *(see Procedure)*. Answer the client's questions, or refer the questions to appropriate health professionals.
- Assess communications for verbal-nonverbal expressions of anxiety and fear about tests and/or the potential or actual problem.
- Monitor pulse and blood pressure during procedure. Baseline vital signs should be recorded. Report irregularity of pulse rate immediately to the health care provider. Check for signs of respiratory distress during catheter insertion.

Client Teaching

- Inform the client that food and fluids are restricted for 8 to 12 hours before the test. Alcoholic beverages should be avoided for 24 hours prior to test.
- Explain to the client that certain drugs taken (i.e., antacids, anticholinergics, adrenergic blockers, cholinergics, cimetidine) may be withheld for 24 hours. If these drugs are not withheld, the drug name and dose and the last time the drug was taken should be recorded on the laboratory slip.
- Instruct the client to sit in the high Fowler's position for insertion of the catheter.

Esophageal Activity—Client Teaching

- Inform the client that a catheter (with electrode) will be swallowed, and the pH of the esophagus secretions are recorded.
- Tell the client to perform the Valsalva's maneuver (bear down and hold breath) or to lift legs to stimulate gastric acid reflux as directed by the health care provider.
- Instruct the client to inform the health care provider of any pain or discomfort.

Esophageal Acidity: 24-Hour pH Monitoring—Client Teaching

- Instruct the client that he or she can have a regular diet during the 24 hours of recording unless otherwise indicated.
- Inform the client that a catheter (with electrode) will be inserted through the nostril and the pH of the esophageal secretions will be recorded.
- Inform the client that the catheter will be attached to a recording device. He or she will wear the recorder for 24 hours.
- Instruct the client that a diary will be provided. Symptoms and activities should be noted in the diary at the time they occur.
- Instruct the client not to operate the microwave oven during the 24 hours.
- Inform the client that the recorder should not get wet. A sponge bath rather than a shower is suggested.
- Instruct the client to return to the department in 24 hours to have the probe removed.

Esophageal Manometry—Client Teaching

- Inform the client that a manometric catheter is to be swallowed. The esophageal pressure and peristaltic contractions are recorded.
- Tell the client that drinking water will be requested.

Acid Perfusion (Bernstein Test)—Client Teaching

- Inform the client that a catheter is to be inserted through the nose into the esophagus.
- Tell the client there will be two IV solutions and that only one will be dripping into the catheter at a time.
- Instruct the client to inform the health care provider immediately when pain or discomfort occurs during the procedure.

Esophagogastroduodenoscopy, esophagogastroscopy

Gastroscopy, Esophagoscopy, Duodenoscopy, Endoscopy

Normal Finding

Normal mucous membranes of the esophagus, stomach, and duodenum; absence of pathology.

Description

Esophagogastroscopy includes gastroscopy and esophagoscopy. If duodenoscopy is included with the endoscopic examination, the term is *esophagogastroduodeno-scopy*. A flexible fiberoptic endoscope is used for direct visualization of the internal structures of the esophagus, stomach, and duodenum. Biopsy forceps or a cytology brush can also be inserted through a channel of the endoscope. Suction can be ap-plied for the removal of secretions and foreign bodies.

This test is performed under local anesthesia or IV sedation (benzodiazepine or narcotics), in a gastroscopy room of a hospital or clinic, usually by a gastroenterolo-gist. This procedure can be done on an emergency basis for removal of foreign ob-jects (a bone, a pin, etc.) and for diagnostic purposes. The major complications that can occur from esophagogastroduodenoscopy are perforation and hemorrhage.

Purposes

- To visualize the internal esophagus, stomach, and duodeneum.
- To obtain a cytologic specimen.
- To confirm the presence of gastrointestinal pathology.

Clinical Problems

Esophageal: Esophagitis, hiatal hernia, esophageal stenoses, achalasia, esophageal neoplasms (benign or malignant tumors), esophageal varices, Mallory-Weiss tear.

Gastric: Gastritis, gastric neoplasm (benign or malignant), gastric ulcer (acute or chronic), gastric varices.

Duodenal (Small Intestine): Duodenitis, diverticula, duodenal ulcer, neoplasm (benign or malignant).

Procedure

- A consent form should be signed.
- The client should be NPO for 8 to 12 hours before the test. When this procedure is used during an emergency and NPO cannot be enforced, the client's stomach is lavaged (suctioned) to prevent aspiration.

- The client may take prescribed medications at 6 AM on the day of the test. Check with laboratory or health care provider for any changes.
- A sedative/tranquilizer, a narcotic analgesic, and atropine may be given an hour before the test, or they can be titrated intravenously immediately prior to the procedure and during the procedure as needed.
- A local anesthetic may be used.
- Dentures, jewelry, and clothing should be removed from the neck to the waist.
- Record baseline vital signs. The client should void before the procedure.
- Specimen containers should be labeled with the client's name, the date, and the type of tissue.
- Emergency drugs and equipment should be available for hypersensitivity to medications (premedications and anesthetic) and for severe laryngospasms.
- The test takes approximately 1 hour or less.
- The client should not drive self home following the test because of possible aftereffects of sedation.

Factors Affecting Diagnostic Results

- Barium from a recent gastrointestinal imaging series can decrease visualization of the mucosa. This test should not be performed within 2 days after such tests. An x-ray film of the abdomen can be taken to see if barium is in the stomach or duodenum.

NURSING IMPLICATIONS WITH RATIONALE

- Recognize that a gastroscopy test for visualizing the esophageal, gastric, and duodenal mucosa is actually an esophagogastroduodenoscopy. These names are frequently used interchangeably.
- Check that the client's dentures, eyeglasses, and jewelry are removed. Give the client a hospital gown.
- Have the client void. Take vital signs.
- Check that a consent form has been signed before giving the client premedications. Once the sedative and the narcotic analgesic are given, the client should remain in bed with the bed sides up. Tell him or her that these medications will cause drowsiness.
- Be a good listener. Allow the client time to ask questions and to express concerns or fears. Refer questions you cannot answer to the gastroenterologist or health care provider.

Client Teaching
Posttest

- Explain the procedure to the client. Inform the client that the instrument is flexible; the procedure will be done under local anesthesia (the throat will be sprayed); premedications will be given before the test and usually IV sedation is given with the test; dentures and jewelry should be removed; and food and fluids will be restricted for 8 to 12 hours before the test.

- Explain to the client that he or she may feel some pressure with the insertion of the endoscope and may feel some fullness in the stomach when air is injected for better visualization of the stomach and intestine areas.
- Check the gag reflex before offering food and fluids by asking the client to swallow or by touching the posterior pharynx with a cotton swab or tongue blade if the throat was sprayed with an anesthetic.
- Keep the client NPO for 2 to 4 hours after the test or as ordered.
- Monitor vital signs (blood pressure, pulse, respirations) as ordered.
- Give the client throat lozenges or analgesics for throat discomfort. Inform the client that he or she may have flatus or "burp-up gas," which is normal. This is caused by the instillation of air during the procedure for visualization purposes.
- Observe the client for possible complications (e.g., perforation in the gastrointestinal tract from the endoscope). Symptoms could include pain (epigastric, abdominal, back pain), dyspnea, fever, tachycardia, and subcutaneous emphysema in the neck.
- Be supportive of the client and family.

Fetal nonstress test (NST) and contraction stress test (CST)*

Normal Finding

Normal (negative) result

NST: Expressed as a *reactive* (reassuring) NST; evidenced by acceleration in fetal heart rate (FHR) occurring either spontaneously or in response to fetal movement in utero. The American College of Obstetricians and Gynecologists (ACOG) criteria for a *reactive* NST is the presence of 2 or more accelerations of fetal heart rate of at least 15 beats per minute (bpm) or more. Above the baseline FHR of 120–160 bpm (each acceleration having a duration of at least 15 seconds) within a 20-minute period of monitoring.

 Reactive (reassuring) NST implies presence of adequate fetal oxygenation and an intact central and autonomic nervous system.

CST: Expressed as a *negative* (reassuring) test; evidenced by detecting NO late decelerations during a 10-minute period when 3 "good" quality contractions of

*Prepared by Jane Purnell Taylor, Associate Professor, Neumann College, Aston, PA.

40 seconds or more occur. Additionally, the CST result is expressed as negative if contractions are 3 minutes apart, of palpable intensity, and of 40- to 60-second duration, and the fetus shows no late decelerations.

Negative (reassuring) CST implies presence of uteroplacental sufficiency such that the fetus is considered likely to be able to withstand the stressors associated with labor contractions with decreased risk for intrauterine asphyxia.

Description

The fetal nonstress test (NST and the contraction stress test (CST) are two diagnostic tests used to help evaluate fetal functioning and well-being in response to either fetal movement (NST) or to spontaneous or induced uterine contraction (CST). The **NST** is inexpensive, rapidly accomplished, lacks side effects, and is helpful in identifying at-risk fetuses of mothers who exhibit high-risk pregnancy conditions, including diabetes, intrauterine growth retardation, pregnancy induced hypertension, report by mother of decreased fetal movements, among others. Only minimal equipment is required (external transducer for fetal heart rate monitoring); testing occurs 1 to 2 times per week depending on the reason for doing the testing. The **CST** is also employed at 32 to 34 weeks in evaluating high-risk preganancies, particularly pregnancy condition which may place the fetus at risk if there is poor placental perfusion including diabetes, intrauterine growth retardation, and postterm gestation over 42 weeks. In addition, certain fetuses who exhibit a nonreactive NST in the presence of additional data may also have a CST performed. Contraindications to CST testing include presence of a classical uterine incision, presence of placenta previa, multiple gestation, and vaginal bleeding, among others. Equipment required for CSTs includes an external transducer (for FHR monitoring), together with a tocodynamometer (toco) for monitoring uterine contractions. The NST and CST are able to be performed in hospital, office, and clinic settings; the NST may also be conducted in the home care setting with supervision.

Fetal Nonstress Test (NST): NST is a noninvasive test that monitors FHR with fetal movement. According to the ACOG, the FHR should increase by 15 bpm within a 20-minute interval. If there is no fetal movement or increased FHR in 20 minutes, the mother's abdomen may be rubbed or a loud noise made close to the abdomen to stimulate fetal movement. If after 40 minutes there is no acceleration of FHR, the NST is nonreactive and a CST may be ordered. With a nonreactive NST after 40 minutes, fetal distress may be considered; however, the fetus may be in a sleep cycle or the mother may have taken a CNS depressant drug. The NST is usually performed at 30 weeks of gestation to allow for sufficient CNS maturation after which heart rate accelerations in response to movement become more fully established.

Contraction Stress Test (CST): There are two types of CST; the nipple stimulation test and the oxytocin challenge test (OCT). The nipple stimulation test is a noninvasive test that stimulates the hypothalamus which promotes the release of oxytocin. This can cause uterine contractions, and a normal result would be that the FHR does not show late deceleration. The OCT is somewhat noninvasive but could induce labor in some clients. Oxytocin, a uterine stimulant, is well diluted in IV fluids and thus does not cause continuous contractions. There should be 3 moderate contractions occurring within 10 minutes, and the FHR should not show any late deceleration. If there is a late deceleration of FHR with contractions, the test indicates that hypoxia may result during labor due to insufficient placental function. The CST with oxytocin is performed at 32 weeks, preferably 34 weeks of gestation. In case this test would induce labor, the fetus would have a better chance to survive.

Purposes

- To evaluate fetal functioning and well-being.
- To evaluate sufficiency of uteroplacental function to support the fetus in labor.
- To screen high-risk pregnancies.

Clinical Problems

Abnormal Findings: Fetal distress, fetal death, placental dysfunction.

Procedure

- A signed consent form is required.
- Baseline vital signs are taken for future comparison.
- Position mother in semifowler or lateral position with roll/wedge under right hip to displace uterus to the left slightly.
- Apply transducer (NST) or transducer and toco (CST).
- Monitor maternal blood pressure during the procedure for occurrence of hypotension.

Nonstress Test (NST)

- The client presses the pressure transducer when she feels the body move.
- Monitor for FHR acceleration. There should be 15 bpm that last for 15 seconds. If the FHR does not increase, rub the mother's abdomen or thump/hit a pan that is close to her abdomen to stimulate fetal movement. If there is no fetal movement in 40 minutes and no acceleration in FHR, the test indicates a nonreactive fetus.

Contraction Stress Test (CST)

Nipple Stimulation:

- The client stimulates one nipple with water-soluble ointment until a contraction occurs. Contraction should occur within 2 minutes, and if not, nipple stimulation could continue for 15 minutes.
- If there is no late deceleration in FHR, the test result is considered normal with deceleration of FHR during contractions, and the appropriate health care provider should be notified. It can indicate that the fetus is receiving insufficient blood supply from the placenta.

Ocytocin Challenge Test (OCT)

- Vital signs and FHR are taken at frequent intervals.
- NPO may be suggested in case labor begins.
- Administer oxytocin by IV infusion pump, dosage will be ordered. The oxytocin rate may be slowly increased until the client has a moderate contraction. If contraction occurs before the oxytocin infusion, withhold the drug.
- A normal test result is no late deceleration of FHR. If late deceleration occurs, it could indicate placental dysfunction that could cause the fetus to receive insufficient oxygen during labor.
- Test should be conducted in a health facility.
- Monitor FHR for 30 to 60 minutes after oxytocin infusion has been stopped.
- Test takes approximately 1 to 2 hours.

Factors Affecting Diagnostic Results

- NST is often nonreactive before 30–32 weeks due to central nervous system immaturity.
- NST may be classified as falsely nonreactive because of the occurrence of fetal sleep cycles;
- NST may be more commonly classified as falsely reactive in diabetic clients, postterm pregnancies, and pregnancy-induced hypertension associated with intrauterine growth retardation.
- NST may be falsely nonreactive when smoking has occurred prior to the NST; also in the event of CNS depressant drugs or beta blockers taken by the client.
- NST and CST's equipment difficulties and/or inexperienced operators may have difficulty obtaining or accurately interpreting tracings.

NURSING IMPLICATIONS WITH RATIONALE

- Obtain a gestation history from the client.
- Determine mother's knowledge level related to high-risk pregnancy condition and purposes of NST/CST testing and what these measure.
- Incorporate family into discussion and testing process as much as possible and desired.
- Remain with the client during testing as often as possible if other supports are lacking.
- Attempt to schedule testing times at client's convenience; follow-up on missed appointments.
- Position client correctly to prevent hypotension.
- Monitor blood pressure and other vital signs at stated intervals consistent with agency protocols.
- Report abnormal changes.

Client Teaching

- Use testing opportunity (NST) to teach importance of observing fetal movement.
- Encourage the client to rest following the test procedure.
- Inform the client to report bleeding, continuous contractions, and lack of fetal movement.

Fetoscopy*

Percutaneous Umbilical Blood Sampling (PUBS); cordocentesis

Normal Findings

Absence of abnormalities as presented in Clincial Problems, Abnormal Findings.

Description

Fetoscopy: Fetoscopy is the direct visualization of the fetus by means of an endoscope inserted through the maternal abdominal wall into the uterine cavity for the purpose of obtaining blood or skin sample or for visualization of external developmental abnormalities. It is rarely used now for blood sampling due to 2 to 5% risk of serious complications. As a result of possible complications, this technique has evolved (particularly in high-risk perinatal center) into the increased use of ***percutaneous umbilical blood sampling or PUBS,*** which is known as ***cordocentesis.***

Cordocentesis or PUBS: It is a technique in which an ultrasound-guided 22–26 gauge needle is used to puncture the umbilical cord to obtain fetal blood samples. Reports indicate that many operators find a site about 1 cm from the placenta to be an optimal site for obtaining fetal blood from the umbilical vein. Cordocentesis has been done as early as 12 weeks, but more commonly after 18 weeks until 36 weeks. Early procedures carry a higher risk to the fetus. The amount of blood removed is between 1 to 4 ml; after 20 weeks of gestation, 5 ml may be safely removed. Ultrasound is used to ascertain gestational age of the fetus, position of the fetus, the thickness and location of the placenta, position of tissues to be visualized or sampled, and placement of the needle tip used to obtain the sample. While fetoscopy is less used today for purposes of fetal blood sampling, the endoscopic technique does allow for direct visualization of aspects of the fetus determined at risk for external abnormalities involving the spine, extremities, face, and genital areas; also for visual access to preferred skin biopsy sites including the back, thighs, or scalp to aid in diagnosis of selected skin disorders of genetic origin

---

*Prepared by Jane Purnell Taylor, MS, RN, Associate Professor, Neumann College, Aston, PA.

unable to be otherwise detected. In the event that fetal blood sampling is desired but the umbilical cord is unable to be punctured to obtain fetal blood, a safe alternative for consideration is ultrasound needle-guided *fetal heart puncture*. These procedures, their benefits and risks for fetoscopy, cordocentesis (PUBS), or fetal heart puncture, should be discussed with the client and family.

Purposes

(Overall purpose is to aid in diagnosis, treatment, and monitoring fetal disease)

- To detect inherited blood disorders, including hemophilia A or B, hemoglobinopathies (measurement of hemoglobin concentration to assess fetal anemia), and fetal thrombocytopenia (measurement of fetal platelet count to assess and treat potential risks for perinatal cerebral bleeding).
- To perform rapid fetal karotyping.
- To detect fetal chromosome abnormalities.
- To detect fetal infection (including CMV, toxoplasmosis, rubella).
- To validate suspected fetal hypoxia or acidosis.
- To treat fetal anemia by transfusion.
- To assess and treat isoimmunization.

Clinical Problems

Abnormal Findings: Hemophilia A and B, fetal anemia, fetal thrombocytopenia, chromosome abnormalities, fetal hypoxia, fetal acidosis, fetal infection, isoimmune hemolytic disorders.

Procedure (Cordocentesis)

- A consent form should be signed and witnessed.
- Health care providers should schedule this diagnostic test within ready access to a room suitable for delivery if necessity should arise whether to employ steroid therapy to the mother prior to the procedure.
- Should the need arise, respiratory support (anesthesiologist/anesthetist) should be quickly available in the setting.
- Monitor maternal vital signs prior to and throughout the test.
- Position mother to reduce opportunity for occurrence of supine hypotension; she must remain still during the procedure.
- Ultrasound scanning of abdomen is performed to visualize chosen area and identify an approach that will protect fetal parts and avoid maternal vessels.
- Skin insertion site is cleansed with agency protocol specificd antiseptic.
- Local anesthetic is injected into the skin and onto the abdominal and uterine peritoneum.
- Use of prophylactic antibiotics varies by setting; rationale for use generally is to avoid amnionitis (infection to amniotic fluid). It has been suggested that this invasive procedure to the fetus might be avoided in the case of a known infected mother depending on benefit to risk ratio.

- A paralytic drug, intravascular pancuronium bromide, may be used to prevent the fetus from moving during the samplying procedure.
- The mother may be given medication to assist her to relax during the procedure; however, it is important that the mother not become sedated to the point she exhibits deep breathing. Deep breathing could, as a result of the movement created by her diaphragm, interfere with the puncture of the umbilical vein during the procedure.
- Real-time ultrasound is used for confirmation that the needle tip is correctly placed in the umbilical vein (approximately 1 cm from the placenta cord insertion site). This allows for removal of the stylet from the needle and subsequent aspiration of designated quantity of blood into a syringe containing anticoagulant.

Posttest

- Observe the puncture site (using ultrasound) for bleeding after removal of the needle.
- Employ fetal heart rate (FHR) monitoring for 30 minutes (minimal) postprocedure, followed by an additional ultrasound 1 hour postprocedure to verify no evidence of bleeding/hematoma.

Factors Affecting Diagnostic Results

- Degree of experience of operator and with ultrasound-guided needle procedures.
- Incorrect placement of needle tip resulting in need for additional manipulation; aspiration of sample at wrong time; amniotic fluid contamination of sample (which the amniotic fluid has a coagulation effect), or failure to actually obtain a sample.
- Amount of sedation received by mother; degree of hyperventilation; adequacy of placental perfusion (as related to incorrect maternal positioning with resultant supine hypotension). These factors may affect fetal oxygenation levels and outcome of diagnostic studies.
- Placement of sample into incorrect container or container having insufficient or incorrect anticoagulant; loss of portion of the sample; sample contamination; improper labeling of sample.

NURSING IMPLICATIONS WITH RATIONALE

- Obtain a history of the client's health problems, familial health disorders, medications, and any pregnancy past or present problems.
- Monitor vital signs. Monitor fetal heart rate (FHR).
- Monitor maternal anxiety level.
- Check medical record to determine if the mother is Rh negative and not sensitized and if the father is Rh positive or negative or unknown. Plan to administer an IM injection of Rh IgG globulin (RhoGAM) following cordocentesis unless the mother is found to be previously sensitized.

- Discuss the benefits and risks to this procedure by the health care provider or an appropriate health professional. Genetic counselor should also be included.
- Be available to answer questions and concerns, and if unable, refer the questions to other health professionals.
- Assist mother with proper positioning for the test; assist mother to relax using relaxation exercises and guided imagery.
- Prevent oversedation of the mother for the procedure to reduce chance of occurrence of deep breathing with diaphragm movement that may interfere during the puncture procedure.

Posttest

- Monitor the mother's vital signs, and fetal heart rate.

Client Teaching

- Instruct client that she will be ultrasonically monitored for bleeding once the needle is removed.
- Instruct mother to expect to have fetal monitoring for 30 minutes or more postprocedure.
- Instruct the mother that if intravascular pancuronium bromide (Pavulon) is used during the procedure she may not detect the amount of fetal movement she has become accustomed to for a few hours.
- Instruct Rh negative mother to expect, if not sensitized previously, that she will receive an injection of RhoGAM postprocedure.
- Instruct the client to report any pain or bleeding that might occur.
- Instruct her to rest for at least a day following the procedure and no heavy lifting.
- Encourage her to increase fluid intake.
- Inform her to notify the health care provider with any questions or concerns.

Fluoroscopy

Fluoroscopic Examination

Normal Finding

Normal size, structure, and physiologic function of the organ(s) being examined (chest, heart, intestines).

Description

The fluoroscopic examination allows the radiologist and health care provider to view in motion the physiologic function of organs on a fluorescent screen. Usually the client is between the x-ray tube and the fluorescent screen. The x-ray beam penetrates the client and then strikes the screen. Unfortunately, the client can receive substantially more radiation than he would receive from standard radiography. Today fluoroscopy is used with many diagnostic tests for visualization and for guidance.

During cardiac catheterization, the fluoroscopic procedure is essential for visualizing the coronary arteries. The moving images can be recorded on videotape and can be a valuable aid to diagnosis.

During fluoroscopic examination, the room is darkened for contrast and visualization purposes. If the radiologist and assistant remain in the room, aprons should be worn.

Purpose

- To view the functions of organs in motion.

Clinical Problems

Test Area	Indications/Purposes
Thorax	To visualize lung expansion, diaphragm movement or paralysis, bronchiolar obstruction
Abdomen	To detect bowel obstruction (stricture or tumor), filling defects, active bleeding and ulceration (peptic ulcer), Meckel's diverticulum, intra-abdominal hernias
Heart	To detect coronary occlusion (partial or total)

Procedure

Thorax

- Food and fluids are usually not restricted.
- Jewelry should be removed. A gown should be worn.
- The client should breathe deeply and cough as instructed.

Abdomen

- The client should be NPO after midnight.
- A gown should be worn.
- The client swallows a chalky substance, barium sulfate.
- Food and fluids are permitted after the examination.
- A laxative is usually ordered after the test or that evening.

Heart

- The client should be NPO after midnight.
- Follow the procedure for cardiac catheterization *(see Cardiac Catheterization).*

Factors Affecting Diagnostic Results

- Jewelry and metal objects.
- Nausea and vomiting.
- Medications: Narcotics, barbiturates.

NURSING IMPLICATIONS WITH RATIONALE

Client Teaching

- Explain the procedure to the client.
- Inform the client that the fluoroscopic examination should *not* cause discomfort.
- Discuss the client's anxiety and fears. Refer questions you cannot answer to other appropriate health professionals.
- Explain to the client that the chest fluoroscopy should take approximately 10 minutes and the abdominal fluoroscopy 30 minutes to 1 hour.
- Determine if the client is pregnant or if pregnancy is suspected. Report findings immediately. Fluoroscopy should not be done during pregnancy.
- Inform the client that the radiologist or x-ray personnel will give step-by-step instructions during the procedure. Tell the client to ask questions if he or she has any.
- Determine if the client has had extensive exposure to x-rays in the last few years or during his or her lifetime. Excessive radiation can be cumulative. Notify the health care provider of previous prolonged exposure to radiation.

Gastric analysis (basal and stimulation with tube), tubeless gastric analysis

Normal Finding

Fasting: 1.0–5.0 mEq/l/h.

Stimulation: 10–25 mEq/l/h.

Tubeless: Detectable dyes in the urine.

Description

The gastric analysis test examines the acidity of the gastric secretions in the basal state (without stimulation) and the maximal secretory ability (with stimulation; i.e., with histamine phosphate, betazole hydrochloride [Histalog], pentagastrin). An increased amount of free hydrochloric acid (HCl) could indicate a peptic ulcer (stomach or duodenal), and an absence of free HCl (achlorhydria) could indicate gastric atrophy (possibly caused by gastric malignancy) or pernicious anemia. In addition, gastric contents can be collected for cytologic examination.

Gastric analysis by tube (basal and stimulation) and tubeless gastric analysis (urine examination after a resin dye and stimulant are administered) are the methods used for evaluating gastric secretions.

Basal Gastric Analysis (Tube): Gastric secretions are aspirated through a nasogastric tube after a period of fasting. Specimens are obtained to evaluate the basal acidity of the gastric content first and the gastric stimulation test follows.

Stimulation Gastric Analysis (Tube): The stimulation test is usually a continuation of the basal gastric analysis. After samples of gastric secretions are obtained, a gastric stimulant (i.e., Histalog or pentagastrin) is administered, and gastric contents are aspirated every 15 to 20 minutes until several samples are obtained.

Tubeless Gastric Analysis: This test is for screening purposes to detect the presence or absence of HCl; however, it will *not* indicate the amount of free acid in the stomach. A gastric stimulant (caffeine, Histalog) is given, and an hour later a resin dye (Azuresin, Diagnex Blue) is taken orally by the client. The free HCl releases the dye from the resin base; the dye is absorbed by the gastrointestinal tract and is excreted in the urine. Absence of the dye in the urine 2 hours later is indicative of gastric achlorhydria. This test method saves the client the discomfort of being intubated with a nasogastric tube; however, it does lack accuracy.

There is controversy over the usefulness of gastric acid secretory tests; however, they are still used to document gastric acid hypersecretions (e.g., Zollinger-Ellison syndrome and hypergastrinemia).

Purposes

- To evaluate gastric secretions.
- To detect an increase or decrease of free HCl.

Clinical Problems

Decreased Level: Pernicious anemia, gastric malignancy (atrophy), atrophic gastritis.

Elevated Level: Peptic ulcer (duodenal), Zollinger-Ellison syndrome.

Procedure

Basal Gastric Analysis (Tube)

- The client should be NPO for 8 to 12 hours prior to the test. Smoking should be restricted for 8 hours.
- Certain groups of drugs (i.e., anticholinergics, cholinergics, adrenergic blockers, antacids, steroids) and alcohol and coffee should be restricted for at least 24 hours before the test. It should be noted on the request slip if the drugs cannot be withheld.
- Baseline vital signs should be recorded.
- Loose dentures should be removed.
- A lubricated nasogastric tube is inserted through the nose or mouth.

- A residual gastric specimen and four additional specimens taken 15 minutes apart should be aspirated and labeled with the client's name, the time, and a specimen number. The nasogastric tube may be attached to low intermittent suction.

Stimulation Test: A continuation of the basal gastric analysis.

- A gastric stimulant is administered (i.e., betazole hydrochloride [Histalog] or histamine phosphate intramuscularly; pentagastrin subcutaneously).
- Several gastric specimens are obtained over a period of 1 to 2 hours (histamine four 15-minute specimens in 1 hour and Histalog eight 15-minute specimens in 2 hours). Specimens should be labeled with the client's name, the date, the time, and specimen numbers.
- Vital signs should be monitored. Emergency drugs such as epinephrine (Adrenalin) should be available.
- The test usually takes $2\frac{1}{2}$ hours for both parts (basal and stimulation).

Tubeless Gastric Analysis

- The client should be NPO for 8 to 12 hours before the test.
- The morning urine specimen is discarded.
- Certain drugs are withheld for 48 hours before the test (i.e., antacids, electrolyte preparations [potassium, calcium, sodium, magnesium], quinidine, quinine, iron, vitamin B complex), with the health care provider's permission.
- Give the client caffeine sodium benzoate 500 mg in a glass of water.
- Collect a urine specimen 1 hour later. This is the control urine specimen.
- Give the client the resin dye agent (Azuresin or Diagnex Blue) in a glass of water.
- Collect a urine specimen 2 hours later. The urine may be colored blue or blue-green for several days. Absence of color in the urine usually indicates absence of HCl in the stomach.

Factors Affecting Diagnostic Results

- Incorrect labeling of specimens could affect test results.
- Drugs—antacids, anticholinergics, and histamine blockers (cimetidine, ranitidine) could decrease HCl levels; adrenergic blockers, cholinergics, steroids, and alcohol could elevate HCl levels; antacids, electrolyte and iron preparations, vitamin B complex, and quinidine could falsely elevate the Diagnex Blue level.
- Stress, smoking, and sensory stimulation could increase HCl secretion.

NURSING IMPLICATIONS WITH RATIONALE

- Notify the health care provider if the client is receiving the following categories of drugs: antacids, antispasmodics, anticholinergics, adrenergic blockers, cholinergics, and steroids. Drugs from the above groups and a few others should be withheld for 24 to 48 hours before the gastric analysis. Drugs that cannot be withheld should be listed on the request slip.
- Monitor vital signs. Observe for possible side effects from use of stimulants (i.e., dizziness, flushing, tachycardia, headache, and a lower systolic blood pressure).

■ Label the specimens (gastric or urine) with the client's name, the date, the time, and the specimen number.

■ Be supportive of the client. Encourage the client to express his or her concerns or fears. Answer questions or refer them to appropriate health professionals.

Client Teaching

■ Explain the purpose and procedure of the tube or tubeless gastric analysis test to the client. Check with the health care provider before you give your explanation to find out whether he or she will perform both basal and stimulation gastric analysis *(see Procedure)*. List the steps of the test on paper for the client, if needed.

■ Tell the client how the nasogastric tube is inserted (i.e., the tube is lubricated and passes through the nose or mouth) and that he or she will be asked to swallow or will be given sips of water as the tube is passed into the stomach. The end of the tube may be attached to low intermittent suction.

Gastrointestinal (GI) series, upper GI series, barium swallow, small bowel series, hypotonic duodenography

Normal Finding

Normal structure of the esophagus, stomach, and small intestine, and normal peristalsis.

Description

Upper gastrointestinal (GI) and small-bowel series are fluoroscopic and x-ray examinations of the esophagus, stomach, and small intestine. Oral barium meal (barium sulfate) or a water-soluble contrast agent, Gastrografin (meglumine diatrizoate), is swallowed. By means of fluoroscopy, the barium is observed as it passes through the digestive tract, and spot films are taken. Inflammation, ulcerations, and tumors of the stomach and duodenum can be detected through this procedure.

Upper GI series are performed in hospitals or in private laboratories. A preparation sheet is given or sent to the client prior to the test.

If increased peristalsis, a spastic duodenal bulb, or a space-occupying lesion is observed or suspected in the duodenal area during the GI series, a *hypotonic duodenography* procedure can be performed by giving glucagon, atropine, or propantheline (Probanthine) to slow down the action of the small intestine. Preparations for the hypotonic duodenography are similar to those for the upper GI series. Because of the anticholinergic effect of the drug, the client should be observed closely for urinary retention.

Purposes

- To detect an esophageal, gastric, or duodenal ulcer.
- To identify polyps, tumor, or hiatal hernia in the GI tract.
- To detect foreign bodies, esophageal varices, or esophageal or small bowel strictures.

Clinical Problems

Abnormal Findings: Hiatal hernia; esophageal varices; esophageal or small-bowel structures; gastric or duodenal ulcer; gastritis or gastroenteritis; gastric polyps; benign or malignant tumor of the esophagus, stomach, or duodenum; diverticula of the stomach and duodenum; pyloric stenosis; malabsorption syndrome; volvulus of the stomach; foreign bodies.

Procedure

- The client should be NPO (food and fluids) and should refrain from smoking for 8 to 12 hours before the test. A low-residue diet may be ordered for the 2 and 3 days before the test.
- Withhold medications 8 hours before the test unless otherwise indicated. Narcotics and anticholinergic drugs are withheld for 24 hours to avoid intestinal immobility.
- Laxatives may be ordered the evening before the test.
- The client swallows a chalk-flavored (chocolate, strawberry) barium meal or meglumine diatrizoate (Gastrografin) in the calculated amount (16 to 20 oz).
- Spot films are taken during the fluoroscopic examination. The procedure takes approximately 1 to 2 hours but could take 4 to 6 hours if the test is to include the bowel series. A 24-hour x-ray film (post-GI series) may be requested.
- A laxative is usually ordered after the completion of the test to get the barium out of the GI tract.

Factors Affecting Diagnostic Results

- Barium in the GI tract from a recent barium study.
- Retention of foods and liquids, which would decrease visualization.
- Excessive air in the stomach and small intestine.

NURSING IMPLICATIONS WITH RATIONALE

- Record vital signs. Note in the chart of any epigastric pain or discomfort.

Client Teaching

- Explain the procedure to the client concerning diet and medication restrictions; no smoking; the length of time required to complete the procedure; and the post-test laxative, if ordered *(see Procedure)*.
- Inform the client that all of the chalk-flavored liquid must be swallowed. Tell the client the tests should not cause pain or any significant discomfort.
- Encourage the client to ask questions or to express any concerns. Refer questions you cannot answer to other appropriate health professionals.

Posttest

- Check with the radiology department that the upper GI series and/or small bowel studies are completed before giving the late breakfast or late lunch. Usually the x-ray department will send a slip with the client stating that the test is finished or that a 24-hour x-ray film will be needed.
- Administer the ordered laxative (e.g., milk of magnesia) after the test.

Client Teaching

- Inform the client that the stools should be light in color for the next several days. Instruct the client to notify the health care provider if he or she does not have a bowel movement in 2 to 3 days. Barium can cause fecal impaction.

Gastroscopy

See Esophagogastroduodenoscopy

Holter monitoring*

Ambulatory Electrocardiography, Dynamic Electrocardiography

Normal Finding

No abnormal electrocardiographic findings.

Description

Holter monitoring (ambulatory electrocardiography) evaluates the client's heart rate and rhythm during normal daily activities, rest, and sleep over 24 hours (occasionally 48 hours). The Holter monitor consists of a continuous electrocardiogram (ECG) recording on a cassette tape that is boxed inside an approximately 1-lb monitor. After 24 hours, the monitor with the tape is returned to the cardiac center and is scanned or reviewed for abnormal findings such as cardiac dysrhythmias.

Holter monitoring began 30 years ago and it is widely used today. The Holter recorder contains a clock that is coordinated with the tape recorder and an event marker for the client to use when having symptom(s). The client is given a diary to record the symptoms such as palpitations, chest pain, shortness of breath, syncope, vertigo, and the time of the symptoms.

The primary purpose for Holter monitoring is to identify suspected and unsuspected cardiac dysrhythmias, which can be correlated between the recorder, event marking of symptoms, and transient symptoms marked in the diary. It is infrequently ordered for clients having Prinzmetal's variant angina, a form of myocardial ischemia that results from spasms of the coronary arteries. Holter monitoring is more sensitive for identifying the cause of the symptoms than a routine ECG.

Purpose

■ To identify cardiac dysrhythmias related to cardiac symptoms as marked on the monitor and recorded in the diary.

Clinical Problems

Indications: Suspected and unsuspected cardiac dysrhythmias (supraventricular and ventricular), correlation of symptoms with the ECG tape, mitral valve prolapse causing dysrhythmia, hypertrophic obstructive cardiomyopathy causing atrial and ventricular dysrhythmias, pacemaker malfunction.

---

*Revised by Frank DiGregorio, CNMT, RDMS, Director, Community Imaging Center, Wilmington, DE.

Procedure

- A signed consent form may be required.
- There is no food or fluid restriction.
- The skin is cleansed and shaved as needed, and electrodes are placed over bony areas to eliminate artifacts that could be caused by skeletal muscle movements.
- Five to seven electrode patches are placed on the chest. For a five-lead electrode placement, two negative electrodes are secured at the upper right and left manubrial border of the sternum, and two positive electrodes are placed below the sternum, one placed at 2 cm right of the xiphoid process on the rib margin and the second at the left anterior axillary line—6th rib. A ground electrode is secured at the lower right rib margin over the bone.
- The client is given a diary to record what he or she was doing when symptom(s) such as palpitations, chest pain, and shortness of breath occured.
- The client should not shower, take a bath, or swim until the electrodes are removed.

Posttest

- The client returns the Holter monitor the next day (24 hours later) with the diary.
- The nurse/technician reviews the diary with the client for any needed clarification.
- The tape is scanned (reviewed) and the cardiologist submits a written report to the personal health care provider. The client's health care provider explains the ECG monitoring results to the client.

Factors Affecting Diagnostic Results

- The client does not record activities correlated with symptoms in the diary.
- The electrodes fall off the chest.

NURSING IMPLICATIONS WITH RATIONALE

- Review client's history of cardiac disorders and/or symptoms.
- Check that a baseline ECG has been received. A comparison of the baseline ECG with the 24 hour ECG monitoring could be requested.

Client Teaching

- Explain to the client that this test does not cause pain or any major discomfort. Tell the client that the monitor device weighs approximately one pound.
- Instruct the client that the monitor device will be attached either by a shoulder strap or as a belt.
- Review the procedure for Holter monitoring with the client *(see Procedure)*. Answer questions the client may have or refer the questions to appropriate health professional.

- Emphasize the importance of pushing the event marker button on the monitor when symptoms occur and recording in the diary the time, symptoms, and activity that is taking place at the time of symptoms.
- Inform the client that the monitor should *not* get wet. Bathing, showering, and swimming should be avoided. The client should not use an electric razor or electric toothbrush during the 24 hours of monitoring to avoid possible ECG artifacts.
- Instruct the client to return the Holter monitor approximately the same time that the test was started. The electrodes will be removed. The diary should be given to the nurse or technician, and the client should not leave until the diary has been briefly reviewed for any needed clarifications.
- Explain to the client that the cardiologist will submit a written report to his or her health care provider. The health care provider or other health care providers will notify the client of the findings.

Hysterosalpingography (hysterosalpingogram)

Normal Finding

Normal structure of the uterus and patent fallopian tubes.

Description

Hysterosalpingography is a fluoroscopic and x-ray examination of the uterus and fallopian tubes. A contrast substance, either oil-base Ethiodol or Lipiodol or water-soluble Salpix, is injected into the cervical canal. It flows through the uterus and into the fallopian tubes and spills into the abdominal area, allowing visualization of the uterus, the fallopian tubes, and the body of the uterus. Usually the procedure is performed by the radiologist and the health care provider (gynecologist).

The hysterosalpingogram should be done on the seventh to the ninth day after the menstrual cycle. The client should not be pregnant or have active bleeding, or an acute infection; if any of these conditions exists, the test should be canceled.

There may be some abdominal cramping, and sometimes there are chills and transient dizziness as the contrast substance spills into the abdominal area. Normally the spillage is not harmful and is expected.

The amount of radiation exposure is high because of the fluoroscopic examination. Today ultrasonography is replacing hysterosalpingography, except that the latter test is more effective in determining tubal patency.

Purposes

- To identify uterine fibroids, tumor, or fistula.
- To identify fallopian occlusion.
- To evaluate repeated fetal losses.

Clinical Problems

Abnormal Findings: Uterine masses (i.e., fibroids, tumor), uterine fistulas, fallopian tubal occlusion (i.e., adhesions, stricture), extrauterine pregnancy, evaluation of repeated fetal losses.

Procedure

- A consent form for hysterosalpingography should be signed by the client.
- Food and fluids are not restricted.
- A cleansing enema and douche may be ordered prior to the test.
- A mild sedative (e.g., diazepam [Valium]) may be ordered prior to the test.
- The client lies on an examining table in the lithotomy position. The gynecologist, health care provider, or radiologist inserts the speculum into the vaginal canal, and the contrast substance is injected into the cervix under fluoroscopic control. X-rays are taken throughout the 15- to 30-minute procedure.

Factors Affecting Diagnostic Results

- Tubal spasm may cause tubal stricture, which could give the appearance of a partial or complete tubal obstruction in a normal fallopian tube.

NURSING IMPLICATIONS WITH RATIONALE

- Check to see that the consent form is signed.
- Administer pretest orders—enema, douche, or sedative. If the client comes from home, check that she has prepared herself as ordered.

Client Teaching

- Explain to the client that the purpose of the test is to visualize the uterus and tubes for any abnormalities or to determine the patency of the fallopian tubes.
- Explain the procedure to the client. The procedure may slightly differ in your institution, so check before explaining to the client.
- Ask the client when she had her last menstrual period. Record the information. If pregnancy is suspected, the procedure should not be done.
- Inform the client that the test takes about 15 to 30 minutes.
- Encourage the client to ask questions and to express concerns. Be a good listener. Refer questions and concerns you cannot handle adequately to other appropriate health professionals.

Posttest

- Check for signs and symptoms of infection following the test, such as fever, increased pulse rate, and pain. Notify the health care provider.

Client Teaching

- Inform the client that she may experience some abdominal cramping and some dizziness. Explain that this is normal but that if there is continuous and severe cramping, she should tell the examiners.
- Inform the client that there may be some bloody discharge for several days following the test. If it continues beyond 3 to 4 days, she should notify her health care provider.
- Instruct client to call the health care provider if a high fever is present.

Hysteroscopy

Normal Finding

Normal uterine cavity; normal endometrial uterine tissue.

Description

Hysteroscopy allows visualization of the entire endometrial cavity of the uterus. This test is considered to be more effective for viewing and obtaining endometrial pathology than the D & C (dilatation and curettage) or hysterosalpingography. With D & C, scraping of the endometrial tissue is done without visualization, which may result in failure to harvest the pathologic tissue. With the use of the hysteroscope, a biopsy could be taken and polyp(s) removed.

Hysteroscopy is contraindicated if there is cervical or vaginal infection, pelvic inflammatory disease, or purulent vaginal discharge, or if cervical surgery had been performed previously. Risks of hysteroscopy include perforation of the uterus or infection.

Purpose

- To visualize the uterine cavity.
- To obtain a biopsy of the endometrial lining of the uterus.
- To remove a uterine polyp.

Clinical Problems

Abnormal Findings: Hyperplasia of the endometrial tissue in the uterus; endometrial cancer; polyps.

Procedure

- A consent form should be signed.
- Restrict food and fluid for 8 hours prior to the test.
- Have the client void before the procedure.
- The client is placed in the lithotomy position.
- A hysteroscope is placed through the cervical os into the endometrial cavity of the uterus. Carbon dioxide is usually instilled to distend the uterine cavity.
- Biopsy of tissue can be obtained.
- The test takes approximately 30 minutes.

Factors Affecting Diagnostic Results

- None reported.

NURSING IMPLICATIONS WITH RATIONALE

- Obtain a signed consent form from the client.
- Obtain a menstrual history. The test should be performed after menstruation and prior to ovulation.

Client Teaching

- Explain the procedure to the client.
- Explain that discomfort following the carbon dioxide instillation is possible. Lower abdominal distention (uterus) and bloating can result.

Posttest

- Monitor vital signs.
- Check for excessive bleeding or discharge.

Client Teaching

- Inform the client that cramping may occur following the test. Use of a mild analgesic decreases discomfort.
- Sexual intercourse or douching should be avoided for 2 weeks or as instructed by the health care provider.
- Instruct the client to report severe discomfort or shortness of breath immediately to the health care provider.

Intravenous pyelography (IVP)

Intravenous Pyelogram, Excretory Urography

Normal Finding

Normal size, structure, and function of the kidneys, ureters, and bladder.

Description

Intravenous pyelography (IVP) is more properly called *excretory urography,* because it visualizes the entire urinary tract and not just the kidney pelvis. A radiopaque substance (sodium diatrizoate or meglumine diatrizoate [Renografin-60]) is injected intravenously and a series of x-rays are taken at specific times. The test usually takes 30 to 45 minutes.

Excretory urography is useful for locating stones and tumors and for diagnosing kidney diseases (i.e., polycystic kidney, renovascular hypertension). A few clients may be hypersensitive to the radiopaque iodine dye, especially if they have a history of allergy to many substances. Emergency drugs (epinephrine, vasopressors, etc.), a tracheostomy set, a suction machine, and oxygen should be available for treating anaphylactoid reaction if it should occur.

Purposes

- To identify abnormal size, shape, and functioning of the kidneys.
- To detect renal calculi, tumor, cyst.

Clinical Problems

Abnormal Findings: Renal calculi, neoplasm (tumor) of the kidney or bladder, kidney diseases (polycystic kidney, hydronephrosis, renovascular hypertension).

Procedure

- A consent form for IVP should be signed by the client or an appropriate member of the family.
- The client should be NPO for 8 to 12 hours before the test. In the morning the client may be slightly dehydrated; however, this will help the kidney to concentrate the dye.
- A laxative is ordered the night before, and a cleansing enema(s) is ordered the morning of the test. These preparations may vary, so check with the radiology department for exact preparations.
- An antihistamine or a steroid may be given prior to the test to clients who are hypersensitive to iodine, seafood, and contrast dye used in other diagnostic tests as well as to those who have histories of asthma and severe allergies.

- Baseline vital signs should be recorded.
- The client lies in the supine position on an x-ray table. X-rays are taken 3, 5, 10, 15, and 20 minutes after the dye is injected.
- Emergency drugs and equipment should be available at all times.
- The test takes approximately 30 to 45 minutes. A delay in visualizing the kidneys could indicate kidney dysfunction.
- The client voids at the end of the test and another x-ray is taken to visualize the residual dye in the bladder.

Factors Affecting Diagnostic Results

- Feces, gas, and barium in the intestinal tract can decrease visualization of the kidney, ureters, and bladder.

NURSING IMPLICATIONS WITH RATIONALE

- Obtain a client history of known allergies. Notify the health care provider (HCP) if the client is allergic to seafood, iodine preparations, or contrast dye. As a precaution, an antihistamine or a steroid drug may be ordered if the client has an allergic reaction to drugs. A skin test may be performed to determine how hypersensitive the client is to the radiopaque contrast dye.
- Check the blood urea nitrogen (BUN). If BUN levels are >40 mg/dl, notify the HCP. Normally the test would not be done.

Client Teaching

- Explain to the client that the purpose of the test is to detect any kidney disorder or to observe the size, shape, and structure of the kidney, ureters, and bladder.
- Explain the procedure to the client. As a reminder, the procedural steps could be listed for the client.
- Instruct the client that he or she is not to eat or drink after dinner. Mild dehydration usually occurs. This could be harmful to clients with poor renal output, especially the aged and the debilitated. Sips of water or a glass of water may be indicated to avoid complications.
- Inform the client that he or she may feel a transient flushing or burning sensation and a salty or metallic taste during or following the IV injection of the contrast dye.
- Encourage the client to ask questions and to express any concerns before and during the procedure to the nurse, radiologist, and technician.

Posttest

- Monitor vital signs and urinary output.
- Observe, report, and record possible delayed reactions to the contrast dye (i.e., dyspnea, rashes, flushing, urticaria [hives], tachycardia, and others).

- Check the site where the dye was injected (usually it is in the antecubital fossa vein). If pain, warmth, or redness at the injection site is present, apply warm compresses, with permission.
- Administer oral antihistamines or steroids as ordered to treat dye reactions.

Laparoscopy

Pelviscopy, Peritoneoscopy

Normal Findings

Normal abdominal and pelvic organs; no pathology noted.

Description

Laparoscopy is the insertion of a laparoscope through the abdominal wall into the peritonium to visualize the abdominal and pelvic organs. A light camera is usually attached to the scope for visualization, and the peritoneal cavity is filled with liters of carbon dioxide gas to increase the view and separate the abdominal wall from the organs.

The **laparoscopy and pelviscopy** are useful for diagnosing endometriosis, ovarian cyst, tubal pregnancy, uterine fibroids, benign and malignant tumors, pelvic inflammatory disease (PID), salpingitis, cause of infertility, and adhesions. Surgical procedure can be performed with laparoscopy, such as biopsy specimens, tubal ligation, release of adhesions, and laser treatment for endometriosis.

Peritoneoscopy is primarily prescribed to view the liver and to stage cancers including lymphomas. It can be used for surgical procedures such as cholecystectomy, appendectomy, hernia repairs including hiatal hernia, bowel resection, and biopsies. Laparoscopy and peritoneoscopy overlap somewhat with their surgical procedures. These tests are usually performed with general anesthesia.

Contraindications for a laparoscopy include advanced abdominal wall cancer, severe bleeding disorder, and severe respiratory and/or cardiac disorders.

Purposes

- To visualize the abdominal and pelvic organs.
- To perform surgical procedures within the abdominal and pelvic region.

Clinical Problems

Abnormal Findings: Endometriosis, ovarian cysts, tumors, abscesses, ectopic pregnancy, uterine fibroids, liver nodules, cirrhosis, adhesions in the abdominal area, PID.

Procedures

Pretest

- A signed consent form is required.
- Nothing by mouth after midnight or 8 to 12 hours prior to the test procedure.
- Anticoagulant therapy should be discontinued 5 to 7 days prior to the test.
- Laboratory tests ordered prior to the test.
- Cleansing enemas as ordered the night before the procedure and/or in the morning.
- Client should void before the procedure.
- IV infusion started. IV medications may be given through the IV line.

Test Procedure

- Small surgical incision is made below the umbilicus.
- The peritoneal cavity is filled with carbon dioxide gas so that the organs can easily be visualized.
- Laparoscope is inserted through a trocar.
- After the procedure, carbon dioxide escapes; however, not all of the gas is removed but will be slowly eliminated from the body over a period of 24 hours.

Posttest

- Vital signs are monitored and bleeding from the small incisional area is checked periodically.
- Analgesics for pain and for shoulder or subcostal discomfort caused by carbon dioxide gas may be given every 4 to 6 hours.
- Physical activity should be minimized for 4 to 7 days posttest or as instructed by the health care provider.

Factors Affecting Diagnostic Results

- Excessive adhesions.
- Severely obese.

NURSING IMPLICATIONS WITH RATIONALE

- Obtain a history of the client's health problem. Relate findings with other health professionals.
- Check baseline vital signs. These vital signs are compared with those during the test procedure and during the posttest time.
- Report gas pains that remain beyond 24 to 36 hours and any frank bleeding from incision site.

■ Follow the posttest procedure.

Client Teaching

■ Explain to the client to take analgesics as ordered to relieve pain and discomfort due to the gas that was inserted in the abdomen. Inform the client that all the gas in the abdomen is not always released from the procedure; it may take at least 24 hours.

■ Instruct the client to report pain that lasts for 48 hours or more and any bright bleeding that occurs at the incisional site.

■ Answer the client's questions and if unable to, refer the questions to the primary health care provider or other professionals.

Lymphangiography (lymphangiogram)

Lymphography

Normal Finding

Normal lymphatic vessels and lymph nodes.

Description

Lymphangiography is an x-ray examination of the lymphatic vessels and lymph nodes. A radiopaque iodine contrast oil substance (e.g., Ethiodol) is injected into the lymphatic vessels of each foot; the dye can also be injected into the hands to visualize axillary and supraclavicular nodes. Fluoroscopy is used with x-ray filming to check on lymphatic filling of the contrast dye and to determine when the infusion of the contrast dye should be stopped. The infusion rate is controlled by a lymphangiographic pump, and approximately 1½ hours are required for dye to reach the level of the third and fourth lumbar vertebrae.

This test is useful to identify malignant lymphoma (Hodgkin's disease) and metastasis to the lymph nodes. Lymphangiograms are also used for staging malignant lymphoma, from stage I (a single lymph node area of involvement) to stage IV (diffuse extranodal involvement). Other tests, such as ultrasonography, computed tomography, and/or biopsy, may be used to confirm the diagnosis and to stage lymphoma involvement.

Lymphangiography is usually contraindicated if the client is hypersensitive to iodine or has severe chronic lung disease, cardiac disease, or advanced liver or kidney disease. Persons with possible allergies to iodine and/or contrast dye used in other diagnostic tests (e.g., IVP) should receive antihistamines or steroids before the test, and emergency drugs should be available during the test. Lipid pneumonia may occur if the contrast dye flows into the thoracic duct and sets up microemboli in the lungs. The small emboli that can occur will gradually disappear after several weeks or months.

Purposes

- To detect metastasis of the lymph nodes.
- To identify maliganant lymphoma.
- To determine the cause of lymphedema.
- To assist with the staging of malignant lymphoma.

Clinical Problems

Indications: Malignant lymphoma (Hodgkin's disease), metastasis to the lymph nodes, lymphedema (primary [decreased number of lymphatic vessels] or secondary [tumor or surgical removal]), staging of malignant lymphoma.

Procedure

- A consent form should be signed by the client.
- Food and fluids are not restricted.
- Antihistamines and a sedative may be ordered prior to the test.
- Contrast dye (blue) is injected intradermally between several toes of each foot, staining the lymphatic vessels of the feet in 15 to 20 minutes. This is for visualization of the lymphatic vessels.
- A local skin anesthetic is injected, and small incisions are made on the dorsum of each foot.
- A 30-gauge lymphangiographic needle with polyethylene tubing is inserted carefully into the identified lymphatic vessel. The contrast dye is slowly infused with the aid of the infusion pump over a period of $1\frac{1}{2}$ hours until it reaches the third and fourth lumbar vertebrae. The client should remain still during the procedure. X-rays are taken of the lymphatics in the leg, pelvic, abdominal, and chest. The entire test takes $2\frac{1}{2}$ to 3 hours.
- Twenty-four hours later, a second set of films is taken to visualize the lymph nodes. X-ray filming usually takes 30 minutes. The contrast dye remains in the lymph nodes for 6 months to a year; thus repeated x-rays can be taken to determine the disease process and the response to treatment.

Factors Affecting Diagnostic Results

- None known.

NURSING IMPLICATIONS WITH RATIONALE

- Explain the purpose and procedure to the client. Be available to answer questions, and be supportive of the client and family.

- Check that the consent form was signed by the client before giving the sedative for the test.
- Obtain a client history of allergies to seafood, iodine preparations, or contrast dye used in another x-ray test.
- Record baseline vital signs, and have the client void before the test.

Client Teaching

- Instruct the client to remain still during the test. Inform the client that there may be some discomfort with the injection of the local skin anesthetic into each foot. The sedative is given to promote relaxation and to decrease movement during the test.
- Inform the client that the blue contrast dye will discolor the urine and stool for several days and could cause the skin to have a bluish tinge for 24 to 48 hours.
- Inform the client that the test takes 2½ to 3 hours and that he or she will be told to return the next day for additional x-rays. Tell the client that the procedure will *not* be repeated the next day; only x-rays will be taken.

Posttest

- Keep the client on bed rest for 24 hours or as ordered.
- Monitor vital signs until stable and as indicated.
- Observe for dyspnea, pain, and hypotension, which could be due to microemboli from the spillage of the contrast dye.
- Assess the incisional site for signs of an infection (i.e., redness, oozing, and swelling). Report and record findings. The dressing is usually not changed for the first 48 hours.
- Check for leg edema. Elevate lower extremities as indicated.

Magnetic resonance imaging (MRI)

Nuclear Magnetic Resonance (NMR) Imaging

Normal Findings

Normal tissue, structure, and blood flow.

Description

Magnetic resonance imaging (MRI) produces images similar to those produced by computed tomography (CT), however, unlike CT, it does not use ionizing radiation and thus is free of the hazards presented by exposure to x-rays. The cost of MRI is approximately one-third more than the cost of CT.

The MRI scanner consists of a magnet encased in a large, doughnut-shaped cylinder. The client lies on a narrow table and is guided into the cylinder until the body part to be imaged is within the magnetic field. The anatomic nuclei of the cells of the body respond like magnets to the magnetic field and align. When a radio frequency wave is applied, the protons in the nuclei resonate, and when the radio frequency wave is removed, the energy released by the protons as they relax is detected as a radio signal. This signal is interpreted by a computer and translated into cross-sectional images.

Since the introduction of MRI in 1983, the quality of images produced by this technique has greatly improved, and MRI is now the most sensitive technique for defining the structure of internal organs and for detecting edema, infarction, hemorrhage, blood flow, tumors, infections, and plaques on the myelin sheath that cause Multiple Sclerosis. Many of these conditions would be difficult to distinguish using CT or conventional x-rays. It can differentiate between edema and tumor. MRI excels in diagnosing pathologic problems associated with the central nervous system (CNS), such as degenerated discs, tumors, hemorrhage, edema, cerebral infarction, and subdural hematoma. Early after an ischemic stroke, imaging can detect the stroke's location and extent, and can determine the severity of the damage to the brain tissue. MRI can visualize bone, joint, and soft tissue injuries. Bone artifacts do not occur and MRI can identify a tumor adjacent to or within bony structures (e.g., pituitary gland tumor).

Pacemakers, wires left in the chest from a previous pacemaker, aneurysm or surgical clips, certain hearing aids, and metallic heart valves are contraindications to undergoing an MRI procedure. Jewelry, watches, keys, credit cards, and hair clips must be removed prior to the procedure. When an emergency situation occurs during imaging, the client must be moved from the MRI room so that resuscitation equipment can be used. MRI is difficult to use to study critically ill clients on life-support systems because of the effect of the magnet on the equipment.

MRI and CT can be used for similar tissue studies. MRI involves use of contrast media in certain circumstances, but the IV contrast for MRI is chemically unrelated to the iodinated contrast used in CT and conventional radiography. Presently the only commercially available contrast for MRI is gadolinium-DTPA. Gadolinium (Magnavist) and Ferodax are frequently used to evaluate problems of the brain, base of the skull, and spine. This contrast agent can cross the abnormal blood-brain barrier. Imaging can occur 5 to 60 minutes after the start of the gadolinium infusion.

Magnetic Resonance of the Brain and Spine (Intracranial [IC] MRI):
Intracranial MRI gives cross-sectional images of the brain and spine. It can detect neuropathology through the bone such as visualizing fluid (edema) within soft tissues. The IC-MRI can identify cerebral thrombosis caused by cerebral vascular accident (stroke), cerebral tumors, abscesses, or aneurysms, cerebral hemorrhage, and demyelinated nerve fibers (myelin sheaths) causing multiple sclerosis (MS). It can also detail the abnormalities of the spinal cord.

Magnetic Resonance of the Heart and Coronary Arteries: Cine MRI, or ultrafast MRI, is a fast-moving MRI procedure that can image the heart in a continuous

motion. It is useful for perfusion imaging, and it can determine the patency of coronary arteries following coronary grafts. Also, it is used to detect the viability of the myocardium and to assess cardiac volumes. The echo-planar MRI (EPI), like cine MRI, is used for rapid imaging of the heart and coronary arteries.

Magnetic Resonance Angiography: Magnetic resonsance angiography (MRA) is a noninvasive means of displaying vessels by imaging. It maximizes the signals in structures containing blood flow and reconstructs only the structures with flow. It is useful for evaluating vascular lesions. Other structures of lesser interest are subtracted from the image by the computer.

Magnetic Resonance Spectroscopy: This MRI is a scanner that can evaluate and detect ischemic heart disease and the effects of cancer treatment on tumors. It is used to "rule out" Alzheimer's disease, to determine the extent of head injury due to trauma and stroke, and to identify the cause of coma.

Purpose

- To detect a central nervous system lesion, vascular problem (blood flow, hemorrhage), cardiac perfusion problem, injury, tumor, or edema.

Clinical Problems

Abnormal Findings: Tumors, blood clots, cysts, edema, hemorrhage, abscesses, infarctions, aneurysms, demyelinating disease (multiple sclerosis), dementia including Alzheimer's disease, muscular disease, skeletal abnormalities, congenital heart disease, intervertebral disc abnormalities, spinal cord compression, acute renal tubular necrosis, blood flow abnormalities.

Procedure

- A consent form should be signed.
- Inform the client that there will be no exposure to radiation.
- Empty bladder prior to the test.
- Remove all jewelry, including watches, glasses, hairpins, cosmetics that may contain metallic fragments, and any metal objects. The magnetic field can damage watches. Those with pacemakers are not candidates for MRI; some with metal prosthetics, especially heart valves, and those with nerve stimulating devices may not be candidates for MRI. Remove dentures and hearing aids as advised.
- Occupational history is important. Metal in the body, such as shrapnel or flecks of ferrous metal in eye, may cause critical injury, such as retinal hemorrhage.
- Contraindications include pregnancy and clients with epilepsy. MRI could cause excess heat in the amniotic fluid.
- With the closed MRI, the client must lie absolutely still on a narrow table with a cylinder-type scanner around the body area being scanned.
- Sedation may be needed if the client, receiving closed MRI, is extremely claustrophobic. A client receiving a sedative should not drive home, therefore, a family member or friend should be available to drive.

- Opened MRI may be ordered for clients who are claustrophic, obese, confused, or a child; a family member or friend may be present. A mirror is available to see outside during the procedure. Clients need to remain still during the opened MRI. Open MRI uses a lower-field magnet, whereas the close MRI uses a higher-field magnet.
- Certain MRI studies require a noniodinated contrast media (gadolinium Magnevist) which may be injected intravenously. Use of MR contrast media may be contraindicated for those with kidney dyfunction; the contrast media is excreted by the kidneys.
- There is no food or fluid restriction for adults. NPO for 4 hours for children.
- The procedure takes approximately 45 minutes to $1\frac{1}{2}$ hours.

Blood Flow: Extremities

- The limb to be examined is rested in a cradlelike support. Reference sites to be imaged are marked on the leg or arm, and the extremity is moved into a flow cylinder.
- The procedure takes approximately 15 minutes for arms and 15 minutes for legs.

Factors Affecting Diagnostic Results

- Movement during the procedure will distort the imaging.
- Ferrous metal in the body could cause critical injury to the client.
- Nonferrous metal may produce artifacts that degrade the images if in close proximity to the area being scanned.

NURSING IMPLICATIONS WITH RATIONALE

- Elicit any problems with claustrophobia. Relaxation techniques or a sedative might be used.
- Ascertain from the client the presence of a pacemaker, wire left in the body from a previous pacemaker, heart valve, any metal prosthetics, or shrapnel left in the body which could cause serious tissue injury as the result of the magnetic pull.
- Alert the physician or health care provider if client is on an IV pump. MRI can disrupt IV flow.
- Provide emotional support.

Client Teaching

- Explain the procedure. Inform the client that various noises (clicking, thumping) from the scanner will be heard. Ear plugs are available. Inform the client that the MRI personnel will be in another room but can communicate via an intercom system. With the open MRI, a family member or friend may be in the room with the client while the MRI scanning is taking place.
- Explain to the client that there is no exposure to radiation. The contrast media that might be used is not iodinated contrast.

- Instruct the client to remove watches, credit cards, hairpins, jewelry, and makeup. The magnetic field can damage a watch.
- Inform the client that the MRI procedure is painless. Encourage the client to relax during the testing.
- Caution clients with cardiac pacemakers not to approach the MRI unit.
- Inform the client who has metal fillings in teeth that a "tingling sensation" may be felt during imaging.

Mammography (mammogram)

Normal Finding

Normal ducts and glandular tissue; no abnormal masses.

Description

Mammography is an x-ray examination of the breasts to detect cysts or tumors. Benign cysts are seen on the mammogram as well-outlined, clear lesions and tend to be bilateral, whereas malignant tumors are irregular and poorly defined and tend to be unilateral. A breast mass (neoplasm) cannot be clinically palpable until it is 1 cm in size, so it may take 5 years or longer to grow and be detectable. A mammogram can detect a breast lesion approximately 2 years before it is palpable.

The second most common cause of cancer deaths in women in the United States is breast cancer (cancer of the lung being the most common cause). Eighty to 85% of breast cancer occurs in women over 50 years of age. The majority of those women do not have any other identifiable risk factors.

There is much controversy on how often a woman should receive a mammogram and whether this x-ray test should be only for symptomatic women having a palpable mass, nipple discharge, skin thickening of the breast, or a markedly asymmetric breast, rather than for those who are asymptomatic.

The American Cancer Society and the American College of Radiologists have suggested that women between 35 and 40 years of age have a mammogram every 2 years, and women over 40 years have an annual mammogram. Radiation received is very low dose.

The mammogram can detect approximately 90% of breast malignancies; however, the test carries a 10% false-positive rate. A positive test should be confirmed by biopsy.

There have been technical improvements in the equipment, mammographic units, and the recording system used for mammography. The use of radiographic grids has improved the imaging quality of mammograms by decreasing image density. With the use of grids, the visibilty of small cancers is increased. Also, the use of magnification mammography has improved the capability to identify cancers; however, the magnification increases the client's radiation dose by prolonging exposure time.

Purposes

- To screen for breast mass(es).
- To detect breast cyst or tumor.

Clinical Problems

Indications: A breast mass (cyst or tumor); peroidic examination of the breast, as indicated by the health care provider.

Procedure

- Food and fluids are not restricted.
- The client removes clothes and jewelry from the neck to the waist and wears a paper or cloth gown that opens in the front. Powder and ointment on the breast should be removed to avoid false-positive results. No deodorants should be used.
- The client is standing, and each breast (one at a time) rests on an x-ray cassette table. As the breast is compressed, the client will be asked to hold her breath while the x-ray is taken. Two x-rays are taken of each breast.
- The procedure usually takes 15 to 30 minutes.

Factors Affecting Diagnostic Results

- Previous breast surgery can affect the reading of the x-ray film.
- Jewelry, metals, ointment, and powder could cause false-positive results.

NURSING IMPLICATIONS WITH RATIONALE

- Ascertain whether the client is pregnant or is suspected of being pregnant. A mammogram is contraindicated during pregnancy.
- Ask the client to identify the lump in the breast if one is present.
- Be supportive of the client. Allow the client time to express her fears and concerns. Notify the health care provider of her concerns, especially if they cause her great anxiety.
- Answer the client's questions when possible or refer the question(s) to other health care professionals.

Client Teaching

- Explain the procedure to the client. Explain that the test will not hurt but may cause a little discomfort when the breast is compressed during the x-ray.

- Inform the client that the test takes 15 to 30 minutes; however, the client will be asked to wait until the x-rays are developed and readable. Inform the client not to be alarmed if an additional x-ray is needed.
- Instruct the client not to use ointment, powder, or deodorant on the breast or under the arms on the day of the mammogram.
- Instruct the client to perform a self-examination of the breast after each menstrual period. Demonstrate breast examination, if necessary.

Mediastinoscopy

Normal Finding

Normal mediastinal structure and lymph nodes; absence of disease process.

Description

This is a surgical procedure in which a mediastinoscope is inserted through a small incision at the suprasternal notch. The purpose is to visualize mediastinal structure and lymph nodes and to obtain lymph node biopsy. These mediastinal lymph nodes receive lymphatic drainage from the lungs. They are examined to detect lymphoma (e.g., Hodgkin's disease, sarcoidosis, lung metastasis, and for staging of lung cancer).

Mediastinoscopy is an invasive procedure and usually is performed when x-rays, sputum cytology, and lung scans (computed tomography and nuclear) have not confirmed a diagnosis. Complications from this test may include perforation of the trachea, esophagus, aorta, or other blood vessels; pneumothorax; laryngeal nerve damage; and infection.

Purposes

- To view mediastinal structure and lymph nodes.
- To obtain lymph node biopsy.

Clinical Problems

Abnormal Findings: Lymphoma (e.g., Hodgkin's disease), sarcoidosis, lung metastasis to mediastinal lymph nodes, granulomatous infection, mediastinal tuberculosis.

Procedure

- Food and fluids are restricted 8 to 12 hours prior to the test.
- Consent should be signed by the client before premedication or by the designated family member.

- Obtain baseline vital signs and have client void prior to the surgical procedure.
- Complete a preoperative checklist.

Factors Affecting Diagnostic Results

- None known.

NURSING IMPLICATIONS WITH RATIONALE

- Check that the consent form is signed before the client is premedicated for surgery.
- Record baseline vital signs. Check to be sure that the preoperative checklist is completed.
- Encourage the client to express concerns about the mediastinoscopy. Answer questions; refer questions you cannot answer to appropriate health professionals.
- Be available to family members and provide time for them to express concerns and ask questions.

Client Teaching

- Explain the procedure to the client. It is a surgical procedure and the client will receive general anesthesia. Ask the client if he or she is allergic to any anesthetic. Explain that this test procedure will take approximately 1 hour.

Posttest

- Monitor vital signs until stable and as indicated. Report changes (i.e., increase in pulse rate [tachycardia], increase in respirations and dyspnea, decrease in blood pressure).
- Check breath sounds. Report absence of breath sounds if noted.
- Check dressing for bright blood or increased blood on dressing.
- Report if crepitus is detected at chest or neck area. This could be due to air leaking into the subcutaneous tissue as the result of perforated lung.
- Be supportive to client and family members. Provide comfort measures as needed (i.e., position change, medication).

Myelography (myelogram)

Normal Finding

Normal spinal subarachnoid space; no obstructions.

Description

Myelography is a fluoroscopic and radiologic examination of the spinal subarachnoid space (spinal canal) using air or a radiopaque contrast agent (oil and water soluble). With clients who are hypersensitive to iodine and seafood, air is the contrast agent used. This procedure is performed in an x-ray department by a radiologist, a neurologist, and/or a neurosurgeon. After the contrast dye is injected into the lumbar area, the fluoroscopic table is tilted until the suspected problem area can be visualized, and spot films are taken.

If the contrast agent is an oil (i.e., Pantopaque or isophendylate), then the contrast agent must be removed at the end of the test. Because oil is heavier than spinal fluid, it does not mix and tends to sink to the lower part of the spinal canal. Water-soluble contrast agents (e.g., metrizoate sodium [Amipaque]) do not have to be removed; however, after the procedure the client should remain in a high Fowler's position (60-degree elevation of the head) for 8 hours.

The myelogram is usually performed to detect spinal lesions (i.e., intervertebral disks, tumors, or cysts). This procedure is contraindicated if increased intracranial pressure is suspected.

Purposes

- To identify herniated intervertebral disks.
- To detect cysts or tumor at or within the spinal column.
- To detect spinal nerve root injury.

Clinical Problems

Abnormal Findings: Herniated intervertebral disks, metastatic tumors, cysts, astrocytomas and ependymomas (within the spinal cord), neurofibromas and meningiomas (within the subarachnoid space), spinal nerve root injury, arachnoiditis.

Procedure

- A consent form should be signed.
- The client should be NPO for 4 to 8 hours before the test. If the myelogram is scheduled for the afternoon, then the client may have a light breakfast or clear liquids in the morning, as ordered.
- A cleansing enema may be ordered the night before or early in the morning of the test to remove feces and gas for improved visualization.
- Premedications include a sedative and/or narcotic analgesic and usually atropine. The drugs are prescribed by the health care provider.
- The client is placed in the prone position on a fluoroscopic table and is secured to the table with the use of several straps. A spinal puncture is performed, and contrast dye is injected. As the dye enters the spinal canal, the table is tilted.
- The myelogram takes approximately 1 hour.

Posttest

- After the test the radiopaque oil is removed, and the client should remain flat for 6 to 8 hours. If a water-soluble radiopaque agent was used, then the client's head should be elevated at 60 degrees for 8 hours.

Factors Affecting Diagnostic Results

- Gas or fecal material in the gastrointestinal tract.

NURSING IMPLICATIONS WITH RATIONALE

- Obtain a client history of allergies to iodine, seafood, and radiopaque dye used in other x-ray tests. Inform the health care provider, because air or oxygen can be used as the contrast agent instead of the dye. A skin test may be performed.
- Follow the prescribed pre-test regimen (i.e., NPO, a cleansing enema, and pre-medications [sedative or narcotic analgesic]). Check that the consent form has been signed before giving a sedative or narcotic.
- Allow the client the time to ask questions and to express concerns or fears. Refer questions you cannot answer to other health professionals.
- Recognize conditions in which myelography would be contraindicated (i.e., multiple sclerosis [could cause an exacerbation] and increased intracranial pressure [↑ ICP]). The radiologist and/or neurosurgeon should be notified if they are unaware of the client's condition.
- Record base-line vital signs.

Client Teaching

- Explain the procedure to the client. Inform the client that he or she will most likely lie on the abdomen and will be strapped to a table. The health care provider will tilt the table as the dye circulates in the spinal canal.
- Inform the client that he or she may have a transient burning sensation and/or a flushed, warm feeling as the dye is injected; the sensation may last for a short time afterwards.
- Instruct the client to let the health care provider know of any discomfort (i.e., pain down the legs). The test takes about 1 hour.

Posttest

- Monitor vital signs until stable and as indicated.
- Monitor urinary output. The client should void in 8 hours.
- Observe for signs and symptoms of chemical or bacterial meningitis (i.e., severe headache, fever, stiff neck, irritability, photophobia, and convulsions).

Client Teaching

- Instruct the client to lie in the prone and/or supine position for 6 to 8 hours, as ordered. If the client received a water-soluble contrast agent or if all the contrast oil was not removed, the head of the bed should be elevated at a 60-degree angle for 8 hours or longer.

- Encourage the client to increase fluid intake. The fluids will help restore the cerebrospinal fluid loss. Increased fluid intake may decrease a post-lumbar-puncture headache, which could be due to a loss of spinal fluid.
- Instruct the client about prevention measures for avoiding back injury (i.e., principles of good body mechanics, such as flexing the knees and keeping the back straight when lifting).

Nephrotomography

Normal Finding

Normal size and shape of kidney; no abnormality noted in kidney tissue.

Description

Nephrotomography visualizes the kidney in detail by combining the use of tomography and intravenous pyelography. Tomography is a radiographic examination in which each sequence of x-ray film represents a slice of a single layer of tissue. Flat-plate x-ray cannot give detailed visualization of tissue from various angles and depth as can tomography. Contrast medium is injected prior to the tomographic examination. The purpose of this test is to differentiate between a solid renal tumor and a renal cyst. The thickness of the mass and its interior are recorded on film.

Purpose

- To differentiate between a renal tumor and a renal cyst.

Clinical Problems

Abnormal Findings: Solid renal tumors, renal cysts, renal sinus-related lesions, adrenal tumors, renal trauma, renal areas of nonperfusion.

Procedure

- Food and fluids are restricted for 8 hours before the test.
- A consent form should be signed.
- Check that the client is not allergic to contrast medium used in other x-ray tests, iodine, or seafood. Notify the health care provider if the client has allergies to these substances.

- During the test changes in positions to prone, supine, and lateral might be requested. The x-ray tube moves rapidly during the test procedure.
- Contrast medium is injected intravenously (by infusion or bolus), and tomographic filming takes place while the dye is perfusing the kidney and while kidney is excreting dye.

Factors Affecting Diagnostic Results

- Recent use of barium sulfate for a gastrointestinal series or barium enema might decrease detailed visualization of the kidney.

NURSING IMPLICATIONS WITH RATIONALE

- Obtain baseline vital signs prior to the test.
- Check client's history for allergy to contrast dye, iodine, or seafood. The health care provider should be notified of any past allergic reaction or sensitivity to the above substances.

Client Teaching

- Explain the procedure to the client *(see Procedure)*. Inform the client that the test takes approximately 1 hour and that there should be no discomfort except for lying on the x-ray table.
- Inform the client that several x-rays are taken first, then dye is injected, and more x-rays are taken.
- Tell the client that a flush may be felt as the dye is injected. The contrast medium can be given as an infusion or as a bolus injection.
- Inform the client that changing body positions, such as back to side, may be requested by the radiologist.
- Allow time for the client to express concern about the test and unknown findings. Answer the client's questions or refer the questions to appropriate health professionals.

Posttest

- Monitor vital signs and urine output. Changes in pulse rate (tachycardia) should be reported immediately to the health care provider.
- Observe for allergic reaction to contrast medium (i.e., rash, itching, dysphagia, or urticaria [hives]).

Nuclear scans (bone, brain, brain perfusion, heart, kidney, liver and spleen, colon and ovary, gastroesophageal reflux, gastrointestinal bleeding, gastric emptying, gallbladder, lung, and thyroid studies)*

Radionuclide Imaging, Radioisotope Scans

Normal Finding

Adult: Normal; no observed pathology.

Description

Nuclear medicine is the clinical field concerned with the diagnostic and therapeutic uses of radioactive materials or isotopes (one or more atoms of the same chemical element but with different atomic weights). A radioactive isotope is an unstable isotope that decays or disintegrates, emitting radiation or energy. Radioisotopes are referred to as *radionuclides*. Radioactive materials are concentrated by certain organs of the body, and their distribution in normal tissue differs from the distribution in diseased tissues. Equal or uniform gray distribution is normal, but lighter areas, referred to as *hot spots,* indicate hyperfunction and darker areas, *cold spots,* indicate hypofunction. ***Note:*** The hot spots can be lighter or darker areas which depends on the equipment, display of the images, and the film. Hyperfunction or hot spots mean that more of the tracer is concentrated in the area and can be displayed as light spots on a black screen or dark spots on a white screen.

Nuclear medicine imaging began in the early 1950s with the use of a rectilinear scanner. This type of scanner was replaced in the late 1960s by the gamma scintillation camera, also called the Anger camera, after its inventor, Hal Anger. The gamma scintillation camera converts photons emitted by the radionuclide to a signal which forms an image of the distribution of radionuclide.

The two types of imaging systems are planar imaging which projects images acquired from two or three different angles, and single photon emission computed tomography (SPECT), in which the scintillation camera rotates and projects images in an arc of 180° (for cardiac imaging) to 360°, acquiring 32 or more images. SPECT became available in the 1980s. The advantage of SPECT over planar imaging is that with SPECT the images are not obscured by overlying organs, tissue, or bone. SPECT uses a conventional Anger camera detector head with parallel hole collimator (the part of the camera that absorbs photons) which fits in a rotating gantry. This

*Revised by Frank Di Gregorio, CNMT, RDMA, Director, Community Imaging Center, Wilmington, DE.

camera orbits around a client lying on a special table. Also with SPECT, the images are enhanced with computer processing. The use of a two- or three-headed imaging gamma camera increases the sensitivity and specificity of the SPECT system. With the use of filtering and three-dimensional computer reconstruction of the images, the data analysis can be of great diagnostic value. Nuclear medicine imaging is moving toward a new era with the use of high-speed computers.

The use of radionuclides as radiopharmaceuticals is considered safe. Reactions are uncommon and adverse reactions are rare (occurring 1 to 10 per 100,000 administrations). The radionuclide used in most studies is technetium 99m (Tc-99m), which accounts for 70% of the nuclear imaging procedures. Other radionuclides used for studying the function, anatomy, and morphology of organs include Iodine 123 and 125 (I-123, I-125), thallium (T-201), xenon (Xe-133), indium 111 (In-111)-labeled white blood cells, and gallium (Ga-67) citrate.

The purposes and methods of various imaging organs are discussed in detail below. Positron emission tomography (PET) is discussed separately elsewhere in this text.

Clinical Problems

Organ/Study	Indications/Purposes
Bone	To detect early bone disease (i.e., osteomyelitis, ankylosing spondolysis); carcinoma metastasis to the bone; bone response to therapeutic regimens (i.e., radiation therapy, chemotherapy [antineoplastic agent])
	To determine unexplained bone pain
	To detect fractures and abnormal healing of fractures; degenerative bone disorders
Brain	To detect an intracranial mass (i.e., tumors [malignant or benign], abscess, cancer metastasis to the brain, head trauma [subdural hematoma], cerebral vascular accident [stroke] after the third or fourth week, aneurysms)
Brain perfusion	To diagnose Alzheimer's disease, brain death, AIDS dementia
	To locate seizure foci
	To determine the location and size of cerebral ischemia
Heart (cardiac) (MUGA*)	To identify cardiac hypertrophy (cardiomegaly)
	To quantify cardiac output (ejection fraction), wall motion
	To detect congestive heart failure (CHF), and aneurysm
Kidney (renal)	To detect parenchymal renal disease (i.e., tumor, cysts, glomerulonephritis), obstruction of the urinary tract
	To assess the function of renal transplantation
Liver and spleen	To detect tumors, cysts, or abscesses of the liver or spleen; hepatic metastasis; splenic infarct
	To assess liver response to therapeutic regimens (i.e., radiation therapy, chemotherapy)
	To identify hepatomegaly and splenomegaly
	To identify liver position and shape

Organ/Study	Indications/Purposes
Colon and ovary (monoclonal antibodies for cancer)	To detect colon and ovarian cancer cells in the body
Gastrointestinal reflux	To detect esophageal reflux syndrome
Gastrointestinal bleeding	To detect the localization of gastrointestinal (active and occult) and non-gastrointestinal bleeding sites
Gastric emptying	To diagnose gastric obstruction and the cause of dysmotility
Gallbladder (cholecytokinin hepatobiliary)	To diagnose acute or chronic cholecystitis, common duct obstruction To detect hypercholestosis conditions
Lung	To detect pulmonary emboli; tumors; pulmonary diseases with perfusion changes (i.e., emphysema, bronchitis, pneumonia) To assess arterial perfusion changes secondary to cardiac disease
Thyroid	To detect thyroid mass (i.e., tumors); diseases of the thyroid gland (i.e., Graves', Hashimoto's thyroiditis) To determine the size, structure, and position of the thyroid gland To evaluate thyroid function resulting from hyperthyroidism and hypothyroidism

*For nuclear stress tests see the Procedure for Heart (Cardiac) Scanning section, below.

Procedure

The radionuclide (radioisotope) is administered orally, inhaled, or intravenously. The interval from the time the radioactive substance is given to the time of the imaging can differ according to the radionuclide and organ in question. The scintillation camera detects the radiation that comes from the organ. Normally masses such as tumors absorb more of the radioactive substance than does normal tissue.

For diagnostic purposes the dose of radionuclide is low (<30 mCi) and should have little effect on visitors, other clients, and nursing and medical personnel. Usually food and fluids are not restricted unless the studies are to diagnose the gallbladder.

The procedures for the organ scans are listed according to the radionuclides used, the method of administration, the waiting period after injection, the food and fluids allowed, and other instructions.

1. **Bone:** Bone scanning can detect abnormalities weeks to months before conventional skeletal radiography. The use of SPECT improves the sensitivity and specificity of the bone scan.
   a. *Radionuclides:* TC-99m–labeled phosphate compounds (Tc-99m diphosphonate, pyrophosphate, medronate sodium).
   b. *Administration:* Intravenously.
   c. *Waiting period after injection:* Waiting periods can differ according to the radionuclides used (e.g., for Tc-99m the period is 2 to 3 hours [3 hours for an edematous person]).
   d. *Food and fluids:* No restrictions; for Tc-99m, water is encouraged during the waiting period (at least 6 glasses).

e. *Other instructions:* The client should void before the imaging begins and be well hydrated. Any metal objects, such as jewelry or keys, should be removed. Scanning usually occurs 2 to 4 hours after IV injection of the radionuclicide and takes $\frac{1}{2}$ to 2 hours to complete. A sedative may be ordered if the client has difficulty lying quietly during imaging. Both anterior and posterior view are obtained.

2. **Brain:** Scanning is done for cerebral blood-dynamic or static imaging flow study. Many abnormalities of the central nervous system alter the blood-brain barrier and permit localization of the radioactive tracer dose. Radionuclide brain scanning is very effective for identifying metastatic disease, strokes, subdural abscesses, and hematomas.

a. *Radionuclides:* Tc-99m glucoheptonate, Tc-99m-O_4, Tc-99m diethylenetri-amine penta-acetic acid, (Tc-99m-DTPA), Tl-201 NaCl.

b. *Administration:* Intravenously.

c. *Waiting period after injection:* Tc-99m-O_4, 1 to 3 hours; Tc-99m-DTPA, 45 minutes to 1 hour. Frequently a few photo scans are taken before the waiting period is over.

d. *Food and fluids:* No restrictions.

e. *Other instructions:* When Tc-99m-O_4 is used, the client may be given 10 drops of Lugol's solution the night before or at least 1 hour before the injection of potassium perchlorate, 200 mg to 1 g, 1 to 3 hours before the scheduled scan. These drugs block the uptake of Tc-99m-O_4 in the salivary glands, thyroid, and choroid plexus. With Tc-99m-DTPA, blocking agents are not necessary. The client should remain still during the imaging (for $\frac{1}{2}$ to 1 hour).

3. **Brain Perfusion Study:** The perfusion study is done to diagnose Alzheimer's disease and extrapyramidal disorders (e.g., Parkinson's disease), and locate seizure foci and cerebral ischemia.

a. *Radionuclides:* Tc-99m-hexamethylpropyleneamineoxime (Tc-99m-HM-PAO).

b. *Administration:* Intravenously.

c. *Waiting period after injection:* Scanning begins 15 minutes, but no longer than 30 minutes, after the injection.

d. *Food and fluids:* No restriction.

e. *Other instructions:* The imaging room should be quiet and lights dimmed. The IV line should be inserted before the test. The client lies still 15 minutes before the Tc-99m-HM-PAO injection. During imaging the client is in the supine position with the head in a head holder. The entire brain including the cerebellum is imaged.

4. **Heart (Cardiac) MUGA:** (*For myocardial perfusion imaging studies with stress imaging, see Stress/Exercise Testing.*)

Multigated acquisition (MUGA) scanning is a rapid, safe method to evaluate the heart size, ventricle wall motion, and ejection fraction. The client's blood is tagged with a radioactive tracer, such as technetium-99m, which permits the heart and its function to be visualized. There is multiple imaging during MUGA scanning. MUGA identifies changes occurring with contraction and expansion of the ventricles of the heart. With cardiac disease, the heart's ability to pump blood sufficiently may be reduced. The amount of radiation exposure is comparable to that of a CT scan. MUGA may be performed with the stress test.

a. *Radionuclides:* Tc-99m-O_4 tagged red blood cells (RBCs).

b. *Administration:* Intravenously.

c. *Waiting period after injection:* None.

d. *Food and fluids:* None.

e. *Other instructions:* The electrocardiogram is monitored. The client is in a supine position with a gamma camera over the chest. The radioactive tracer (containing no dye) allows visualization of the heart and its function.

5. **Kidney (Renal):** The renal scan is performed to evaluate renal function and perfusion and to detect renovascular diseases associated with glomerular filtration problems. This test can identify renal obstruction, trauma, acute and chronic renal failure, renal artery stenosis, and renal transplant rejection. Two drugs may be used with renal imaging: furosemide (Lasix), for determining renal excretory function, and Captopril, for identifying renovascular hypertension.

a. *Radionuclides:* Tc-99m pertechnetate and Tc-99m-glucoheptomate for renal cortical and tubular disorders; Tc-99m diethylenetriamine penta-acetic acid (Tc-99m-DTPA) for evaluating renal function and perfusion disorders; Tc-99m glucoheptonate and I-131 hippuran (for renal perfusion studies); Tc-99m mercaptylacetyltriglycine (Tc-99m-MAG3) for evaluating renal clearance related to renal insufficiency.

b. *Administration:* Intravenously.

c. *Waiting period after injection:* Renal perfusion study: Imaging is done immediately after the radiopharmaceutical is given intravenously. Renogram curves are plotted. Kidney disorders: 3 to 30 minutes after Tc-99m-DTPA is injected.

d. *Food and fluids:* No restrictions. The client should be well hydrated. He or she should drink at least two or three glasses of water 30 minutes before the scheduled scan. Dehydration could lead to false test results.

e. *Other instructions:* The client should void before the scan. If the client has had an IVP or renogram, the scan should be delayed 24 hours. The client should lie quietly 30 minutes to 1 hour during imaging. Usually there are a combination of diagnostic renal tests performed along with radionuclide renal scanning to determine the cause of the renal disorder. Radionuclide renal scanning is useful for clients allergic to contrast.

6. **Liver and Spleen:** Liver imaging can detect 90% of hepatic metastases and 85% of hepatocellular diseases. It is useful for screening the liver and spleen for lacerations and hematomas following trauma. SPECT improves lesion/mass detection.

a. *Radionuclides:* Tc-99m compounds: Tc-99m sulfur colloid.

b. *Administration:* Intravenously.

c. *Waiting period after injections:* Tc-99-sulfur colloid, 15 minutes. A spleen scan can be done at the same time.

d. *Food and fluids:* No restrictions.

e. *Other instructions:* The client should lie quietly for 30 minutes to 1 hour during the imaging. The client may be asked to turn from side to side and onto his or her abdomen during the imaging.

7. **Colon and Ovary:** Colorectal cancer is the third most common malignancy. Ovarian cancer is the fourth most frequent cause of cancer death in women. Radiolabeled monoclonal antibodies are used to identify colon and ovarian cancer cells in areas of the body. The radiolabeled monoclonal antibodies attach to cancer cells and the cancer cells can then be detected with use of a gamma camera.

a. *Radionuclides:* Monoclonal antibodies labeled with indium 111 (111-In).

b. *Administration:* Intravenously. Infusion takes 5 to 30 minutes.

c. *Waiting period after injection:* 3 to 5 days after radiolabeled monoclonal antibodies. Usually two sets of images are taken at different times using the nuclear gamma camera.

d. *Food and fluids:* Light breakfast or lunch.

e. *Other instructions:* Regular medications can be taken. Client voids prior to the test. Allergic reaction to the monoclonal antibodies, though uncommon (<4%), may occur. Monoclonal antibodies are obtained from mice (human cancer cells are injected into the mice to produce antibodies).

8. **Gastroesophageal Reflux:** Esophageal clearance is determined following a swallowed radioactive tracer. Numerous esophageal tests, such as endoscopy, barium esophagoscopy, and acid reflux testing may be performed to detect esophageal reflux syndrome. The radionuclide gastroesophageal reflux scan is highly sensitive (99%) for esophageal reflux.

a. *Radionuclides:* Solution containing 150 ml of orange juice, 150 ml of 0.1 N hydrochloric acid, and 300 µCi Tc-99m sulfur colloid (Tc-99m-SC). Child: 250 µCi Tc-99m-SC in 10 ml of sterile water via a feeding tube.

b. *Administration:* Orally.

c. *Waiting period:* 30 seconds.

d. *Food and fluids:* Fasting for at least 4 hours prior to the study.

e. *Other instructions:* The client is in an upright or supine position. The procedure may require that the client perform a Valsalva maneuver.

9. **Gastrointestinal (GI) Bleeding:** Upper GI bleeding sites can be more easily detected than lower GI bleeding sites. Tc-99m-labeled (tagged) RBCs are most effective for detecting active bleeding sites. The radionuclide GI bleeding study is more sensitive than angiography. For a positive test result the client must be actively bleeding at the time of imaging for accurate identification of the bleeding site.

a. *Radionuclides:* Tc-99m-labeled RBCs.

b. *Administration:* Intravenously by bolus injection. For Tc-99m-labeled (tagged) RBCs, withdraw 5 to 8 ml of whole blood into a shielded syringe containing Tc-99m sodium pertechnetate. After processing the blood, Tc-99m-labeled RBCs are injected as a bolus.

    c. *Waiting period after injection:* Imaging begins immediately after injection or until the site of bleeding is located. If negative after 2 hours, imaging may be repeated when client begins active bleeding or imaging at different time periods during the 24 hours after injection.

    d. *Food and fluids:* NPO unless otherwise indicated.

    e. *Other instructions:* The client is in the supine position. Imaging is usually over the abdominal and pelvic areas. This test may be done as an emergency study, before surgery to locate the site of gastric bleeding, or before angiography. Sequential images are acquired for 90 minutes. If the test is negative for bleeding sites, imaging can be taken within 2 to 4 hours or when active bleeding is suspected.

10. **Gastric Emptying:** Delayed gastric emptying could be due to acute disorders, such as trauma, postoperative ileus, gastroenteritis, or chronic disorders, such as diabetes gastroparesis, peptic ulcers, pyloric stenosis, and Zollinger-Ellison syndrome.

    a. *Radionuclides:* In-111 DTPA or Tc-99m-labeled juice and Tc-99m sulfur colloid-labeled eggs.

    b. *Administration:* The client ingests a scrambled egg sandwich and juice (all radiolabeled). Tc-99m-sulfur colloid-labeled instant oatmeal may be ordered instead of eggs.

    c. *Waiting period after oral meal:* Immediately after ingesting the oral meal and continuously for 1 hour. A 2-hour imaging may also be requested following the oral meal.

    d. *Foods and fluids:* NPO for at least 4 hours and no smoking prior to the test.

    e. *Other instructions:* The client is in a mid-Fowler's position for the meal and during imaging. The test should be performed in the morning because during the day the gastric emptying time can vary.

11. **Gallbladder (Hepatobiliary Scan):** Hepatobiliary radioactive scanning is more sensitive for diagnosing acute cholecystitis than other standard gallbladder diagnostic tests. With hepatobiliary scanning, accurate imaging of the biliary tract can be performed even when there is marked hepatic dysfunction and jaundice.

    a. *Radionuclides:* Tc-99m disofenin, Tc-99m mebrofenin, or other Tc-IDA derivatives.

    b. *Administration:* Intravenously, cholecytokinin (CCK), a hormone that stimulates the gallbladder (GB) to contract and empty, may be used with normal saline solution as an infusion to promote GB emptying for imaging purposes.

    c. *Waiting period after injection:* Immediate after CCK and radionuclide infusions.

    d. *Foods and fluids:* NPO for at least 4 hours before the test with use of CCK.

    e. *Other instructions:* Usually CCK is given before the radiopharmaceutical injection to stimulate the gallbladder or clients who have not eaten. CCK is short-acting (20 to 30 minutes). The normal value for gallbladder ejection fraction (GBEF%) is >35%. Lower values indicate chronic cholecystitis. Higher values usually indicate hypercholestosis conditions. Nausea and abdominal discomfort may occur for a few minutes after the CCK infusion.

12. **Lung (Pulmonary):** Lung perfusion and ventilation scannings are sensitive for detecting pulmonary emboli (PE), obstructive pulmonary disease, and lung carcinoma. Both types of lung scans may be performed to identify the pulmonary disorder.
    a. *Radionuclides:* Perfusion study: Tc-99m compounds: macroaggregated albumin (Tc-99m-MAA), Tc-99m human albumin microspheres (Tc-99m-HAM). Ventilation study: Xe-133 (more commonly used), Xe-127 (not commonly used), krypton (Kr) 81m, and Tc-99m-DTPA aerosol.
    b. *Administration:* Intravenously (perfusion) or inhaled (ventilation).
    c. *Waiting period after injection:* Tc-99m compounds, 5 minutes after the injection of the radionuclide.
    d. *Food and fluids:* No restrictions.
    e. *Other instructions:* A chest radiograph is usually ordered for comparison with the nuclear medicine study. The client should lie quietly for 30 minutes during the imaging; however, for the inhaled test, the client is seated. Usually the camera is positioned behind the client.

13. **Thryoid:** Thyroid scintigraphy is effective for determining the functional status of the thyroid nodules, and for differentiating between primary thyroid carcinoma and metastases to the thyroid gland. Radioactive iodine is the most frequently used radionuclide because iodine is easily taken up in the thyroid gland. Iodine is a precursor in thyroid hormone synthesis.
    a. *Radionuclides:* I-131 sodium iodide, I-123, I-125, Tc-99m-pertechnetate.
    b. *Administration:* I-123, I-125, I-131 (oral: liquid or capsule), Tc-99m-pertechnetate (intravenously).
    c. *Waiting period after injection:* I-123, I-125, I-131—2 to 24 hours. I-123 is the radionuclide most commonly used because it has a shorter half-life. Tc-99m-pertechnetate, 30 minutes.
    d. *Food and fluids:* No breakfast and NPO for 2 hours following oral iodine.
    e. *Other instructions:* Three days before the scan (imaging), iodine preparations, thyroid hormones, phenothiazines, corticosteroids, aspirin, sodium nitroprusside, cough syrups containing iodides, and multivitamins are usually discontinued with the health care provider's permission. Seafoods and iodized salt should be avoided. If the drugs cannot be withheld for 3 days, the drugs should be listed on the nuclear medicine request slip. The client should lie quietly for 30 minutes during the imaging procedure.

Factors Affecting Diagnostic Results

- Antihypertensives may affect results.
- Two radionuclides administered in 1 day may interfere with each other.

- Movement by the client may distort the image.
- A distended bladder could decrease visibility of the pelvic (bone) area.
- Diet and drugs containing iodine could interfere with the results of the thyroid scan *(see Procedure for the Thyroid)*.
- Too short or too long a waiting period after injection of the radionuclide could affect the results.
- Dehydration prior to imaging.

NURSING IMPLICATIONS WITH RATIONALE

- Explain to the client the procedure for the ordered study. Procedures will differ according to the type of study *(see Procedure)*. In most cases, food and fluids are not restricted. For the bone scan (Tc-99m), water is encouraged during the waiting period. For the renal scan the client should be well hydrated before the scheduled scan. Blocking agents (i.e., Lugol's solution and potassium perchlorate) are usually ordered before studies that use radioiodine, except for the thyroid scan.
- Obtain a signed consent form, if required.
- Obtain a brief health history in regard to recent exposure to radioisotopes (radionuclides), allergies that could cause an adverse reaction, being pregnant, breastfeeding, and drugs.
- Adhere to the instructions from the nuclear medicine laboratory concerning the client and the radionuclide procedure. The client should arrive on time. This is especially true if he or she has received the injection. The waiting periods for each study have specified times.
- Be supportive of the client and family. Answer questions, or refer questions you cannot answer to appropriate health care personnel.
- Advise the client to ask questions and to communicate any concerns. Be available when the client wishes to discuss concerns and fears.
- Report to the health care provider (HCP) if the client is extremely apprehensive. The HCP may wish to see the client and/or order a sedative.
- Notify the dietitian and/or dietary department not to send foods high in iodine content for 3 days to the client who is to receive a thyroid scan, unless otherwise indicated. This also includes iodized salt. Instruct the client not to eat foods rich in iodine (i.e., seafood, table salt).
- List restricted drugs containing iodine that the client is taking on the nuclear medicine slip *(see Procedure for the Thyroid)*. This is important if the radionuclide is iodine.

Client Teaching

- Explain to the client that the dose of radiation he or she will receive from radionuclide imaging is usually less than the amount of radiation received from diagnostic x-rays.

- Inform the client that the injected radionuclide should not affect the family, visitors, other clients, or staff members. The radioactive substance usually leaves the body in 6 to 24 hours. The dose of radionuclide is very low.
- Inform the client that there could be a waiting period after the injection of the radioactive substance. Some of the tissues take longer than others to concentrate the substance.
- Instruct the client to void before the study. Voiding will diminish bladder activity and increase visibility.
- Explain to the client that the detection equipment will be moved over a section or sections of the body; however, there should not be any discomfort from the imaging equipment.
- Inform the client that he or she may be asked to change body positions during the test. Other than that, he or she should lie still during the procedure. Cardiac imaging requires the left arm be raised, which can be uncomfortable, for approximately 25 minutes.
- Inform the client that the imaging may take 30 minutes to 1 hour, depending on which organ is being studied. The client should be informed that he or she may need to return for additional imaging at specified intervals.
- Instruct the client to remove jewelry or any metal object in the area of the study.
- Inform the client that the personnel in nuclear medicine will give step-by-step directions concerning the procedure. Tell the client to ask questions if he or she does not understand.
- Inform the client that heart (cardiac) imaging may be done during the stress test as part of the testing for ischemic heart disease.

Papanicolaou smear (pap smear)*

Cytology Test for Cervical Cancer

Normal Finding

No abnormal or atypical cells.

Description

The Pap (Papanicolaou) smear became nationally known and used in the early 1950s for detecting cervical cancer and precancerous tissues. Dr. George Papanicolaou developed the cytology test in 1928 after spending 18 years in research. Today

*Updated with the assistance of Ellen K. Boyda, RN, MS, CRNP, Family Nurse Practitioner, PA.

he is referred to as the father of modern cytology. As the result of his work, there are many cytology studies done on body tissues and secretions.

Because malignant tissue changes usually take many years, yearly examination of exfoliative cervical cells (cells that have sloughed off) allows detection of early, precancerous conditions. It is suggested that women from the age of 18 to 40 years have Pap smears every 2 years and that women from the age of 40 years on have yearly smears. How often the Pap smear test should be performed is determined by the client's health care provider.

The Pap smear (cytology) results are reported by the Bethesda system. General categories of The Bethesda System (TBS) are as follows:

I. Within normal limits.
II. Abnormal changes
    A. Benign cellular changes
        1. Differentiates reactive or inflammatory changes from true dysplastic changes.
        2. Most important features of TBS. *Management:* Repeat smears yearly.
    B. Epithelial abnormalities
        1. Atypical cells of undetermined significance (ASCUS): favoring a neoplastic process or a reactive process. *Management:* Repeat smears at closer intervals, recall for colposcopy and/or combine repeat cytology with cervicography or HPV-DNA type.
        2. Low-grade squamous intraepithelial lesion (LGSIL): shows the earliest abnormal nuclear changes; combines diagnosis of HPV and mild dysplagia. *Management:* Repeat cytology at close intervals, recall for colposcopy.
        3. High-grade squamous intraepithelial lesion (HGSIL): includes moderate and severe dysplastic changes. *Management of HGSIL:* Recall for colposcopy.
        4. Squamous cell carcinoma: changes consistent with cancer. *Management:* Recall for colposcopy.
        5. Glandular cell abnormalities
            a. Atypical cells of undetermined significance, atypical endocervical cells. *Management:* In young women, check for endocervicitis, repeat smear, refer to colposcopy; in older women; refer for colposcopy with endocervical sample.
            b. Cancer *Management:* Refer for colposcopy.

For suggestive or positive Pap smears, colposcopy and/or a cervical biopsy are frequently ordered to confirm the test results. Atypical cells can occur following cervicitis and after excessive or prolonged use of hormones.

Purposes

- To detect precancerous and cancerous cells of the cervix.
- To assess the effects of sex hormonal replacement.

- To identify viral, fungal, and parasitic conditions.
- To evaluate the response to chemotherapy or radition therapy to the cervix.

Clinical Problems

Precancerous and cancerous cells of the cervix; cervicitis; viral, fungal, and parasitic conditions.

Procedure

- Food and fluids are not restricted.
- The client should not douche, insert vaginal medications, or have sexual intercourse for at least 24 hours (preferably 48 hours) before the test. The test should be done between menstrual periods.
- The client is generally asked to remove all clothes, because the breasts are examined after the Pap smear is taken. A paper or cloth gown is worn.
- Instruct the client to lie on the examining table in the lithotomy position (heels in the stirrups).
- A speculum is inserted into the vagina. The speculum may be lubricated with warm running water.
- A curved spatula (Pap stick) is used to scrape the cervix. The obtained specimen is transferred onto a slide and is immersed immediately in a fixative solution or sprayed with a commercial fixation spray. Label the slide with the client's name and date.
- The Pap smear procedure takes approximately 10 minutes.

Factors Affecting Diagnostic Results

- Allowing cells to dry on the slide before using the fixative solution or spray.
- Douching, use of vaginal suppositories, or sexual intercourse within the 24 hours before the test.
- Menstruation can interfere with the test results.
- Drugs (i.e., digitalis preparations, tetracycline, female hormones) could change cellular structure.
- Lubricating jelly on the speculum can interfere with test results.
- Inadequate specimen.

NURSING IMPLICATIONS WITH RATIONALE

- Explain the procedure to the client. Emphasize to the client that she should not douche, insert vaginal suppositories, or have sexual intercourse for at least 24 hours (some say 48 hours) before the Pap smear. Douching could wash away the cervical cells.
- Obtain a client history regarding menstruation and any menstrual problems (i.e., the last menstrual period, bleeding flow, vaginal discharge, itching, and whether she is taking hormones or oral contraceptives).

- Answer the client's questions, and refer questions you cannot answer to other health professionals. Try to alleviate the client's anxiety, if at all possible. Be a good listener.
- Label the slide with the client's name and the date. The laboratory slip should include the client's age and the specimen site(s).

Client Teaching

- Inform the client that a manual examination of the vagina, lower abdomen, rectum, and breast may or will follow the Pap smear.
- Explain to the client that the test should be done yearly or more as determined by her health care provider. High-risk clients with a familial history of cervical cancer or dysphagia should have a Pap smear taken twice a year. Usually women over 40 years old should have a Pap smear once a year.
- Inform the client that test results should be back in 5 to 7 days. Physicians and health care providers differ in the way they report test results; some send cards to the client stating that the Pap smear is normal, while other send cards only if the test is abnormal.

Positron emission tomography (PET)*

Normal Findings

Normal brain, heart, lung, gastrointestinal, activities and blood flow.

Description

Positron emission tomography (PET), a relatively noninvasive test, measures areas of positron-emitting isotope concentration. Myocardial perfusion abnormalities can be determined at rest and after administration of dipyridamole (Persantine). Devices for imaging positron-emitting radioactivity was in existence as early as the 1950s; however, it was not until the mid-1970s that tomographic imaging of positron-emitting radiotracers began. PET scanning has greatly improved since the 1970s.

Early use of PET was primarily to study the brain and heart. Today PET is also used to study the lungs and abdominal organs, and for oncologic purposes. In oncology, PET has recently been approved for lung nodules and colorectal cancer imaging. PET's greatest advances have been in oncology. For brain studies, PET assesses normal brain function; regional cerebral blood flow and volume; glucose, protein, and oxygen metabolism; blood-brain barrier function, neuroreceptor-

---

*Revised by Frank DiGregorio, CNMT, RDMS, Director, Community Imaging Center, Wilmington, DE.

neurotransmitter systems; and the pathophysiology of neurologic and psychiatric disorders. For heart studies, PET assesses cardiac perfusion or blood flow; glucose and oxygen metabolism; and receptor functions. PET perfusion imaging provides information concerning the severity of coronary artery disease (CAD).

Most PET imagers have several radiation detector rings. Each detector group represents a profile or one-dimensional projection of the radioactivity distribution in a tomographic slice. These profiles are combined to produce a cross-sectional (tomographic) image. The two-dimensional (2D) PET images are reconstructed from projection data derived from the detector rings. Three-dimensional (3D) PET imaging is a new approach in which images are generated from the 2D images.

The client receives a substance tagged with a radionuclide (i.e., radioactive glucose, rubidium 82, oxygen 15, nitrogen 13). Flurodeoxyglucose (FDG) is the most common radioisotope used in PET. Tomographic slices from crosssections of tissue are detected and visually displayed by computer. PET is most effective in determining blood flow to the brain and heart. Radiation from PET is a quarter of that received from computed tomography.

Purposes

- To detect a decreased blood flow or perfusion with coronary artery disease.
- To determine the size of infarct and myocardial viability.
- To detect transient ischemia.
- To detect decreased oxygen utilization and decreased blood flow with brain disorders such as cerebral vascular accident (CVA).
- To differentiate between types of dementia, for example, Alzheimer's disease and other dementia such as parkinsonism.
- To identify stages of cranial tumors.
- To identify lung nodules and colorectal metastasis.
- To differentiate between benign and malignant lesions.
- To stage malignant lesions and disease.
- To monitor a response to therapy.

Clinical Problems

Abnormal Findings: Hypoperfusion to brain and heart, stroke, epilepsy, migraine, Parkinson's disease, dementia, Alzheimer's disease, acute myocardial infarction (AMI) for first 72 hours, malignant lesions.

Procedure

- A consent form should be signed.
- Nothing by mouth (NPO) 4 to 6 hours prior to the study.
- No coffee, alcohol, or tobacco is allowed for 24 hours before the test.
- CT or MRI scans of less than 6 weeks should be available for purpose of comparison.
- Any laboratory or biopsy reports should be available.

- Start two IVs, one for radioactive substance and the second to draw blood gas samples.
- For certain brain studies, a blindfold may be used to keep the client from being distracted.
- For brain studies, the client's head is placed in a holder to restrict movement. For heart or abdominal studies, Velcro straps are used to restrict body motion.
- No sedatives are given, since client needs to follow instructions.
- Empty the bladder 1 to 2 hours before the test if imaging the pelvis.
- Test takes 1 to 2 hours.

Factors Affecting Diagnostic Results

- Anxiety could interfere with test results.
- Sedatives given might prevent client from following directions.

NURSING IMPLICATIONS WITH RATIONALE

Pretest

- Check that a consent form has been signed.
- Assess the IV site, monitor vital signs.
- Listen to the client's concerns.

Client Teaching

- Inform the client that instructions given during test should be followed.
- Inform the client that a head holder or velcro straps could be used for the restriction of body movement during imaging.

Posttest

- Continue to monitor vital signs.
- Avoid postural hypotension by slowly moving the client to upright position.
- Increase fluid intake to remove radioisotope from the bladder.

Client Teaching

- Explain to the client that the radiation from the test is short lived and that the test is considered to be a relatively noninvasive test.
- Encourage the client to remain relaxed and to avoid stress. The client should not sleep but should remain quiet and still.
- Instruct the client to take fluids posttest to help eliminate the radioactive substance.

Proctosigmoidoscopy, proctoscopy, sigmoidoscopy

Normal Finding

Normal mucosa and structure of the rectum and sigmoid colon.

Description

Proctosigmoidoscopy is the term for proctoscopy (an examination of the anus and rectum) and sigmoidoscopy (an examination of the anus, rectum, and sigmoid colon). There are three types of instruments used: (1) a 7-cm rigid proctoscope or anoscope, (2) a 25- to 30-cm rigid sigmoidoscope, and (3) a 60-cm flexible sigmoidoscope used to visualize the descending colon. A proctosigmoidoscopy can be performed in the hospital, in a clinic, or in the health care provider's office.

With this procedure the rectum and distal sigmoid colon can be visualized, and specimens can be obtained by a biopsy forceps or a snare, cytology brush, or culture swab. This test is usually indicated when there are changes in bowel habits, chronic constipation, or bright blood or mucus in the stool; or it can be done as part of an annual physical examination in clients over 40 years old. With asymptomatic clients, proctosigmoidoscopy is usually performed every 5 years.

Purposes

- To examine the anus, rectum, and sigmoid colon.
- To detect blood or tumor in the sigmoid colon.
- To obtain a culture of tissue or secretion for cytologic study.

Clinical Problems

Abnormal Findings: Hemorrhoids; rectal and sigmoid colon polyps; fistulas, fissures; rectal abscesses; neoplasms (benign or malignant); ulcerative or granulomatous colitis; infection and/or inflammation of the rectosigmoid area.

Procedure

- A consent form should be signed.
- The client is allowed a light dinner the night before the test and a light breakfast or else is NPO for 8 hours prior to the test. Usually heavy meals, vegetables, and fruits are prohibited within 24 hours of the test.
- The client may take prescribed medications by 6 AM the morning of the test with the health care provider's permission.
- No barium studies should be performed within 3 days of the test.
- A saline or warm tap water enema(s) or hypertonic salt enema(s) (Fleet enema) is given the morning of the test. If enemas are contraindicated, then a rectal suppository, such as bisacodyl (Dulcolax), could be given. Fecal material must be

evacuated before the examination. Preparation with Golytely could be used. Oral cathartics are seldom used, because they may increase fecal flow from the small intestine during the test.

- The client should assume either a knee-chest position or Sims (side-lying) position for the proctosigmoidoscopy. The client will be properly draped to avoid embarrassment and strapped to table if needed.
- As the lubricated endoscope (proctoscope, sigmoidoscope, or proctosigmoidoscope) is inserted into the rectum, the client should be instructed to breathe deeply and slowly. Sometimes air is injected into the bowel to improve visualization. The air can cause gas pains. Cotton swabs and suction should be available.
- Specimens can be obtained during the procedure. Tissue specimen(s) should be placed in a bottle containing a preservative or on a slide and sprayed with a fixative solution. The commercial fixative sprays may cause distortion of cells.
- The procedure takes approximately 15 to 30 minutes.

Factors Affecting Diagnostic Results

- Barium can decrease the visualization, and so barium studies should be performed a week before the test or afterward.
- Fecal material in the lower colon can decrease visualization.
- Placement of tissue and cell specimens in solutions without preservative solutions can cause false results. Fixative sprays could distort the cells.

NURSING IMPLICATIONS WITH RATIONALE

- Explain to the client that the purpose of the test is to determine the cause of symptoms (i.e., bright blood or mucus in stools, constipation, bowel changes), or tell the client that it is part of the routine physical examination for preventive health care.
- Explain the procedure to the client in regard to body position, pre-test preparation (enema and diet), and the time required for the procedure.
- Check the chart to determine if the client has had a barium study within 3 days before the scheduled proctosigmoidoscopy. If so, the health care provider should be notified.
- Obtain a client history in regard to being pregnant or having ulcerative colitis. Frequently enemas and suppositories are contraindicated during pregnancy and with ulcerative colitis.
- Record baseline vital signs before the test. Vital signs may be monitored during the examination.
- Allow the client time to ask questions and express concerns. Refer questions you cannot answer to a physician or to the appropriate health professional.

Client Teaching

- Inform the client that the procedure may cause some discomfort but should not cause severe pain. Encourage the client to breathe deeply and slowly and to relax during the test. Explain that there may be some gas pains if a small amount of air is injected during the procedure for better visualization.

Posttest

- Monitor vital signs as indicated or at least every 30 minutes for the first 2 hours.
- Observe the signs and symptoms of bowel perforation (i.e., pain, abdominal distention, and rectal bleeding). This problem rarely occurs. Also observe for shock-like symptoms (i.e., paleness, diaphoresis, tachycardia, and later a drop in blood pressure). Report all symptoms immediately to the health care provider.
- Be supportive of the client and his or her family.

Client Teaching

- Encourage the client to rest for several hours after the test if possible. This procedure may be done in a clinic, in a physician's office, or in the hospital. If the test is done on an outpatient basis, the client should rest for 1 hour before leaving.

Pulmonary function tests*

Pulmonary Diagnostic Tests

Normal Findings

Normal values according to patient's age, sex, and height; >80% of the predicted value. 95% confidence levels are also being used, these confidence ranges give a normal and a low or minimal normal value. This is done to account for physiologic differences in body types.

Description*

Pulmonary function tests (PFTs) are useful in differentiating between obstructive and restrictive lung diseases and in quantifying the degree (mild, moderate, or severe) of obstructive or restrictive lung disorders. Other purposes for PFTs include establishing baseline test results for comparison with future tests; evaluating pulmonary status before surgery; determining pulmonary disability for insurance; tracking the progress of lung disease; assessing the response to therapy; pulmonary evaluation; and determining pulmonary status before rehabilitation.

---

*David C. Sestili, CRTT, RPFT, Manager of the Pulmonary Laboratories, Medical Center of Delaware, Christiana Hospital, Newark, DE, 1978.

In pulmonary physiology testing, the lungs are monitored by many complex devices and tests. The most basic device is the spirometer; it is used to measure flows, volumes, and capacities.

A number of pulmonary tests are conducted, because no single measurement can evaluate pulmonary performance. The most frequently performed PFTs are the slow vital capacity tests; lung-volume tests; forced vital capacity, flow-volume loop, and diffusion-study tests; bronchodilator response studies; exercise studies; and nutritional studies.

Pulmonary Rehabilitation

Many pulmonary laboratories incorporate pulmonary rehabilitation into their outpatient programs because it is important for clients with pulmonary diseases to keep active. Activities and exercises prescribed in the pulmonary rehabilitation program have been demonstrated to reduce the amount of oxygen required for muscle use. Other benefits gained from exercise for clients with pulmonary disease include a decrease in the sedentary life style that can lead to depression, decrease in dyspnea, increase in activities of daily living, lesser dependence on significant others to assist in basic care; a decrease in complications and increase in the recovery time for clients having transplant and lung reduction surgery (pre- and postoperatively); and improvement in respiratory status for clients with interstitial fibrosis, cystic fibrosis, asthma, emphysema, primary pulmonary hypertension, or alpha-1-antitrypsin deficiency.

Pulmonary rehabilitation incorporates a multidisciplinary approach. Specialists in the program include the dietitian; exercise physiologist; nurse; occupational, physical, and respiratory therapists; and social worker.

Purposes

- To assess pulmonary/respiratory function.
- To detect the occurrence of pulmonary dysfunction.
- To differentiate between obstructive and restrictive lung diseases.
- To evaluate the response of drug therapy for decreasing lung dysfunction.
- To be informed of program(s) for improving respiratory status for clients with pulmonary dysfunction or for clients prior to or following lung surgery.

Pulmonary Function Tests

1. Slow Vital Capacity (SVC) Tests
   - *Tidal volume (TV, V_t):* The amount of air inhaled and exhaled during rest or quiet respiration or normal breathing.
   - *Inspiratory capacity (IC):* The maximal inspired amount of air from end-expiratory tidal volume in normal breathing.
   - *Expiratory reserve volume (ERV):* The maximal amount of air that can be exhaled from end-expiratory tidal volume in normal breathing.
   - *Inspiratory reserve volume (IRV):* The maximal amount of air that can be inspired from end-inspiratory tidal volume in normal breathing.

- *Vital capacity (VC):* The maximal amount of air exhaled after a maximal inhalation:

$$VC = ERV + IC$$

Note: These pulmonary measurements are done slowly, without force. Individuals with obstructive lung disease will be able to expire more volume with this test than during the forced vital capacity maneuver.

2. Lung Volume Studies
   - *Lung volume using indicator gas:* Lung volumes are special studies that use data generated in the slow vital capacity test. To obtain lung volumes, a tracer gas such as helium or nitrogen is required. Using one of the gases in a small quantity, the person breathes in and out as the tracer gas is equilibrated in the lung; the functional residual capacity (FRC) is calculated from the changes. This method will tend to underestimate persons with advanced obstructive lung disease.
   - *Lung volumes by plethysmography method:* Lung volumes can be obtained by total body plethysmography. Body plethysmography is a device that resembles an air-tight telephone booth in which the subject sits. This method is a more accurate means to measure total volume of the lungs than the tracer gas method. Volumes measured in the box will be larger than by the indicator gas method.
   - *Lung volume measurements:* See Figure 2.
   - *Residual volume (RV):* The amount of air that remains in the lungs after maximal expiration.

$$RV = FRC - ERV$$

   - *Functional residual capacity (FRC):* The amount of air left in the lungs after tidal or normal expiration.

$$FRC = ERV + RV$$

In obstructive disorders FRC is increased because of hyperinflation of the lungs due to air trapping. In restrictive disorders FRC and RV can be normal or decreased.

   - *Total lung capacity (TLC):* The total amount of air that is in the lungs at maximal inspiration.

$$TLC = VC + RV \quad \text{or} \quad TLC = FRC + IC$$

3. Lung Volumes and Capacity
   See Figure 2.
   - *Forced vital capacity (FVC):* In obstructive lung disease the FVC is decreased; in restrictive lung disease, the FVC is normal or decreased.

$$FVC = IC + ERV$$

   - *Forced inspiratory volume (FIV):* The greatest amount of air inhaled after a maximal expiration.

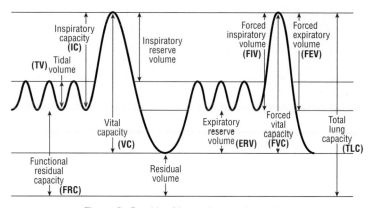

Figure 2. Graphic of lung volume and capacity.

- *Forced expiratory volume timed (FEV$_T$):* The greatest amount of air exhaled in 0.5 second FEV$_{0.5}$, 1 second FEV$_1$, 2 seconds FEV$_2$, and 3 seconds FEV$_3$. See Figure 3. FEV$_1$ is considered the parameter of choice to evaluate asthmatics and other obstructive lung disease and to evaluate the response to bronchodilator therapy. An improvement of >15% after bronchodilator therapy is considered significant and indicates the presence of reversible airway obstruction, such as bronchospasm.

4. Flow-Volume Loop (FVL)

   Another method to visualize FVC measurement is by graphing flow versus volume, as seen in Figure 4. Abnormal FVLs in Figure 5 indicate types of pulmonary problems. This test yields the same basic information as the FVC test but in addition provides the following useful visual information, such as

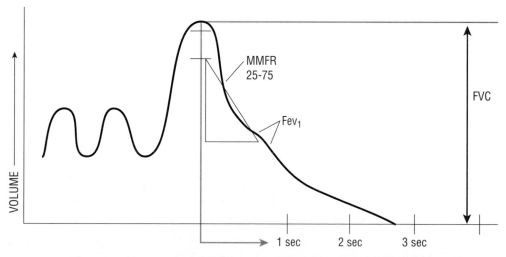

Figure 3. Graphic of forced expiratory volume timed. *(Courtesy of David C. Sestilli, CRTT, RPFT.)*

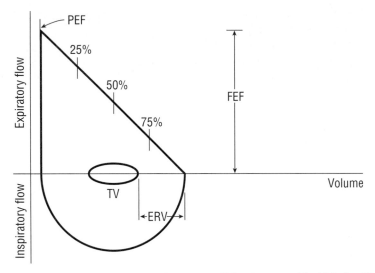

Figure 4. Flow-volume loop (FVL); and forced expiratory flow (FEF). *(Courtesy of David C. Sestilli, CRTT, RPFT.)*

small-airway disease and upper-airway obstruction. Its usefulness in screening people with some types of sleep disorder problems has been recently documented.

■ *Peak expiratory flow (PEF):* The highest flow rate achieved at the beginning of the FVC; reported in liters per second. *Note:* Peak flow meters measure in liters per minute.

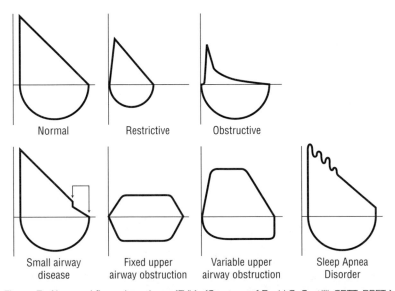

Figure 5. Abnormal flow-volume loops (FVL). *(Courtesy of David C. Sestilli, CRTT, RPFT.)*

- *Peak inspiratory flow (PIF):* The highest flow rate achieved at the beginning of the forced inspiratory capacity.
- *Forced expiratory flow (FEF):* Figure 4 demonstrates the rate of flow at selected points on the flow-volume loop. The FEF looks at flow at the 25%, 50%, and 75% of the FVC and evaluates flow in various size airways. It can evaluate the effectiveness of bronchodilator therapy. FEF 25% reflects flow through large airways; FEF 50% reflects flow through medium airways; and FEF 75% reflects flow through small airways. Decreased FEF 75% indicates small-airway disease.

5. Diffusion Capacity Test

   Diffusion tests can be done using a number of techniques. The most commonly used one is the single breath test. This requires the client to inspire from RV to TLC. The gas inhaled is a mixture of helium 10%, carbon monoxide 0.3%, oxygen 21%, and nitrogen 68.7%. The client holds his breath for 10 seconds prior to expiraton. After the first 750 ml is discarded to wash out dead-space gas, an alveolar sample is collected and analyzed for helium and carbon monoxide (CO) concentration. Results of this reflect the state of the alveolar capillary barrier. Decreased diffusing capacity occurs in such disease states as interstitial fibrosis, interstitial edema, and emphysema. It will also decrease in persons with abnormal hemoglobin, such as occurs in anemias and carboxyhemoglobinemia, and in smokers. Cardiac output can effect result.

6. Bronchial Provocation Studies

   Inhalation of pharmacologic and antigenic substances is used to test the sensitivity of the airways. Serial spirometry tests are performed to document the amount or degree of reactivity (a drop in FEV_1 >20% of baseline spirometry). A bronchoconstrictor is given first followed by a bronchodilator. Indications for these tests are (1) normal spirometric test, (2) a history of symptoms such as wheezing, or coughing without a cause, and (3) symptoms related to exposure to industrial substances.

   Methacholine chloride is usually the testing drug of choice because it causes bronchoconstriction rapidly. The client inhales progressively larger doses of the drug until all levels are administered without change in FEV_1 or a drop of 20% of baseline FEV_1 is reached. The drug is then reversed by administration of a bronchodilator.

7. Exercise Studies

   Pulmonary function studies are done at a resting state. Exercise studies allow evaluation during an active state. These tests are performed by having the subject walk on a treadmill or pedal an ergometer to a set protocol to stimulate activity at progressive work loads. During the test, the heart rate and rhythm will be monitored by a 12-lead electrocardiogen (ECG). The client will be breathing through a mouthpiece during the test, to measure ventilation, expired carbon dioxide (CO_2) and oxygen (O_2) consumption. Blood gases may be drawn at rest and at peak exercise. Pulse oximetry may also be monitored, as well as blood pressure. These tests are used to determine the amount of disability and to evaluate persons with exertional dyspnea. This allows the client to have an exercise prescription for activities for pulmonary and cardiac rehabilitation.

Types of exercise testing can be designed to simulate various activity-related problems, of which *exercise induced bronchospasm* (EIB) is an example. A common complaint of clients active in sport activities is bronchospasm. Several theories suggestive of the cause include allergy-triggered airway hyper-reactivity in association with physical activity, and mouth breathing required when the participant increases activity. When the participant breathes rapidly in and out through the mouth, the nose, which warms and filters air, is bypassed. This dry air causes chilling of the airway, leading to instability of the airways and bronchoconstriction in some persons.

8. Pulse Oximetry

This is a noninvasive procedure to measure the oxygen saturation (SaO_2) of the blood. The device measures the SaO_2 by passing two wavelengths of infrared light through an extremity such as a finger. The device (sensor probe) measures the saturation of oxyhemoglobin in the pulsatile fraction of blood. This method is an excellent noninvasive trending device; when values vary, a blood gas analysis of the partial pressure of oxygen (PO_2) and/or CO-oximetry to measure oxyhemoglobin ($\%HbO_2$) and SaO_2 should be done to validate the results. A note of caution: Blood gas analyses normally do not measure SaO_2; they are calculated. Check with your blood gas laboratory for this information.

Pulse oximetry is a very useful test but it has some drawbacks. It should be trusted after direct comparison to CO-oximetry is done. Abnormal hemoglobin levels (i.e., carboxyhemoglobinemia, methemoglobinemia, and sulfhemoglobinemia) could fool the device. These abnormal levels are detected at the same infrared wavelengths and may falsely be interpreted by the oximeter to be oxygen. Impeded blood flow to an area will also affect the pulse oximetry. Correlation with the client's true pulse will assist in correcting this problem. Light sources may also affect the results; thus the area should be guarded against external light sources.

9. Nutritional studies

Indirect calorimetry is the measurement of CO_2 production and O_2 consumption. The respiratory quotient (RQ), obtained from the calorimetry ($PO_2 + CO_2 = RQ$), yields the type of substrate used in metabolism (carbohydrate, fat, protein).

This noninvasive test gives useful information as to the energy expenditure (EE), the amount of calories needed for minimal existence expressed in kilocalories per 24 hours. The RQ will indicate the type of fuel being metabolized. For example, RQ 1.0 indicates carbohydrates, RQ 0.80 indicates mixed carbohydrates and fats, and RQ 0.75 indicates lipids.

10. Body Plethysmography (body box)

Body plethysmograph is a method to measure the exact amount of air in the thorax. This is accomplished by having the subject sit inside an airtight box and breathe through a flow measuring device. A panting maneuver is done, and a shutter is closed to measure pressure at the mouth and pressure changes of the box. By knowing these measurements and applying Boyle's Law, the thoracic gas volume (TGV), which correlates to functional residual capacity, (FRC) can be measured. The compliance and resistances to the lung can also be measured by this device. Advantages are that the body box measures all air in the chest. Volumes tend to be larger in box studies. Disadvantages to the body box test are that some clients have claustrophobia, and persons with perforated eardrums will tend to have readings higher than normal, which could be misleading. This test requires total client cooperation.

Clinical Problems

Obstructive Diseases: Emphysema, chronic bronchitis, bronchiectasis, bronchospasm, bronchial secretions, airway inflammation caused by bacterial or viral infections, asthma.

Restrictive Diseases: Pulmonary fibrosis, pneumonia, lung tumors, kyposcoliosis, neuromuscular diseases, chest trauma, obesity, scleroderma, pulmonary edema, surgical removal of lung tissue, high abdominal incisions.

Procedure

- Eating a heavy meal before the test should be discouraged.
- Smoking should be avoided 4 to 6 hours before the test.
- The client should wear nonrestrictive clothing.
- Record the client's age, height, and weight, which may be used to predict the normal range.
- Bronchodilators are restricted prior to the test, because they are usually administered in the pulmonary function laboratory with tests. Usually sedatives and narcotics are not given. Other medications are given prior to the test unless otherwise indicated by the health care provider.
- Postpone procedure if the client has an active cold or is under the influence of alcohol.
- Dentures may be left in during testing.
- The test can be performed with the client in a sitting or standing position (children in a standing position only). A nose clip is applied and the client is instructed to breathe in and out through the mouth.
- Practice sessions on fast-and-deep breathing are given. Normally the test is repeated twice and the best tracing is used. The test may be repeated after using a bronchodilator.

Bronchial Provocation Studies

- The client inhales varied doses of methacholine chloride, a short-acting bronchoconstrictor, until all doses, approximately five, are administered without a change in FEV_1 or a drop of 20% of baseline FEV_1. The drug is then reversed by administration of a bronchodilator.
- There should be no exercise, smoking, or caffeine (coffee, cola, or chocolate) consumption for a minimum of 6 hours before testing. Any bronchodilator or

antihistamine therapy (PO or inhaled) should be discontinued for at least 48 hours prior to testing. Avoid testing during pregnancy and breastfeeding.

Nutritional Studies

- The client should be NPO for 12 hours prior and until completion of test.
- There should be no activity before test. Nutritional studies are usually formed $1/2$ hour after awakening.
- The client's exhalation is analyzed for oxygen consumption and CO_2 production. Clients on ventilators, hyperalimentation, or tube feeding can be tested as long as there are no changes in the diet or ventilator settings until the test is completed.

Exercise Studies

Exercise induced bronchospasm (EIB) stress testing is a form of bronchoprovocation testing that can be performed by one of the two methods.

In the first method:

- The client refrains from pulmonary medications, caffeine, exposure to cold air, and physical exercise for 24 hours prior to testing.
- A 12-lead ECG is applied.
- A baseline spirometer test is done, which acts as the control.
- The client exercises on a treadmill or a bicycle ergometer until the target heart rate of 85% of maximum is met or the client has symptoms limiting the exercise.
- Exercise is terminated and spirometry is performed after 1, 3, 5, and 10 minutes and then every 5 minutes for a period of 45 minutes postexercise. A drop of 10% of the FEV_1 indicates a positive test.

In the second method:

- The procedures of the first method are followed.
- The client inhales cold (-20°C), dry air, which is generated by a chilling device driven by compressed air during exercise test. The cold, dry air is thought to cause hyperactivity in the bronchial tubes.
- Spirometry is performed at 1-minute intervals; see the first method.

Factors Affecting Diagnostic Results

- Use of bronchodilators 4 hours before the pulmonary function test may produce falsely improved pulmonary results.
- Sedatives and narcotics given before the test could decrease test results.
- Lack of cooperation by the client due to not understanding the specific test procedure may affect results.

NURSING IMPLICATIONS WITH RATIONALE

- List on the request slip oral/inhaled bronchodilators and steroids the client is taking. Record client's age, height, and weight.
- Record vital signs.

- Assess for signs and symptoms of respiratory distress (i.e., breathlessness, dyspnea, tachycardia, severe apprehension, and gray or cyanotic color).
- Be supportive of client, and answer client's questions if you can.

Client Teaching

- Instruct the client to eat a light breakfast, except in nutritional studies; to take medications, except for bronchodilators, sedatives, narcotics, and others as stated by health care provider orders; and to avoid smoking for 4 to 6 hours before test.
- Tell the client that the test should not be performed if he or she has an active cold or other communicable disease unless approved by the health care provider and the pulmonary function laboratory chief.
- Practice breathing patterns for pulmonary function tests with the client (i.e., normal breathing, rapid breathing, and forced deep inspiration and forced deep expiration).

Radioactive iodine (RAI) uptake test

I-131 Uptake Test, Radioiodine Thyroid Uptake Test

Normal Finding

Adult: *2 hours:* 1–13% (thyroid gland). *6 hours:* 2–25% (thyroid gland). *24 hours:* 15–45% (thyroid gland).

Description

The radioactive iodine (RAI) uptake test is used to determine the metabolic activity of the thyroid gland by measuring the absorption of I-131 or I-123 in the thyroid. The uptake test is one of the tests used in diagnosing hypothyroidism and hyperthyroidism. It is also useful for differentiating between hyperthyroidism (Graves' disease) and an overactive adenoma. This test tends to be more accurate for diagnosing hyperthyroidism than for diagnosing hypothyroidism.

A calculated dose of I-131 or I-123 (in capsule or liquid form) is given orally. The client's thyroid is scanned at three different times. The tracer dose has small amount of radioactivity and is considered harmless. The client's urine output may be checked for radioactive iodine excretion.

Purposes

- To determine the metabolic activity of the thyroid gland.

- To diagnose hypothyroidism and hyperthyroidism.
- To differentiate between hyperthyroidism and an overactive adenoma.

Clinical Problems

Decreased Level: Hypothyroidism (myxedema). *Drug Influence:* Lugol's solution, vitamins, expectorants (i.e., SSKI), antithyroid agents, cortisone preparation, ACTH, aspirin, antihistamines, phenylbutazone (Butazolidin), anticoagulants (i.e., warfarin [Coumadin]), thiopental sodium (Pentothal). *Foods:* Seafood, cabbage, ionized salt.

Elevated Level: Hyperthyroidism (Graves' disease), thyroiditis, cirrhosis of the liver. *Drug Influence:* Barbiturates, estrogens, lithium carbonate, phenothiazines.

Procedure

- The client should be NPO for 8 hours prior to the test. The client can eat an hour after the radioiodine capsule or liquid has been taken.
- The amount of radioactivity in the thyroid gland is measured three times (after 2, 6, and 24 hours).
- The client should return to the nuclear medicine laboratory at specified times to allow measurement of the I-131 uptake level with the scintillation counter.

Factors Affecting Diagnostic Results

- Certain drugs can affect test results *(see Drug Influence)*. Foods containing iodine (seafood, ionized salt) could cause a false-negative result.
- Drugs and foods *(see Clinical Problems)*.
- Severe diarrhea, intestinal malabsorption, and x-ray contrast media studies may cause a decreased I-131 uptake level, even in normal thyroid glands.
- Rapid diuresis during the test could cause iodine excretion and a low iodine uptake in the thyroid gland.
- Renal failure could cause an increased iodine uptake.

NURSING IMPLICATIONS WITH RATIONALE

- Explain to the client the purpose and procedure for the test.
- Ask the client if he or she is allergic to iodine products.
- Inform the client that a technician from the nuclear medicine laboratory will give the radioactive substance and that he or she must go to the laboratory 2, 6, and 24 hours after taking the iodine preparation. Explain to the client that the procedure is to determine the percentage of I-131 or I-123 uptake, that the test should not be painful, and that the amount of radiation received should be harmless. Emphasize the importance of being on time for each determination.
- List on the request slip for the I-131 uptake test the x-ray studies and drugs the client has received in the last week that could affect test results. These drugs should, if possible, be discontinued for 3 or more days before the test *(see Drug Influence)*.

- Draw blood for thyroid hormone (T_3 and/or T_4) tests, if ordered, before the client takes the radioiodine capsule or liquid.
- Answer the client's questions. Encourage the client to communicate concerns.
- Observe for signs and symptoms of hyperthyroidism (i.e., nervousness, tachycardia, excessive hyperactivity, exophthalmos, mood swings [euphoria to depression], and weight loss). Report these to the health care provider, and record them in the client's chart.

Client Teaching

- Inform the client that he or she may eat an hour after the radioiodine capsule or liquid has been taken, according to the nuclear medicine laboratory's procedure.
- Instruct the client to return to the nuclear medicine laboratory at specified times. The testing should be done on time.
- Inform the client that the radioactive substance should not harm family members, visitors, or other clients, since the dosage is low and gives off very little radiation. Women who are pregnant definitely should not be given this test or any other radioactive tests.

Retrograde pyelography (retrograde pyelogram)

Retrograde Ureteropyelography

Normal Finding

Normal size and structure of the bladder, ureters, and kidneys.

Description

A retrograde pyelography test may be performed after or in place of intravenous pyelography (IVP). The contrast dye is injected through a catheter into the ureters and the renal pelvis. The visualization of the urinary tract is exceptionally good because the dye is injected directly. Usually this test is done in conjunction with cystoscopy.

Although retrograde pyelograms are not done too frequently today, this test is still performed when there is a suspected nonfunctioning kidney, an unlocated calculus, or an allergy to IV contrast dye. Only a small amount of the dye that is injected directly into the ureters will be absorbed through the membranes.

Purposes

- To view the urinary tract.
- To check for a nonfunctioning kidney.

Clinical Problems

Abnormal Findings: Renal calculi, neoplasm (tumor), renal stricture, nonfunctioning kidney.

Procedure

- A consent form should be signed.
- The client should be NPO for 8 hours before the retrograde pyelography. The client should not be dehydrated before the test.
- Laxatives and cleansing enemas may be ordered prior to the test.
- Baseline vital signs should be recorded.
- Sedatives/tranquilizers and narcotic analgesics are given approximately 1 hour before the test.
- The client is usually placed in the lithotomy position (feet and legs in stirrups).
- Radiopaque contrast dye is injected through a ureteral catheter into the renal pelvis and x-rays are taken. As the catheter is removed, additional x-rays may be taken.
- This procedure is usually done under local or general anesthesia, and the test takes approximately 1 hour.

Factors Affecting Diagnostic Results

- Barium in the gastrointestinal tract could interfere with good visualization. Barium studies should be done after a retrograde pyelogram.

NURSING IMPLICATIONS WITH RATIONALE

Pretest

- Record baseline vital signs.
- Obtain a client history of allergies to seafood, iodine, and/or radiopaque dye used in other diagnostic tests.
- Administer laxatives, cleansing enemas, and premedications as prescribed. If the client is not hospitalized, check that the prescribed orders were completed at home or in another institution. Check that the consent form has been signed before giving premedications.

Client Teaching

- Explain to the client that the purpose of the test is to identify kidney stones or to determine the cause of his or her kidney problems, or give a similar response related to the symptoms.
- Explain the procedure to the client. Explain to the client that he or she will be placed in stirrups. If the client is having the test done under local anesthesia, tell

the client that he or she will most likely feel pressure and the urge to urinate with insertion of the cystoscope.

- Inform him or her that there should be little to no pain or discomfort. Tell the client that the test takes about 1 hour.
- Inform the client that food and fluids are restricted for 8 hours before the test. Some health care providers may not restrict water unless the client is to have general anesthesia. Check for symptoms of dehydration (i.e., dry mouth and mucous membranes, poor skin turgor, decreased urine output, and fast pulse and respirations). Report symptoms to the health care provider and record them on the client's chart.

Posttest

- Monitor vital signs until stable or as ordered.
- Observe for allergic reactions to the contrast dye (i.e., skin rash, urticaria [hives], flushing, dyspnea, and tachycardia).
- Monitor urinary output. Report and record gross hematuria. Blood-tinged urine usually is normal. Report to the health care provider if the client has not voided in 8 hours or the urinary output is <200 ml in 8 hours.
- Give an analgesic for discomfort or pain. Report severe pain.
- Observe for signs and symptoms of infection (sepsis; i.e., fever, chills, abdominal pain, tachycardia, and, later, hypotension).
- Be supportive of the client and family. Answer the client's questions, or refer them to urologist or appropriate health professional.

Scans

See Nuclear Scans

Schilling test (urine)

Co-57-Tagged Vitamin B_{12}, (Cobalt-57-Tagged Cyanocobalamine)

Reference Values

Adult: >7% excretion of radioactive Vitamin B_{12} within 24 hours. Usual range is

10–40% of Vitamin B_{12} excretion. *Pernicious Anemia:* Excretion of Vitamin B_{12} is <3%. *Intestinal Malabsorption:* Excretion is 3–5%.

Description

The Schilling test is primarily ordered to diagnose pernicious anemia, a macrocytic anemia. The test determines if the client lacks the intrinsic factor in the gastric mucosa that is necessary for the absorption of Vitamin B_{12} from food. With impaired absorption due to the lack of intrinsic factor or from intestinal malabsorption, little to no Vitamin B_{12} is absorbed and therefore less is excreted in the urine.

A Vitamin B_{12} deficiency affects the bone marrow, the gastrointestinal tract, and the neurologic system. The bone marrow becomes hyperplastic, having many bizarre red blood cell forms. The leukocytes (white blood cells) are large but reduced in number; likewise, the platelets are bizarre in form and reduced in number. The gastrointestinal mucosa atrophies and there is a decrease in hydrochloric acid. Classic symptoms of pernicious anemia include a beefy red tongue, indigestion, abdominal pain, diarrhea, and tingling and numbness of the hands and feet.

The test consists of collecting a 24-hour urine specimen after the client has taken a radioactive capsule of Vitamin B_{12} administered by a technician from the nuclear medicine laboratory and an injection of intramuscular Vitamin B_{12} given by the nurse. The intramuscular Vitamin B_{12} will saturate the liver and the protein-binding sites, thus permitting the absorption of the capsule cobalt-tagged Vitamin B_{12} by the small intestines and its excretion in the urine. There are various types of radioactive cobalt (Co-57, Co-56, Co-60), but Co-57 is preferred because of its shorter half-life and its low-energy gamma radiation. Usually a Schilling test is performed after a plasma Vitamin B_{12}, RIA assay test; however, the Schilling test aids in diagnosing pernicious anemia.

Purposes

- To determine if there is a vitamin B_{12} deficiency.
- To detect pernicious anemia and intestinal malabsorption syndrome.

Clinical Problems

Decreased Level: Pernicious anemia, intestinal malabsorption syndrome, liver diseases, hypothyroidism (myxedema), pancreatic insufficiency, sprue.

Procedure

- Obtain a signed consent form.
- The client should be NPO for 8 to 12 hours before the test. Food and fluids are permitted after the IM Vitamin B_{12} dose.
- Avoid ingestion of B vitamins for 3 days prior to the test and no laxatives for 1 day prior to the test.
- A sample of urine (25–50 ml) should be collected before cobalt-tagged Vitamin B_{12} is given to determine if there are radionuclide contaminants.

- The radioactive Co-57-tagged Vitamin B_{12} capsule(s) of liquid is/are administered orally by a technician from nuclear medicine.
- Vitamin B_{12} (usually 1 mg) is given IM by the nurse 1 to 2 hours after the radioactive dose.
- Collect urine in a large container for 24 hours, according to the institution's procedure. No preservative is needed in the urine container. The container may or may not be iced or refrigerated; check with the laboratory's policy.
- Label the urine container with the client's name, the room number, the date, and the time.
- Rubber gloves should be worn to handle the urine for the 24-hour specimen.

Factors Affecting Laboratory Results

- A recent radionuclide scan within 7 days prior to the test.
- Food and fluid taken within 1 to 8 hours before the test.
- Inadequate urine output due to renal insufficiency or old age.
- Partial gastrectomy can decrease the amount of intrinsic factor, so less Vitamin B_{12} could be absorbed.
- If IM Vitamin B_{12} is not given on time, the Co-57-Vitamin B_{12} can be absorbed in the liver.

NURSING IMPLICATIONS WITH RATIONALE

- Obtain a history of chronic diseases or conditions that could decrease renal function or gastrointestinal absorption of the radioactive capsule, such as diabetes mellitus, hypothyroidism, liver disease, or pancreatic insufficiency.
- Assess for signs and symptoms of pernicious anemia, such as beefy red tongue, indigestion, abdominal pain, diarrhea, tingling numbness of the hands and feet.
- Assess urine output; low urine output affects test results. If the urine output is <25 ml/hour or 600 ml/day, the health care provider should be notified.
- Do not administer laxatives the night before the test. Laxatives could decrease the absorption rate.
- Determine the time of administration of the radioactive vitamin B_{12} capsule. The nurse administers the IM Vitamin B_{12} 1 to 2 hours after the technician administers the capsule.
- Observe the client for at least 1 hour for possible anaphylactic reaction to radionuclide.
- Administer the nonradioactive Vitamin B_{12} injection at the *specified* time.
- Notify the dietary department to release the breakfast tray after the nonradioactive Vitamin B_{12} is given.
- Label the urine container and laboratory slip with the exact dates and times of collection (e.g., 2/3/04 at 8:00 AM to 2/4/04 at 8:00 AM).

Client Teaching

- Explain the procedure to the client. Tell the client that he or she is to have nothing by mouth for 8 to 12 hours before the test. Breakfast will be given after the IM injection is given. Urine will be collected for 24 hours.
- Instruct the client to avoid putting feces or toilet paper in the urine. Inform the client that the hands should be washed thoroughly with soap and water after handling the urine.
- Tell the client's family or visitors not to throw away the urine. Inform the family that hands should be washed thoroughly with soap and water after handling the urine.
- Explain to the client that the radioactive substance should not be harmful to family members, visitors, or self unless the person is pregnant. Notify the nursing staff when urine needs to be emptied.
- Instruct the client that foods high in Vitamin B_{12} are mostly animal products such as milk, eggs, meat, and liver. Vegetables are low in Vitamin B_{12}. Discuss dietary needs with the client and refer the dietitian to the client as needed.

Sex chromatin mass, buccal smear, Barr body analysis

Normal Finding

Barr body in 25% to 50% of the female buccal mucosal cells.

Description

The sex chromatin test is a screening method to detect the presence or absence of Barr chromatin body (an inactivated X chromosome in a mass lying at the periphery of the cell nucleus) in the buccal mucosal cells. Buccal smears are used to check for Barr body when chromosomal abnormalities are suspected (e.g., Turner's syndrome [absent or <20% Barr body in females] and Klinefelter's syndrome [presence of Barr body in males]). This test is also indicated if amenorrhea or abnormal sexual development is present.

Abnormal findings should be followed up by chromosome analysis (karyotype). The sex chromatin test should not be used for sex determinations.

Purposes

- To detect Barr chromatin body.
- To check for the presence of Turner's syndrome or Klinefelter's syndrome.

Clinical Problems

Abnormal Findings: Turner's syndrome (female): absence of Barr body, amenorrhea, sterility, underdeveloped breasts; Klinefelter's syndrome (male): presence of Barr body, small penis and testes, sparse facial hair, gynecomastia, sterility.

Procedure

- There is no food or fluid restriction.
- The client should rinse his or her mouth well.
- A wooden or metal spatula is used to scrape the buccal mucosa twice; the first scraping is discarded, and the second is spread over a glass slide. The slide should be sprayed with a fixative solution and sent to the laboratory for identifying a Barr body in the cells. The specimen should be labeled with the client's name, sex, and age, as well as the date and the specimen site.
- Check that the specimen is not saliva. The smear is stained and examined under a microscope.
- The procedure usually takes 10 to 20 minutes.

Factors Affecting Diagnostic Results

- If the specimen is saliva and not cells, the test result could be inaccurate.
- Failure to use a preservative spray on the buccal smear specimen will cause cell deterioration.

NURSING IMPLICATIONS WITH RATIONALE

- Record in the chart any abnormal sexual characteristics or problems and note them on the request slip (e.g., amenorrhea, gynecomastia).
- Be supportive of the client and his or her family. Be a good listener. Answer questions or refer them to the appropriate health professionals.

Client Teaching

- Explain to the client and/or parents that the purpose of the test is to determine the cause of abnormal sexual development. Inform them that this is a screening test and that other tests, such as chromosome analysis, may be indicated.
- Explain the procedure to the client and parents. Inform the client that the cells from inside the mouth (buccal smear) are used because they are easy to obtain. Tell them that the test has a high percentage of accuracy. The procedure usually takes 10 to 20 minutes; however, the results from the test may take several weeks.
- Inform the client that there should be a minimal amount of discomfort. Light pressure will be applied when scraping the mucosa.

Sinus endoscopy

Normal Finding

Normal sinuses; no infection or structural abnormalities noted.

Description

Sinus endoscopy examines the anterior ethmoids and the middle meatus of the sinuses. The primary purposes are to correct structural abnormalities and alleviate an infectious process. Sinus endoscopy is frequently prescribed for clients with chronic sinusitis who are nonresponsive to antibiotic therapy.

The sinus endoscopy may be performed in the health care provider's office or in an outpatient department.

Purpose

- To diagnose the presence of a chronic sinus infection or structural abnormality.

Clinical Problems

Acute or chronic sinusitis, cysts, sinus erosion, structural abnormality.

Procedure

- A consent form should be signed.
- Food and fluids are restricted after midnight or for 12 hours prior to the procedure.
- Dentures, jewelry, and hairpins, if present, should be removed.
- Intravenous fluids are usually started prior to the procedure.
- Eye pads may be used to protect the eyes from injury during the procedure.
- The nostrils are sprayed with a topical anesthetic.
- A fiberoptic endoscope is frequently used.
- Computed tomography may be needed during the procedure to visualize the sinus area.
- Nasal packing may be inserted into the nostril(s) following the procedure.

Factors Affecting Diagnostic Results

- Severe nasal septal defect.

NURSING IMPLICATIONS WITH RATIONALE

- Obtain a history of the sinus problem(s) from the client.
- Check that the consent form is signed.
- Monitor vital signs.

Client Teaching

- Explain the procedure for sinus endoscopy *(see Procedure)*. Answer questions that the client may have or refer questions to appropriate health professionals.

Posttest

- Continue monitoring the client's vital signs until stabilized.
- Check for excessive bleeding or discharge.

Client Teaching

- Instruct the client to call the health care provider if excessive bleeding or discharge occurs and if body temperature becomes elevated.
- Instruct the client to take prescribed drugs (antibiotic and pain medication). Discuss posttest care as indicated by the health care provider.

Skin tests (tuberculin, blastomycosis, coccidioidomycosis, histoplasmosis, trichinosis, and toxoplasmosis)

Normal Finding

Negative results.

Description

Skin testing is useful for determining present or past exposure to an infectious organism: bacterial (tuberculosis), mycotic (blastomycosis, coccidioidomycosis, histoplasmosis), or parasitic (trichinosis and toxoplasmosis). The types of skin tests include scratch, patch, multipuncture, and intradermal. The antigen of the organism is injected intradermally (under the skin), and if the test is positive in 24 to 72 hours, the injection site becomes red, hard, and edematous.

Bacterial Organism and Disease: *Tuberculosis:* The tuberculin (antigen) skin test indicates whether a person has been infected by the tubercle bacilli. A negative test usually rules out the disease.

The methods for skin testing include:

1. *Mantoux test:* Purified protein derivative tuberculin (PPD) is injected intradermally. PPD has several strengths, but the intermediate strength is usually used unless the client is known to be hypersensitive to skin tests. The client

should not receive PPD if there has been a previous positive test. The test is read in 48 to 72 hours.

2. *The tine test or Mono-Vacc test:* These are multipuncture tests that use tines impregnated with PPD. This method is used for mass screening. The tine test is read in 48 to 72 hours, and the Mono-Vacc Test is read in 48 to 96 hours.

3. *Vollmer's patch test:* This patch resembles a Band-Aid; however, the center piece is impregnated with concentrated old tuberculin (OT). The patch is removed in 48 hours, and the test is read 48 hours later.

Mycotic Organisms and Diseases: *Blastomycosis:* The organism *Blastomyces dermatitidis* causes blastomycosis. The antigen blastomycin is injected intradermally, and if an erythematic area >5 mm in diameter developes, the test is positive. The skin test should be read in 48 hours. Positive sputum and tissue specimens will confirm the blastomycin skin test. *Coccidioidomycosis:* The coccidioidin skin test is useful for diagnosing coccidioidomycosis, a fungus disease caused by *Coccidioides immitis*. The antigen coccidioidin is injected intradermally, and the skin test should be read in 24 to 72 hours. A client treated for coccidioidomycosis may remain positive during his or her life span. *Histoplasmosis:* Histoplasmosis is caused by the organism *Histoplasma capsulatum,* which on a lung x-ray resembles tuberculosis. The histoplasmin skin test for histoplasmosis is not always reliable. The antigen is injected intradermally and should be read in 24 to 48 hours. A positive test result occurs when an erythematic area is over 5 mm in diameter. To confirm the skin test results, sputum and tissue specimens should be obtained.

Parasites: *Trichinosis:* The parasitic organism *Trichinella spiralis* causes trichinosis. This organism is present in uncooked meat, especially pork. Symptoms occur approximately 2 weeks after ingesting the organism; the client complains of nausea, diarrhea, pain, colic, fever, and swelling of the muscles. The antigen is injected intradermally, and the test should be read in 15 to 20 minutes. A positive test is a blanched wheal with an erythematic area surrounding it. *Toxoplasmosis:* *Toxoplasma gondii* is the organism causing toxoplasmosis. This organism is found in the eye ground and brain tissue of humans. It can cause blindness and brain damage. The antigen toxoplasmin is injected intradermally and the test result should be read in 24 to 48 hours. A positive test is an erythematic area >10 mm in diameter.

Purposes

- To determine the present or past exposure to an infectious organism.
- To determine if the client has been infected by the tubercle bacilli using the tuberculosis skin test.

Clinical Problems

Antigen Skin Test	Organism	Disease
Tuberculin	Tubercle bacilli	Tuberculosis
Blastomycin	*Blastomyces dermatitidis*	Blastomycosis
Coccidioidin	*Coccidioides immitis*	Coccidioidomycosis
Histoplasmin	*Histoplasma capsulatum*	Histoplasmosis
Trichinellin	*Trichinella spiralis*	Trichinosis
Toxoplasmin	*Toxoplasma gondii*	Toxoplasmosis

Procedure

- Food and fluids are not restricted.
- Cleanse the inner aspect of the forearm with alcohol and let it dry.
- Inject intradermally 0.1 ml of the antigen into the inner aspect of the forearm.
- Record the client's name, the name of the test, the site of the arm of the skin test, the date, and the time it should be read *(see Description for readings of individual tests)*.

Factors Affecting Diagnostic Results

- Steroids and immunosuppressants given within 4 to 6 weeks can cause false-negative skin test results.
- A skin test performed before the body's incubation period (infectious process) can cause a false-negative result.
- Test results read several days after the designated time can give an inaccurate reading.

NURSING IMPLICATIONS WITH RATIONALE

- Obtain a client history about hypersensitivity to skin tests. Ask the client if the skin test was performed before and, if so, whether the skin test result was positive or negative. The skin test should be repeated only if it was negative.
- Report if the client is taking steroids (e.g., cortisone) or immunosuppressant drugs in the last 4 to 6 weeks, because false test results could occur.
- Record the client's abnormal signs and symptoms. Ask the client about his or her contact with bacterial, fungal, or parasitic organisms, if known.
- Be supportive of the client and family, and allow them time to express their concerns.

Client Teaching

- Explain to the client that the purpose of the skin test is to determine the presence of an organism. The organism and the type of skin test should be discussed.
- Explain the procedure to the client. Tell the client that a pin prick will be felt as a small needle with a small amount of solution is injected under the skin.

■ Inform the client that the result of the skin test must be read during the stated time.

■ Inform the client that a positive skin test does not always indicate active infectious disease. However, the positive test does indicate that the organism is present in the body in either an active or a dormant state. If the results are positive, other studies are performed (i.e., x-rays, sputum and tissue cultures, and serum tests).

Sleep studies

Polysomnography (PSG)

Normal Findings

Normal sleep pattern with normal ECG, EEG, EMG, O_2 saturation.

Description

Sleep studies, primarily called polysomnography (PSG), determine the cause of sleep disorders, including daytime sleepiness, obstructive sleep apnea (OSA) which is also called sleep disordered breathing, insomnia, nocturnal awakening, and snoring problems. OSA occurs when there is no ventilation for 10 seconds. It may be attributed to oxygen desaturation, cardiac dysrhythmia, or sleep interruption. Also PSG is indicated for persons having difficulty staying awake during the day who fall asleep at inappropriate times.

Testing for sleep disorders is performed in a sleep laboratory at night over an 8-hour period of time. The client is monitored during the night by electrocardiogram (ECG or EKG), pulse oximetry to determine heart rate and oxygen saturation, electroencephalogram (EEG), electrooculogram (EOG), electromyogram (EMG), airflow monitoring, and snoring sensor. All these testing devices may not be indicated.

Purpose

■ To determine the cause of the sleep disorder.

Clinical Problems

Abnormal Findings: Obstructive sleep apnea (OSA), insomnia, noctural awakening, and snoring.

Procedure

■ A consent form should be signed.

- Keep a sleep log for 1 to 2 weeks prior to the PSG test.
- Avoid caffeine products, alcohol, sedatives, and naps 1 to 2 days before testing.
- Omit prescribed medications until the sleep studies are completed, if indicated.
- Sleep studies are scheduled in the sleep laboratory at night usually 10 or 11 PM until 6 or 7 AM (8-hour period of time).
- Attach electrodes for ECG, EEG, EMG.
- Attach the pulse oximetry.
- Place a commode by the bedside. Electrode leads may inhibit bathroom use.
- Lights are turned off.
- In the AM, have the client evaluates his/her sleep experience.

Factors Affecting Diagnostic Results

- Defective electrodes or those that become loose or fall off.
- Inability to sleep.
- Drugs such as sedatives, caffeine taken prior to the test.

NURSING IMPLICATIONS WITH RATIONALE

- Obtain a history from the client in regards to medications, past stroke, head injury, headaches, seizures.
- Review the sleep log that the client has given.
- Check vital signs. Note if there is respiratory distress.

Client Teaching

- Explain to the client that electrodes will be attached to the head, chest and legs.
    ECG: selected leads attached
    EEG: 2 sets of electrodes to the scalp.
    EOG: 1 electrode to canthus eye.
    EMG: electrodes attached to the leg muscles.
    Pulse oximeter: attached to the finger to determine heart rate and oxygen saturation.
- Answer clients questions or refer the questions to other health professionals.

Stress/exercise tests: treadmill exercise electrocardiology, exercise myocardial perfusion imaging test (thallium/technetium stress test), nuclear persantine (dipyridamole) stress test, nuclear dobutamine stress test*

Normal Finding

Normal electrocardiogram (ECG) with little or no ST-segment depression with exercise. Normal myocardial perfusion.

Description

Treadmill stress testing is based on the theory that clients with coronary artery disease (CAD) will have marked ST-segment depression on the ECG when exercising. Depression of the ST segment and depression or inversion of the T wave indicate myocardial ischemia. In 1928 Fiel and Siegel reported on the relationship of exercising and ST-segment depression in clients complaining of angina. Master used an exercise test (two-step) in 1929 to demonstrate ischemia but used only pulse and blood pressure (BP) to note changes. In 1931 Wood and Wolferth felt exercise was a useful tool for diagnosing coronary disease but that it could be dangerous. Later it was discovered that ST-segment depression usually occurred before the onset of pain and was still present for some time after the pain had subsided. Mild ST-segment depression after exercise can occur without CAD.

Treadmill and Bicycle Electrocardiology: In 1956 Bruce established guidelines for performing stress testing on a treadmill. Master's Step Test (1955) was also accepted as a method for stress testing. Another method used today is the bicycle ergometer test; however, the treadmill seems to be the choice for testing cardiac status. The body muscles do not seem to tire with the treadmill method as much as leg muscles do with the bicycle ergometer. For clients who cannot walk (i.e., paraplegics, amputees), an arm ergometer or pharmacologic stress testing (to be discussed later) can be used. With the treadmill stress test, the work rate (load) is changed every 3 minutes by increasing the speed slightly and the degree of incline (grade) by 3% each time (3%, 6%, 9%). The clients will exercise until they are fatigued, develop symptoms, or reach their maximum predicted heart rate (MPHR).

Exercise Thallium Perfusion Test: The radioisotope thallium 201, which accumulates in the myocardial cells, is used during the stress test to determine myocar-

---

*Revised by Frank Di Gregorio, CNMT, RDMS, Director, Community Imaging Center, Wilmington, DE.

dial perfusion during exercise. With severe narrowing of the coronary arteries, there is less thallium accumulation in the heart muscle. If a coronary vessel is completely occluded, no uptake of thallium will occur at the myocardial area that the vessel supplies. Thallium is most effective for assessing myocardium viability.

Clients with coronary artery disease (CAD) may have normal thallium perfusion scans at rest; however, during exercise, when the heart demands more oxygen, myocardial perfusion decreases. The client returns in 2 or more hours to take a second scan of the heart at rest. Frequently second scans are done to differentiate between an ischemic area and an infarcted or scarred area of the myocardium. This test could be normal even with moderately narrowed coronary arteries when adequate collateral circulation to the heart is present.

Uses for the stress/exercise test or the exercise myocardial perfusion test include screening for CAD, evaluating myocardial perfusion, evaluating the work capacity of cardiac clients, and developing a cardiac rehabilitation program.

Exercise Technetium Perfusion Test: For detection of myocardial ischemia, technetium Tc-99m-laced compounds, such as Tc-99m-sestamibi (Cardiolite), are commonly used for perfusion scanning because they are trapped in the myocardium and does not redistribute. Technetium compounds provide more clinical information by allowing the assessment of perfusion, wall motion, and ejection fraction in one test procedure. Other technetium agents approved by the U.S. Food and Drug Administration (FDA) are Tc-99m-teboroxime and Tc-99m-tetrofosmin. Tc-99m-furifusion is a new technetium agent whose approval by the FDA is pending.

Cardiolite imaging is perhaps the most useful noninvasive test for diagnosing and following CAD at the present time. Positive stress Cardiolite scanning should be considered strong presumptive evidence of CAD. The more markedly abnormal the scan, the more likely the client has serious CAD. It is important to correlate the scan findings with the ECG, the exercise stress test, and the client's symptoms. The use of gated single positron emission (SPECT) (gated refers to the synchronizing of images with the computer and the client's heart rhythm) greatly improves the sensitivity and specificity of the Cardiolite scan.

Nuclear Persantine (Dipyridamole) Stress Test: This is an alternative stress test usually ordered when the client is not physically able to exercise or to walk on a treadmill. Persantine is administered intravenously to dilate the coronary arteries and increase blood flow to the myocardium. Arteries that have become narrowed because of CAD cannot expand like normal arteries. Thallium, cardiolite, or other Tc-based compounds, administered intravenously, detects decreased blood flow to the heart muscle (myocardium). The isotope is administered 3 minutes after the 4-minute IV Persantine infusion.

The client must avoid foods, beverages, and medications containing xanthines (caffeine and theophyllines), such as colas, chocolate, and tea, 24 hours prior to the test, and theophylline preparations 36 hours prior to the test.

Nuclear persantine stress testing is contraindicated for clients who have severe bronchospastic lung disease, such as asthma, or advanced atrioventricular heart block. Additional unfavorable conditions in which this test is not indicated includes acute myocardial infarction within 48 hours of the test, severe aortic or mitral stenosis, resting systolic blood pressure <90 mm Hg, and allergy to dipyridamole.

Nuclear Dobutamine Stress Test: Dobutamine is an adrenergic (sympathomimetic) drug that increases myocardial contractility, heart rate, and systolic blood pressure, which increases the myocardial oxygen consumption and thus increases coronary blood flow. If the client has heart block or asthma and takes a theophylline preparation daily, this test may be ordered instead of the nuclear Persantine (dipyridamole) stress test. Dobutamine is an alternative stressor test.

Nuclear dobutamine stress testing can identify clients with CAD, and identify those who are at high risk for severe ischemic changes prior to vascular surgery. Currently this test is not FDA approved; it is considered an investigational drug test.

Contraindications for nuclear dobutamine stress testing include clients having acute myocardial infarction within 10 days, acute myocarditis or pericarditis, unstable angina pectoris (prolonged episodes, episodes at rest), ventricular or atrial dysrhythmias, severe hypertension or hypotension, severe aortic or mitral stenosis, hyperthyroidism, and acutely severe infections. Propranolol (Inderal) should be available for any possible adverse reaction to the dobutamine infusion.

Purposes

- To screen for CAD.
- To evaluate myocardial perfusion.
- To differentiate between an ischemic area and an infarcted or scar area of the myocardium.
- To develop a cardiac rehabilitation program.
- To evaluate cardiac status for work capability.
- To evaluate drug efficacy.

Clinical Problems

Abnormal Findings: Positive: >2 mm ST depression, coronary artery disease, myocardial hypoperfusion.

Procedure

- A consent form should be signed by the client.
- The client should be NPO 2 or 3 hours before the test. The client should not consume alcoholic and caffeine-containing drinks and should avoid smoking for 2 to 3 hours before the test. Milk could cause nausea.
- Medications should be taken, unless otherwise indicated by the health care provider.
- Comfortable clothes should be worn (i.e., shorts or slacks with a belt and sneakers or tennis shoes with socks). Most bedroom slippers are not suitable.
- The chest is shaved as needed, and the skin is cleansed with alcohol.
- Electrodes are applied to the chest according to the lead selections.

- Baseline ECG, pulse rate, and BP are taken and then are monitored throughout the test.
- The test is stopped if the client becomes dyspneic, suffers severe fatigue, complains of chest pain, has a rapid increase in pulse rates and/or BP, or develops life-threatening arrhythmias (i.e., ventricular tachycardia, premature ventricular contractions [PVCs] >10 PVC in 1 minute).
- Usually the test is not stopped abruptly unless this is necessary. Vital signs and ECG tracings are recorded at the end of the testing or the recovery stage.
- The test takes approximately 30 minutes, which includes up to 10 to 15 minutes of exercising.

Treadmill Stress Test: Usually there are five stages. In the first stage the speed is 2 mph at a 3% grade or incline for 3 minutes. In the second stage the speed is 3.3 mph at a 6% grade for another 3 minutes. Normally the speed does not go beyond 3.3 mph. With each stage the grade is increased 3% and the time is increased by 3 minutes, unless fatigue or adverse reactions occur. The power-driven treadmill has support rails to help the client maintain balance.

Bicycle Ergometer Test: The client is instructed to pedal the bike against an increased amount of resistance. The bike handlebars are for maintaining balance and should not be gripped tightly for support. The client should not shower or take a hot bath for 2 hours after testing.

Exercise Thallium Perfusion Test: An IV line is inserted. Exercise time for the stress test is determined. The client obtains the maximal exercise level, and thallium is injected intravenously 1 minute before the test ends. The client continues to exercise for 1 to 2 more minutes. A scan is then taken by gamma camera, which visualizes thallium perfusion of the myocardium.

Client returns in 2 or more hours for a second scan.

Exercise Technetium Perfusion Test: With the Cardiolite stress test, the client receives two injections intravenously, one at rest and one at stress. The client should be NPO for 2 to 3 hours prior to the test. Any medications that may affect the blood pressure or heart rate should be discontinued 24 to 48 hours prior to the test (unless the test is being performed to evaluate the efficacy of cardiac medications). The client should be physically able to exercise on a treadmill. The total time for the test is 3 hours, which is shorter compared to thallium imaging.

Persantine (Dipyridamole) Stress Test: The client remains NPO after midnight except for water. A diabetic client may have a light breakfast of juice and toast and one-half of the insulin dose, but should first check with the health care provider. Caffeine-containing drugs, food, and beverages such as colas must be avoided 24 hours prior to the test. Decaffeinated beverages should also be avoided. Theophylline preparations (TheoDur, Theolair-SR, Bronkodyl, Elixophyllin SR, and others) should be stopped 36 hours before the test.

The client is in a supine position during the test. The client receives a total of 0.56 mg/kg/dose of IV Persantine (dipyridamole) over a period of 4 minutes. Three minutes after the Persantine infusion, the isotope (thallium, Cardiolite, or other

Tc-based compound) is injected intravenously. Aminophylline should be available to reverse any adverse reaction to Persantine. Imaging procedure begins 15 to 30 minutes after the isotope infusion. Heart rate, blood pressure, and ECG will be monitored before and during the test.

The test is terminated if any of the following occur: ventricular tachycardia, second degree (heart block, severe ST-segment depression, severe hypotension (<90 mm Hg), and severe wheezing). The asthmatic client may use the beta-agonist inhaler if necessary during the procedure.

Nuclear Dobutamine Stress Test: The client remains NPO after midnight except for water. Beta blockers, calcium channel blockers, and angiotensin-converting enzyme (ACE) inhibitors should be discontinued for 36 hours prior to the test. Nitrates should not be taken 6 hours before the test. Dobutamine is administered intravenously using an infusion pump. The dobutamine is mixed in a liter of normal saline solution and the dose and infusion rate is increased until the client heart rate reaches approximately 85% of his or her maximum predicted heart rate. If the heart rate is <110 beats/min, IV atropine sulfate may be given. The isotope is injected when the maximum heart rate is achieved.

The test is terminated if any of the following occur: atrial or ventricular tachycardia, atrial flutter or fibrillation, severe ST-segment depression, progressive anginal pain, severe hypotension (<90 mm Hg systolic), and severe hypertension (>220 mm Hg systolic or >120 mm Hg diastolic). Nitroglycerin may be given for angina pain. Propranolol (Inderal) should be available for adverse reaction to dobutamine. Imaging procedure occurs 15 minutes after the completion of the dobutamine infusion.

Factors Affecting Diagnostic Results

- Certain drugs (e.g., digitalis preparations) can cause a false-positive test result.
- Leaning on support rails of the treadmill or the handlebars of the bicycle.

Nuclear Persantine (Dipyridamole) Stress Test

- Taking theophylline preparations within 24 hours of the test.
- Ingesting caffeine products (beverages, chocolates) 6 hours before the test.
- Ingesting decaffeinated beverages 4 hours before the test.

Nuclear Dobutamine Stress Test

- Taking beta blockers, calcium channel blockers, ACE inhibitors, 24 hours before the test.
- Taking nitrates 4 hours before the test.
- Ingesting a full meal 4 hours before the test.

NURSING IMPLICATIONS WITH RATIONALE

- Recognize when the stress/exercise test is contraindicated (i.e., with recent myocardial infarction; severe, unstable angina; uncontrolled cardiac dysrhythmias; congestive heart failure; or recent pulmonary embolism).

- Check that the consent form has been signed.
- Recognize whether a treadmill stress test or pharmacological stress test is appropriate.
- Review medications that may interfere with test, for example, beta blockers to decrease heart rate.

Client Teaching—Treadmill Stress Test

- Explain the procedure to the client in regard to NPO 2 to 3 hours prior to test; not smoking, continuing with medications; the clothing and shoes that should be worn; shaving and cleansing the chest area; electrode application; continuous monitoring the ECG, pulse rate, and BP; and not leaning on the rails of the treadmill or the handlebars of the bike.
- Instruct the client to inform the cardiologist or technician if he or she experiences chest pain, difficulty in breathing, or severe fatigue. The risk of having a myocardial infarction during the stress test is less than 0.2%.
- Inform the client that after 10 to 15 minutes of testing or when the heart rate is at a desired or an elevated rate, the test is stopped. It will be terminated immediately if there are any severe ECG changes (i.e., multiple PVCs, ventricular tachycardia).
- Allow the client to ask questions. Refer questions you cannot answer to other appropriate health professionals (i.e., a cardiologist, a specialized technician, or a nurse in the stress test laboratory).
- Instruct the client to continue the walking exercise at the completion of the test for 2 to 3 minutes to prevent dizziness. The treadmill speed will be decreased. Tell the client that he or she may be perspiring and may be "out of breath." Profuse diaphoresis, cold and clammy skin, severe dyspnea, and severe tachycardia are not normal and the test will be terminated.
- Inform the client that an ECG and vital signs are taken 5 to 10 mintes after the stress test (recovery stage).
- Encourage the client to participate in a cardiac/exercise rehabilitation program as advised by the health care provider/cardiologist. Tell the client of the health advantages—constant heart monitoring, improved collateral circulation, increased oxygen supply to the heart, and dilating coronary resistance vessels.
- Discourage the client over 35 years of age from doing strenuous exercises without having a stress/exercise test or a cardiac evaluation.
- Inform the client that he or she can resume activity as indicated.
- Explain to the client that a written report is submitted to the client's personal physician from the cardiologist. The client should check with the health care provider for the test results.

Exercise Thallium Perfusion Test—Client Teaching

- Explain the procedure for the test (see Procedure). Explain that the difference between the routine stress test and the exercise thallium perfusion test is an injection of thallium 201 during the routine stress test followed by scans and/or x-rays. Nursing implications are the same for both tests.

- Instruct the client to return for additional pictures in 2 to 4 hours as indicated by the technician or cardiologist.

Exercise Technetium Perfusion Test—Client Teaching
- Explain the procedure *(see Procedure)*
- The client should lie quietly for approximately 30 minutes during the imaging.
- Inform the client that the test should last no more than 3 hours.
- Instruct the client taking medications that affect the blood pressure or heart rate to check with the health care provider as for discontinuing the medications for 24 to 48 hours prior to testing.

Nuclear Persantine (Dipyridamole) Stress Test—Client Teaching
- Explain the procedure for the test to the client *(see Procedure)*. The client should be NPO after midnight except for water.
- Instruct the client to avoid food, beverages, and drugs that contain caffeine. Beverages and foods rich in caffeine include colas (Coke and Pepsi), Dr. Pepper, Mountain Dew, Tab, chocolate (syrup and candy), tea, and coffee. Decaffeinated coffee and tea should also be avoided. Drugs containing caffeine include Anacin, Excedrin, NoDoz, Wigraine, Darvon compound, cafergot, fiorinal. Theophylline preparations should be avoided 36 hours before the test; the client should check with the health care provider in case it is not possible to discontinue the theophylline drug for that period of time.
- Explain to the client that first Persantine will be given intravenously and then an isotope. The client is positioned under a camera with his or her left arm over the head. The camera will be moving very close to the chest for taking pictures (imaging). The imaging takes approximately 20 to 30 minutes.
- Instruct the client to return for additional pictures in 2 to 4 hours as indicated by the technician or cardiologist.
- Explain to the client that a written report is submitted to the client's personal health care provider from the cardiologist.

Nuclear Dobutamine Stress Test—Client Teaching
- Explain the procedure for the test to the client *(see Procedure)*. The client should be NPO after midnight except for water.
- Instruct the client to discontinue drugs that are beta blockers, calcium channel blockers, ACE inhibitors for 36 hours prior to the test with the health care provider's approval. Give the client the date and time for stopping the drug. Nitrates should not be taken 6 hours before the test unless necessary (check with the health care provider).

Thermography (breast)

Mammothermography

Normal Finding

No hot "white" spots; symmetric appearance of the breasts (photograph).

Description

Mammothermography (breast thermography), an infrared photographic test, measures and records heat energy from the skin surface of the breast. Lesions of the breast, especially cancerous ones, cause increased breast metabolism, resulting in an increased breast surface temperature and vascularity. If hot spots are recorded, then additional tests (such as low-dose mammography, ultrasonography, and/or biopsy) should be performed to confirm breast cancer.

Approximately 80% of positive thermograms are accurate for diagnosing lesions of the breast (35% of positive thermograms show benign breast lesions). The remaining 20% of the tests give false-positive results. Because one-fifth of the results are false positive, mammothermography is not commonly used, except for screening purposes. Usually it cannot detect small or deep breast cancer lesions. Mammothermography should be used in conjunction with a physical examination of the breast.

Purpose

- To aid in the diagnosis of a breast lesion.

Clinical Problems

Indications: Cancer of the breast, abscesses of the breast, fibrocystic disease of the breast.

Procedure

- Food and fluids are not restricted. Immediately before the test, hot or very cold drinks should be avoided.
- The client should remove jewelry and clothes from the neck to the waist. The client is given a cloth or paper gown, and the gown should be worn with the opening in the front.
- Ointment or powder on the breast should be removed before the test.
- The client usually sits in a cool room (68°F) for 10 to 15 minutes before the test. This helps to equalize body temperature.
- The client is seated and will be asked to place her hands over her head or on her hips.

- Usually three photographs of different angles are taken of each breast. The procedure takes about 15 minutes.
- The films are checked for readability before the client dresses.

Factors Affecting Diagnostic Results

- Ointment, powder, and recent sunburn could change skin temperature and cause false-positive results.
- Fluctuations in room temperature could affect the test results.
- Menstruation (immediately before or during) could increase vascular engorgement of the breasts.

NURSING IMPLICATIONS WITH RATIONALE

- Obtain a menstrual history. Ask the client when she had her last menstrual period. She should not have the thermogram if she is pregnant or if she is menstruating or close to her period. The vascularity of the breasts increases at these times.

Client Teaching

- Explain the procedure to the client. Procedure in hospitals and in private laboratories may differ slightly, so check before discussing the procedure with the client. Tell the client the test is not painful.
- Instruct the client not to use ointment or powder on the breast the day of the test. These could cause false-positive results. Check the skin for recent exposure to sunlight.
- Inform the client that the test takes about 15 minutes; however, she will be asked to wait for several minutes after the pictures are taken to be sure they are readable. Tell the client not to be alarmed if one of the pictures needs to be repeated.
- Encourage the client to express her concerns. Answer questions, if possible, or refer questions to other appropriate health professionals.
- Inform the client that the mammothermography is generally a screening test and that if the test is positive, other tests will be conducted to confirm the test results. Inform the client that approximately one third of the positive results are benign lesions and one fifth of the positive results could be false positives.
- Encourage the client to perform breast examination after each menstrual period and to keep routine medical appointments. If necessary, demonstrate the breast examination technique.

Thoracoscopy

Normal Findings

Free of pleural and lung disease.

Description

With thoracoscopy, an endoscope (thoracoscope) tube is inserted into the thoracic cavity to visualize the pleural space, thoracic wall, pericardium, and the mediastinum. This test is replacing the thoracotomy procedure. Biopsies and fluid can be obtained with this procedure; also fluid can be drained. Wedge resection to remove blebs or disease tissue, and laser procedure may be performed during this test.

Purposes

- To obtain biopsy specimens.
- To assess tumor growth, pleural effusion, pleural and pulmonary infections, emphysema.
- To perform laser procedure to the thoracic area.

Clinical Problems

Abnormal Findings: Pleural or lung tumors, metastatic cancer in the lungs and/or pleura, emphysema, empyema, inflammatory process in the thoracic cavity.

Procedure

- A signed consent form is required.
- Nothing by mouth (NPO) for 8 to 12 hours prior to the test.
- ***Pretest Requirements:*** Pulmonary function tests, chest X-ray, ECG (EKG), selected laboratory tests. These tests should be completed before the thoracoscopy.
- IV line is inserted for IV medications.
- Client is anesthetized, and an endobronchial tube is inserted.
- The lung on the operative side is collapsed.
- The thoracoscope is inserted through a trocar to view the thoracic cavity.
- Following the thoracoscopic procedure, the lung is reexpanded, and a chest tube is placed in the thoracic cavity with a water-sealed drainage tube attached (closed drainage system).
- The thoracoscopy takes approximately 1 hour.

Factors Affecting Diagnostic Results

- Previous thoracic surgery can inhibit the test procedure.

NURSING IMPLICATIONS WITH RATIONALE

- Obtain a history of the client's health problems and drugs that are taken daily.
- Obtain vital signs.
- Check that the client has completed the pretest orders. Report any abnormal findings.

Client Teaching

- Explain the procedure to the client and refer unknown questions to other health professionals.
- Inform the client that pain medication will be available if the client has discomfort following the procedure.
- Inform the client that he/she will have a chest tube with a drainage system after the test. The chest tube is to assure that any fluid left in the chest will be removed.

Posttest

- Monitor vital signs every 15 minutes X 1 hour; then every 30 minutes X 2 hours, and then hourly for 2 more hours.
- Check frequently or as ordered for patency of the drainage tube.
- Assess respiratory status.
- Report frank bleeding that appears in the drainage tube.
- Administer analgesics for pain as ordered and as needed.
- A chest X-ray will be ordered to determine if the lung has expanded. Chest tube remains in the thoracic cavity until the lungs have expanded.

Ultrasonography (abdominal aorta, brain, breast, carotid, doppler—arteries and veins, eye and eye orbit, gallbladder, heart, kidney, liver, pancreas, pelvis [uterus, ovaries, pregnant uterus], prostate, scrotum, spleen, thoracic, and thyroid)*

Ultrasound, Echography (Echogram), Sonogram

Normal Finding

A normal pattern image of the organ or normal Doppler analysis.

Description

Ultrasonography (ultrasound or sonogram) is a diagnostic procedure used to visualize body tissue structure or wave-form analysis of Doppler studies. An ultrasound probe called a transducer is held over the skin surface or in a body cavity to produce an ultrasound beam in the tissues. The reflected sound waves or echoes from the tissues can be transformed by a computer into either scans, graphs, or audible sounds (Doppler).

Ultrasonography diagnostic, a dynamic, non-ionizing test, is relatively inexpensive and fast, and does not cause any known harm to the patient. It is also referred to as a *sonogram.* There are limitations, because it cannot be used to determine bone abnormalities or for air-filled organs. The ultrasound beam cannot penetrate air. In obese persons it is difficult for sound waves to pass through fat layers.

Ultrasound can detect tissue abnormalities (i.e., masses, cysts, edema, stones). Most ultrasound studies (e.g., gallstones) do not need other modalities for confirmation; however, computed tomography (CT), magnetic resonance imaging, or radionuclide scanning may be used to confirm certain ultrasound results.

Some of the body structures that this procedure examines are the abdominal aorta, the brain, the arteries and veins (Doppler), the gallbladder, the heart, the kidney, the liver, pregnant uterus (pelvic), the pancreas, the spleen, and the thyroid.

Abdominal Aorta: The area for abdominal scanning includes the xyphoid process to the umbilicus. Ultrasonography can detect aortic aneurysms with 98% accuracy and determine whether they are fusiform, saccular or dissecting types.

Arteries and Veins with Doppler: An arterial study is indicated for clients with symptoms of claudication, rest pain, or a persisting open wound in the lower

*Revised by Frank Di Gregorio, CNMT, RDMS, Director, Community Imaging Center, Wilmington, DE.

extremity. Doppler ultrasonography can determine the presence or absence of flow, flow direction, and flow character. The doppler effect can detect decreased blood flow caused by partial arterial occlusion or by deep-vein thrombosis. It can be used in fetal monitoring during labor and delivery. The doppler instrument is available to nurses for monitoring blood flow for those who have altered circulation. Low-frequency waves usually indicate low-velocity blood flow. This procedure may also be used to evaluate the patency of a graft.

Brain: Echoencephalography is an ultrasound of the brain. Neonatal neurosonography is also ultrasound of the brain. If the ventricles are dilated and/or shifted to one side, then pathologic findings, such as intracranial lesions or intracranial hemorrhage, may be suspected. This test is most useful for evaluating hydrocephalus and intracranial hemorrhage in newborns. *(See echoencephalography for detailed data).*

Breast: Ultrasonography of the breast is helpful for (1) diagnosing breast lesions in women who have dense breasts, (2) differentiating between cystic and solid lesions, (3) follow-up of fibrocystic breast disease, and (4) evaluating women with silicone breast implants for breast lesions. Breast ultrasonography may be suggested for pregnant women as well as any woman with a palpable breast mass. X-ray mammography remains the *screening* examination of choice as ultrasonography cannot detect microcalcification. Still, ultrasonography serves as a valuable adjunctive tool.

Carotid Artery with Doppler: Blood flow in the cartoid artery can be measured by using doppler technique to determine carotid stenosis. During a carotid sonogram, vertebral arties can be visualized by this doppler technique to determine antegrade or retrograde blood flow through these vessels.

Eye and Eye Orbit: Ultrasonography of the eye and eye orbital area may be used to (1) determine abnormal tissue of the eye (vitreous adhesions, retinal detachment) when opacities within the eye are present, and (2) detect orbital lesions. With this test, orbital lesions can be distinguished from orbital inflammation.

Gallbladder and Bile Ducts: Gallbladder ultrasonography is accurate in delineating the anatomy of the gallbladder and biliary system. It can evaluate the size, structure, and position of the gallbladder and can determine the presence of gallstones. It may be used in conjunction with nuclear medicine.

Heart (Cardiac): Echocardiography is ultrasound of the heart. It can determine the size, shape, and position of the heart and the movement of heart valves and chambers. The methods commonly used are the M-mode method, which records the motion of the intracardiac structures, such as valves, and the two-dimensional method, which records a cross-sectional view of cardiac structures. The echocardiogram is useful in detecting mitral stenosis, pericardial effusion, congenital heart disease, and enlargement of a heart chamber. *(See echocardiography for detailed data.)*

Intravascular Ultrasonography: An ultrasound transducer mounted on a catheter is used to obtain pathologic changes to the arterial wall and to evaluate vascular procedures such as angioplasty placement. This test is usually performed in large medical centers.

Kidneys (Renal): Ultrasonography is a reliable method of identifying and differentiating renal cysts and tumors. Cysts are echo free, and tumors and renal calculi record multiple echoes. This test is highly recommended when the client is hypersensitive to iodinated contrast dye used in x-ray tests (e.g., intravenous pyelography). This test is most useful for depicting anatomic changes in the kidneys.

Liver (Hepatic): The liver was one of the first organs examined by ultrasound, because it is large and difficult to x-ray. Ultrasonography is useful for distinguishing between cysts and tumors and for determining the size, structure, and position of the liver. With cysts, the sonogram reflects an echo-free response, whereas with a tumor, multiple echoes are recorded. Ultrasonography is very helpful in differentiating obstructive from nonobstructive jaundice. The client may have abnormal liver laboratory values, and the liver may still appear within normal limits.

Pelvis: *Uterus:* Ultrasonography may be used to distinguish between cystic, solid, and complex masses as well as to localize free fluid and inflammatory processes. *Ovaries:* The dimensions of the ovaries, as well as ovarian cysts and solid lesions, can be identified by pelvic sonography. Pelvic ultrasonography is a valuable tool but should not replace a gynecologic examination. *Pregnancy:* In pregnancy the amniotic fluid enhances reflection of sound waves from the placenta and fetus, thus revealing their size, shape, and position. Echoes from the pregnancy may be seen after as few as 4 weeks of amenorrhea. For visualization of pelvic structures, a full bladder is indicated in the nongravid and first-trimester pregnancy. The uterus is sometimes evaluated with a transvaginal transducer with the bladder empty.

Pancreas: The pancreas is a more difficult organ to examine and may require distending the stomach with water to create an acoustic window. Ultrasonography does not measure pancreatic function, but it can determine overall size of the gland and detect pancreatic abnormalities, such as pancreatic tumors, pseudocysts, and pancreatitis. This test is useful for clients who are too thin for adequate CT scanning.

Prostate (Transrectal): Ultrasonography of the prostate gland is used to (1) evaluate palpable prostate nodules and seminal vesicles, (2) determine if urinary problems may be related to benign prostatic hypertrophy (BPH), (3) detect early small prostatic tumors, and (4) identify tumor location for biopsy and/or radiation purposes. A rectal examination and the laboratory test, prostate-specific antigen (PSA), should be included for diagnosing prostatic lesions.

Scrotum/Testes: Ultrasonography of the scrotum sac contents is helpful in diagnosing abscesses, cysts, hydroceles, spermatoceles, varicoceles, testicular tumors, torsion and, chronic scrotal swelling. This type of sonogram does not determine blood flow or lack of blood flow.

Spleen: Ultrasonography can be used for determining the size, structure, and position of the spleen. This procedure can identify splenic masses. In some cases it is a useful tool for evaluating the need for splenectomy, and follow-up of pathologies such as hematoma or abscess.

Thoracic: Ultrasonography is useful in identifying lesions, but it is not diagnostic in the air-filled lungs unless there is a lesion adherent to the chest wall. It may be used to identify pleural fluid, malposition of the diaphragm, and the presence of an abscess. Ultrasound of the thoracic area may be used in combination with x-ray and thoracic scans.

Thyroid: Ultrasonography of the thyroid is 85% accurate in determining the size and structure of the thyroid gland. This procedure can differentiate between a cyst and a tumor and can determine the depth and dimension of thyroid nodules. Nuclear imaging is the choice test for thyroid pathology.

Purposes

- To evaluate the size, structure, and position of body organs.
- To evaluate the blood flow in arteries and veins.
- To detect cysts, tumors, and calculi.

Clinical Problems

ORGAN	ABNORMAL FINDINGS
Abdominal aorta	Aortic aneurysms, aortic stenosis
Arteries and veins (Doppler)	Arterial occlusion (partial or complete), deep-vein thrombosis, chronic venous insufficiency, arterial trauma
Brain	Intracranial hemorrhage, lesions (tumors, abscess), hydrocephalus
Breast	Cysts, tumors (benign or malignant), metastasis to the lymph nodes and muscle tissue
Carotid artery	Carotid plaque, thrombus, degree of stenosis
Eye and eye orbit	Vitreous opacities, detached retina, foreign bodies, orbital lesion, orbital inflammation, meningioma, glioma, neurofibroma, cyst, keratoprosthesis
Gallbladder	Acute cholecystitis, cholelithiasis, biliary obstruction
Heart (Cardiac)	Cardiomegaly, mitral stenosis, aortic stenosis and insufficiency, pericardial effusion, congenital heart disease, left ventricular hypertrophy, ischemic heart disease, septal defects
Kidney (Renal)	Renal cysts and tumors, hydronephrosis, perirenal abscess, acute pyelonephritis, acute glomerulonephritis
Liver (Hepatic)	Hepatic cysts, abscesses, tumor; hepatic metastasis; hepatocellular disease, congenital abnormalities
Pelvis	
Uterus	Uterine tumor, fibroids, hydatiform mole, endometrial changes
Ovaries	Ovarian cysts or tumor
Pregnancy	Fetal age, fetal death, placenta previa, abruptio placenta, hydrocephalus, breech fetal presentation
Pancreas	Pancreatic tumors, pseudocysts, acute pancreatitis
Prostate	Cancer of the prostate gland, benign prostatic hypertrophy (BPH), prostatitis
Scrotum	Hydrocele, spermatocele, varicocele, testicular tumors, torsion, orchitis, acute/chronic epididymitis, cyst, abscess, chronic scrotal swelling

ORGAN	ABNORMAL FINDINGS
Spleen	Splenomegaly; splenic cysts, abscesses, tumor, congenital anomalies
Thoracic	Pleural fluid, abscess formation, malposition of the diaphragm
Thyroid	Thyroid tumors (benign or malignant), thyroid goiters or cysts

Procedure

- Obtain a signed consent form.
- Restrict food and fluids for 4 to 8 hours before test for abdominal aorta, gallbladder, liver, spleen, and pancreas ultrasound studies.
- The client should eat a fat-free meal the night prior to the test for abdominal, gallbladder, liver, pancreas, and kidney sonograms.
- Premedications are seldom given unless the client is extremely apprehensive or has nausea and vomiting.
- Mineral oil or conductive gel is applied to the skin surface at the site to be examined. The transducer is hand-held and is moved smoothly back and forth across the oiled or gel-skin surface.
- The client's position may vary from supine to oblique, prone, semirecumbent, and erect.
- The average time for a procedure is 30 minutes.
- The client should not smoke or chew gum prior to the examination to prevent swallowing air.

Brain

- Remove jewelry and hairpins from neck and head.

Breast

- Hand-held, real-time contact scanning over the palpable mass is the most widely used method for breast imaging.
- The automated system utilizing full-breast water immersion and a reproducible, systematic survey is less widely used because of its higher cost, space requirements, and lack of real-time capability.
- No lotion or powder should be applied under the arm or on the breasts the day of the test.

Doppler

- The blood pressure will be taken at certain limb sites.

Eye and Eye Orbit

- Anesthetize the eye and eye area.
- With the contact method, the probe touches the corneal surface.

Heart and Liver

- Ask the client to breathe slowly and to hold breath after deep inspiration.

Obstetrics (First Trimester), Pelvic and Renal

- The client should drink 24 ounces of water 1 hour prior to the examination, or three to four 8-ounce glasses of clear liquid 90 minutes prior to the test. The client should not void until the test is completed. Second and third trimester clients need not drink large amount of water *unless* bleeding has occurred, in which case the above procedure is followed.

Prostate

- Administer an enema 1 hour prior to the test.
- The client should drink two 8-ounce glasses of clear fluid 1 hour prior to the test.
- The client should *not* void 1 hour prior to the test.
- The client lies on his left side.
- Rectal examination is usually performed before the transducer is inserted into the rectum. Lubricate the rectal probe and insert it into the rectum. The test takes approximately ½ hour.

Scrotum

- The penis is strapped back to the abdominal area.
- Gel is applied and the transducer is passed over the scrotum.

Factors Affecting Diagnostic Results

- Residual barium sulfate in the GI tract from previous x-ray studies will interfere with ultrasound results. Ultrasonography should be performed before barium studies.
- Air and gas (bowel) will not transmit the ultrasound beam.
- Excess fecal material in the colon and rectum (prostate).

NURSING IMPLICATIONS WITH RATIONALE

Client Teaching

- Explain the purpose and procedure to the client *(see Description and Procedure above)*. Tell the client that an oil or lubricant is applied to the skin surface at the site of the organ and that a probe will move with light pressure back and forth over the area.
- Inform the client that this is a painless procedure unless there has been trauma (injury) to the area. Tell the client that there will be no exposure to radiation, and that the ultrasound test is considered to be safe and fast.
- Instruct the client to remain still during the procedure. Inform him or her that the test usually takes 30 minutes or less, except for a few ultrasound tests (e.g., arterial, venous, and carotid ultrasonography), which could take 1 hour.
- Encourage the client to ask questions and to express any concerns. Refer questions you cannot answer to the ultrasonographer or the health care provider.
- Be supportive of the client and the family.

Eye

- Avoid rubbing the eyes until the anesthetic effect has worn off in order to avoid corneal abrasion.
- Inform the client that blurred vision may be present for a short time until the anesthetic has worn off.

Abdominal Studies

- Inform the client that she/he should be NPO for 6 hours prior to all abdominal studies.
- Confirm that the client has not had other tests that may interfere with the ultrasonography, such as upper GI series.

Venography (lower limb)

Phlebography

Normal Finding

Normal, patent deep leg veins.

Description

Lower-limb venography is a fluoroscopic and/or x-ray examination of the deep leg veins after injection of a contrast dye. This test is useful for identifying venous obstruction caused by a deep-vein thrombosis (DVT). A thrombus formation usually occurs in the deep calf veins and at the venous junction and its valves. If DVT is not treated, it can lead to femoral and iliac venous occlusion, or the thrombus can become an embolus and cause pulmonary embolism.

This procedure is frequently done after doppler ultrasonography to confirm a positive or questionable DVT. *Radionuclide venography* using iodine 125 (I-125)-tagged fibrinogen with scintillation scanning may be done for clients who are too ill for venography or are hypersensitive to contrast dye. The tagged fibrinogen, given intravenously, collects at the site of the thrombus. It may take 6 to 72 hours for the isotope to collect at the thrombus site; thus the scanner will be used to check the leg daily for 3 days. This test should not be performed for screening purposes.

Purposes

- To detect DVT.
- To identify congenital venous abnormalities.
- To select a vein for arterial bypass grafting.

Clinical Problems

Abnormal Findings: DVT, congenital venous abnormalities.

Procedure

- A consent form should be signed.
- The client should be NPO for 4 hours before the test; some hospitals permit clear liquids before the test.
- Anticoagulants may be temporarily discontinued.
- A skin test, antihistamine, and/or steroids may be ordered for patients who have a history of allergies to iodine, seafood, or x-ray dye from other tests (e.g., intravenous pyelography).
- The client lies on a radiographic table tilted at a 40- to 60-degree angle. A tourniquet is applied above the ankle, a vein is located in the dorsum of the foot, a small amount of normal saline is administered intravenously into the vein, and then the contrast dye is injected slowly over a period of 2 to 4 minutes. A cutdown may be necessary if a vein in the foot cannot be located or is not suitable. Fluoroscopy may be used to monitor the flow of the contrast dye, and spot films are taken.
- Normal saline is used after the procedure to flush the contrast dye from the veins.
- A sedative may be indicated prior to the test for clients who are extremely apprehensive and for those who have a low threshold of pain.
- The test takes 30 minutes to 1 hour.

Factors Affecting Diagnostic Results

- Weight on the leg being tested can cause a decrease in the flow of the contrast dye.
- Movement of the leg being tested can interfere with the clarity of the film.

NURSING IMPLICATIONS WITH RATIONALE

Pretest

- Obtain a client history of allergies to iodine, iodine substances (x-ray dye), and seafood. Antihistamines or steroids (e.g., cortisone) may be given for 2 to 3 days before the test.
- Record baseline vital signs. Have the client void before the test.

Client Teaching

- Explain the purpose and procedure to the client.
- Inform the client that he or she may have a slight burning sensation when the dye is injected. Inform the client not to move the leg being tested during the injection of the dye or during x-ray filming.

Posttest

- Monitor vital signs until stable and as ordered.
- Check the pulse in the dorsalis pedis, popliteal, and femoral arteries for volume intensity and rate.

- Observe for signs and symptoms of latent allergic reaction to the contrast dye (i.e., dyspnea, skin rash, urticaria [hives], and tachycardia).
- Observe the injection site for bleeding, hematoma, and signs and symptoms of infection (i.e., redness, edema, and pain). Report abnormal changes and problems to the health care provider, and record the observations on the client's chart.
- Elevate the affected leg as ordered. If the venogram is positive for DVT, the health care provider most likely will order bed rest, blood laboratory tests, heparin infusion, leg elevation, and warm, moist compresses.
- Be supportive of the client. Answer the client's questions, or refer them to the health care provider.

Ventilation scan

Pulmonary Ventilation Scan

Normal Finding

Normal lung tissue with normal gas distribution in both lungs.

Description

The ventilation scan is a nuclear scan of the lungs. The client inhales a mixture of air, oxygen, and radioactive gas (xenon [Xe-127 or Xe-133] or krypton 85 [Kr-85]). A single-breath scan is taken first. Then three phases of scanning follow: (1) the wash-in phase, which is the build-up of gas distribution in the lungs; (3) the equilibrium phase, in which radioactive gas reaches a steady state; and (3) the washout phase, in which room air is breathed to remove radioactive gas from the lungs.

The pulmonary ventilation scan is usually performed with the pulmonary perfusion scan to differentiate between a ventilatory problem and vascular abnormalities in the lung. The pulmonary perfusion scan indirectly evaluates problems related to blood flow to the lungs (e.g., pulmonary embolism). The radioactive substance used is technetium or iodine, and images are displayed by a scintillator. A ventilation scan can reveal decreased ventilation (uptake of radioactive gas) caused by chronic obstructive lung disease, atelectasis, and pneumonia, although the pulmonary perfusion scan is normal. However, pulmonary embolus can cause an abnormal perfusion scan and a normal ventilation scan.

Purposes

- To differentiate between a ventilatory problem and vascular abnormalities in the lung.
- To detect lung cancer, sarcoidosis, or tuberculosis.
- To determine hypoventilation due to excess smoking or chronic obstructive pulmonary disease (COPD).

Clinical Problems

Abnormal Findings: COPD, pulmonary emboli, tuberculosis, sarcoidosis, lung cancer.

Procedure

- Obtain a signed consent form.
- There is no food or fluid restriction.
- Remove all metal objects (jewelry) from around the neck and chest.
- The client inhales gas (radioactive xenon or krypton). The client will be asked to take a deep breath and to hold it for a short time (single breath) while the scanner takes an image of the lung. Other images will be recorded during three phases of the test; wash-in, equilibrium, and washout.

Factors Affecting Diagnostic Results

- Metal objects could cause inaccurate recorded images.

NURSING IMPLICATIONS WITH RATIONALE

- Assess respiratory status. Note and report changes in rate and difficulty in breathing. Check breath sounds.
- Assess communications for verbal and nonverbal expressions of anxiety and fear about tests and/or potential or actual problem.
- Report if the client is having chest pain, especially if pulmonary embolism is suspected.
- Be supportive of the client and family members prior to the test. Answer questions, or refer the questions to appropriate health professionals.

Client Teaching

- Explain the procedure to the client *(see Procedure)*. Tell the client that the amount of radioactive gas is minimal.
- Instruct the client to remove all jewelry from the chest and neck area.

Water loading test

Water Loading ADH Suppression Test

Normal Finding

1000 ml of Water Intake: *Urine Output:* >600 ml in 4 hours. *Abnormal:* <500 ml in 4 hours. *Urine Osmolality:* <180 mOsm/kg. *Abnormal:* >230 mOsm/kg. *Serum Osmolality:* >280 mOsm/kg. *Abnormal:* <280 mOsm/kg. *Plasma ADH: See Antidiuretic Hormone.*

Description

Water loading test is a diagnostic test for determining the presence of excess secretion of antidiuretic hormone (ADH), also called syndrome of inappropriate ADH secretion (SIADHs). This test is to suppress the secretion of ADH from the posterior pituitary gland or neurohypophysis through water loading. Normally, as fluid intake increases, urine output increases and urine osmolality decreases. With SIADHs, as water intake increases the urine output does not increase and the urine osmolality could be higher than serum osmolality *(see above, Abnormal Findings)*. Caution in administering this test should be taken for clients with a history of congestive heart failure (CHF).

SIADHs may be the result of ectopic hormone production caused by tumors, such as bronchogenic carcinoma, pancreatic carcinoma, brain tumors, and lymphoma. Other conditions that can cause SIADHs include tuberculosis, pneumonia, meningitis, thyroid and adrenal disorders, and certain drugs (thiazide diuretics, vincristine).

Purpose

- To detect the presence of SIADHs.

Clinical Problems

Abnormal Findings: SIADHs from ectopic hormone production due to malignant tumors (lung, pancreas, brain), respiratory conditions (pneumonia, tuberculosis), certain CNS disorders, and certain thyroid and adrenal disorders.

Procedure

- The client should be NPO after midnight. Check with institution's policy.
- Hold diuretics for 12 hours prior to the test.
- Collect 7 ml of venous blood in a red-top tube. This blood specimen is for baseline serum osmolality. Collect a urine specimen for a baseline urine osmolality.
- Have the client drink 1 liter (1000 ml) of water in 15 to 30 minutes.

- Collect 7 ml of venous blood and urine specimen every hour after water ingestion for 4 to 5 hours. (This may be a 4- or a 5-hour test; check with the institution). Refrigerate blood samples and urine specimens until test is completed.
- Blood specimens may also be ordered for serum sodium and plasma ADH. Check with the health care provider.

Factors Affecting Diagnostic Results

- Diuretics can dilute urine and cause a false test result. Diuretics should be held for at least 12 hours before the test and until the test is completed.
- Lithium carbonate can dilute the urine.
- Not collecting all blood and urine specimens.

NURSING IMPLICATIONS WITH RATIONALE

- Obtain a history of cardiac condition, including CHF.
- Assess for fluid retention, chest rales, peripheral edema.
- Administer 1 liter (1000 ml of water) in 15 to 30 minutes.
- Collect blood samples and urine specimens hourly. Measure the urine output hourly and total after 4 to 5 hours.

Client Teaching

- Explain the procedure to the client. It may be necessary that the procedure be written, step by step, for the client to follow. Emphasize the importance of collecting urine samples and blood specimens on time.
- Listen to the client's concern.

X-ray (chest, heart, flat plate of abdomen, kidney, ureter, bladder, and skull)

Roentgenography, Radiography

Normal Finding

Chest: Normal bony structure and normal lung tissue.

Heart (Cardiac): Normal size and shape of the heart and vessels.

Flat Plate of Abdomen: Normal abdominal structures.

Kidney, Ureter, Bladder (KUB): Normal kidney size and structure.

Skull: Normal structure.

Description

In November of 1895, Wilhelm Konrad Roentgen, a German physicist, discovered x-radiation for diagnosing diseases. Adequate control of the rays (roentgen rays) for the client and the operator did not occur until 1910, and it was then when the machines and techniques were greatly improved. Today x-ray studies cause only small amounts of radiation exposure because of the high quality of x-ray film and procedure.

There are four densities in the human body—air, water, fat, and bone—that will absorb varying degrees of radiation. Air has less density, causing dark images on the film, and bone has high density, causing light images. Bone contains a large amount of calcium and will absorb more radiation, thus allowing less radiation to strike the x-ray film; thus a white structure is produced.

The chest x-ray is one of the diagnostic tests most often ordered by the health care provider. A skull x-ray is usually ordered following head trauma. The requests for cardiac, flat plate of abdomen, and kidney-ureter-bladder (KUB) x-rays have increased in the last two decades. X-ray studies are requested primarily for screening purposes and then are followed by other extensive diagnostic tests.

Purposes

- To identify bone structure and tissue in the body.
- To detect abnormal size, structure, and shape of bone and body tissues.

Clinical Problems

Test	Abnormal Findings
Chest	Atelectasis, pneumonias, tuberculosis, tumors, lung abscess, pneumothorax, sarcoma, sarcoidosis, scoliosis/kyphosis
Heart	Cardiomegaly, aneurysms, anomalies of the aorta
Abdominal (flat plate)	Abdominal masses, small bowel obstruction, abdominal tissue trauma, ascites
KUB	Abnormal size and structure of KUB, renal calculi, kidney and bladder masses
Skull	Head trauma (intracranial pressure, skull fractures), congenital anomalies, bone defects
Skeletal	Fractures, arthritic conditions, osteomyelitis

Procedure

Chest

- Food and fluids are not restricted.
- PA chest film is usually ordered with the client standing. An anteroposterior (AP) chest film may be ordered when PA film cannot be obtained. With an AP chest film, the client is sitting or lying down. A lateral chest film may also be ordered.
- Clothing and jewelry should be removed from the neck to the waist, and a paper or cloth gown should be worn.
- The client should take a deep breath and hold it as the x-ray is taken.

Heart

- Food and fluids are not restricted.
- Posteroanterior (PA) and left-lateral chest films are usually indicated for evaluating the size and shape of the heart. The left anterior oblique (LAO) 60-degree rotation with the PA position may be ordered for cardiac evaluation.
- Clothing and jewelry should be removed from the neck to the waist, and a paper or cloth gown should be worn.
- Client instructions will include body position (usually standing) and when to take a deep breath and hold it.

Abdomen and KUB

- Food and fluids are usually not restricted.
- X-rays should be taken before an intravenous pyelogram or gastrointestinal studies.
- Clothes are removed, and a paper or cloth gown is worn.
- The client lies in the supine position with his or her arms away from the body on a tilted x-ray table.
- The testes should be shielded as an added precaution.

Skull

- Food and fluids are not restricted.
- The client should remove hairpins, glasses, and dentures before the x-ray tests.
- The client will be asked to assume various positions so that different areas of the skull can be x-rayed. X-rays may include the facial bones and sinuses.

Skeletal

- The client should be NPO if a fracture is suspected.
- Immobilize suspected fracture site.

Factors Affecting Diagnostic Results

- Radiopaque materials for IVP and GI studies administered within 3 days of routine x-rays (ie, chest, flat plate of abdomen, and KUB) could distort the pictures.
- Incorrect positioning of the client could produce distorted pictures.
- Obesity and ascites could affect the clarity of the x-ray film.

NURSING IMPLICATIONS WITH RATIONALE

- Describe the x-ray procedure to the client.

Client Teaching

- Inform the client that the x-ray test usually takes 10 to 15 minutes.
- Inform the client that there may be several x-rays taken, one or two chest films, or five skull films. The client may be asked to remain in the waiting room for 10 to 15 minutes after x-rays are taken to be sure the films are readable.

- Encourage the client to ask questions or to express his or her concerns to the nurse, physician, and the technician. Also, if the client does not understand the directions, he or she should ask to have them repeated.
- Ask the female client if she is pregnant or if pregnancy is suspected. X-rays should be avoided during the first trimester of pregnancy. If x-ray of the chest is necessary, the female client should wear a lead apron covering the abdomen and pelvic areas. Some dentists have women of childbearing age (12 to 48 years old) wear lead aprons.
- Explain to the client that the x-ray equipment and film today are of good quality and decrease the exposure to radiation.

PART THREE

Laboratory/ Diagnostic Assessments of Body Function

3

Numerous laboratory and diagnostic tests are ordered to assist in the diagnosis of disease entities and to determine organ function. The purpose of Part III is to provide a listing of groups of tests, with explanations, used for diagnosing body dysfunction. Twelve categories related to organ, body structure, and clinical condition are presented. In each categoric section, the laboratory and diagnostic tests frequently performed are explained as they relate to the disorder. Nursing processes follow with nursing diagnoses, nursing implications, and evaluation at the end of each of the 12 categories. Nursing diagnoses are stated according to the North American Nursing Diagnosis Association (NANDA), 2001–2002.

For a more detailed description, procedure, and specific nursing implications of each test, the nurse should refer to Parts I and II of the text.

Cardiac function

Laboratory Tests	Diagnostic Tests
Cardiac Enzymes:	ECG/EKG
CK/CPK	Echocardiography
AST/SGOT	Phonocardiography
LD	X-ray
High Sensitivity C-Reactive Protein (hs CRP)	Exercise/Stress Tests
Myoglobin (Serum & Urine)	Thallium Perfusion
Electrolytes (Serum)	Persantine
Lipoproteins (Serum Lipids)	Dobutamine
Clotting Times	Holter Monitoring
PT	Cardiac Catheterization (Cardiac
PTT, APTT	Arteriography)
Coagulation Time	Nuclear Heart Scan
ESR	Magnetic Resonance Imaging (MRI)
Antimyocardial Antibody (Serum)	Positron Emission Tomography (PET)
Anticardiolipin Antibody (ACA)	
Atrial Natriuretic Hormone (ANH)	
Hydroxybutyric Dehydrogenase (HBD)	
Glucose (Blood, Serum)	
Leukocytes (WBC)	
ABGs	
TDM	

Introduction

Numerous laboratory and diagnostic tests are performed to detect cardiac problems and the extent of myocardial injury. Serum enzyme levels are generally ordered immediately upon complaint of cardiac discomfort. Enzyme levels are frequently repeated later to determine if significant changes have occurred. Other tests ordered include serum electrolytes, blood glucose, blood lipids, sedimentation rate, PT, PTT, ECG, cardiac x-ray, and cardiac catheterization, among others.

Laboratory Tests

Cardiac Enzymes: Because serum cardiac enzyme levels might be normal immediately following cardiac trauma, the first set of enzyme levels acts as the baseline measurement for comparison of changes. Following heart injury, creatine kinase (CK/CPK) and isoenzyme CK-MB band, lactate dehydrogenase (LD/LDH) and LD isoenzymes with an LD_1:LD_2 shift, and aspartate aminotransferase (AST/SGOT) increase in the blood in proportion to the extent of the injury. Each enzyme has its own time course of release after injury. Table 1 is a list of cardiac enzymes including significant changes that can occur.

TABLE 1   CARDIAC ENZYME TESTS

Enzyme	Reference Values	Changes	Comments
Creatine kinase (CK) or Creatine phosphokinase (CPK)	*Norms:* Male: 5–35 μg/ml 30–180 IU/l 55–170 U/l at 37°C Female: 5–25 μg/ml 25–150 IU/l 30–135 U/l at 37°C CPK-MB: 0%–6%	Early detection after heart damage: 4–6 hours. Maximal levels for 24 hours. Maximum level rise is five to eight times normal. CK-MB: 5–15 times normal. Return to normal 3–4 days.	Increased CK is an indicator of muscle damage (cardiac or skeletal). Differentiation between cardiac and skeletal involvement is determined by the CK isoenzymes: CK-MB (heart) CK-MM (skeletal muscle) CK-BB (brain)
Asparatate aminotransferase (AST) or SGOT	*Norms:* Average: 8–38 U/l Adult: 0–35 U/l 5–40 U/ml (Frankel) 4–36 IU/l 16–60 Karmen U/ml 30°C 8–33 U/l at 37°C, SI units	AST/SGOT increases within 6–10 hours after heart damage. Peak within 24–48 hours. Returns to normal in 4–6 days. Rise is three to five times normal.	AST/SGOT is not the first enzyme to rise after severe heart damage.
Lactic dehydrogenase (LD/LDH)	*Norms:* Adult, total: 100–190 IU/l, 70–250 U/l 70–200 IU/l	LD elevation occurs 6–12 hours after heart damage. Peak 2–5 days. Returns to normal 6–12 days.	Rise in LD is later than CK/CPK and AST/SGOT. The prolongation of serum level makes it valuable for diagnosing a late MI.
Isoenzymes: LD_1, LD_2	Isoenzymes: LD_1 14%–26% LD_2 27%–37%	Isoenzymes: 12–24 hours after heart damage. Flipped LD ratio $LD_1:LD_2$.	Normally LD_2 has a higher level than LD_1 with a ratio $LD_2:LD_1$. After acute myocardial infarction, LD_1 increase is greater than LD_2.

High Sensitivity C-Reactive Protein (hs CRP): *Norms:* Adult: <0.175 mg/l.
It is a highly sensitive test in detecting the risk of cardiovascular and peripheral vascular diseases. A positive hs CRP may indicate that the client is at a high risk for coronary artery disease (CAD).

Myoglobin (Serum): *Norms:* 12–90 ng/ml; 12–90 μg/l.
Myoglobin is a protein found in the skeletal and cardiac muscle cells. After an injury, this protein is released into circulation. After an acute myocardial infarction (AMI), it peaks in approximately 8 to 12 hours.

Electrolytes (Serum): *Norms:* Potassium: 3.5–5.3 mEq/l. Sodium: 135–145 mEq/l.
Serum electrolyte levels could be normal immediately following myocardial damage. Cellular potassium is lost, and so the serum potassium level might be elevated if urinary output is decreased. It could be normal or decreased if urinary output is increased. Serum sodium level could be normal or decreased if sodium shifts into heart cells. Potassium-wasting diuretics (i.e., hydrochlorothiazide [HydroDIURIL], furosemide [Lasix]) used for treating congestive heart failure could cause a loss of potassium and sodium.

Lipoproteins (Serum Lipids): *Norms:* Adult: Total: 400–800 mg/dl, 4–8 g/l (SI units). Cholesterol: 150–240 mg/dl. Triglycerides: 30–39 years: 20–150 mg/dl; 40–49 years; 30–160 mg/dl; >50 years: 40–190 mg/dl. Phospholipids: 150–325 mg/dl. There could be laboratory differences with these ranges.
Elevated lipid levels (cholesterol, triglycerides, and phospholipids) could be the major factor in the cause of coronary artery disease (CAD). Because most lipids are bound to protein (lipoproteins), electrophoresis is used to separate the lipoproteins. Low-density lipoprotein (LDL) is composed of 45% cholesterol, and very-low-density lipoprotein (VLDL) is composed of 70% triglycerides. Both LDL and VLDL are strongly associated with CAD.

Clotting Times: The tests frequently used to monitor clotting time are prothrombin time (PT), partial thromboplastin time (PTT), activated partial thromboplastin time (APTT), and coagulation time (CT) or Lee-White clotting time (LWCT). Table 2 explains these tests, gives the reference values, and their purposes.

Sedimentation (Sed) Rate, Erythrocyte Sedimentation Rate (ESR): *Norms:* Adult: Under 50 years (Westergren method): 0–10 mm/hr; female: 0–20 mm/hr. Over 50 years (Westergren method): male: 0–20 mm/hr; female: 0–30 mm/hr.
An elevated sedimentation rate might occur after MI or bacterial endocarditis.

Antimyocardial Antibody (Serum): *Normal:* None detected.
Antimyocardial antibodies occur because of a specific antigen in the heart muscle. This antigen can cause autoimmune damage to the heart.

Anticardiolipin Antibody (ACA) (Serum): *Normal:* Negative result.
ACA is an autoantibody found in some clients with systemic lupus erythematosus.

TABLE 2 TESTS FOR MONITORING CLOTTING TIMES

Test	Reference Values	Purpose
Prothrombin time (PT)	*Norms:* 11–15 seconds or 70% Anticoagulant therapy: 2 to 2.5 times control in seconds or 20%–30% INR 2.0–3.0	PT is used to monitor clot formation and oral anticoagulant therapy. The PT is kept 2 to 2.5 times the control for anticoagulant therapy.
Partial thromboplastin time (PTT) or Activated partial thromboplastin time (APTT)	*Norms:* 60–70 seconds Anticoagulant therapy: 1.5 to 2.5 times the control *Norms:* 20–35 seconds	PTT and APTT are primarily used to detect clotting factor defects and to monitor heparin therapy. Following MI, many clients receive heparin therapy, and later some take oral anticoagulants.
Coagulation time (CT) or Lee-White clotting time (LWCT)	*Norms:* 3-tube method: 5–15 minutes	An infrequently used test to determine coagulation problems. It can be used to regulate heparin therapy. It is a time-consuming test.

Atrial Natriuretic Hormone (ANH) (Plasma): *Norm:* 20–77 pg/ml.

ANH, secreted from the atrium of the heart, acts as an antagonist to renin and aldosterone. It has antihypertensive effects, lowering blood pressure.

Hydroxybutyric Dehydrogenase (HBD) (Serum): *Norm:* 140–350 IU/l. 114–290 U/l.

HBD, an enzyme primarily in heart muscle, is similar to LD_1. Levels rise 8 to 10 hours following MI.

Blood Glucose: *Norms:* 60–100 mg/dl.

Serum or Plasma Glucose (Fasting): *Norms:* 70–110 mg/dl.

A slight to moderate increase in blood or serum glucose level (blood 150 mg/dl or serum 160 to 180 mg/dl) could be the result of stress caused by release of glucogen and catecholamines. A continuous elevation in blood or serum glocose level is a risk factor for CAD.

Leukocytes, White Blood Cells: *Norms:* 5000–10000 mm^3; (μl) 5–10 × 10^3/μl; 5–10 × 10^9/l (SI units).

An elevated WBC count could occur after MI because of an inflammatory response secondary to the infarction or could occur as the result of bacterial endocarditis.

Arterial Blood Gases (ABGs): *Norms:* Adult: pH: 7.35–7.45; $PaCO_2$: 35–45 mm Hg; PaO_2: 75–100 mm Hg; HCO_3: 24–28 mEq/l; BE: +2 to −2.

Abnormal ABGs could occur after an acute myocardial infarction; PaO_2 decreased, $PaCO_2$ decreased because of hyperventilation, normal or increased because of hypoventilation, HCO_3 and base excess (BE) decreased.

Therapeutic Drug Monitoring (TDM): Drugs taken for cardiac conditions should be closely monitored through blood samples to determine therapeutic levels and peak time to avoid drug toxicity. Most drug levels should be checked after serum drug level is at a steady state, approximately in 12 to 72 hours. Lidocaine is usually checked in 12 hours after administration and then daily. Propranolol (Inderal), procainamide (Pronestyl), and quinidine are checked 24 to 72 hours after administration; digoxin after 5 days. A schedule for TDM is suggested to maintain therapeutic levels and to prevent drug toxicity.

Name of Drug	Therapeutic Range	Peak Time	Toxic Level
Digitoxin	10–25 ng/ml	12–24 hours	>30 ng/ml
Digoxin	0.5–2 ng/ml	6–8 hours	2.5 ng/ml
Lidocaine	1.5–5.0 µg/ml	10 minutes	>6 µg/ml
Propranolol (Inderal)	50–100 ng/ml	1–2 hours	>150–1000 ng/ml
Procainamide (Pronestyl)	4–10 µg/ml	1 hour	>10 µg/ml
Procainamide + NAPA	5–20 µg/ml		>30 µg/ml
Disopyramide (Norpace)	2–5 µg/ml	2 hours	>7 µg/ml
Quinidine	2–5 µg/ml	1–3 hours	>5–6 µg/ml
Diazepam (Valium)	400–600 ng/ml	1–2 hours	>1000 ng/ml
Verapamil (Isoptin)	100–300 ng/ml	1–2 hours	>300 ng/ml
Nifedipine (Procardia)	50–100 ng/ml	30 minutes	100 ng/ml
Diltiazem (Cardizem)	50–200 ng/ml	2–3 hours	>200 ng/ml

Diagnostic Tests

Electrocardiography (ECG, EKG): Electrocardiography records the electrical impulses of the heart by means of electrodes attached at appropriate sites on the chest. Abnormal P waves, QRS complexes, ST segments, and/or T waves indicate a possible cardiac problem. A depressed ST segment and an inverted T wave could indicate myocardial ischemia.

Echocardiography, Ultrasound Cardiography: This test is useful in detecting enlargement of a heart chamber, changes in heart dimensions during cardiac cycle, valvular disease (e.g., mitral stenosis, pericardial effusion, and congenital heart disease). It is considered a noninvasive test.

Phonocardiography, Phonocardiogram: Phonocardiography is the graphic recording of sounds from the heart. The phonocardiogram is considered superior to examination by stethoscope in that it can record low-frequency sounds (e.g., gallop sounds). It is useful to detect cardiac valvular damage and to record the shape of various murmurs heard.

X-ray of Heart and Chest: X-rays of the chest to determine heart size are taken in posteroanterior (PA) and left-lateral positions. The x-ray films from these positions are helpful for identifying cardiomegaly and anomalies of the aorta.

Exercise/Stress Testing: Stress testing is a diagnostic tool that provides information about the cardiac function during exercise (stress). From the results of the test, decisions can be made about the degree of work level considered safe and how soon the individual should return to work after the MI.

Thallium Perfusion Stress Test: The radioisotope thallium-201 is used during the stress test to determine myocardial perfusion during exercise. With severe narrowing of the coronary arteries, there is less thallium accumulation in the heart muscle.

Persantine (Dipyridamole) Stress Test: If the client is unable to exercise or to walk on a treadmill, Persantine (dipyridamole) is administered intravenously to dilate the coronary arteries. Narrowed coronary arteries respond poorly to the Persantine.

Dobutamine Stress Test: Dobutamine, an adrenergic or sympathomimetic, increases the myocardial contractility, myocardial oxygen consumption, heart rate, and systolic blood pressure. Dobutamine-thallium is an alternative stress test. This test can identify clients with CAD and those who are at high risk for severe ischemic changes prior to vascular surgery.

Holter Monitoring: Holter monitoring is a type of continuous ECG recorded on tape within a device known as the monitor. This test evaluates the heart rate and rhythm during normal daily activites, rest, and sleep for 24 to 48 hours.

Left Cardiac Catheterization, Cardiac Angiography/Arteriography: This is an invasive procedure to determine the patency of the coronary arteries and functions of aortic and mitral valves. Dye is injected to determine left ventricular functioning while video film is recording the activity of the coronary arteries and heart valves.

Nuclear Heart Scan: The radionuclides technetium 99m and thallium-201 are used to detect cardiomegaly, cardiac output, ischemic heart disease, and the presence of an aneurysm.

Magnetic Resonance Imaging (MRI): MRI, a noninvasive test, is useful for evaluating the cardiovascular system. It can detect atrial and ventricular septal defects, MI, aortic and ventricular aneurysms, plaque formation, and blood flow through coronary branches and through extremities.

Positron Emission Tomography (PET): This test is useful for studying myocardial perfusion imaging. It can evaluate myocardial perfusion 72-hour after MI; it can also be used to determine if the ischemic area in the myocardium is viable or is infarcted after an acute MI.

NURSING DIAGNOSES

- Anxiety related to pain and the unknown.
- Deficient knowledge related to lack of understanding of the laboratory or diagnostic procedure, disease process, and/or outcome.
- Noncompliance to prescribed laboratory test related to lack of adequate explanation.
- Ineffective tissue perfusion related to coronary artery insufficiency.
- Acute pain related to chest pain secondary to cardiac tissue ischemia.
- Ineffective coping with disease process and laboratory and diagnostic test procedures.
- Impaired physical mobility related to perceived or actual chest pain.
- Disturbance in self-esteem related to dependence and/or role change.

NURSING IMPLICATIONS WITH RATIONALE

- Explain the purpose of the laboratory and diagnostic tests.
- Give a detailed explanation concerning the laboratory and diagnostic procedures and the need for the client's compliance with the procedure(s). Explanation might be brief or in-depth depending upon the individual's unfamiliarity with the test.
- Explanation of the tests and procedures to the family members could be helpful with test compliance.
- Inform the client of any food, beverage, or drug restrictions (see Parts I and II).
- Listen to the patient's expressed anxiety or fear concerning the tests and potential clinical problems. Clarification of test procedure might alleviate fear and anxiety and promote test compliance.
- Assess the patient's chest discomfort by eliciting the intensity, duration, and location of the pain from the client. Check skin color and vital signs. Report findings immediately to the health care provider (HCP).
- Provide care to the client as prescribed by the HCP (i.e., oxygen, drugs).
- Suggest to the client and family members the community resources available to them (e.g., American Heart Association).

Evaluation

- Determine if the test was completed correctly according to the procedure. Notify the laboratory of any changes that occurred during the test.
- Check to see that the client's discomfort was alleviated. If not, notify the HCP.
- Evaluate the status of the client's anxiety and fear in regard to the test(s) and clinical problem.
- Assist the client and family member in making changes regarding activity, recreation, future tests, and health care.
- Contact the dietitian and social service agency to secure their participation in the client's health care in the hospital and at home.

Respiratory function

Laboratory Tests	Diagnostic Tests
ABGs	Chest X-Ray
Sputum Culture	Pulmonary Function Studies
α-1-Antitrypsin (Serum)	Tomography
Angiotensin-Converting Enzyme	Thoracic Computed Tomography (CT)
(ACE) (Serum)	Bronchoscopy
TDM	Bronchography
Skin Tests	Mediastinoscopy
	Radionuclide Thoracic Scan
	Lung Scan
	Ventilation Scan
	Pulmonary Angiography/Arteriography
	Lung Biopsy
	Thoracentesis
	Thoracoscopy
	Magnetic Resonance Imaging (MRI)
	Sinus Endoscopy

Introduction

Chest x-ray, arterial blood gases (ABGs), and pulmonary function studies are usually ordered for respiratory problems. If abnormalities are reported, other diagnostic tests are performed (i.e., thoracic computed tomography [CT], radionuclide thoracic scan, bronchoscopy, and others).

Laboratory Tests

Arterial Blood Gases (ABGs): *Norms:* pH: 7.35–7.45; $PaCO_2$: 35–45 mm Hg; PaO_2: 75–100 mm Hg; HCO_3: 24–28 mEq/l.

A decreased $PaCO_2$ <35 mm Hg, and an elevated pH >7.45 indicate respiratory alkalosis. An increased $PaCO_2$ >45 mm Hg and a decreased pH <7.35 indicate respiratory acidosis. The latter acid–base imbalance is the result of many respiratory problems (i.e., chronic obstructive lung disease, pneumonia, drug-induced respiratory depression).

Culture (Sputum): Sputum specimens are useful for diagnosing microorganisms causing respiratory infection and for detecting malignant cells in lung tissue. Table 3 explains three studies conducted on sputum that are associated with respiratory problems.

α-1-Antitrypsin (Serum): *Norms:* Adult: 78–200 mg/dl; 0.78–2.0 g/l. Child: same as adult.

TABLE 3 USES OF SPUTUM CULTURE

Sputum Test	Comments
Culture and sensitivity (C&S)	Sputum specimens are useful for diagnosing microorganisms causing respiratory infection and the appropriate antimicrobial sensitive to the pathogens.
Acid-fast bacilli (AFB)	When tuberculosis is suspected, sputum specimens are checked (over 3 days) to determine the presence of *Mycobacterium tuberculosis*.
Cytology	Cytologic examination of slough cells from the lung are checked. If malignant cells are *not* present, this means lung cancer is unlikely. However, the malignancy may be in its early stage and not shedding cancer cells.

Antitrypsin inhibits proteolytic enzymes in destroying lung tissue. With a lack of this protein, the alveoli are damaged, resulting in chronic obstructive lung disease (e.g., emphysema). A nonsmoker with a decreased antitrypsin level could develop pulmonary emphysema.

Angiotensin-Converting Enzyme (ACE) Serum: *Normal:* 11–67 U/l.

ACE is found primarily in the lung epithelial cells and renal cells. ACE is elevated in pulmonary conditions such as pulmonary embolism, pulmonary fibrosis, tuberculosis, and sarcoidosis.

Therapeutic Drug Monitoring; Theophylline: *Serum Theophylline: Therapeutic Range:* Adult: 5–20 μg/ml; 28–112 μmol/l (SI units). *Toxic Level:* Adult: >20 μg/ml; >112 μmol/l (SI units). Child: same as adult.

Clients with bronchoconstriction (e.g., asthma) are usually given one of the theophylline preparations (i.e., aminophylline, Theo-dur, Slo-phyllin). Serum theophylline levels should be closely monitored to maintain therapeutic levels and to avoid toxic levels.

Skin Tests: Skin tests are useful for determining the presence of suspected bacterial or mycotic organisms that can infect lung tissue. This test is one of the methods used to diagnose tuberculosis and histoplasmosis.

Diagnostic Tests

Chest X-Ray: Chest x-ray is a frequently ordered diagnostic test. It is useful in diagnosing pneumonia, neoplasms (malignant and benign tumors), lung abscess, tuberculosis, atelectasis, and pneumothorax.

Pulmonary Function Studies: These tests are routinely ordered for clients with respiratory disorders or for those suspected of having a respiratory problem. Pulmonary function studies are helpful for assessing the progression of lung disease and for evaluating the response to drug and rehabilitative therapies.

Tomography, Laminography, Planigraphy: Tomography is used to detect lung tumors and mediastinal lesions. The x-ray machine or tube and film moves around

the client. Because it emits high radiation levels, this test is not used as a routine screening test to diagnose lung disorders.

Thoracic Computed Tomography (CT): CT scanning is useful for detecting questionable chest masses—lesions and tumors. It identifies metastasis in the lung. Contrast media (dye) may or may not be used.

Bronchoscopy: Either a standard metal or flexible fiberoptic bronchoscope is inserted into the tracheobronchial tree to visualize the larynx, trachea, and bronchi for abnormalities (i.e., strictures, inflammation, tumors). Also bronchial secretions may be aspirated for bacteriologic, cytologic, and histologic examination. To remove a foreign object or to excise a small lesion or growth, a large metal bronchoscope would be necessary. Complications as a result of the test procedure might be bleeding, infection, and pneumothorax.

Bronchography: A bronchography may be done in conjunction with bronchoscopy. Contrast media (radiopaque iodine dye) is injected through a catheter into the tracheobronchial tree, followed by x-rays. This test is not frequently performed because of newer, more effective diagnostic tests (e.g., CT scan). However, the purposes for the test are to detect bronchial obstruction, tumors, cysts, and bleeding sites.

Mediastinoscopy: The mediastinoscope is inserted through a small incision at the suprasternal notch for the purposes of examining mediastinal lymph nodes and of obtaining biopsy specimen(s). This test is frequently indicated when other diagnostic tests (i.e., chest x-ray, sputum cytology, bronchoscopy) fail to confirm a diagnosis. It is also useful to determine if the lung cancer is inoperable because of metastatic spread to the lymph nodes. Other uses of this test include detecting lymphoma (e.g., Hodgkin's disease and sarcoidosis).

Radionuclide Thoracic Imaging (Scan): *Lung Scan:* Radionuclide imaging is useful for evaluating pulmonary blood perfusion and for diagnosing perfusion obstruction (e.g., pulmonary embolism). A radionuclide, such as technetium tagged with macroaggregated albumin or technetium tagged with human albumin microspheres, is injected into the client's peripheral vein. *Ventilation Scan:* When the perfusion problem is due to an airway obstruction causing decreased ventilation, a ventilation scanning may be ordered. The client inhales radioactive gas, such as xenon. A nuclear scanner checks the distribution of the gas in the lungs at intervals.

Pulmonary Angiography/Arteriography: Contrast medium (radiopaque dye) is injected into the pulmonary arteries to detect vascular abnormalities (e.g., pulmonary embolus). Usually pulmonary angiography/arteriography is performed when other diagnostic tests fail to confirm a diagnosis.

Lung Biopsy: Biopsy specimens from the tracheobronchial tree and lymph nodes are usually obtained during bronchoscopy (if ordered) and mediastinoscopy. A transbronchial lung biopsy may be obtained through the use of a bronchoscope by wedging a small biopsy forcep into the lung tissue.

Thoracentesis; Pleural Fluid Aspiration: This test is used to remove fluid from the pleural cavity and to examine the fluid for the cause of pleural effusion.

Thoracoscopy: This endoscopic test is a tube that is inserted into the thoracic cavity to visualize the pleural space, thoracic wall, pericardium, and the mediastinum and to also obtain a biopsy or fluid sample as ordered. It can detect pleural and lung tumors, emphysema, and empyema.

Magnetic Resonance Imaging (MRI): MRI helps to supplement CT examination of the chest in lung cancer. It can evaluate recurrent or residual lung masses.

Pulmonary Function Tests (PFTs): Various pulmonary studies evaluate pulmonary function. These include slow vital capacity groups, lung-volume groups, forced vital capacity, diffusion study, bronchodilator response studies, exercise studies, and nutritional studies.

Sinus Endoscopy: Sinus endoscopy examines the anterior ethmoids and the middle meatus sinus areas. The primary purposes are to correct structural abnormalities and alleviate an infectious process.

NURSING DIAGNOSES

- Anxiety related to breathlessness.
- Deficient knowledge related to lack of understanding of laboratory and diagnostic procedures, disease process, and/or outcome.
- Noncompliance to prescribed laboratory and diagnostic tests related to lack of adequate explanation.
- Activity intolerance related to breathlessness and/or fatigue.
- Impaired gas exchange related to obstructive lung disease (e.g., chronic obstructive lung disease).
- Impaired verbal communication related to dyspnea.
- Risk for infection related to excessive, tenacious, mucous secretions.
- Disturbed sleep pattern related to dyspnea secondary to chronic lung disease.
- Risk for injury related to allergic reactions to contrast medium (dye) secondary to diagnostic test (i.e., bronchography, radionuclide scan, pulmonary angiography).
- Situational low self-esteem related to dependence and/or role change.

NURSING IMPLICATIONS WITH RATIONALE

- Explain the purpose of the laboratory and diagnostic tests.
- Give detailed explanation concerning the test procedures and the need for client's compliance. Explanation may be brief or in-depth, depending upon the client's familiarity with the test.
- Inform the client of any food, beverage, or drug restrictions (see Parts I and II).
- Elicit from the client or family member a history of any allergies, especially to contrast medium (dye), iodine, or seafood.
- Assess respiratory status in regard to breathlessness and dyspnea caused by acute and chronic lung diseases.

- Be supportive of the client with dyspnea during the procedure. Remain with the client and provide adequate time; this reduces anxiety and increases test compliance.
- Assist the client with breathing difficulty as needed.
- Check bleeding sites at incisional areas (e.g., mediastinoscopy test).
- Monitor vital signs before, during, and following invasive tests (i.e., bronchoscopy, pulmonary angiography).
- Listen to the client's expressed anxiety or fear concerning the tests and potential clinical problems. Clarification of the test procedure might alleviate fear and anxiety and promote compliance.

Evaluation

- Determine if the test was correctly performed according to the procedure. Notify the laboratory and health care provider of any changes that occur during the test.
- Check the client's vital signs for changes.
- Evaluate the client's activity in regard to breathlessness.
- Determine if support measures to client and family have been effective.
- Clarify or answer any questions the client and family members might have.
- Encourage the client to use resources for information and support, such as the American Lung Association.
- Reinforce the importance of seeking health care assistance whenever changes in health status occur.

Renal function

Laboratory Tests	Diagnostic Tests
Urinalysis	Kidney, Ureter, Bladder (KUB) x-ray
BUN	IVP
BUN/Creatinine Ratio (Serum)	Retrograde Pyelography
Creatinine (Serum)	Cystoscopy
Inulin Clearance	Cystography
Protein (24-Hour Urine)	Cystometry
Electrolytes (Serum & Urine)	Computed Tomography
Osmolality (Serum & Urine)	Nephrotomography
Antidiuretic Hormone (Plasma)	Renal Ultrasound
Complement C_3 (Serum)	Radionuclide Renal Scan
Complement C_4 (Serum)	Renal Angiography
Aldosterone (Serum)	Renal Biopsy
Renin (Plasma)	
Urine Culture	
Antiglomerular Basement Membrane Antibody (Serum)	
Uric Acid (Serum and Urine)	

Introduction

The first set of laboratory tests performed to determine renal function are urinalysis, blood urea nitrogen (BUN), and serum creatinine. These tests are ordered routinely when renal insufficiency is suspected. If any of these are abnormal, other laboratory and diagnostic tests would be necessary (i.e., creatinine clearance, inulin clearance, serum and urine osmolality, serum and urine electrolytes, intravenous pyelography [IVP], kidney, ureter, bladder [KUB] x-ray, renal ultrasound, renal computed tomography [CT] scan, and others).

Laboratory Tests

Urinalysis: A urinalysis is routinely performed in a variety of settings (hospitals, clinics, and health care provider's office) for checking kidney and endocrine function. The components it measures are color, pH, specific gravity (SG), protein, glucose, and blood cells. Table 4 shows the components that are usually checked during urinalysis and their significant results. For more comprehensive data on urinalysis, *see Part I*.

TABLE 4   URINALYSIS

Components	Results
Color	Color can indicate lack of body fluids (dark yellow), excess of body fluids (pale yellow), or the result of blood, drugs, and food (red, red-brown).
pH	Urine pH is usually 4.5–8. The urine would be acidic if pH is 4.5 and alkalotic if pH is >7.5. Bacteria multiply rapidly in alkalotic urine.
Specific gravity (SG)	A low SG is related to diluted urine, and a high SG is associated with concentrated urine.
Protein	Urine protein >8 mg/dl could indicate renal disorder. However, an athlete's urine protein (single sample) level might be 10–20 mg/dl. This could be normal after strenuous activity.
Glucose	Glycosuria could indicate diabetes mellitus. Normally glucose is not a measurable quantity in urine.
Blood cells (BCs)	Urine should not contain BCs. The presence of BCs in urine could indicate a renal disorder.

Blood Urea Nitrogen (BUN): *Norms:* 5–25 mg/dl. Child: 5–20 mg/dl.

Urea is a by-product of protein metabolism excreted by the kidneys. If the BUN is slightly elevated, 25 to 35 mg/dl, the cause could be dehydration caused by hemoconcentration. Elevated BUN that remains elevated after hydration is an indicator of renal disorder.

BUN/Creatinine Ratio (Serum): 10:1 to 20:1.

The BUN/creatinine ratio is useful for determining renal function. An increased ratio could be due to reduced renal perfusion, glomerular disease, or obstructive uropathy.

Creatinine (Serum): *Norms:*

Adult	Infant	2–6 Years	Older Child
0.5–1.5 mg/dl 45–132.5 μmol/l (SI units)	0.7–1.7 mg/dl	0.3–0.6 mg/dl	0.4–1.2 mg/dl 36–106 μmol/l (SI units)

Creatinine, a by-product of muscle creatinine phosphate, is excreted entirely by the kidneys. Serum creatinine is a more reliable test to determine renal function, because it is less affected, if at all, by dehydration or malnutrition than BUN. After renal damage or insult, the serum creatinine would rise because the kidneys could not excrete this by-product. Monitoring serum creatinine is important for determining kidney function.

Creatinine Clearance: *Norms:*

Person	Creatinine Clearance	Urine Creatinine
Adult:		
Male	85–135 ml/min	20–26 mg/kg/24 h 0.18–0.23 mmol/kg/24 h
Female	somewhat lower values	14–22 mg/kg/24 h 0.12–0.19 mmol/kg/24 h
Child:		
Male	98–150 ml/min	
Female	95–123 ml/min	

The creatinine clearance test (12- or 24-hour) is performed to determine glomerular filtration rate (GFR) and renal insufficiency. Usually this test includes serum creatinine level on the morning of or at the beginning of the test. Serum and urine creatinine levels are assessed, and creatinine clearance rate is calculated (*see Part I*). If <40 ml/min, the test is suggestive of moderate to severe renal impairment.

Inulin Clearance: *Norms:* Male: 125 ml/min/1.73 m^2, 124 ± 15 ml/min. Female: 110 ml/min/1.73 m^2, 110 ± 15 ml/min.

Inulin, a small, inert sugar that is not bound to protein, is freely filtered by the glomeruli and can be used to determine GFR. This is not a routine clinical test because it involves an initial IV injection of inulin and a continuous controlled infusion rate to achieve a constant plasma level. It is a reliable test for GFR and is often compared with other urine clearance procedures. Decreased levels are indicative of renal impairment.

Protein (24-hour Urine): *Norms:* 25–150 mg/24 h. Random: 0–5 mg/dl.

If urinalysis report indicated proteinuria, a 24-hour protein-urine test might be ordered. The presence of protein in the urine, >150 mg/24 h, could indicate glomeruli damage or disease.

Electrolytes (Serum and Urine): Both serum electrolytes and urine electrolytes are closely monitored in renal disorders. Table 5 explains the effects of serum and urine potassium and sodium as they relate to renal dysfunction.

TABLE 5 SERUM AND URINE ELECTROLYTES

Electrolytes	Reference Values	Cause and Effect
SERUM		
Potassium (K)	*Norms:* Adults: 3.5–5.3 mEq/l Child: 3.5–5.5 mEq/l Infant: 3.6–5.8 mEq/l	Primary cause of hyperkalemia; >5.5 mEq/l is renal insufficiency.
Sodium (Na)	*Norms:* Adult, child: 135–145 mEq/l Infant: 134–150 mEq/l	Hypernatremia, >145 mEq/l, might be caused by anuria due to acute renal failure. Hyponatremia, <135 mEq/l, might result from tubular disorders when there is an inability to reabsorb sodium.
URINE		
Potassium (K)	*Norms:* Adult: 25–120 mEq/24 h 25–120 mmol/24h (SI units)	Decreased urine potassium level <25 mEq/24 h, with an increased serum potassium level, could be indicative of acute renal failure. Elevated urine potassium level could be due to chronic renal failure. *Note:* Urine potassium range depends on the amount of potassium consumed in the diet.
Sodium (Na)	*Norms:* Adult: 40–220 mEq/24 h 40–220 mmol/24 h (SI units)	A low urine sodium level occurring with oliguria could be due to acute renal failure from decreased perfusion of the kidneys. An increased urine sodium level could result from the inability of the kidney tubules to reabsorb sodium (i.e., polycystic disease, chronic pyelonephritis).

Osmolality (Serum): *Norms:* Adult: 280–300 mOsm/kg. Child: 270–290 mOsm/kg. Serum and urine osmolality are used in assessing distal tubular response to circulating antidiuretic hormone (ADH). An increased serum osmolality could be due to an inadequate ADH release or due to the distal renal tubules' inadequate response to circulating ADH.

Osmolality (Urine): *Norms:* Adult: 50–1200 mOsm/kg (average 200–800 mOsm/kg). Child: same as adult. Newborn: 100–600 mOsm/kg.

Urine osmolality is a more accurate indicator of the kidneys' ability to concentrate and dilute urine than specific gravity. In advanced renal medullary disease, the urine osmolality could be decreased because of the inability of the kidneys to concentrate urine.

Antidiuretic Hormone (ADH) (Plasma): 1–5 pg/ml.

ADH, produced by the hypothalamus, and stored and secreted by the posterior pituitary gland, promotes water reabsorption from the distal renal tubules in response to the serum osmolality. With an increased serum osmolality (dehydration or hypovolemia), there is an increase in ADH secretion. More water is reabsorbed and conserved in the body.

Complement C_3 (Serum): *Norms:* Male: 80–180 mg/dl. Female: 76–120 mg/dl.

Complements contribute about 10% of the total plasma proteins and play an important role in the immunologic system. Serum C_3 (the most abundant complement) is decreased in certain renal conditions (i.e., glomerulonephritis and acute renal transplant rejection).

Complement C_4 (Serum): *Norms:* 15–45 mg/dl.

Serum C_4, the second most abundant component of the complement system, is significantly decreased in lupus nephritis and acute poststreptococcal glomerulonephritis.

Aldosterone (Serum): *Norms:* Adult: 1–9 ng/dl (supine position).

An increased serum aldosterone level can be associated with renal disease and chronic renal failure.

Renin (Plasma): *Norms:* Adult: 1.3–4.0 ng/ml (upright position, normal salt intake).

Renin, an enzyme secreted by the kidneys, is a test used for diagnosing renal vascular hypertension. The result of this hypertension could lead to renal failure.

Urine Culture: Urine cultures are commonly performed to determine the type of microorganism present in the genitourinary tract. To avoid urine contamination, the urine should be obtained using the procedure for midstream specimen collection or by catheterization.

Antiglomerular Basement Membrane Antibody (AGBM): This test detects GBM antibodies that can damage the glomerular basement membrane in the glomeruli. Beta-hemolytic streptococcus is the major organism responsible for antibody response.

Uric Acid (Serum): *Serum:* Male: 3.5–8.0 mg/dl. Female: 2.6–6.8 mg/dl. *Urine:* 250–500 mg/24 h (normal diet).

Serum and urine uric acid level is dependent upon renal function. Elevated serum uric acid can be attributed to renal disease such as glomerulonephritis and renal failure. A decreased urine uric acid is associated with renal disease.

Diagnostic Tests

Kidney, Ureter, Bladder (KUB) X-Ray: The KUB x-ray is a flat plate of the lower abdomen to identify the size, shape, and position of the kidneys, ureters, and bladder. If abnormalities (i.e., tumors, calculi, or malformations) are noted, more extensive diagnostic tests are performed. Usually the x-ray is taken while the client is in the supine position; however, an upright KUB film may be requested for better visualization of the area.

Intravenous Pyelography (IVP): During IVP, radiopaque contrast medium (dye) is injected intravenously. A series of x-rays is taken at specified times as the dye circulates and is collected by the renal glomeruli and passed throughout the urinary tract. The purpose is to visualize the kidneys, kidney pelvis, ureters, and bladder. This test is useful for determining kidney dysfunction and for locating renal tumors and calculi. A test dose of the dye is given first because some clients may be allergic to the dye.

Retrograde Pyelography: During the retrograde pyelography (pyelogram) test, contrast medium (dye) is injected through a ureteral catheter to visualize the ureters and kidneys. X-rays are taken. This test is usually done during cystoscopy to determine the cause of unilateral kidney disease (e.g., ureteral obstruction). The retrograde pyelogram gives better visualization of the ureter and problems than the IVP test.

Cystoscopy: A cystoscope, lighted, telescopic tube, is transurethrally inserted into the bladder for numerous purposes, including the following: to visualize the bladder wall; to obtain tissue biopsy of the bladder, urethra, or prostate; to remove calculi from the bladder or urethra; to remove small lesions and/or growths; or to obtain a urine specimen directly from the kidney(s). If ureter examination is necessary, dye is injected through an ureteral catheter into the ureters and x-rays are taken (retrograde pyelogram).

Cystography: The bladder is instilled with contrast medium (dye) to detect a rupture in the bladder, a neurogenic bladder, fistulas, or tumors. X-rays are taken. The client voids, if able, or the dye is withdrawn through the catheter.

Cystometry: This test evaluates the neuromuscular function of the bladder. Bladder dysfunction can be caused by neurologic disorders such as spinal cord injury, stroke, multiple sclerosis, diabetes mellitus.

Computed Tomography (CT) Scan: CT, also known as computerized axial tomography (CAT), provides an image of the kidneys for the purpose of identifying tumors, malformations, cysts, and calculi. Contrast medium (dye) might be used during the CT scan to enhance visualization of the kidneys. Usually renal CT scan is done after abnormal IVP results have been reported.

Nephrotomography: The nephrotomography test combines IVP and CT. It provides a clearer picture of the kidneys, identifying and differentiating between cysts and solid tumors.

Renal Ultrasound, Ultrasonography: Renal ultrasonography (considered a noninvasive test) passes high-frequency sound waves through a transducer to the kidneys and perirenal area. An image of the kidneys and surrounding structures is displayed on an oscilloscope screen. The purpose of this test is to detect abnormalities (i.e., masses [cyst, tumor]) or to clarify findings from other tests.

Radionuclide Renal Scan: A radionuclide, such as technetium compounds (Tc-99m), Tc-99m–pertechnetate, Tc-99m–diethylenetriamine-penta-acetic acid (Tc-99m–DTPA), and iodine-131 hippuran, is administered intravenously. The purpose of the test is to detect renal lesions or masses and to determine the presence of acute or chronic renal diseases. This test may be used instead of IVP for clients who are allergic to contrast medium (dye).

Renal Angiography: A contrast medium (dye) is injected into the renal artery to visualize renal arterial, capillary, and venous systems. Rapid-sequence x-ray filming detects renal vascular malformations (e.g., stenosis, nonfunctioning kidney, renal masses, and obstructive uropathy).

Renal Biopsy: Microscopic examination of kidney tissue provides data concerning renal disease (e.g., glomerulonephritis caused by streptococcal infection or lupus). The renal biopsy test is useful for diagnosing primary or metastatic cancer of the kidney. Complications that could result are hematuria, uncontrolled bleeding, and kidney damage.

NURSING DIAGNOSES

- Knowledge deficit related to lack of understanding of the laboratory and diagnostic procedures, disease process, and/or outcome.
- Noncompliance with prescribed laboratory and diagnostic tests related to lack of or inadequate explanation.
- Impaired urinary elimination related to decreased urine output secondary to urinary tract obstruction, renal lesions or masses, acute or chronic renal failure.
- Ineffective tissue perfusion, renal, related to renal vascular obstruction, drug toxicity, or tumors.
- Excess fluid volume related to sodium and fluid retention secondary to renal damage or insufficiency.
- Fear related to kidney status, the unknown, and/or dependence on others.
- Risk for impaired skin integrity related to peripheral edema secondary to renal failure.
- Risk for injury related to allergic reactions to contrast medium (dye) secondary to diagnostic test (e.g., IVP).
- Situational low self-esteem related to dependence and/or role change.

NURSING IMPLICATIONS WITH RATIONALE

- Explain the purpose of the laboratory and diagnostic tests.
- Give a detailed explanation of the test procedures and the need for the client's compliance. Explanation might be brief or in-depth, depending upon the client's familiarity with the test.
- Inform the client of any food, beverage, or drug restriction *(see Parts I and II)*.
- Collect specimen(s) at specific times according to the procedures.
- Elicit from the client a history of any allergies, especially to contrast medium (dye) or iodine.
- Assess renal function (i.e., changes in urinary output, abnormal laboratory results—elevated BUN and serum creatinine, hematuria).
- Monitor the client's intake and output and vital signs before and after laboratory and diagnostic tests.
- Listen to the client's expressed anxiety or fear about the tests and potential clinical problems. Clarification of test procedure might alleviate fear and anxiety and promote compliance.

Evaluation

- Determine if the test was correctly performed according to the procedure. Notify the laboratory or health care provider of any changes that occur during the test.
- Check the client's urinary output and vital signs for changes: improvement or deterioration.
- Determine if the client's fear and/or anxiety has been lessened or alleviated.
- Clarify or answer any additional questions client might have.
- Encourage the client to use resources available (e.g., National Kidney Foundation).
- Encourage the client and family members to participate in the decision-making process concerning the patient's long-term needs.

Liver, gallbladder, and pancreatic function

Laboratory Tests	Diagnostic Tests
Liver	
Bilirubin (Serum)	X-ray of Abdomen
Bilirubin (Urine)	Ultrasonography of Liver
Urobilinogen (Urine)	Liver and Spleen Scan
Liver Enzyme Tests	CT, Liver
ALP and Isoenzyme (Serum)	Liver Biopsy
5' N (Serum)	Hepatic Angiography

Laboratory Tests	Diagnostic Tests
ALT SGPT (Serum)	
LDH and Isoenzymes (Serum)	
GGT/GGTP (Serum)	
Protein (Serum)	
Protein Electrophoresis	
Ammonia (Plasma, Blood)	
Antimitochondial Antibody (AMA) (Serum)	
Antismooth Muscle Antibody (Serum)	
PT (Plasma)	
Cholesterol (Serum)	
Hepatitis A Virus (Serum)	
HB_sAg (Serum)	
HB_sAb/anti-HB_s (Serum)	
HB_cAb/anti-HB_c (Serum)	
	Gallbladder
	X-ray of Abdomen
	Cholecystography (Oral)
	Cholangiography
	Intravenous
	Percutaneous
	T tube
	ERCP
	Ultrasonography of
	Gallbladder and Biliary System
	Gallbladder Nuclear Study
	HIDA Scan
	CT: Gallbladder and Biliary System
Pancreas	
Amylase (Serum) & P-type isoenzyme	ERCP
Amylase (Urine)	Ultrasonography of Pancreas
Lipase (Serum)	Hypotonic Duodenography
Secretin Test	CT, Pancreas
	Pancreatic Ultrasonography

Introduction

Because the liver, gallbladder, and pancreas are in close proximity, several diagnostic tests (i.e., computed tomography [CT]; ultrasound of the liver, gallbladder, and pancreas; and endoscopic retrograde cholangiopancreatography [ERCP]) are performed on two or three of these organs at the same time. However, assessment of these organs will be represented separately.

Liver Assessment

Laboratory Tests

Bilirubin (Serum): *Norms:*

Person	Indirect Unconjugated	Direct Conjugated	Total
Adult	0.1–1.0 mg/dl 1.7–17.1 μmol/l (SI units)	0.1–0.3 mg/dl 1.7–5.1 μmol/l (SI units)	0.1–1.2 mg/dl 1.7–20.5 μmol/l (SI units)
Child >6 months	Same as adult	Same as adult	0.2–0.8 mg/dl
Newborn			1–12 mg/dl

Bilirubin is derived from hemoglobin and results from the breakdown of red blood cells (RBCs). There are two forms of bilirubin in the body: indirect or unconjugated, and direct or conjugated.

Indirect or Unconjugated: Elevated indirect bilirubin is related to increased destruction of RBCs.

Erythroblastosis fetalis in newborns results from massive hemolysis of RBCs, resulting in a possible serum indirect bilirubin level of 20 mg/dl or greater. Other causes include sickle cell anemia, drug toxicity, transfusion reaction caused by blood incompatibility, and autoimmune diseases.

Direct or Conjugated: Bilirubin is conjugated (transformed) by the liver and made water soluble. There are smaller amounts of conjugated bilirubin than unconjugated bilirubin in the blood. Only water-soluble bilirubin (conjugated) can be excreted in the urine. Only water-soluble bilirubin (conjugated) can be excreted in the urine. Causes of an increase in direct bilirubin are cirrhosis, biliary obstruction, infectious hepatitis, carcinoma of the pancreas, and drugs (i.e., oral contraceptives, sulfonamides, rifampin, aspirin, morphine, thiazides, and procainamide).

Bilirubin (Urine): *Norms:* Negative to 0.02 mg/dl.

Unconjugated bilirubin (fat soluble) cannot be excreted in the urine because it is not water soluble. If urine bilirubin test is positive, then conditions causing conjugated hyperbilirubinemia are likely to be the cause.

Urobilinogen (Urine): *Norms:* Adult: Random: 0.3–3.5 mg/dl. 24-hour specimen: 0.05–2.5 mg/24 h. 0.09–4.23 μmol/24 h (SI units).

Conjugated bilirubin from bile is changed in the duodenum to urobilinogen. Decreased urobilinogen level might indicate severe liver damage, biliary obstruction, and/or severe inflammatory disease. Elevated levels may be indicative of hemolytic disease, early cirrhosis of the liver, toxic or infectious hepatitis.

Liver Enzyme Tests: As the result of liver damage by insult or disease, most of the liver enzymes are released into the blood stream, resulting in increased enzyme levels. Some of these enzymes are also found in other organs and are considered nonspecific. Examples of the nonspecific enzymes are alkaline phosphatase and lactic dehydrogenase. Usually several liver enzyme tests are performed at the same time to confirm liver disorder. Table 6 compares the enzyme studies that are usually

660

TABLE 6 LIVER ENZYME TESTS

Enzyme (Serum)	Reference Values	Comments
Alkaline phosphatase (ALP) and isoenzyme	*Norms:* Adult: 42–136 U/l ALP$_1$ 20–130 U/l Child: 40–115 U/l Older Child: 50–230 U/l	ALP is found mainly in bone and liver and also in intestine, kidney, and placenta. Because ALP is produced by several systems and cells in the body, its activity is classified as nonspecific; therefore other liver function tests should be performed to confirm the diagnosis. In severe liver damage (i.e., cancer of liver, hepatocellular problems) serum ALP is greatly increased. ALP isoenzymes assist in identifying the origin of the problem. ALP$_1$ is of liver origin, and ALP$_2$ is of bone origin.
5'Nucleotidase (5'NT or 5'N)	*Norms:* <17 U/l	5'NT is specific to liver cells. ALP and 5'NT are measured at the same time, because both enzymes are found in liver cells and are elevated in hepatocellular disease. However, serum ALP will be elevated in bone disease, but 5'NT will *not* be increased.
Leucine aminopeptidase (LAP)	*Norms:* 8–22 mU/ml, 12–33 IU/l, 75–200 U/ml, 20–50 U/l at 37°C (SI units)	LAP enzyme is found mainly in liver tissue. Serum LAP is elevated in liver disease (i.e., cancer of the liver, viral hepatitis, acute necrosis of the liver, and extrahepatic biliary obstruction). LAP, 5'NT, and ALP tests are frequently ordered together to confirm liver disease. If only ALP is elevated and the other two enzymes are not, bone disease would be probable.
Alanine aminotransferase (ALT or SGPT)	*Norms:* Adult: 10–35 U/l 4–36 U/l at 37°C (SI units)	ALT/SGPT is found primarily in liver cells and is effective in diagnosing hepatocellular obstruction. AST/SGOT is found in liver cells; however, it is more specific to cardiac muscle and skeletal muscle. Serum ALT is slightly to moderately increased in cancer of the liver and cirrhosis. It is highly increased during viral hepatitis and drug hepatotoxicity.

(*continued*)

TABLE 6 LIVER ENZYME TESTS (continued)

Enzyme (Serum)	Reference Values	Comments
Lactic Dehydrogenase (LD/IDH) Isoenzymes	*Norms:* Adult: 100–190 IU/l Isoenzyme LDH_5 6%–16% Child: 50–150 IU/l, 110–295 U/l	LDH is elevated in heart, lung, liver, and renal disease. To determine if the increased LDH is due to liver disease, LDH isoenzymes are measured. LDH_5 rises before jaundice occurs and falls before bilirubin level does.
Gamma-glutamyl transferase/ transpeptidase (GGT/GGTP)	*Norms:* Adult: Male: 4–23 IU/l Female: 3–13 IU/l Average: 0–45 U/l	GGT/GGTP is found mostly in the liver and kidney and small amounts in heart muscle, spleen, and prostate gland. It is a more sensitive indicator for liver disease than other liver enzymes (i.e., ALP and AST/SGOT). Elevated GGT/GGTP occurs in cirrhosis of the liver, alcoholism, cancer of the liver, viral hepatitis, and acute pancreatitis.

ordered to evaluate suspected liver diseases: alkaline phosphatase (ALP), alanine aminotransferase (ALT or SGPT), 5' nucleotidase (5'NT), leucine aminopeptidase (LAP), LDH_5, and gamma-glutamyl transferase (GGT).

Protein (Serum), Protein Electrophoresis: *Norms:* Adult: Total protein: 6–8 g/dl. Albumin: 3.5–5.0 g/dl. Globulin: 1.5–3.5 g/dl.

Serum protein is an indirect measure of albumin and globulin. Albumin and globulin are indicators of liver function and diseases. Protein electrophoresis gives the breakdown of albumin and globulin. The albumin level is decreased, and the gamma globulin level is elevated in cirrhosis of the liver. The α_2-globulin fraction is elevated in inflammatory disease of the liver and cancer of the liver. An elevated β-globulin might occur in biliary obstruction. In chronic liver disease the A/G ratio is reversed.

Ammonia (Plasma, Blood): *Norms:* Adult (depends on method used): 15–45 μg/dl, 3.2–4.5 g/dl, or 32–45 g/l; 11–35 μmol/l (SI units). Child: 21–50 μg/dl. Newborn: 64–107 μg/dl.

Ammonia, a by-product of protein metabolism, is converted to urea by the liver. Ammonia levels are elevated in severe liver diseases (i.e., cirrhosis, acute hepatic necrosis, or when blood flow to the liver is altered).

Antimitochondrial Antibody (AMA) Serum: Negative at 1:5 dilution.

This test may be ordered to differentiate between persons having primary biliary cirrhosis and other liver disease.

Antismooth Muscle Antibody (ASTHMA) (Serum): Negative or <1:20; Positive: >1.20.

ASTHMA is associated primarily with autoimmune chronic active hepatitis (CAH). The titer is usually > 1:160 with CAH. Clients with primary biliary cirrhosis may have a slight titer elevation.

Prothrombin Time (PT) (Plasma): *Norms:* Adult: 11–15 seconds or 70–100%. PT levels might differ in institutions.

Prothrombin, factor II of the coagulation factors, is produced by the liver and requires vitamin K for its synthesis. Increase in PT time frequently occurs in liver disease.

Cholesterol (Serum): *Norms:* Adult: 150–240 mg/dl, <200 mg/dl (desired level); 3.90–6.50 mmol/l (SI units). Child: 130–185 mg/dl. Infant: 90–130 mg/dl.

Cholesterol is a blood lipid that is synthesized in the liver. In chronic liver disease, serum cholesterol could be decreased. In biliary obstruction and pancreatitis, serum levels could be increased.

Hepatitis A Virus (HAV) Serum: None detected.

Previously HAV was called "infectious hepatitis." It is usually transmitted by oral–fecal contact.

Hepatitis B Surface Antigen (HB$_S$Ag) (Serum): *Norms:* Negative.

A positive HB$_S$AG is an indicator of acute hepatitis B, chronic active hepatitis, or a carrier of hepatitis B.

Hepatitis B Surface Antibody (HB$_S$Ab/anti-HB$_S$): *Norms:* Negative.

A positive HB$_S$Ab test indicates a *previous* infection of hepatitis B virus. Years after an acute hepatitis B infection, the HB$_S$Ab test might still be positive.

Hepatitis B Core Antibody (HB$_C$Ab/anti-HB$_C$) (Serum): *Norms:* Negative.

This test is performed following negative serum HB$_S$Ag and HB$_S$Ab results when hepatitis is suspected. A positive Hb$_C$Ab might indicate a recent hepatitis B infection.

Diagnostic Tests

X-ray of Abdomen: A flat plate x-ray of the abdomen is used to detect abdominal masses in the liver, pancreas, stomach, and intestine. It could indicate small-bowel obstruction and ascites.

Ultrasonography, Ultrasound (Liver): This is a noninvasive procedure useful in locating cysts, abscesses, and tumors. Liver ultrasound can differentiate between obstructive and nonobstructive jaundice. It is useful with liver scanning to define the cold spots. This test is usually ordered for clients with jaundice of unknown cause and unexplained hepatomegaly.

Liver and Spleen Scan: In nuclear liver imaging, a radionuclide (e.g., technetium [Tc] compound [Tc-99m pertechnetate, Tc-99m sulfide]) is administered intravenously to determine the size and structure of the liver and to detect abnormalities. If the liver has less radionuclide uptake than the spleen, cirrhosis or chronic hepatitis could be suspected. If cold spots (areas that do not take up radionuclide) appear, cysts, abscesses, and tumors might be suspected. Follow-up diagnostic tests (i.e., ultrasound, CT scan, and/or biopsy) are needed to confirm diagnosis.

Computed Tomography (CT) (Liver): CT visualizes the liver and biliary tract with or without contrast medium. It can detect hepatic cysts, abscesses, tumors, and can differentiate between obstructive and nonobstructive jaundice. CT should be performed before or four days after barium studies. Ultrasound is cheaper than CT and can detect liver and biliary disorders equally well.

Percutaneous Liver Biopsy: Liver cells can be obtained for microscopic examination by needle biopsy. The needle is inserted through the skin to the liver. It is used to confirm diagnosis of hepatocellular diseases (i.e., cirrhosis, hepatitis, tumors). Liver biopsy should not be performed on clients with bleeding disorders or having obstructive jaundice caused by possible bile leakage.

Hepatic Angiography, Celiac and Mesenteric Arteriography: Hepatic angiography is used to evaluate cirrhosis and portal hypertension and to evaluate vascular damage after abdominal trauma.

Gallbladder Assessment

Diagnostic Tests

X-ray of Abdomen: Flat plate x-ray of the abdomen can visualize gallbladder stones. The stones that are not calcified and are composed of cholesterol will not be seen. Therefore contrast medium tests should be ordered.

Cholecystography (Oral), Gallbladder Series: Oral cholecystography is an x-ray test to visualize stones and to diagnose inflammatory disease and tumors of the gallbladder. The client ingests radiopaque iodinated dye tablets the night before. This test is concentrated in the gallbladder 12 to 14 hours after ingestion. This test should be performed before or 2 to 4 days after upper gastrointestinal tract and small-bowel series, because the barium would hamper visualization.

Cholangiography (Intravenous, Percutaneous, and T Tube or Postoperative): Cholangiography is an x-ray examination of the bile ducts using contrast medium either intravenously or percutaneously or through the T tube. Table 7 describes the cholangiography tests used for visualizing the biliary ducts.

Endoscopic Retrograde Cholangiopancreatography (ERCP): Through a fiberoptic endoscope, contrast medium (dye) is injected into the duodenal papilla to visualize the biliary tract for cause of obstructive jaundice. The use of ERCP has increased, since the development of the fiberoptic side-view endoscope. This test is used when other diagnostic tests fail to determine cause of jaundice (i.e., stones, tumors).

Ultrasonography, Ultrasound of the Gallbladder, and Biliary System: Ultrasound of the gallbladder and biliary tract is useful for diagnosing cholelithiasis and cholecystitis and to differentiate between obstructive and nonobstructive jaundice. It can detect polyps and tumors. Advantages for the use of ultrasound include the

TABLE 7 CHOLANGIOGRAPHY TESTS

Tests	Comments
IV cholangiography	With IV cholangiography, contrast medium (e.g., meglumine iodipamide) is injected intravenously. The dye is filtered by the liver and passes into the gallbladder and biliary ducts for visualization. There are more reported side effects with the use of IV contrast media than with oral tablets. This test is not indicated if hepatocellular disease is highly suspected or serum bilirubin is >3 mg/dl.
Percutaneous transhepatic cholangiography (PTHC)	A needle is passed through the skin to the liver and into a dilated bile duct. Contrast medium is injected. The purpose is to visualize the biliary tract and to determine the cause of obstructive jaundice.
T-tube or postoperative cholangiography	Dye is injected into the T tube, which was inserted during surgery. Purpose is to check for retained gallstones in the common bile duct.

fact that it is cheaper than CT scan with equal results, there is no risk of radiation, and no contrast media is used.

Gallbladder Nuclear Study: The use of cholecytokinin (CCK) may be used to promote emptying of the gallbladder. Low emptying values can suggest chronic cholecystitis.

HIDA Scan: Technetium 99m dimethyacetanilide iminodiacetic acid (Tc-99m HIDA) is injected intravenously to visualize the hepatobiliary system. It is useful in detecting biliary obstruction and also hepatocellular disease.

Computed Tomography of the Gallbladder and Biliary System: CT of the right upper quadrant includes the visualization of the liver, gallbladder, and biliary tract. It can detect stones in the gallbladder and biliary ducts. Although ultrasound is cheaper, CT is preferred for obese patients and for those who have livers high in the rib cage.

Pancreas Assessment

Laboratory and diagnostic tests for diabetes mellitus will be covered in the section on assessment of endocrine function.

Laboratory Tests

Amylase (Serum): *Norms:* Adult: 60–160 Somogyi U/dl, 30–170 U/l (SI units). Child: usually not done.

Amylase is a pancreatic enzyme that changes starch to sugar. In acute pancreatitis, serum amylase level is elevated in 2 to 12 hours after onset and remains elevated for 2 to 3 days. Levels are also increased in biliary duct obstruction, (e.g., gallstones). P-type isoenzyme is elevated with acute pancreatitis.

Amylase (Urine): *Norms:* Adult: 4–37 U/l/24 h.

When serum amylase is slightly to moderately elevated and pancreatitis is suspected, a 24-hour urine amylase level may be ordered. Urine amylase level is useful to confirm the diagnosis of acute pancreatitis.

Lipase (Serum): *Norms:* Adult: 20–180 IU/l, 114–286 U/l, 14–280 U/l (SI units). Child: 20–136 IU/l at 37°C.

Lipase is a pancreatic enzyme that aids in the digestion of fats in the duodenum. Serum lipase level is elevated early in acute pancreatitis and remains elevated longer than serum amylase level.

Secretin Test: This test assesses pancreatic exocrine function and is helpful in diagnosing pancreatic tumor, obstruction of the pancreatic duct, and chronic pancreatitis. It is a 3-hour test and requires a double-lumen tube; one lumen is inserted into the duodenum for aspiration of duodenal secretions and the other lumen into the stomach for aspiration of gastric secretions. Three samples are collected for baseline determination. Then secretin is administered intravenously and four more samples are collected.

Diagnostic Tests

Endoscopic Retrograde Cholangiopancreatography (ERCP): At the duodenal papilla, ERCP visualizes the biliary tract and the pancreatic duct. This test can detect pancreatic tumor and stricture of the pancreatic duct caused by chronic pancreatitis. A complication that might result from this procedure is pancreatitis.

Ultrasonography, Ultrasound of the Pancreas: Ultrasound is helpful in the detection of pancreatic abscess, cysts, and tumors. It could support the diagnosis of pancreatitis after serum amylase and lipase levels have returned to normal.

Hypotonic Duodenography: The purpose of this test is to detect pancreatic and duodenal diseases (i.e., tumor at the head of pancreas, stricture caused by chronic pancreatitis, and small duodenal lesion). A catheter is passed through the nose to the duodenum, and barium sulfate and air are injected. Spot x-ray films are taken.

Computed Tomography (CT) of the Pancreas: CT of the pancreas is useful to distinguish between pancreatic tumors and cysts and to detect suspected pancreatitis. The use of oral or IV contrast media during the test provides a more detailed visualization of the pancreas. Recent barium studies could hamper visualization of the pancreas.

Pancreatic Ultrasonography: Ultrasound of the pancreas does not measure pancreatic function, but it can detect pancreatic abnormalities, such as pancreatic tumors, pseudocysts, and pancreatitis.

NURSING DIAGNOSES

- Knowledge deficit related to lack of understanding of laboratory and diagnostic procedures, disease process, and/or outcome.
- Noncompliance to prescribed laboratory and diagnostic tests related to lack of or inadequate explanation and/or anxiety about physical condition.
- Altered nutrition: less than body requirements related to anorexia, reduced food intake, and/or impaired metabolism.
- Risk for injury related to bleeding tendencies secondary to decreased prothrombin production.
- Risk for injury related to allergic reactions to contrast medium (dye) secondary to diagnostic tests (i.e., CT with contrast medium, angiography).
- Excess fluid volume (peripheral and peritoneal) related to sodium and fluid retention and fluid volume shift secondary to liver disorders (e.g., cirrhosis).
- Impaired skin integrity related to peripheral edema.
- Risk for activity intolerance related to peripheral edema and ascites.
- Ineffective coping related to disease process and laboratory and diagnostic test procedures.
- Disturbed body image related to body changes (e.g., ascites).
- Interrupted family processes related to social problems from alcoholism.

NURSING IMPLICATIONS WITH RATIONALE

- Explain that the purpose of the laboratory and diagnostic tests is to aid in diagnosing liver, gallbladder, and pancreatic disorders. Be specific with the explanation as indicated.
- Give an explanation, in detail if indicated, about the laboratory and diagnostic procedures. Provide a written instruction sheet to reinforce verbal instructions. Emphasize the importance of the client's compliance to the test procedures. Stress that tests might need to be repeated if the procedure is improperly performed.
- Inform the client of any food, beverage, or drug restrictions. Each test should be checked for specific restrictions (see Parts I and II).
- Inform the health care provider if the client has had recent barium studies or if ultrasonography, CT, or ERCP is ordered. Barium sulfate can hinder visualization, and a 2- to 4-day waiting period after barium studies is usually required.
- Listen to the client's expressed anxiety concerning the tests and potential client problems. Clarification of test procedure might alleviate fear and anxiety and promote test compliance.
- Be prepared to repeat information to the client and family if the anxiety and/or fear level is determined to be high.
- Elicit from the client awareness or knowledge of any allergies to contrast medium (dye), iodine, or seafood.
- Monitor the client's vital signs before and following laboratory and diagnostic tests.

- Assess lower extremities and abdomen for signs of or changes in peripheral edema and/or ascites.
- Notify the health care provider if the client's serum bilirubin is >3 mg/dl prior to cholecystography or intravenous cholangiography. An elevated serum bilirubin can prevent contrast medium uptake and excretion.
- Check the laboratory results, and notify health care provider of abnormal test reports.
- Assess for bleeding from the nose, rectum, and skin. Liver disorders can cause prolonged prothrombin time resulting in bleeding tendencies.
- Check gag reflex for endoscopic procedures (e.g., ERCP, before giving fluids and food).

Evaluation

- Determine if the test was correctly performed according to the procedure. Notify laboratory and/or health care provider of any changes that occur during the test.
- Check the client's vital signs for changes, worsening and deterioration, or improvement.
- Check lower extremities and abdomen for a decrease in pitting edema and ascites.
- Provide ongoing assessment (before, during, and after procedure) of critical changes; document them; and report them to the health care provider.
- Clarify or answer any additional questions the client might have.
- Encourage the client to seek health care assistance whenever changes in health status occur.
- Encourage the client and family members to participate in the decision-making process concerning long-term plans.

Gastrointestinal function

Laboratory Tests	Diagnostic Tests
Upper GI	
Electrolytes (Serum)	Esophageal Studies
Gastrin (Serum)	Acid Perfusion (Bernstein Test)
Pepsinogen-I (Serum)	Esophageal Acidity
Prealbumin Antibody (Serum)	Esophageal Manometry
	Gastric Analysis Studies
	Basal Gastric Secretion
	Gastric Cytologic Examination
	Gastric Acid Stimulation

Laboratory Tests	Diagnostic Tests
	Esophagogastroduodenoscopy
	Esophagoscopy
	Gastroscopy
	Barium Swallow
	Fluoroscopy
	Cineradiography
	Upper GI Series and Small Bowel
	Celiac and Mesenteric Angiography/
	Arteriography
Lower GI	
CEA	X-ray of Abdomen
Carotene (Serum)	Barium Enema
Electrolytes (Serum)	Proctosigmoidoscopy
Antiparietal Cell Antibody	Proctoscopy
D-Xylose Absorption	Sigmoidoscopy
Lactose Intolerance	Biopsy
Galactose-1-Phosphate Uridyl Transferase (GPUT)	Colonoscopy
Fecal Analysis	Peritoneal Analysis/Paracentesis
Occult Blood	Gastric Emptying Nuclear Study
Fat Content	Gastrointestinal Bleeding
Ova and Parasites	Nuclear Test
Trypsin (Fecal) Norm: positive	
in small amounts	
Rotavirus Antigen (Feces)	

Introduction

There are numerous gastrointestinal (GI) tests performed for assessing GI disorders. When the problem is of the esophagus, stomach, or duodenum, a series of upper GI tests (i.e., gastric analysis, upper GI series, and/or esophagogastroduodenoscopy) might be performed. When the problem is of the colon, a series of lower GI tests (i.e., fecal analysis, barium enema, proctosigmoidoscopy, and/or colonoscopy) might be performed.

Endoscopy is a method using an endoscope, a metal or fiberoptic tube, for visualizing abnormalities of the GI tract. Many upper and lower GI tests are classified as endoscopic tests or procedures. Tests for GI disorders are classified as upper GI and lower GI.

Upper GI Assessment

Laboratory Tests

Electrolytes: Potassium, Sodium, Magnesium (Serum): *Norms:* Adult: Potassium: 3.5–5.3 mEq/l. Sodium: 135–145 mEq/l. Magnesium: 1.5–2.5 mEq/l. Child: *See individual tests.*

Electrolytes are plentiful in the GI tract. Continuous vomiting or gastric intubation can cause a loss of the cations (i.e., potassium [K], sodium [Na], and magnesium [Mg]). Electrolyte replacement through IV fluids is essential to restore electrolyte balance and to prevent life-threatening problems (e.g., cardiac dysrhythmias). Serum electrolyte levels should be monitored, and any changes, decreases, or elevations, should be reported immediately.

Gastrin (Serum): *Norms:* Adult: Fasting: <100 pg/ml. Nonfasting: 50–200 pg/ml.

Gastrin is a hormone secreted from the distal part of the stomach. This hormone stimulates the secretion of gastric juices, mainly hydrochloric acid (HCl). Serum gastrin levels are slightly to moderately elevated in clients having gastric ulcer or pernicious anemia and are highly elevated in clients with Zollinger-Ellison syndrome (pancreatic islet-cell tumor that secretes excess gastrin).

Pepsinogen-I (PG-I) Serum: *Normal:* 124–142 ng/ml.

Elevated pepsinogen-I is frequently present with duodenal ulcer. High PG-I level can be inherited as an autosomal dominant trait.

Prealbumin (PA) Antibody (Serum): 17–40 mg/dl.

This test is used primarily for nutritional assessment.

Diagnostic Tests

Esophageal Studies: One or more esophageal studies are usually performed for determining the cause of heartburn (pyrosis) and swallowing difficulty (dysphagia). Most of these tests check for the pH in the esophagus and esophageal sphincter pressure. Table 8 explains the purposes of three esophageal tests with abnormal results.

TABLE 8 ESOPHAGEAL STUDIES

Test	Reference Values	Results
Acid perfusion (Bernstein test)		Epigastric or retrosternal pain that radiates to the back or arms is usually associated with myocardial infarction; however, these symptoms could be due to juices from the stomach backflowing into the esophagus. This test is useful to determine if chest pain or epigastric discomfort is caused by a cardiac condition or by esophagitis. Normal saline and hydrochloric acid (HCl) are dripped at different times into the esophagus. If the client has pain during the HCl drip, the test is a positive for esophagitis.
Esophageal acidity	*Norms:* pH >5.0	This test measures the pH level of fluid in the lower esophagus. When clients complain of frequent heartburn, a pH electrode attached to a catheter is inserted through the mouth into the esophagus. If the intra-esophageal pH is 1.0–3.0, gastroesopha-

TABLE 8 ESOPHAGEAL STUDIES (continued)

Test	Reference Values	Results
Esophageal manometry	*Norms:* 15–25 mm Hg (lower esophageal sphincter [LES])	geal reflux (backflow of gastric acid into esophagus) caused by an incompetent sphincter is highly probable. Esophageal manometry measures esophageal sphincter and intraluminal pressures and records the sequence and duration of esophageal peristaltic contractions. When LES pressure is 0–5 mm Hg, incompetent or hypotensive sphincter is likely to be the cause; gastroesophageal reflux results. High LES pressure (>50 mm Hg) could indicate hypertensive sphincter caused by achalasia, esophageal diverticula, or tumor.

Gastric Analysis Studies: *Norms:* Basal (fasting): 1–5 mEq/h. Stimulation: 10–25 mEq/h.

Gastric analysis studies determine the quantity of gastric acid secreted between meals or feedings and during gastric acid stimulation. Stimulants used include histamine phosphate, betazole HCl (Histalog), pentagastrin, and caffeine. Table 9 describes the two tests performed for gastric analysis.

TABLE 9 GASTRIC ANALYSIS TESTS

Test	Reference Values	Result
Basal gastric secretion	Basal (fasting): 1–5 mEq/h	No fluid or food for 8–12 hours before the test. High gastric acid levels suggest peptic ulcer (gastric or duodenal), and very high levels could be indicative of Zollinger-Ellison syndrome. Low levels might suggest gastric carcinoma.
Gastric acid stimulation	Stimulation: 10–25 mEq/h	Usually this test follows the basal gastric test. A stimulant such as betazole HCl (Histalog) or pentagastrin is administered. After 15 minutes, four to eight 15-minute specimens are taken. High levels suggest duodenal ulcer and very high levels indicate Zollinger-Ellison syndrome. Low levels might suggest gastric carcinoma.

Gastric Cytologic Examination: Gastric aspiration for cytologic examination is obtained either during gastroscopy or after nasogastric catheter/tube insertion. If secretions aspirated through the tube are insufficient, then 100 ml of saline is instilled to facilitate specimen collection.

Esophagogastroduodenoscopy, Gastroscopy, Esophagoscopy: These endoscopic tests examine the esophagus, stomach, and duodenum to determine cause of epigastric or substernal pain and hematemesis. They are among the most effective methods in diagnosing GI disorders (i.e., peptic ulcer [gastric or duodenal], esophageal varices, tumors, inflammatory conditions, hiatal hernia, Mallory-Weiss syndrome), and for obtaining biopsy, foreign body, cells for cytology, or gastric acid secretions. Esophagogastroduodenoscopy should be done before or 2 days after an upper GI series, because the barium sulfate retention would inhibit visualization. This test is useful to confirm a diagnosis, especially when contrast radiography procedures (e.g., upper GI series) fail to detect the GI problem.

Gastroscopy: This test, part of the esophagogastroduodenoscopy, can detect gastric disorders. A metal gastroscope could be used instead of the fiberoptic endoscope.

Esophagoscopy: It is used to visualize only the esophagus.

Barium Swallow: This diagnostic procedure is ordered to assess the pharynx and the esophagus for abnormalities. Usually it is part of the upper GI series, although it could be a separate test. The client swallows a thick mixture of barium sulfate, and the cineradiographic examination of the pharynx and fluoroscopic examination of the esophagus is performed. Barium swallow is useful for detecting esophageal strictures, tumors, polyps, ulcers, hiatal hernia, diverticula, and motility disorders.

Fluoroscopy: This can be part of the upper GI series. It is x-ray viewing from the time barium sulfate or meglumine diatrizoate (Gastrografin) is ingested and passes from the esophagus to the stomach. Fluoroscopic viewing can also take place during the barium enema test as the contrast agent goes through the large bowel.

Cineradiography: This is a filming method used for detecting esophageal motility problems.

Upper GI Series: The upper GI series uses barium sulfate or meglumine diatrizoate (Gastrografin) as the contrast medium to visualize abnormalities in the esophagus and stomach. Usually barium sulfate is more effective for visualizing the mucosa, and meglumine diatrizoate is preferred when perforation is suspected because it is a water-soluble agent. This test is useful for detecting causes of dysphagia (difficulty in swallowing), epigastric pain and discomfort, hematemesis, and melena. It is primarily used to diagnose gastric or duodenal ulcers, strictures, and tumors. Double-contrast studies (barium and air) give a better view of the mucosa for detecting polyps, early carcinoma, and gastritis.

Angiography, Celiac and Mesenteric Arteriography: This is an invasive procedure in which a catheter is threaded from the femoral artery to the celiac or mesenteric artery to detect the site of GI bleeding or to detect ischemic areas. Contrast medium is injected for visualization. When the GI bleeding site is identified, vasopressin is infused slowly to the site of bleeding. If vasopressin is not effective in stopping bleeding, then arterial embolization might be necessary. This test is performed when endoscopy and barium studies fail to determine the cause of a GI bleeding problem.

Lower GI Assessment

Laboratory Tests

Carcinoembryonic Antigen (CEA) (Plasma): *Norms:* Nonsmokers: <2.5 ng/ml. Smokers: <3.5 ng/ml.

High plasma CEA levels are found in clients with colorectal cancer. The test should not be the sole criterion for diagnosing colon cancer, because this antigen is relatively nonspecific. The usefulness of this test is to monitor plasma CEA levels following surgical intervention or therapeutic treatment for colon cancer. A decreased CEA level indicates effective response to surgery or treatment. A rise in plasma CEA later might indicate a recurrence of the cancer.

Carotene (Serum): *Norms:* Adult: 60–200 µg/dl, 0.74–3.72 µmol/l (SI units). Child: 40–130 µg/dl.

A decreased serum carotene could be a result of intestinal fat malabsorption. This could affect the absorption of fat-soluble vitamins.

Electrolytes: Potassium, Sodium, Magnesium (Serum): *Norms:* Adult: Potassium: 3.5–5.3 mEq/l. Sodium: 135–145 mEq/l. Magnesium: 1.5–2.5 mEq/l. Child: *See individual tests.*

Potassium, sodium, and magnesium are plentiful in the intestine as well as the stomach. Loss of intestinal secretions because of diarrhea or intestinal intubation could cause serum electrolyte deficits (i.e., hypokalemia, hyponatremia, hypomagnesemia).

Antiparietal Cell Antibody (APCA): Negative or <1:120 titer; Positive: 1:180 titer.

Parietal cells in the stomach secrete hydrochloric acid (HCl) which is needed for protein catabolism. This test is effective for detecting pernicious anemia and chronic gastritis.

D-Xylose Absorption (Serum and Urine): *Norms:* Adult: Serum: 25–40 mg/dl/2 h. Urine: >3.5 g/5 h and >5 g/24 h. Older Adult: Serum: 25–40 mg/dl/2 h. Urine: >4g/5 h. Child: Serum: 30 mg/dl/1 h.

Good urine function is needed for this test. It evaluates absorption of D-xylose, a pentose sugar, in the small intestine. Eighty to 95% of the D-xylose dose is excreted in 5 hours. Decreased serum and urine levels could indicate malabsorptive disorder of the small intestine, jejunal enteritis, or jejunal diverticula.

Lactose Tolerance: *Norms:* Adult: blood glucose increase of 20 mg/dl/2 h.

This test is to identify clients who have a deficiency of the intestinal enzyme lactase. With a decreased intestinal lactase activity, lactose ingested (e.g., milk products) is inadequately absorbed. As a result of lactose deficiency, diarrhea,

TABLE 10 FECAL ANALYSIS STUDIES

Fecal Substances	Values	Comments
Occult blood	Negative	When bleeding from the GI tract is not evident but is suspected, a stool sample is examined for occult (hidden) blood. Either microscopic examination or chemical tests (i.e., guaiac or orthotolidine) are used for identifying fecal occult blood.
Fat content	*Norms:* <6 g/24 h	This can be a screening test when malabsorption syndrome is suspected. If fecal fat content is >6 g/24 h, then malabsorption syndrome is the probable cause. A very small stool could cause false test results.
Ova and parasites	Negative	Ova and parasites (O&P) may be present in the intestine. Usually three stool specimens are evaluated to identify and to confirm the organism present, so that appropriate treatment can be ordered.

abdominal cramps, and flatus occur, especially after ingestion of milk and/or milk products.

Galactose-1-Phosphate Uridyl Transferase (GPUT): Negative: Quantitative: 18.5–28.5 U/g in Hb. Deficiency of the enzyme: <5 U/g in Hb; Carrier of the deficiency: 5–18 U/g in Hb.

The galactose enzyme is needed to convert galactose to glucose during lactose metabolism. A deficiency of this enzyme can lead to galactosemia.

Fecal Analysis: Various studies can be performed on stool specimens (i.e., occult blood, fat content, and ova and parasites). Table 10 shows substances that are analyzed in feces.

Trypsin (Feces): Positive in small amounts.

With pancreatic insufficiency, the stool trypsin test is usually negative.

Rotavirus Antigen (Feces):

The rotavirus can cause infectious diarrhea in infants and young children less than 2 years old. Adults can also be infected with this virus.

Diagnostic Tests

X-ray of Abdomen: Flat x-ray films of the abdomen are ordered to identify abdominal masses of the stomach, liver, and intestine. Suspected abnormal findings are confirmed with other GI tests.

Barium Enema: This is a test that has been used for years in diagnosing lower bowel disorders. Barium sulfate is the contrast agent used and when a more detailed visualization is needed, barium sulfate and air (double contrast) is given. Barium enema is ordered when clients complain of abnormal bowel habits, lower abdominal pain or cramps, blood in the stool, or changes in stool formation. This test is useful for diagnosing polyps and intestinal masses (e.g., tumors, diverticula, strictures, and ulcerations). Barium should not be used when perforation of the bowel is strongly suspected.

Proctosigmoidoscopy: This is an endoscopic procedure for visualizing the anus, rectum, and sigmoid colon. Usually a flexible fiberoptic proctosigmoidoscope is used instead of a rigid metal sigmoidoscope. Abnormalities detected by this procedure include polyps, tumors, hemorrhoids, and inflammatory process.

Proctoscopy: Usually this test is performed during a proctosigmoidoscopy; however, the conventional rigid proctoscope, 3 in. in length, could be used to examine the lower rectum and anal canal.

Sigmoidoscopy: For years, the sigmoidoscope (a rigid 10- to 12-inch instrument) was used to examine the rectum and sigmoid colon. The proctosigmoidoscope (fiberoptic endoscope) is the instrument of choice today for this test procedure.

Biopsy and Cytologic Examination: During a proctosigmoidoscopy, specimens can be obtained by the use of biopsy forceps, cytology brush, or culture swab.

Colonoscopy: This is another endoscopic procedure, and its use has markedly increased in recent years. It is an inspection of the large intestine (colon) using a long, flexible fiberscope (colonoscope). Colonoscopy can detect lesions in the proximal colon that would be missed by sigmoidoscopy. Biopsy forceps and cytologic brush can be used during this test. It should not be done before or 2 days after a barium enema because the barium sulfate would inhibit visualization.

Colonoscopy is effective in detecting early cancerous lesions, which have a good prognosis. It can detect advanced cancerous tumors and determine the extent of inflammatory tissue. Polyps can be removed with the use of an electrocautery snare during the colonoscopy.

Peritoneal Analysis/Paracentesis: Draining copious amounts of fluid from the peritoneal cavity is not done unless the large abdominal fluid volume is causing respiratory distress. Loss of large quantities of peritoneal fluid could cause severe fluid and electrolyte imbalance. Fluid samples may be requested for analyzing the fluid content (i.e., electrolytes, blood cells, sugar, protein, organisms, and cancer cells).

Gastric Emptying Nuclear Study: The radionuclide, Tc-99m Ac-labeled eggs and juice, is ingested by the client. This study is useful for diagnosing gastric obstruction and the cause of dysmotility.

Gastrointestinal Bleeding Nuclear Test: This nuclear test is used to detect the localization of gastrointestinal and nongastrointestinal bleeding sites.

NURSING DIAGNOSES

- Deficient knowledge related to lack of understanding of the laboratory and diagnostic procedures, disease process, and/or outcome.
- Noncompliance with the prescribed laboratory and diagnostic tests related to lack of or inadequate explanation and/or anxiety about physical condition.

- Altered nutrition: less than body requirements related to anorexia, nausea, vomiting, and/or diarrhea.
- Impaired skin integrity related to poor nutritional intake.
- Altered comfort related to endoscopic examination(s).
- Ineffective coping with laboratory and diagnostic test procedures.
- Altered pattern of bowel elimination related to diarrhea, constipation, or barium sulfate.
- Deficient fluid volume related to vomiting, diarrhea, or gastric/intestinal intubation.
- Disturbed body image related to body changes (e.g., colostomy).

NURSING IMPLICATIONS WITH RATIONALE

- Explain that the purpose for the laboratory and diagnostic tests is to aid in the diagnosis of esophagus, stomach, or colon disorders. Be more specific in the explanation if indicated.
- Give an explanation (in detail if indicated) about the laboratory and diagnostic procedures. Emphasize the importance of the client's compliance to the test procedures. Stress that tests might need to be repeated if the procedure was improperly performed.
- Inform the client of any food, beverage, or drug restrictions. Each test should be checked for specific restrictions *(see Parts I and II).*
- Inform the health care provider if the client has had recent barium studies (i.e., upper GI series, barium enema), especially if esophagogastroduodenoscopy, proctosigmoidoscopy, and colonoscopy are ordered. Barium sulfate can hinder visualization and a 2- to 4-day waiting period after barium studies is usually required.
- Listen to the client's expressed anxiety and fear concerning the tests and potential client problems. Clarification of the test procedure might alleviate fear and anxiety and promote test compliance.
- Monitor the client's vital signs before and after laboratory and diagnostic tests. Report significant changes.
- Obtain a stool specimen for occult blood analysis. Determine frequency of bowel movements.
- Assess for throat discomfort (i.e., soreness, swallowing difficulty after oral endoscopic procedure).
- Check gag reflex before giving fluids and food after endoscopic procedures.
- Check laboratory results, and report abnormal test findings.

Evaluation

- Determine if the test was correctly performed according to the procedure. Notify the laboratory and/or health care provider of any changes that occur during the test.
- Check the client's vital signs and frequent bowel movements for changes and improvement.
- Evaluate the status of the client's anxiety and fear in regard to the test(s) and clinical problem.

- Clarify or answer any additional questions the client may have.
- Encourage the client to seek health assistance when changes in health status occur. Continue with assessing the client's state of health.

Neurologic and musculoskeletal function

Laboratory Tests	Diagnostic Tests
Neurologic	
CSF	X-rays
Pressure, Cells, Protein, Glucose,	Skull
Culture, Cytology	Lumbosacral Spine
Amyloid Beta Protein Precursor	EEG
TDM—Anticonvulsants	Echoencephalography
	Electronystagmography (ENG)
	Brain Scan
	Brain Perfusion Nuclear Scan
	CT, Brain
	Cerebral Angiography
	MRI
	PET
	Electroneurography
	Myelography
	Thermography of Spine
	Oculoplethysmography
Musculoskeletal	
Muscle Enzymes	X-ray, Bone and Joints
ALD (Serum)	Synovial Fluid Aspiration
AST/SGOT (Serum)	Arthrography
CPK/CK (Serum)	Bone Scan
Bone Enzymes—ALP	Bone Densitometry
Electrolytes (Ca)	Arthroscopy
(Serum)	EMG
	Muscle Biopsy
	MRI

Introduction

With suspected neurologic disorders, a group of diagnostic tests is performed to confirm a diagnosis. When there are frequent headaches, the tests usually ordered to determine their origin include cerebrospinal fluid (CSF) examination, skull x-rays, and electroencephalography (EEG). If headaches intensify and persist, echoencephalogram, computed tomographic (CT) scan of the head, brain scan, or

677

cerebral angiogram or MRI or PET might be requested. For seizure disorders, EEG, echoencephalography, and CT scan of the head usually are ordered. After acute head injury, skull x-rays are immediately taken. CT scan and MRI of the head might be requested. Musculoskeletal disorders are evaluated by using various diagnostic procedures (i.e., synovial fluid analysis, electromyography [EMG] arthrography, bone scan, and arthroscopy). Neurologic assessment will be presented first, then musculoskeletal.

Neurologic Assessment

Laboratory Tests

Cerebrospinal Fluid (SCF): *Norms: See reference values in Part I.*
Analysis of CSF usually includes color, pressure, white blood cell (WBC) count, protein, chloride, glucose, culture, cytologic cells. Table 11 lists the components found in CSF and the result of the analysis.

Amyloid Beta Protein Precursor (CSF): *Norms:* 450 units/l.
This CSF test aids in diagnosing Alzheimer's disease. The amyloid beta protein is present in the senile plaques within the brain. It is believed that this type of protein may have neurotoxic effects to the brain cells.

Therapeutic Drug Monitoring (TDM): Anticonvulsants are ordered for seizure disorders (i.e., grand mal, psychomotor, and/or petit mal), and therapeutic drugs levels should be closely monitored. The following drug outline gives the name of anticonvulsant, type of seizure, therapeutic range, and toxic level for adults (child as indicated).

Diagnostic Tests

X-rays: *Skull:* Skull x-rays are usually ordered after head trauma to detect fracture of the skull. Skull x-rays are also useful to visualize primary and metastatic tumors of the skull, to confirm the existence of increased intracranial pressure, and to diagnose pituitary tumors. *Lumbosacral Spine:* Spinal x-rays are frequently ordered to determine the cause of pain radiating from back to leg(s). Spinal x-rays could show narrowed intervertebral disk spaces and/or calcified spurs in intervertebral foramina, which could be indicative of degenerated disks.

Electroencephalography, Electroencephalogram (EEG): EEG measures the electrical activity of the brain cells to determine abnormalities (e.g., cerebral lesions [tumor, hemorrhage, abscess]). It is useful in locating the cause of seizure disorders. Another use is to confirm cerebral death. It is not the test of choice for evaluating head injuries.

Echoencephalography, Ultrasonography of the Brain, Brain Echogram: Ultrasound of the brain, a noninvasive procedure, is helpful in detecting cerebral midline shifts characteristic of an intracranial hemorrhage. It is used in neonatal intensive care units, checking infants suspected of having intracranial hemorrhage. Follow-up studies using CT and radionuclides might be indicated.

Drug Name	Seizure Disorder	Therapeutic Range	Toxic Level
Carbamazepine	Grand mal	4–12 µg/ml	>12–15 µg/ml
Ethosuximide	Petit mal	40–100 µg/ml	>100 µg/ml
Phenytoin	Grand mal	Adult: 10–20 µg/ml	Adult: >20 µg/ml
		Child: 4–8 mg/kg/day	Child: 15–20 µg/ml
Primidone	Grand mal and psychomotor	Adult: 5–12 µg/ml	Adult: >12–15 µg/ml
		Child: 7–10 µg/ml	Child: >12 µg/ml
Valproic acid	Grand mal and petit mal	Adult: 50–100 µg/ml	Adult: >100 µg/ml
		Child: Same as adult	Child: Same as adult

TABLE 11 ANALYSIS OF CSF

Component of CSF	Abnormal Results
Pressure	A pressure >200 mm H_2O is considered abnormal and could be due to increased intracranial pressure caused by meningitis, subarachnoid hemorrhage, and tumors.
Color	Pink or red color could be due to subarachnoid or cerebral hemorrhage or a traumatic spinal tap. Yellow color might indicate old blood (4 to 5 days after cerebral hemorrhage).
WBC	WBC differential count may be ordered. An increased number of neutrophils could be indicative of bacterial meningitis or cerebral abscess. An increased number of lymphocytes could be indicative of viral meningitis or encephalitis.
Protein	In acute bacterial meningitis, protein levels could be >250 mg/dl. Increased protein levels indicate infections or inflammatory processes (i.e., meningitis, encephalitis, and tumors).
Glucose	Glucose levels in CSF are 40–80 mg/dl, two-thirds of blood/plasma levels. When there is a decrease in CSF glucose, there is usually an increase of other cells (i.e., bacterial, tumor cells in the spinal fluid). A decrease in glucose, <40 mg/dl, might be indicative of bacterial meningitis, leukemia, or tumors.
Culture	A culture specimen of spinal fluid is withdrawn to determine the type of organism present.
Cytology	Slough cells from tumor sites in the brain or spinal column could flow into the spinal fluid. Examination of CSF for cancerous cells might be requested.

Electronystagmography (ENG): This test helps to determine if the problem/abnormality that occurs is in the brain stem, the temporal lobe of the cerebral cortex, auditory nerve, or vestibular-cochlear areas. If nystagmus does not cocur with stimulation, the ENG test aids in determining the neurologic problem.

Brain Nuclear Scan: Brain scans may be ordered for clients complaining of severe headaches or having frequent seizures. This test can detect intracranial lesions (i.e., abscess, tumors [benign or malignant], metastasis to the brain, subdural hematoma, aneurysms, and cerebrovascular accident [CVA]). A technetium compound, Tc-99m-O_4 or Tc-99m-DTPA, is given intravenously prior to cranial scanning. The blood-brain barrier is disrupted at the pathologic lesion site, thus increasing the amount of radionuclide agent uptake.

Brain Perfusion Nuclear Test: This test may be used for diagnosing Alzheimer's disease, brain death, and AIDS dementia. It helps to locate the seizure foci and locate the size of the cerebral ischemia.

Computed Tomography (CT) of the Head: CT of the head is useful for diagnosing cerebral lesions (i.e., tumors, hematomas caused by intracranial bleeding, abscess, cerebral infarction [obstruction], hydrocephalus, and cerebral edema). For detailed visualization of the lesion, IV contrast medium (iodinated dye) is used. CT scan of the head is replacing more invasive procedures (i.e., pneumoencephalography, cerebral angiography).

Cerebral Angiography, Arteriography: Iodinated contrast medium is injected into the carotid or vertebral artery, usually through the femoral or brachial artery, to visualize the cerebral blood vessels for abnormalities (i.e., occlusions, aneurysms, abnormal vascularization resulting from neoplasms [tumors]). This is an invasive procedure, and there are clients who are allergic to the contrast medium.

Magnetic Resonance Imaging (MRI): This is a sensitive test for detecting edema, hemorrhage, blood flow, tumors, and infection sites in the brain tissue. MRI is useful in detecting demyelinating diseases, such as multiple sclerosis.

Positron Emission Tomography (PET): PET is an effective test in determining blood flow to the brain. Radiation from PET is about one fourth of that received by CT. It is useful in studying the epilepsy focal areas, viable brain tissue after a CVA (stroke), brain tumor, migraine headaches, and parkinsonism, and in differentiating between Alzheimer's disease and other types of dementia.

Electroneurography, Nerve Conduction Studies: *Norms:* Normal conduction velocity: 50–60 meters/sec.

This test is useful in determining peripheral nerve injury. It measures the time required for a nerve impulse to travel from the proximal site to the distal site. The distance per time the nerve impulse takes to travel from the proximal site of stimulation (shock) the muscular contraction is known as the *conduction velocity*. The conduction velocity frequently varies with different nerves.

Myelography, Myelogram: Myelography is a fluoroscopic and radiologic examination of the spinal subarachnoid space (spinal column). The purpose of this test is to identify herniated intervertebral disks, cysts, metastatic tumors, neurofibromas, and meningiomas and to detect spinal nerve root injury.

Thermography (Lumbar, Thoracic, and Cervical): Irritated nerve root and musculoligamentous spasm may be detected by the use of thermography. An abnormal thermogram could include asymmetrical heat patterns that would be indicative of nerve root injury. This test might be ordered for clients with severe or chronic back pain. Usually other diagnostic tests are ordered to aid in the diagnosis (i.e., electromyography [EMG], myelography).

Oculoplethysmography: This is a noninvasive test to evaluate carotid blood flow to the ophthalmic artery. It may be used in clients with CVA to determine size of carotid occlusion. Oculoplethysmographic techniques could also be used in clients with asymptomatic bruits, symptoms of transient ischemic attacks (TIA) and syncope, for detecting occlusions, and for preventing CVA.

Musculoskeletal Assessment

Laboratory Tests

Muscle and Bone Enzyme Tests: Certain enzymes are present in muscles, such as aldolase, creatine phosphokinase (CPK/CK), and aspartate aminotransferase (AST or SGOT) and in bones, such as alkaline phosphatase (ALP) and isoenzyme ALP_2. Table 12 explains the uses of these enzyme tests.

Electrolyte (Calcium) (Serum): *Norms:* Adult: 4.5–5.5 mEq/l, 9–11 mg/dl, 2.3–2.8 mmol/l (SI units). Child: 4.5–5.8 mEq/l, 9–11.5 mg/dl. Infant: 5.0–6.0 mEq/l.

Calcium is found abundantly in bones. Frequently in bone disorders, calcium leaves bones and becomes plentiful in circulating body fluid; thus serum calcium level is elevated (hypercalcemia). Elevated calcium levels occur as the result of bone tumors, multiple myeloma, multiple fractures, and prolonged immobilization.

Diagnostic Tests

X-Rays of Bone and Joint: X-rays are frequently taken of bones and joints to determine presence of disease (i.e., arthritis, spondylitis, bone lesions, and fractures).

Synovial Fluid Aspiration, Arthrocentesis: Samples of synovial fluid are aspirated from a joint cavity for analysis of cells (WBCs, rheumatoid arthritic cells, lupus cells), protein, glucose, uric acid, and for culture.

Arthrography, Arthrogram: Arthrography uses contrast medium and/or air (both: double contrast) to visualize joint structure. This test is able to detect tears, derangements of joints, and synovial cysts. X-rays are taken during the procedure.

Bone Scan: Radionuclide, technetium-labeled phosphate compounds (e.g., Tc-99m diphosphonate, given intravenously) are absorbed into bone tissue and concentrated in abnormal bone cells. The scanner can pick up hot spots months before x-rays can note abnormal bone area. This procedure is primarily used to diagnose metastatic bone disease. Bone scans are also useful to monitor bone response to radiation therapy and/or chemotherapy. This test may be used for early detection of osteomyelitis and for detection of degenerative bone disorders.

TABLE 12 ENZYME TESTS OF MUSCLES AND BONES

Enzyme (Serum)	Reference Values	Results
MUSCLE:		
Aldolase (ALD)	Norms: Adults: <6 U/l 3–8 U/dl (Sibley-Lehninger) 22–59 mU/l at 37°C (SI units) Child: 6–16 U/dl	Aldolase is abundant in skeletal and cardiac muscles. Serum aldolase is elevated in muscular dystrophy but not in muscle diseases of neural origin (i.e., multiple sclerosis, myasthenia gravis).
Aspartate aminotransferase (AST or SGOT)	Norms: Adult: 8–38 U/l	AST/SGOT is less sensitive than CPK/CK for determining muscle disorder. This enzyme is assessed in suspected myopathic diseases.
Creatine phosphokinase (CPK/CK)	Norms: Adult: Male: 5–35 μg/ml 30–180 IU/l; Female: 5–25 μg/ml 25–150 IU/l Child: Male: 0–70 IU/l at 30°C Female: 0–50 IU/l at 30°C	CKP/CK is more sensitive than AST/SGOT for determining muscle disorder. Actually CPK/CK is a better indicator of cardiac diseases than muscle diseases; however, this enzyme is assessed in suspected myopathic diseases.
ISOENZYME: (CPK-MM)	94%–100%	
BONE: Alkaline phosphatase (ALP)	Adult: 42–136 U/l Child: 50–230 U/l Infant: 40–300 U/l	ALP is an enzyme produced primarily in the bone and liver. In bone disorders, ALP level is increased because of abnormal osteoblastic activity (bone cell production). High ALP levels can be found in children during prepuberty and puberty ages because of bone growth. Elevated ALP levels are found in cancer of the bone, Paget's disease (osteitis deformans), healing fractures, multiple myeloma, osteomalacia.
Isoenzyme ALP$_2$	20–120 U/l	Isoenzyme ALP$_2$ is of bone origin.

Bone Densitometry: The bone density test is used to detect early osteoporosis by determining the density of the bone mineral content.

Arthroscopy: This is an endoscopic procedure usually performed in an operating room. An incision is made into the knee joint cavity, and a fiberoptic endoscope is inserted for visualization and/or removal of loose particles. It is an invasive procedure, but the findings are more inclusive than with other diagnostic tests. Biopsy of the synovium could be taken during this procedure.

Electromyography (EMG): EMG measures the electrical activity of muscles at rest and during voluntary muscle contraction. When the muscle is at rest, normally there is no electrical activity. Abnormal EMG results occur in neuropathic and myopathic disorders (i.e., peripheral neuropathy [diabetes mellitus, alcoholism], myasthenia gravis, muscular dystrophy, amyotropic lateral sclerosis [ALS]).

Muscle Biopsy: The purpose for the muscle biopsy is to provide histopathologic information that could be used in the diagnosis of myopathic disorders. EMG is usually performed at the affected muscle site prior to the biopsy.

Magnetic Resonance Imaging (MRI): MRI can be used to identify muscle disease and skeletal abnormalities.

NURSING DIAGNOSES

- Deficient knowledge related to a lack of understanding of laboratory and diagnostic procedures, disease process, and/or outcome.
- Noncompliance with prescribed laboratory and diagnostic tests related to a lack of adequate explanation and/or anxiety about physical condition.
- Risk for injury related to allergic reactions to contrast medium (dye) secondary to the diagnostic test (i.e., CT of the head with contrast medium, angiography).
- Impaired physical mobility related to neuromuscular impairment.
- Deficient diversional activity related to an inability to move freely.
- Social isolation related to impaired mobility, or an inability to communicate.
- Altered patterns of bladder and bowel elimination related to lack of bladder and bowel control secondary to neurologic impairment.
- Impaired thought process related to impaired cerebral circulation.
- Impaired verbal communication related to aphasia or brain damage.
- Powerlessness related to an inability to communicate, dependence on others.
- Ineffective coping with the disease process and laboratory and diagnostic test procedures.
- Situational low self-esteem related to dependence and/or role change.

NURSING IMPLICATIONS WITH RATIONALE

- Explain that the purpose of the laboratory and diagnostic tests is to aid in the diagnosis of brain, muscle, and/or bone disorders. Be specific with the explanation as indicated.

- Give an explanation of the test procedures, and emphasize the need for the client's compliance. Explanation might be brief or in-depth, depending upon the client's ability to comprehend.
- Inform the client of any food, fluid, or drug restrictions *(see Parts I and II).*
- Elicit from the client or family member information about any allergies to dye (contrast medium), iodine, or seafood.
- Listen to the client's expressed anxiety about the tests and potential client problems. Clarification of the test procedure might alleviate fear and anxiety and promote test compliance.
- Assess muscle strength in all extremities. Weak or lacking muscle strength might indicate a neurologic (e.g., CVA) or muscular problem.
- Assess the client's ability to talk. Inability to communicate could hinder the client's compliance to the test regimen.
- Assist the client with ambulation as needed.
- Observe for seizures prior to or after test procedure.
- Monitor the client's vital signs before and following diagnostic procedures (i.e., cerebral angiography, myelography, lumbar puncture, pneumoencephalography, arthroscopy).

Evaluation

- Determine if the test was correctly performed according to the procedure. Notify the laboratory and health care provider of any changes that occur during the test.
- Check the client's vital signs for changes.
- Monitor changes in muscle strength, ambulation, and speech. Report changes and abnormal findings.
- Clarify or answer any additional questions the client or family member might have.
- Encourage clients to use resources available (e.g., National Muscular Dystrophy Society).
- Reinforce the importance of seeking health care assistance whenever changes in health status occur.

Endocrine function

Laboratory Tests	Diagnostic Tests

Thyroid

T_4 (Serum) — RAIU Test
T_3 (Serum) — Thyroid Scan
T_3 Resin Uptake — Ultrasonography of Thyroid
Free T_4 Index
Calcitonin (Serum)
TA (Serum)
TSH (Serum)
Provocative Tests
  TSH Stimulation Test
  Thyroid Suppression Test
  TRH Stimulation Test

Parathyroid

Electrolytes (Ca, P) (Serum) — Ultrasonography of Parathyroid
PTH (Serum)
cAMP (Urine)
Prednisone Suppression Test

Adrenal

Electrolytes (K, NA, Ca) (Serum) — X-ray of Sella Turcica
Adrenocorticotropic Hormone (Plasma) — Adrenal Arteriography
Cortisol (Plasma) — Adrenal Venography
Cortisol (Urine) — Ultrasonography of Adrenal
Aldosterone (Serum) — CT Scan
Aldosterone (Urine)
Catecholamines (Plasma)
17-OCHS (Urine)
17-KS (Urine)
17-KGS (Urine)
Pregnanetriol (Urine)
VMA (Urine)
Provocative Tests
  ACTH Stimulation Test
  ACTH Suppression Test
  Dexamethasone Suppression Test
  Metyrapone Suppression Test
  Aldosterone Stimulation Test
  Aldosterone Suppression Test

Pancreas (Beta Cell)

Electrolytes (K, Na) (Serum)
BUN (Serum)

(continued)

Laboratory Tests	Diagnostic Tests
Pancreas (Beta Cell) (*cont.*) Creatinine (Serum) Acetone/Ketone Bodies (Serum, Plasma, Urine) Chemstrip bG and Dextrostix Glucose: FBS and PPBS (Blood) Glucose Self-Monitoring Glucose Tolerance Test Insulin (Serum) Tolbutamide Tolerance Test	

Introduction

Usually there is a battery of laboratory and diagnostic tests ordered for suspected endocrine disorders of the thyroid, parathyroid, adrenal, and pancreas (beta cell) glands. Laboratory tests include serum, plasma, blood, urine, and provocative tests. Provocative tests assess glandular function by stimulating or suppressing secretions. Diagnostic tests are ordered to confirm suspected glandular disorders.

Thyroid Assessment

Laboratory Tests

Thyroxine (T_4) (Serum): *Norms:* Adult: T_4 (RIA); 5–12 µg/dl; T_4 by column: 4.5–11.5 µg/dl; free T_4: 1.0–2.3 ng/dl. Child: 1–6 Years: T_4: 5.5–13.5 µg/dl; 6–10 years: T_4: 5–12.5 µg/dl.

T_4, a major hormone secreted by the thyroid gland, is an effective indicator of thyroid function. Elevated serum T_4 levels are found in clients with hyperthyroidism, acute thyroiditis, and thyrotoxicosis. Decreased levels are found in clients with hypothyroidism. Most thyroxine is bound to thyroxin-binding globulin (TBG).

Triiodothyronine (T_3) (Serum): *Norms:* Adult: 80–200 ng/dl. Child: 6–12 years: 115–190 ng/dl.

T_3, a hormone of the thyroid, is more potent, shorter acting, and of less quantity than T_4. It is helpful in diagnosing thyrotoxicosis, especially when serum T_4 is in normal range. In hypothyroidism, serum T_3 levels may be within normal range; therefore T_4 would be more reliable.

T_3 Resin Uptake: *Norms:* 25–35%.

This test indirectly measures free T_4 levels by determining protein-binding sites present for T_4. T_3 resin uptake and serum T_4 (RIA) give free T_4 index. In hyperthyroidism there is a high T_3 resin uptake and the percentage is increased; in hypothyroidism, there is a low T_3 resin uptake and the percentage is decreased.

Free T_4 Index: *Norms:* Adult: 0.9–2.2 ng/dl.

Free T_4 index is unaffected by TBG and correlates more with the true hormonal status. It is difficult to measure T_4 directly, so T_3 resin uptake and serum T_4 give the free thyroxine index.

Calcitonin, Thyrocalcitonin (Plasma): *Norms:* Basal: Adult: Male: <40 pg/ml; Female: <25 pg/ml. Child: <70 pg/ml.

Calcitonin is a hormone secreted by the C cells of the thyroid gland. Calcitonin lowers calcium levels. Elevated plasma calcitonin levels could indicate medullary carcinoma of the thyroid.

Thyroid Antibodies, Thyroglobulin Antibodies (TA) (Serum): *Norms:* Adult: negative to 1:20, 0–50 ng/ml (RIA). Child: same as adult.

A high titer of thyroglobulin antibodies is indicative of thyroid autoimmune disease. In Hashimoto's thyroiditis, the titer is high, 1:5000. Titer can also be elevated in carcinoma of the thyroid and thyrotoxicosis.

Thyroid-Stimulating Hormone (TSH) (Serum): *Norms:* Adult: 0.35–5.5 μIU/ml, <10 μU/ml (RIA), <3 ng/ml.

TSH is secreted from the anterior pituitary gland in response to thyroid-releasing hormone (TRH) from the hypothalamus. Secretion of TSH is dependent on a negative feedback system that promotes the release of TRH when the level of T_4 is decreased; this in turn stimulates TSH secretion. An elevated TSH level and a decreased T_4 indicate hypothyroidism.

Thyroid Provocative Tests: These tests are useful for evaluating thyroid function.

TSH Stimulation Test, Thyroid Stimulation Test: This test is useful in distinguishing between *primary,* or thyroidal, hypothyroidism and *secondary,* or hypothalamic-pituitary, hypothyroidism. After an injection of TSH, radioactive iodine uptake (RAIU), serum TSH, and/or serum T_4 are measured. In primary hypothyroidism, the RAIU will remain about the same, TRH and TSH will be increased, and T_4 will show no response. In secondary hypothyroidism, the RAIU will increase about 10%, TRH and TSH will not be increased, and T_4 will rise >1.5 μg/dl.

Thyroid Suppression Test: Norms: Adult: 25% decrease in RAIU; T_4 <50% of baseline.

This test is useful to confirm borderline hyperthyroidism. Baseline RAIU and T_3 or T_4 levels are first obtained. The client is given T_4 or T_3 for 7 days. Normally TSH production should be depressed, thus decreasing RAIU and T_4. In hyperthyroidism, the RAIU and T_4 will *not* be decreased.

Thyrotropin-Releasing Hormone (TRH) Stimulation Test: The purpose of the TRH stimulation test is to differentiate between hypothalamic and pituitary insufficiency in clients with hypothyroidism with low serum TSH levels. This test can be used to confirm equivocal thyrotoxicosis, because free thyroid hormone suppresses pituitary production of TSH. A baseline value for serum TSH is obtained. TRH is injected intravenously, followed by serum TSH measurements. A serum TSH increase is indicative of hypothalamic disorder; however, no response in serum TSH is indicative of a pituitary disorder. Decreased TRH and TSH levels occur when aspirin and steroids are being taken.

Diagnostic Tests

Radioactive Iodine Uptake Test (RAIU): *Norms:* Adult: 2 hours: 1–13%; 6 hours: 2–25%; 24 hours: 15–45%.

The RAIU test is primarily used in detecting hyperthyroidism. I-131 or I-123 is given orally or I-125 is given intravenously. The client's thyroid gland is scanned at three different times to determine the concentration of radioactive iodine uptake in the thyroid gland. An elevated RAIU indicates hyperthyroidism or Graves' disease. A low RAIU could mean hypothyroidism; however, if T_3 and T_4 are elevated, then it could be caused by thyrotoxicosis or chronic thyroiditis.

Thyroid Scan: The purpose for thyroid scanning is to determine size, structure, and position of thyroid gland, to detect thyroid masses (e.g., tumors), and to evaluate thyroid function. Thyroid nodules are easily detected; cold spots could indicate hypofunction and thyroid tumor, and hot spots could indicate hyperfunction (i.e., Graves' disease, thyrotoxicosis).

Ultrasonography of Thyroid, Thyroid Echogram, Thyroid Sonography: Ultrasound of the thyroid gland is helpful in distinguishing between solid and cystic nodules. It is a noninvasive procedure and considered safe for pregnant women.

Parathyroid Assessment

Laboratory Tests

Electrolytes: Calcium and Phosphorus (Serum): *Norms:*

Person	Calcium	Phosphorus
Adult	4.5–5.5 mEq/l	1.7–2.6 mEq/l
	9–11 mg/dl	2.5–4.5 mg/dl
Child	9–12 mg/dl	2.5–6.0 mg/dl
		7.0 mg/dl during bone growth

Parathyroid hormone (PTH) promotes calcium absorption from the gastrointestinal tract and promotes a release of calcium from bone when there is a deficit. If the client is in renal failure, the serum calcium level is usually low, and the serum phosphorus (phosphate) is elevated. Secondary hyperparathyroidism can occur because of low calcium levels stimulating the secretion of PTH. Decreased serum phosphorus level (hypophosphatemia) is associated with hyperparathyroidism and hypercalcemia. An elevated phosphorus level (hyperphosphatemia) is associated with hypoparathyroidism, hypocalcemia, and renal failure.

Parathyroid Hormone (PTH) (Serum): *Norms:* Adult: Intact PTH: 11–54 pg/ml, 50–330 pg/ml (C-Terminal); 8–24 pg/ml (N-Terminal).

PTH is released according to serum calcium levels. Decreased circulating calcium stimulates PTH release, and elevated or normal circulating calcium inhibits PTH release. PTH levels might be elevated as the result of parathyroid hyperplasia or tumor. Decreased PTH level could be due to parathyroid trauma or postparathyroidectomy.

Cyclic Adenosine Monophosphate (Cyclic AMP, cAMP) (Urine): PTH promotes production of cAMP in the kidneys. After an IV infusion of PTH, urine cAMP is measured. In primary hyperparathyroidism, cAMP excretion is increased. Poor renal function can decrease cAMP excretion; thus this test may not be the most accurate one for evaluating parathyroid function.

Prednisone/Cortisone Suppression Test: The purpose of this test is to determine the cause of hypercalcemia. Oral prednisone or cortisone is administered daily for 10 to 14 days. If the serum calcium level is lowered in clients with hypercalcemia, then the cause of elevated calcium level is not hyperparathyroidism but might be bone metastasis, sarcoidosis, or excess vitamin D. In hyperparathyroidism, prednisone or cortisone will not lower calcium levels.

Diagnostic Tests

Ultrasonography of the Parathyroid Gland: In ultrasound of the parathyroid gland the echo pattern is of less amplitude than that of thyroid tissue. Enlargement of the gland(s) might be caused by hyperplasia or tumor growth.

Adrenal Assessment

Laboratory Tests

Electrolytes (Potassium, Sodium, Calcium) (Serum): *Norms:* Adult: Potassium: 3.5–5.3 mEq/l. Sodium: 135–145 mEq/l. Calcium: 4.5–5.5 mEq/l, 9–11 mg/dl.

Steroids (e.g., cortisone, secreted from the adrenal gland) promote sodium retention and potassium excretion. Adrenal hyperfunction causes an elevated serum sodium level (hypernatremia), a decreased serum potassium level (hypokalemia), and a decreased serum calcium level (hypocalcemia). Adrenal insufficiency causes hyponatremia and hyperkalemia.

Adrenocorticotropic Hormone (ACTH) Plasma: 7 AM–10 AM: 8–80 pg/ml; 4 PM: 5–30 pg/ml; 10 PM–Midnight: <10 pg/ml.

Plasma ACTH is performed to determine whether a decreased plasma cortisol is due to adrenal cortex hypofunction or pituitary hypofunction. When the plasma cortisol is increased, ACTH release is inhibited, and when plasma cortisol is decreased, ACTH is released. ACTH stimulation and suppression tests are usually needed to confirm the diagnosis of adrenal disorders. Elevated ACTH could be due to pituitary tumors or nonpituitary ACTH-producing tumor (i.e., of the pancreas, lung, ovary), or it could be due to primary adrenal insufficiency in those with Addison's disease. A decreased ACTH level in Addison's disease could indicate hypofunction of the pituitary gland.

Cortisol (Plasma): *Norms:* Adult: 8 AM–10 AM: 5–23 μg/dl, 138–635 nmol/l (SI units); 4 PM–6 PM: 3–13 μg/dl, 83–359 nmol/l (SI units).

Cortisol is a potent glucocorticoid released from the adrenal gland. Cortisol levels are higher in the morning than in the afternoon. The diurnal variation ceases in early adrenal hyperfunction. In Addison's disease, the plasma cortisol levels are decreased.

Cortisol (Urine): *Norms:* Adult: 24–108 µg/24 h.

Urine cortisol levels usually reflect the secretion of cortisol. With an elevated plasma cortisol level, excess free cortisol enters the urine, increasing urine cortisol level. Elevated plasma and urine cortisol are significant of adrenal hyperfunction.

Aldosterone (Serum): *Norms:* <16 ng/dl (fasting); 4–30 ng/dl (sitting). Child: (3–11 years): 5–70 ng/dl.

Aldosterone, a potent mineralocorticoid, promotes sodium reabsorption from the kidneys and potassium excretion. Thus this hormone affects electrolyte balance, especially sodium and potassium. A 24-hour urine aldosterone level is more reliable than the serum aldosterone test. A decreased serum aldosterone level is indicative of adrenal hypofunction and an elevated level is indicative of adrenal hyperfunction. Serum aldosterone may be checked with serum renin; an elevated aldosterone and a decreased serum renin is usually due to primary hyperaldosteronism. If both serum aldosterone and serum renin are elevated, secondary hyperaldosteronism is suspected.

Aldosterone (Urine): *Norms:* Adult: 6–25 µg/24 h.

The 24-hour urine aldosterone test eliminates diurnal variation that occurs with serum aldosterone. Decreased urine aldosterone levels can indicate adrenal hypofunction and elevated levels can indicate primary or secondary hyperaldosteronism, stress, or adrenal hyperfunction.

Catecholamines (Plasma): *See Plasma Catecholamines in Part I. Epinephrine:* Supine: <50 pg/ml. *Norepinephrine:* Supine: 110–410 pg/ml. Epinephrine, norepinephrine, and dopamine are the major catecholamine hormones secreted by the adrenal medulla. Elevated catecholamines, >1000 pg/ml, indicates pheochromocytoma.

17-Hydroxycorticosteroids (17-OHCS) (Urine): *Norms:* Adult: Male: 5–15 mg/ 24 h. Female: 3–13 mg/24 h. Child: lower than adults.

The 17-OHCS are a group of steroids, cortisone and hydrocortisone, excreted in the urine. Urine 17-OHCS and serum cortisol frequently are the tests of choice for assessing adrenal function. Elevated urine 17-OHCS level is indicative of adrenal hyperfunction (e.g., Cushing's syndrome), and a decreased urine 17-OHCS is indicative of adrenal hypofunction (e.g., Addison's disease).

17-Ketosteroids (17-KS) (Urine): *Norms:* Adult: Male: 5–25 mg/24 h. Female: 5–15 mg/24 h. Adolescent: 3–14 mg/24 h. *For other reference values, see Part I.*

The 17-KS are metabolites of male hormones secreted from the adrenal cortex and testes. Urine 17-KS levels are higher in male than female. An elevated urine 17-KS could indicate adrenal cortical hyperfunction (e.g., hyperplasia, Cushing's syndrome, adrenal tumors), and a decreased urine 17-KS could indicate adrenal cortical hypofunction (e.g., Addison's disease).

17-Ketogenic Steroids (17-KGS) (Urine): *Norms:* Adult: Male: 4–22 mg/24 h. Female: 2–15 mg/24 h. Adolescent: 2–9 mg/24 h.

The 17-KGS are a group of steroids that are used to assess adrenal cortical function. An elevated urine 17-KGS level occurs in adrenal hyperfunction and a decreased level occurs in adrenal hypofunction.

Pregnanetriol (Urine): *Norms:* Adult: Male: 0.4–2.4 mg/24 h. Female: 0.5–2.0 mg/24 h. Child: 0–1.0 mg/24 h.

Pregnanetriol comes from adrenal corticoid synthesis. Elevated level is indicative of adrenal cortical hyperfunction (i.e., congenital hyperplasia, adrenal gland tumor).

Vanillylmandelic Acid (VMA) (Urine): *Norms:* Adult: 1.5–7.5 mg/24 h, 7.6–37.9 μmol/24 (SI units).

VMA is a by-product of catecholamines (epinephrine and norepinephrine). Elevated urine VMA levels might indicate adrenal medulla tumor. Certain foods and drugs can give false-positive test results.

Adrenal Provocative Tests: These tests help evaluate adrenal function.

ACTH Stimulation Test: With the administration of ACTH, the plasma cortisol level should double in 1 hour. If the plasma cortisol level remains the same or is lower, adrenal gland insufficiency or Addison's disease is the cause.

ACTH Suppression Test: When a synthetic, potent cortisol, dexamethasone (Decadron), is given, the ACTH production should be suppressed. If an extremely high dose is needed for ACTH suppression, the cause is of pituitary origin, such as pituitary tumor.

Dexamethasone Suppression Test: Norms: Adult: Plasma Cortisol: 8 AM, <10 μg/dl; 4 PM, <5 μg/dl.

This is an overnight screening test to evaluate the pituitary feedback system and to determine the presence of adrenal hyperfunction (e.g., Cushing's syndrome). Dexamethasone (Decadron), a potent adrenal steroid, is given at 12 midnight, and plasma cortisol levels are measured at 8 AM and 4 PM (17-OHCS may be measured also).

With Cushing's syndrome, the adrenals will continue to secrete cortisone despite the ACTH suppression by the pituitary gland.

Metyrapone Suppression Test: Norms: Adult: 17-OHCS should be twofold.

This test evaluates the pituitary feedback system and determines the presence of adrenal hyperfunction. Metyrapone is a potent blocker of cortisol production. After administration of metyrapone, cortisol production should decline, and a decreased plasma cortisol should increase the ACTH secretion. If urine 17-OHCS levels are markedly increased, adrenal hyperplasia is suspected. If there is not an increase in urine 17-OHCS, adrenal tumor might be suspected. Adrenocortical insufficiency (e.g., Addison's disease) is a complication of this test.

Aldosterone Stimulation Test: Norms: Plasma aldosterone increases twofold to fourfold. Urine aldosterone increases twofold to threefold.

This provocative test using furosemide (Lasix) differentiates between adrenal disorder and essential hypertension. As body fluids deplete, aldosterone secretion increases and so does renin secretion. Increased plasma and urine aldosterone levels suggest primary aldosteronism, and decreased levels suggest hypoaldosteronism.

Aldosterone Suppression Test: Norms: Adult: approximately 50% decrease in secretion or excretion of aldosterone.

IV saline infusion expands extracellular fluid volume, thus decreasing aldosterone secretion. If aldosterone levels are not suppressed, primary hyperaldosteronism is suspected. Deoxycorticosterone (DOCA) may be substituted for saline. After normal saline diet and DOCA injections for 3 to 5 days, the plasma aldosterone level should decrease by approximately 70%.

Diagnostic Tests

X-Ray of Sella Turcica: X-raying this site can detect destruction of the sella turcica, which would be suggestive of an ACTH-producing tumor of the pituitary gland. An overproduction of ACTH caused by the pituitary tumor results in secondary adrenal hyperfunction (e.g., Cushing's syndrome).

Adrenal Angiography, Arteriography: Radiopaque dye is injected into the adrenal arteries to visualize the adrenal gland and adrenal arterial system. This is an invasive test and should not be performed if client is allergic to iodine or dye. This test will detect adrenal tumors and hyperplasia. If pheochromocytoma is suspected, beta- and alpha-adrenergic blockers should be given several days before the test to decrease the chance of hypertensive crisis.

Adrenal Venography: This test detects adrenal vein and adrenal disorders. Plasma cortisol levels from both adrenal glands are obtained to determine the involved gland causing Cushing's syndrome (e.g., unilateral tumor). If cortisol levels are bilaterally elevated, then adrenal hyperfunction is caused by bilateral adrenal hyperplasia. If pheochromocytoma is suspected, then adrenal venous blood is tested for catecholamines.

Adrenal Ultrasonography, Sonography: Ultrasound is useful in detecting adrenal gland abnormalities (e.g., tumors).

Computed Tomography (CT) of the Adrenal Gland: CT scan determines the size and shape of the adrenal gland. It is useful in detecting adrenal abnormalities (e.g., tumors).

Pancreas (Beta Cell) Assessment

Laboratory Tests

Electrolytes (Potassium and Sodium) (Serum): *Norms:* Adult: Potassium: 3.5–5.3 mEq/l. Sodium: 135–145 mEq/l.

In diabetic ketoacidosis, serum potassium could be normal or elevated, depending on the client's state of body fluid balance. If severe dehydration is present because of polyuria and glycosuria, there would be elevated potassium value resulting from hemoconcentration secondary to dehydration.

The serum sodium level could be normal or low, depending on body fluid balance. Frequently sodium is lost with fluid as a result of osmotic diuresis because of increased blood sugar.

Blood Urea Nitrogen (BUN) (Serum): *Norm:* Adult: 5–25 mg/dl.

In diabetic ketoacidosis with dehydration, the BUN is slightly to moderately elevated because of hemoconcentration. After hydration, the BUN should return to normal; if it does not, then renal disorder should be suspected.

Creatinine (Serum): *Norms:* Adult: 0.5–1.5 mg/dl, 53–106 μmol/dl (SI units). Child: 0.4–1.2 mg/dl.

A serum creatinine level >2.5 mg/dl could be indicative of renal impairment. In diabetic ketoacidosis, BUN and creatinine levels are usually compared. If BUN is elevated and serum creatinine is in normal range or <2.5 mg/dl, dehydration is likely to be the problem.

Acetone, Ketone Bodies (Serum, Plasma, Urine): *Norms:* Adult: Serum acetone: 0.3–2.0 mg/dl. Serum ketones: 2–4 mg/dl.

Ketone bodies, by-products of fat metabolism and fatty acids, are greatly increased during uncontrolled diabetes mellitus and starvation. Urine should also be checked with reagent strips or tablets for ketone bodies. Positive acetone and ketone tests are indicative of ketoacidosis.

Chemstrip bG, Dextrostix (Blood): Dextrostix has been a useful screening test for blood sugar for 20 years. With this method a drop of blood is placed on the Dextrostix, and after 1 minute the strip is compared to a color chart with many ranges (40 mg to 240 mg). It is not as accurate as the Chemstrip bG. The use of Chemstrip bG for hospital and home blood-sugar monitoring is popular and is considered accurate. Follow directions on set.

Glucose: Fasting Blood Sugar (FBS) and 2-Hour Postprandial Blood Sugar (PPBS), or Feasting: *FBS:* Serum/plasma: 70–100 mg/dl. Blood: 60–100 mg/dl. *PPBS:* Serum/plasma: <140 mg/dl/2 h. Blood: <120 mg/dl/2 h.

Insulin is needed for transportation of glucose into the cells. A decrease in insulin production increases blood glucose level. A decreased glucose level (hypoglycemia) frequently results from too much circulating insulin. An elevated glucose level >200 mg/dl indicates not enough insulin, the condition known as diabetes mellitus.

Glucose Self-Monitoring (Blood): Glucose monitoring devices are available for accurately checking blood glucose levels.

Glucose Tolerance Test (GTT) (Serum, Blood): GTT is a test to diagnose diabetes mellitus. This test should not be performed if the fasting blood sugar is >200 mg/dl.

Insulin (Serum): *Norms:* Adult: 10–250 μU/ml; 5–25 μU/ml.

Serum insulin and blood glucose levels are compared to determine the glucose disorder. If the serum insulin level is elevated or the insulin:glucose ratio is >0.3, tumor or hyperplasia of the islet cells of the pancreas should be suspected.

Tolbutamide (Orinase) Tolerance Test: This test determines the insulin and glucose response to the hypoglycemic agent tolbutamide. After IV injection of tolbutamide, the blood glucose level should decrease and remain low for 30 minutes. Blood samples are drawn for baseline value and then 5, 10, 20, 30, 60, and 120 minutes after IV injection. Serum insulin may also be drawn. With a high serum insulin level and severe hypoglycemia resulting, insulinoma should be suspected. A diminished response could mean possible diabetes mellitus; thus, further studies would be necessary.

NURSING DIAGNOSES

- Deficient knowledge related to a lack of understanding of laboratory and diagnostic procedures, disease process, and/or outcome.
- Noncompliance to prescribed laboratory and diagnostic tests related to a lack of or inadequate explanation and/or anxiety about physical condition.
- Excess fluid volume and hypokalemia related to increased ADH and aldosterone secretion.
- Risk for injury related to allergic reactions to contrast medium (dye) secondary to diagnostic tests (e.g., angiography).
- Ineffective coping with the disease process and laboratory and diagnostic test procedure.
- Situational low self-esteem related to body changes secondary to hypofunction and hyperfunction of the thyroid gland and adrenal gland.
- Impaired nutrition related to insufficient insulin production and inadequate glucose metabolism secondary to diabetes mellitus.
- Ineffective family processes related to exacerbation of glandular dysfunction and hospitalization.

NURSING IMPLICATIONS WITH RATIONALE

- Explain that the purpose of the laboratory and diagnostic tests is to aid in diagnosing a thyroid, parathyroid, adrenal, or pancreatic disorder. Be more specific with explanation as indicated.
- Give an explanation, in detail if indicated, about the laboratory and diagnostic procedures. Emphasize the importance of the client's compliance with the test procedures. Stress that tests might need to be reordered if the procedure is improperly performed.
- Inform the client of any food, fluid, or drug restrictions. Each test should be checked for specific restrictions *(see Parts I and II)*.
- Listen to the client's expressed anxiety about the tests and potential patient problems. Clarification of the test procedure might alleviate fear and anxiety and promote test compliance.
- Check laboratory results, and notify the health care provider of abnormal test reports.

- Observe for signs and symptoms of fluid volume deficit or excess, hypokalemia or hyperkalemia, and hypocalcemia or hypercalcemia. Fluid-volume deficit could result from hyperglycemia because of osmotic diuresis. Symptoms would be those of dehydration or shocklike symptoms. Fluid-volume excess could occur from excess secretion of antidiuretic hormone (ADH), which reabsorbs water from the the distal renal tubules. Hypokalemia could result from excess aldosterone production. Hypocalcemia or hypercalcemia usually occurs from parathyroid and thyroid disorders.
- Monitor the client's vital signs before and after laboratory and diagnostic tests.
- Provide support to the client and family members during and after test procedure.

Evaluation

- Determine if the test was correctly performed according to procedure. Notify the laboratory and health care provider of any changes that occur during the test.
- Check the client's vital signs and intake and output after the laboratory or diagnostic procedure. Assess for significant changes.
- Clarify or answer any additional questions the client and family members might have.
- Identify resources that would provide information, service, and support to the client and family at home. Be available to answer questions.
- Reinforce the importance of health care to maintain wellness. Assist the client and family with health plans as needed.

Reproductive function

Laboratory Tests	Diagnostic Tests
Female Reproductive	
Estrogen (Serum and Urine)	Colposcopy
Estrone (E$_1$) (Serum and Urine)	Laparoscopy
Estradiol (E$_2$) (Serum)	Hysterosalpingography
FSH (Serum and Urine)	Cytogenetic Studies
LH (Serum)	Sex Chromatin Mass
Progesterone (Serum)	Chromosome Analysis
Pregnanediol (Urine)	PAP Smear
Prolactin (Serum)	Cervical Biopsy
	Mammography
	Thermography
	Cervicography
	Hysteroscopy

(continued)

Laboratory Tests	Diagnostic Tests
Male Reproductive	
Testosterone (Serum)	Prostate Ultrasonography
Semen Examination	Scrotum/Testes Ultrasonography
17-KS (Urine)	
Cytogenetic Studies	
Pregnancy	
HCG	Amniocentesis
Home Pregnancy Test Kits	Pelvic Ultrasonography
HPL (Serum)	Fetal Nonstress Test (NST)
Estriol (E_3) (Serum and Urine)	Fetoscopy
Estetrol (E_4) (Plasma)	External Fetal Monitoring
Progesterone (Serum)	Internal Fetal Monitoring
Pregnanediol (Urine)	Breast Massage Stress Test
Amino Acid Screen (Urine)	Chorionic Villi Biopsy
AFP (Serum and Amniotic Fluid)	
Genetic Defect Tests: Down's Syndrome, Sickle Cell Anemia, Neural Tube Defects, Tay-Sachs Disease	
Rubella Antibody Detection	
Mumps Antibody Test (Serum)	
Maternal Enzymes (Serum)	
Blood Type, Rh Screen	
L/S Ratio (Amniotic Fluid)	
Nitrazine Paper Test	
CK/CPK (Serum)	
Renin (Plasma)	
Albumin (Serum)	
Hormone Changes	
Hematologic Changes	
RPR (Serum)	
Herpes Simplex Virus-2 (Serum)	
Cytogenetic Studies	
Cytomegalovirus Antibody (Serum)	
Chlamydia Test (Serum)	
Neonate	
Glucose (Blood)	
Cord Blood: Type and Rh	
Bilirubin (Blood)	
PKU (Serum and Urine)	
TORCH Test	
Toxoplasmosis Antibody (Serum)	
Trypsin (Feces)	
Herpes Simplex Virus-2 (Serum)	

Introduction

The focus on reproductive function in this section is on reproductive processes and products involving male and female. Certain tests in the discussion of the female reproductive function, such as cytogenetic studies, also apply to the male reproductive function and pregnancy. Laboratory tests for reproductive function include serum, plasma, urine, and amniotic fluid. The number of tests in pregnancy has greatly increased in the last 10 to 20 years.

Female Reproductive Assessment

Laboratory Tests

Estrogen (Serum): *Norms:* Early Menstrual Cycle: 60–200 pg/ml. Midmenstrual Cycle: 100–600 pg/ml. Late Menstrual Cycle: 150–350 pg/ml. Postmenopausal: <30 pg/ml. Male: 40–115 pg/ml.

This test is useful for evaluating gonadal hypofunction in females, timing ovulation, and determining hormonally active tumors. Serum estrogen measures estrone (E_1) and estradiol (E_2), but measures small amounts of estriol (E_3); therefore it is *not* a test used in pregnancy to determine fetal well-being.

Estrogen (Urine): *Norms:* Female: Preovulation: 5–25 µg/24 h. Follicular: 24–100 µg/24 h. Luteal Phase: 22–80 µg/24 h. Postmenopausal: 0–10 µg/24 h. Male: 4–25 µg/24 h.

Urine estrogen test includes estrone (E_1), estradiol (E_2), and estriol (E_3). This 24-hour urine test is useful for diagnosing ovarian disorders, tumors, hypogonadism, hypopituitarism, and adrenal hyperplasia. It is not a test for assessing fetal well-being.

Estrone (E_1) Serum and Urine: *See values for estrone in Part I.*

Estrone is a potent estrogen. A decreased estrone level can indicate ovarian failure or dysfunction.

Estradiol (E_2) (Serum): *Female:* Follicular Phase: 20–150 pg/ml. Midcycle: 100–500 pg/ml. Luteal Phase: 60–260 pg/ml. *Male:* 15–20 pg/ml. *Child:* 3–10 pg/ml.

E_2 evaluates gonadal dysfunction, such as amenorrhea syndromes and testicular tumors. It is decreased in primary amenorrhea and ovarian failure and is elevated in testicular tumors, ovarian tumors, and adrenal tumors.

Follicle-Stimulating Hormone (FSH) (Serum): *Norms:* Female: Preovulation, Postovulation: 4–30 mU/ml. Midcycle: 10–90 mU/ml. Luteal Phase: 4–30 mU/ml. Postmenopausal: 40–170 mU/ml. Male: 4–25 mU/ml. Child: 5–12 mU/ml.

Serum FSH is useful for diagnosing infertility and menstrual disorders. FSH is responsible for developing ovarian follicles for ovulation. A decreased serum FSH can indicate anovulation, causing infertility or secondary hypogonadotropic state caused by panhypopituitarism or anorexia nervosa. Elevated serum FSH might indicate primary hypogonadism (Turner's syndrome) or precocious puberty. It may be elevated in postmenopausal women.

Follicle-Stimulating Hormone (FSH) (Urine): *Norms:* Female: Preovulation, Postovulation: 2–15 IU/24 h. Midcycle: 8–60 IU/24 h. Postmenopausal: 50–150 IU/24 h. Male: 4–18 IU/24 h. Child: <10 IU/24 h.

A decreased urine FSH level might indicate neoplasms of the ovary, adrenal gland, or testes or anorexia nervosa. An elevated level could indicate gonadal

697

failure caused by postmenopause, FSH-producing pituitary tumor, or Klinefelter's syndrome.

Luteinizing Hormone (LH) (Serum): *Norms:* Female: Follicular: 3–30 mIU/ml. Midcycle: 30–100 mIU/ml. Postmenopausal: 40–100 mIU/ml. Male: 5–25 mIU/ml. Child: <10 mIU/ml.

LH may determine cause of menstrual disturbances, gonadal failure, and infertility. The FSH test is ordered with LH to check on causes of anovulation and infertility. An elevated LH level might indicate ovarian failure associated with Stein-Leventhal syndrome (which is polycystic ovary syndrome), Turner's syndrome (ovarian dysgenesis), or postmenopause.

Progesterone (Serum): *Norms:* Preovulation: 20–150 ng/dl, 0.1–1.5 ng/ml. Midcycle: 250–2800 ng/dl, 2–28 ng/ml.

Purposes of this test are to determine ovulation, to evaluate infertility problems, and to assess placental function. Serum progesterone levels are elevated at time of ovulation, including 5 days postovulation, in early pregnancy, and in adrenal tumors.

Pregnanediol (Urine): *Norms:* Female: Preovulation: 0.5–1.5 mg/24 h. Midcycle: 2–7 mg/24 h. Postmenopausal: 0.1–1.0 mg/24 h. Male: 0.1–1.5 mg/24 h. Child: 0.4–1.0 mg/24 h.

Pregnanediol is the major metabolite of progesterone. It is produced by the corpus luteum during the latter half of the menstrual cycle and by the placenta. A decreased level could be due to menstrual disorders, ovarian hypofunction, threatened abortion, tumors of the ovary or breast, lutein cell tumors of the ovary, or preeclampsia. Elevated level could be due to pregnancy, ovarian cyst, choriocarcinoma of the ovary, or adrenal hyperplasia.

Prolactin (Serum): *Norms:* Nonlactating Female: 0–23 ng/dl. Pregnancy: rise of 10- to 20-fold.

This test is useful for detecting a suspected pituitary tumor. High prolactin levels, >100 ng/dl, in a nonpregnant female could indicate pituitary adenoma. Hyperprolactinemia may be due to hypothyroidism, acromegaly, or hypothalamic disorders or may occur in clients with galactorrhea and amenorrhea.

Diagnostic Tests

Colposcopy: A colposcope is used to examine the vagina and cervix for precancerous lesions. Colposcopy is performed after an abnormal PAP test, to monitor treatment for dysplasia and cervical lesions, and to monitor females with vaginal and/or cervical tissue changes caused by their mothers taking diethylstilbestrol (DES) during pregnancy.

Laparoscopy: A laparoscope, a small fiberoptic telescope, is inserted through the abdominal wall for the purpose of detecting cysts, fibroids, adhesions, and pelvic masses, and for diagnosing cause of pelvic pain (i.e., endometriosis, pelvic inflammatory disease [PID]). This procedure may be used for tubal sterilization, ovarian biopsy, and removal of foreign bodies. Laparoscopy has decreased the number of surgical laparotomies performed.

Hysterosalpingography: Ultrasonography has nearly replaced hysterosalpingography. However, this test is still useful for evaluating patency of the fallopian tubes. It is one of the infertility studies. The procedure uses contrast medium and fluoroscopic x-ray filming.

Cytogenetic Studies: Cytogenetic studies for analysis are performed on tissue, blood, bone marrow, and amniotic fluid. Sex chromatin and chromosome analysis are the two tests usually ordered when chromosomal abnormalities are suspected.

Sex Chromatin Mass: Sex chromatin mass or Barr chromatin body (clump of chromatin adhered to nuclear membrane in cells) is represented as an inactive X chromosome in females and not in males. With disturbances of gonadal development or function and/or with disturbance in reproductive function, sex chromosome defect (absence or an increased number of inactivated X chromosomes or Barr chromatin bodies) may be suspected. The purpose of the test is to screen for sex chromosome anomalies such as the following:

- Turner's syndrome: i.e., poorly developed sex characteristics (amenorrhea, undeveloped breast, sterility) in a female due to XO (no Barr body) or XX/XO mosaics (some with Barr body and some without).
- Klinefelter's syndrome: i.e., poorly develped sex characteristics (small penis, testes, sterility) in a male due to presence of chromatin body of the Y chromosome with XXY (mostly), XXXY, or XXYY variants.

Buccal mucosa is obtained for sex chromosome study. If results are abnormal, chromosome analysis (karyotype) is indicated.

Chromosome Analysis: Blood, tissue, bone marrow, and amniotic fluid are used to identify chromosomal abnormalities (e.g., Down's syndrome, congenital anomalies, genetic disorders, and proliferative diseases such as leukemias).

Papanicolaou Smear (PAP): This is a cytologic test to detect precancerous or cancerous cells of the cervix; it is also used to detect some infectious diseases, such as monilia. A positive PAP smear needs further diagnostic test (i.e., colposcopy or cervical biopsy) to confirm the PAP result. PAP smears are generally performed during a pelvic examination and during the first prenatal visit if not done previously.

Cervical Biopsy: A cervical biopsy may be indicated for suspicious cervical lesions.

Mammography, Mammogram: This procedure is an x-ray examination of the breasts to detect cysts or tumors. Usually it can detect breast lesion(s) 2 years before the lesion is palpable.

Thermography: An infrared photographic test records heat energy from the skin surface of the breast. Increased breast surface temperature may be caused by increased vascularity resulting from a cancerous lesion.

Cervicography (Cervigram): Cervigraphy is a photographic method to record an image of the cervix. It can identify some cancerous lesions that were missed by PAP smears.

Hysteroscopy: Hysteroscopy visualizes the entire endometrial cavity of the uterus. It is more effective for viewing and obtaining endometrial pathology than the dilatation and curretage (D&C), in which blind scraping is performed.

Male Reproductive Assessment

Laboratory Tests

Testosterone (Serum): *Norms:* Adult: Male: 0.3–1.0 μg/dl, 300–1000 ng/dl. Child: Male (12–14 years): >0.1 μg/dl, >1000 ng/dl. Female: 0.03–0.1 μg/dl, 30–100 ng/dl.

Testosterone, a male sex hormone, is mostly responsible for male sex characteristics and masculinity. The highest serum testosterone level occurs in the morning.

Decreased level could indicate a testicular disorder, Klinefelter's syndrome, alcoholism, estrogen therapy, or hypopituitarism. An elevated level could indicate adrenal hyperplasia or tumor, benign prostatic hypertrophy (BPH), or adrenogenital syndrome in women.

Semen Examination: Semen content is useful for determining sperm count, volume of fluid, percentage of mature spermatozoa (sperms), and percentage of actively mobile sperm cells. This test is ordered to help identify the cause of infertility or to determine the effectiveness of sterilization after a vasectomy.

17-Ketosteroids (17-KS) (Urine): *Norms:* Adult: Male: 8–25 mg/24 h; over 65 years old: 4–8 mg/24 h. Female: 5–15 mg/24 h. Adolescent: Male: 3–15 mg/24 h.

17-KS are metabolites of male hormones from the adrenal cortex and testes. This test is useful in diagnosing adrenal cortex dysfunction and determining pituitary and gonadal hormone function. A decreased level could be indicative of hypogonadism and hypopituitarism. An elevated level could be indicative of adrenocortical hyperplasia or tumor, testicular tumor, hirsutism, or hyperpituitarism.

Cytogenetic Studies: *See Female Reproductive Assessment.*

Diagnostic Tests

Prostate (Transrectal) Ultrasound: Ultrasound of the prostate gland is used to evaluate palpable prostate nodules and urinary problems related to benign prostatic hypertrophy (BPH), to detect early small prostate tumors, and for use of biopsy and/or radiation.

Scrotum/Testes Ultrasound: Ultrasound of the scrotum sac contents is helpful in diagnosing abscess, cyst, hydrocele, spermatocele, varicocele, testicular tumors, and chronic scrotal swelling.

Pregnancy Assessment

Laboratory Tests

Human Chorionic Gonadotropin (HCG) (Serum and Urine): HCG, glycoprotein hormone, is produced by the trophoblast cell of placental tissue. Serum and urine HCG are early tests for confirming pregnancy. HCG tests are positive in pregnant women only and *not* in nonpregnant women. HCG is present 10 days after egg implantation or 14 to 26 days after conception. It peaks within 8 to 12 weeks.

Home Pregnancy Test Kits: Pregnancy kits were first introduced in 1976, and today there are several commercially prepared kits available for home use (i.e., Gravindex [Ortho Diagnostics], Prognosis [Roche], Early Pregnancy Test [EPT; Warner/Chicott], Daisy 2 [Bio Dynamics Home Healthcare], and First Response [Tambrands]). Some tests can be used to detect pregnancy as soon as the day of the first missed menstrual period. False readings can occur. If tests results are negative and menses has not begun a week later, it is suggested that the home pregnancy test be repeated.

Human Placental Lactogen (HPL) (Serum): *Norms:*

Weeks of Gestation	µg/ml
8–27	<4.6
28–31	2.4–6.0
32–35	3.7–7.7
36–40	5.0–10.0

HPL is produced by the placenta throughout pregnancy. The test is valuable to determine fetal well-being but should not be used as the only test. If HPL value falls below 4 µg/ml after 30 weeks, fetal distress might be present because of impaired placental function. If HPL value falls 50% during late pregnancy, fetal distress is apparent.

Estriol (E_3) (Serum and Urine): *Norms:*

SERUM		URINE	
Weeks of Gestation	ng/dl	Weeks of Gestation	mg/24 Hours
		16–24	2–6
25–28	25–165	25–28	6–28
29–32	30–230	29–32	6–32
33–36	45–370	33–36	10–45
37–38	75–420	37–40	15–60
39–40	95–450		

E_3 is a major estrogenic compound produced largely by the placenta. It increases in maternal serum and urine after 2 months of pregnancy and continues at high levels until term. If toxemia, hypertension, or diabetes is present after 30 weeks of gestation, E_3 levels are monitored. A decline in serum or urine E_3 levels suggests fetal distress caused by placental malfunction. The test may be repeated to confirm a suspected situation. A cesarean section may be indicated.

Estetrol (E_4) Plasma: *Weeks of Gestation:* 20 to 26 weeks: 140–210 pg/ml; 30 weeks: 350 pg/ml; 36 weeks: 900 pg/ml; 40 weeks: >1050 pg/ml.

A decreased estetrol level may indicate fetal distress and fetal malformation. Other tests to determine fetal distress should be done.

Progesterone (Serum): *Norms:* Pregnancy: >2400 ng/dl.

Progesterone is responsible for maintaining pregnancy after fertilization and for placental development. It has little value in evaluating fetal well-being but is useful in assessing placental function during pregnancy.

Pregnanediol (Urine): *Norms:* Pregnancy: 10–19 gestation weeks: 5–25 mg/24 h; 20–28 gestation weeks: 15–42 mg/24 h; 29–32 gestation weeks: 25–49 mg/24 h.

Pregnanediol measures the urinary metabolite of progesterone. At times urine pregnanediol may be of normal range even when fetal distress or fetal death has occurred.

Amino Acid Screen (Urine): Adult: 200 mg in 24 hours.

This test screens for elevated levels of amino acid in the urine (aminoaciduria), which can indicate inborn errors of metabolism.

α-1-Fetoprotein (AFP): *Norms:*

SERUM		AMNIOTIC FLUID	
Weeks of Gestation	**ng/ml**	**Weeks of Gestation**	**μg/ml**
8–12	0–39	14	11.0–32.0
13	6–31	15	5.5–31.0
14	7–50	16	5.7–31.5
15	7–60	17	3.8–32.5
16	10–72	18	3.6–28.0
17	11–90	19	3.7–24.5
18	14–94	20	2.2–15.0
19	24–112	21	3.6–18.0
20	31–122		
21	19–124		

Usually serum AFP is done between 16 and 20 weeks of gestation to detect probability of twins, risk of premature delivery or an infant of low birth weight, or serious birth defects such as open neural tube defect. It is a screening test, and if abnormal results occur, it should be repeated. If a high serum AFP level occurs, amniotic AFP may be done to diagnose neural tube defect in the fetus. Amniocentesis and ultrasound are required to confirm or to rule out the possible condition.

Genetic Defect Tests: Specific laboratory tests are designed to determine genetic disorders. Table 13 shows the defect, specimen, person from whom specimen was obtained, and findings.

Rubella Antibody Detection (Serum): *Norms:* Titer >1:64 protection against rubella or German measles.

TABLE 13 TESTS FOR GENETIC DEFECTS

Defect	Specimen	Person	Findings
Down's Syndrome	Amniotic fluid	Pregnant female	Trisomy 21 chromosome
Neural tube defects	Serum	Pregnant female	Increased serum AFP
	Amniotic fluid		Increased amniotic AFP
Tay-Sachs disease	Blood	Mother and father (as carriers)	Low level of enzyme hexosaminidase A
	Amniotic fluid	Pregnant female	
Sickle cell anemia	Blood	Mother and father (as carriers)	Hemoglobin S cells
	Cord blood	Newborn	
Galactosemia	Amniotic fluid	Pregnant female	Presence of galactose
Thalassemia (Cooley's or Mediterranean anemia)	Blood	Mother and father (as carriers)	Hemoglobin F cells
	Cord blood	Newborn	
Phenylketonuria (PKU)	Blood	Mother and father (as carriers)	Increased serum phenylalanine

The rubella antibody detection test is done prior to pregnancy or to check pregnant women during their first trimester of pregnancy at time of rubella exposure and again in 3 to 4 weeks.

Mumps Antibody Test (Serum): Negative or <1:8.

Mump virus could cause orchitis, oophoritis, or meningoencephalitis. If mumps occurs to the adolescent male, the possibility of sterility could occur.

Maternal Enzymes (Serum): During pregnancy there is an increase in maternal serum enzymes (i.e., heat-stable alkaline phosphatase [HSAP], diamine oxidase [DAO], and oxytocinase). Table 14 describes the maternal enzymes and their uses.

TABLE 14 MATERNAL ENZYMES

Maternal Enzyme	Comments
Heat-stable alkaline phosphatase (HSAP)	HSAP rises in concentration throughout pregnancy. A sudden rise in later pregnancy could indicate placental dysfunction and fetal distress or death. Usually a rise in HSAP occurs before a decrease in E_3.
Diamine oxidase (DAO)	This enzyme protects the pregnant female against histamine produced by the fetus. It rises during early pregnancy but tends to plateau during the third trimester.
Oxytocinase (cystyl-aminopeptidase)	Oxytocinase is produced by the placenta during pregnancy and inactivates oxytocin. It indicates placental function, not fetal well-being.

Blood Type and Rh Screening: Adult: Rh+ (positive); RH− (negative).

The Rh-negative pregnant female who carried a fetus that was Rh positive should receive Rho (D) immune globulin or RhoGAM by 72 hours after delivery or abortion to prevent Rh sensitization or Rh antibodies. This is important for prevention of erythroblastosis in future fetus. If the mother is Rh negative and unsensitized, some suggest that Rh immune globulin should be given at 28 weeks gestation.

Maternal blood type should be checked. If mother's type is O positive and the baby's type is A or B, there may be potential for ABO incompatibility after delivery.

Lecithin/Sphingomyelin (L/S) Ratio (Amniotic Fluid): *Norms:* Before 35 weeks of gestation: 1:1; after 35 weeks of gestation: 4:1. (L: 15–21 mg/dl; S: 4–6 mg/dl).

L/S ratio is a predictor of fetal pulmonary maturity before delivery. Lecithin is primarily responsible for the formation of alveolar surfactant that lubricates the alveolar lining and inhibits alveoli collapse. A marked rise in amniotic lecithin after 35 weeks is normal, thus decreasing chances for having hyaline membrane in respiratory distress syndrome. Pulmonary maturity occurs earlier in blacks than in caucasians.

Nitrazine Test: *Norms:* Intact Membranes: pH 5–6 (yellow to olive green). Ruptured Membranes: pH 6.5–7.5 (blue-green to deep blue).

This is a paper test to determine if the amniotic membrane is intact or has ruptured. The pH of amniotic fluid is 7 to 7.5, whereas the pH of vaginal secretions is 4.5 to 5.5.

Creatine Phosphokinase (CPK/CK) (Serum): *Norms:* Female: 5–25 μg/ml; 10–80 IU/l.

Decreased CPK/CK level might occur during the second trimester of pregnancy.

Renin (Plamsa): *Norms:* Upright: 1.6–4.3 ng/ml/h.

An elevated plasma renin level might occur during the first trimester of pregnancy, preeclampsia, and eclampsia. This could be due to a kidney problem.

Albumin (Serum): *Norms:* 3.5–5 g/dl.

Albumin levels may decrease by 0.5 to 1.0 g/dl. This could be due to increased plasma volume or acceleration of albumin degradation.

Hormone Changes: Thyroid, parathyroid, and adrenal hormone alterations usually accompany pregnancy. Table 15 shows the increases and decreases of these hormones during pregnancy.

Hematologic Changes: Hematologic values should be monitored during pregnancy. Changes in laboratory values are expected. Table 16 shows the expected changes of hematologic tests.

Rapid Plasma Reagin (RPR) (Serum): *Norms:* Nonreactive.

The RPR test is a rapid screening test for syphilis. A positive RPR should be verified by VDRL and/or FTA-ABS tests.

TABLE 15 HORMONAL CHANGES DURING PREGNANCY

Hormone	Changes	Comments
TBG	Increased markedly	Rise begins after fertilization and continues until 12 weeks of gestation. Failure of TBG rise might indicate hypothyroidism or estrogen deficiency.
T_4	Increased	T_4 rise is not as great as that of TBG.
Resin T_3 uptake	Decreased	T_3 uptake decreases slightly during pregnancy.
TSH	Normal	TSH remains normal in the euthyroid pregnant female.
ACTH	Decreased	Markedly decreased during first trimester of pregnancy.
Cortisol	Increased	Cortisol production slightly declines during pregnancy; however, the plasma half-life is increased. If cortisol value is in the normal range, adrenal hypofunction might be suspected.
Aldosterone	Increased	Aldosterone is increased throughout pregnancy, which increases plasma volume and sodium retention.
PTH	Increased	Reason unknown.

Herpes Simplex Virus (Type 2) (HSV-2) (Serum): HSV-2 is sexually transmitted and infects the urogenital tract. It also can be transmitted to the newborn during vaginal delivery. Neonatal herpes can result in minor to severe complications (e.g., from skin rash or eye infection to central nervous disorder). If the mother has active HSV-2 at the time of birth, a cesarean delivery may be indicated.

Cytogenetic Studies: *See Female Reproductive Assessment.*

Chlamydia Test (Serum, Tissue Smear, Culture): Serum: <1:16.

Chlamydia is bacterialike organism that resembles a virus. Chlamydia can be passed to the newborn during birthing and may result in blindness to the newborn if untreated. Untreated genital chlamydia infection could lead to sterility.

Cytomegalovirus Antibody (CMV) Serum: Negative to <0.30.

This virus belongs to the herpes virus family. If the pregnant woman is infected with CMV, the fetus may become infected. In infants this virus could cause cerebral tissue malformation and/or damage.

Diagnostic Tests

Amniocentesis, Amniotic Fluid Analysis: The purposes for analysis of amniotic fluid are to detect chromosomal abnormalities such as Down's syndrome (trisomy 21), neural tube defects, sex-linked disorders, and fetal and pulmonary

TABLE 16 HEMATOLOGIC CHANGES DURING PREGNANCY

Blood Tests	Changes	Comments
Red blood cells (RBCs)	Increased	RBC mass increases slightly during pregnancy even with increased plasma volume.
Hemoglobin and hematocrit	Decreased	Plasma volume increase causes hemodilution.
Platelets	Slightly decreased or normal value	Decreased platelet count could result from increased plasma volume.
Reticulocytes	Increased	There is a slight rise in reticulocytes during the second trimester of pregnancy.
White blood cells (WBCs)	Increased	Slightly elevated WBCs. During the last half of pregnancy, granulocytes increase and lymphocytes remain unchanged.
Fibrinogen	Increased	Fibrinogen level increases throughout pregnancy.
Plasminogen	Increased	Reason unknown.
Prothrombin time (PT) and partial thromboplastin time (PTT)	Slightly decreased or normal	Reason unknown.
Erythrocyte sedimentation rate (ESR)	Increased	ESR increases markedly because of increase in fibrinogen level.
Folate (folic acid)	Decreased	Mother's tissues absorb more folic acid.
Vitamin B_{12}	Decreased	Mother's tissues absorb more vitamin B_{12}.
Iron	Decreased	Fetal use and increased plasma volume (hemodilution).

maturity. *See Female Reproductive Assessment above and Amniotic Fluid Analysis (Part II).*

Pelvic Ultrasonography: The numerous uses for pelvic ultrasound are to detect multiple fetuses or fetal anomalies; to determine the location of the placenta (rule out placenta previa) or fetal and placenta locations during an amniocentesis; and to evaluate fetal viability, gestational age, and fetal growth. This test procedure is considered noninvasive because contrast media is *not* used.

Fetal Nonstress Test (NST): The NST as well as the contraction stress test (CST) are performed to evaluate the viability of the fetus and the function of the placenta to provide adequate blood flow. NST is a noninvasive test that monitors fetal heart rate with fetal movement. The CST can be an invasive test with the use of oxytocin, a uterine stimulant. The CST with oxytocin is usually not performed before 32 weeks.

Fetoscopy: This endoscopic procedure uses a fetoscope that is inserted through the abdominal wall into the uterine cavity for direct visualization and to obtain blood samples from the blood vessel in the umbilical cord. It is usually performed during the 18th week of gestation. This procedure is useful for detecting neural tube defect, sickle cell anemia, and hemophilia.

External Fetal Monitoring: External fetal monitoring records the fetal heart rate and uterine contractions. It is considered a noninvasive test. It can be used as a nonstress test to determine fetal well-being during stressful and nonstressful conditions. Also it can be used as a stress test using oxytocin to determine fetal well-being.

Internal Fetal Monitoring: This is an invasive procedure in which an electrode is attached to the scalp of the fetus to measure fetal heart rate and a catheter is placed in the uterine cavity to measure uterine contractions. Internal fetal monitoring is performed during labor after the membranes have ruptured. It is indicated when external fetal monitoring provides inadequate information.

Breast Massage Stress Test: Breast massage is a relative new contraction stress test (CST) for assessing fetal well-being in high-risk pregnancies. If a nonstress test is *not* effective in determining fetal well-being, then a CST is indicated. CST can be done using the standard stress test with IV infusion of oxytocin or breast massage.

Neonate Assessment

Laboratory Tests

Glucose (Blood): *Norms:* .40 mg/dl.

Neonatal hypoglycemia may occur 4 to 6 hours after birth. Chemstrip bG and Dextrostix are useful for monitoring blood glucose in the newborn. Blood sugar falls rapidly during the first few hours of life but stabilizes in 6 hours in the healthy newborn. Newborns who are at high risk (e.g., born of diabetic mothers, erythroblastotic newborns, or pregnant women taking terbutaline) should have blood glucose monitored closely. In some institutions Chemstrip bG is used as a routine screening test for all newborns.

Cord Blood: At the time of birth a blood sample from the umbilical cord is tested for blood type and Rh (factor) antibody titer.

Bilirubin: Neonatal (Blood): *Norms:* <12 mg/dl. *Critical Range:* 15 mg/dl.

Blood is drawn from the newborn's heel by means of a capillary pipette.

Neonatal jaundice could be due to erythroblastosis fetalis, hemorrhage, or physiologic jaundice (caused by increased RBC breakdown and immature liver cells). Repeated heel stick may be needed to monitor bilirubin levels in the newborn.

Phenylketonuria (PKU) (Urine) or Phenylalanine (Blood): *Norms:* 1–3 mg/dl (blood). *Critical Range:* >4 mg/dl.

Blood phenylalanine is checked 48 to 120 hours after birth following milk or protein feedings. A positive test indicates that the newborn lacks the enzyme needed to metabolize phenylalanine, an amino acid found in protein foods.

PKU testing of the urine is done between 2 and 4 weeks of life. Phenistix (Ames) is a dipstick for testing the infant's urine for PKU. Green color is an indicator of a positive PKU test.

TORCH Test (TORCH Screen, TORCH Battery, TORCH Titer): TORCH stands for toxoplasma, rubella, cytomegalovirus, and herpes virus. It is used to determine the presence or exposure of a TORCH agent that could cause congenital or neonatal infections, which could result in central nervous system (CNS) impairment. The test identifies past infection, immunity, or recent infection. It can be done on pregnant women as well as newborns and infants. The number of TORCH testings has grown, with more than 20 TORCH kits produced for laboratory and health care provider's use. Accuracy of test results has been questioned, as there is often a variation in TORCH titers.

Trypsin (Feces): Positive in small amounts in the stool.
A child with cystic fibrosis, the test result is negative at dilution >1:10.

Herpes Simplex Virus (HSV) Serum: Negative or <1:10.
Herpes simplex virus-2 (HSV-2) is referred to as genital herpes, which primarily infects the genitourinary tract. HSV-2 is transmitted primarily through sexual contact, and the virus can infect the newborn during vaginal delivery. This can cause neonatal herpes.

Toxoplasmosis Antibody (Serum): No previous infection: <1:4.
Congenital form of toxoplasmosis occurs to the fetus when the mother is acutely infected with the *Toxoplasma gondii (T. gondii)* during pregnancy and passes the organism via placenta to the unborn child. *T. gondii* is transmitted via raw or poorly cooked meat or by feces from infected cats (litter box).

NURSING DIAGNOSES

- Anxiety related to health status and the unknown.
- Deficient knowledge related to a lack of understanding of laboratory and diagnostic procedures, disease process, and/or outcome of pregnancy.
- Noncompliance to prescribed laboratory and diagnostic tests related to a lack of or inadequate explanation and/or anxiety about physical condition.
- Ineffective coping with laboratory and diagnostic test procedures.
- Excess fluid volume related to hormonal changes as evidenced by fluid retention.
- Altered comfort related to the procedure as evidenced by back hurting when lying flat for various test procedures.
- Impaired urinary elimination related to bladder compression by enlarged pregnant uterus.
- Anxiety related to the consequences of the tests that could result in alterations in parenting, coping, and self-concept.
- Impaired parenting related to a lack of effective coping mechanisms.

- Risk for sexual dysfunction related to altered body structure or function, including pregnancy, disease process, and/or diagnostic procedure.

NURSING IMPLICATIONS WITH RATIONALE

- Explain that the purpose for the laboratory and diagnostic tests is to aid in establishing baseline data regarding previous male or female disease, existing disease, predisposition to disease, or complications in pregnancy.
- Give an explanation (in detail if indicated) about the laboratory and diagnostic procedures. Emphasize the importance of the client's compliance with the test procedure *(see procedures for individual tests in Parts I and II)*.
- Assess the client's communication for verbal and/or nonverbal expressions of anxiety or fear concerning tests and/or potential sexual problems.
- Determine if the anxiety level needs to be reduced before the client will be able to absorb information concerning test procedure.
- Encourage expression of feelings through provision of private, calm environment; use quiet, steady speech patterns when interacting; and employ touch if appropriate.
- Be prepared to repeat information to the client and family briefly and clearly if the anxiety or fear level is determined to be high. Attempt not to appear irritated with the client's behavior; plan time to be with the client.
- Answer questions, or refer the questions to appropriate health professionals.
- Check laboratory results, and report the abnormal test findings.

Evaluation

- Determine if the test was correctly performed according to the procedure. Notify the laboratory and/or health care provider of any changes that occur during the test.
- Check the client's vital signs and fetal heart rate for changes.
- Provide ongoing assessment before, during, and after the procedure. Document and communicate any alteration.
- Determine if support measures to the client and family have been effective.
- Evaluate the status of the client's anxiety and fear in regard to the tests or problems related to pregnancy or infertility.
- Clarify or answer any additional questions the client and family members might have.

Arthritic and collagen conditions

Laboratory Tests	
Rheumatoid Arthritis	**Lupus Erythematosus**
RA Factor	Lupus Erythematosus (LE) Cells
ESR/Sed Rate	ANA
CRP	Anti-DNA
Complements C_3, C_4	Complements C_3, C_4
ASO	Cryoglobulins
Cryoglobulins	RA Factor
Parvovirus B19 Antibody	Synovial Fluid Analysis
Synovial Fluid Analysis	Hydroxyproline (Urine)

Introduction

The majority of laboratory tests for arthritic and collagen disorders are to confirm the diagnosis or progression of rheumatoid arthritis and lupus erythematosus. Several of the same laboratory tests are ordered for both suspected conditions; these tests are complements C_3, C_4, and rheumatoid arthritis (RA) factor; cryoglobulins; and synovial fluid analysis.

Rheumatoid Arthritis

Laboratory Tests

Rheumatoid Factor (RF), Rheumatoid Arthritis (RA) Factor: *Norms:* Adult: <1:20 titer, >1:80 positive for rheumatoid arthritis.

RA factor is a screening test used to detect antiglobulin antibodies in clients with suspected rheumatoid arthritis. It is not uncommon to have positive RA factor test results in clients with collagen diseases (e.g., lupus erythematosus). Approximately 75% of those with rheumatoid arthritis have a positive RA factor. Other tests are needed to confirm diagnosis.

Erythrocyte Sedimentation Rate (ESR, Sed Rate) (Serum): *Norms: See reference values in Part I.*

Sed rate, or ESR, is a nonspecific test that usually increases during an acute inflammatory process. Frequently the ESR is elevated in clients with rheumatoid arthritis; however, it is not the most reliable test. C-reactive protein (CRP) test is considered more useful than ESR.

C-Reactive Protein (CRP) (Serum): *Norms:* Not usually present; >1:2 titer considered positive.

CRP is a nonspecific test similar to ESR; however, during an inflammatory process, CRP elevates sooner than ESR and returns to normal faster than ESR. This test is useful in monitoring the progression of rheumatoid arthritis.

Complements C_3 and C_4 (Serum): *Norms:* C_3: Adult: 83–177 mg/dl. C_4: Adult: 15–45 mg/dl.

Both C_3 and C_4 could be slightly elevated in clients with rheumatoid arthritis.

Antistreptolysin O (ASO) (Serum): *Norms:* Adult: <100 IU/ml.

Serum ASO levels can be mildly elevated in clients with rheumatoid arthritis.

Cryoglobulins (Serum): *Norms:* Negative.

Cryoglobulins are proteins that are present in the immunoglobulins IgG and IgM. They may be present in rheumatoid arthritis and also in systemic lupus erythematosus.

Parvovirus B 19 Antibody (Serum): *Norms:* Negative.

A positive parvovirus B 19 has been associated with joint inflammation and joint arthritis.

Synovial Fluid Analysis: Examination of the synovial fluid for rheumatoid factor, complements, leukocytes (white blood cells), and glucose gives additional information about the possibility of the presence of rheumatoid arthritis. In rheumatoid arthritis, synovial fluid analysis could include a positive RA factor, decreased complements because of complement binding, slightly elevated leukocyte count, and decreased glucose level.

Lupus Erythematosus

Laboratory Tests

Lupus Erythematosus (LE) Cell Test: The LE cell test is an in vitro procedure used either to aid in the diagnosis of systemic lupus erythematosus (SLE) or to monitor the treatment for this condition. It is not the most reliable test; however, LE cells can be found in 60% to 80% of clients with SLE. If it is used for the purpose of diagnosing SLE, then other laboratory tests, such as antinuclear antibodies (ANA) and anti-DNA, should be ordered to confirm SLE.

Antinuclear Antibodies (ANA) (Serum): *Norms:* Negative.

The ANA test for assessing tissue-antigen antibodies is frequently used for diagnosing SLE. A positive titer can indicate SLE; however, other clinical conditions such as rheumatoid arthritis, scleroderma, myasthenia gravis, and infectious mononucleosis may have positive titers.

Anti-Deoxyribonucleic Acid (Anti-DNA): Anti-DNA, an antinuclear antibody, is almost always present in SLE and is in lupus nephritis 95% of the time. Anti-DNA values may fluctuate according to the remission and exacerbation of the disease.

Complements C_3 and C_4 (Serum): *Norms: See complements under Rheumatoid Arthritis.*

C_3 and C_4 of the complement system (group of 11 serum proteins) are measured during acute and/or chronic inflammatory process. In SLE, both serum C_3 and C_4 will be decreased.

Cryoglobulins (Serum): *Norms:* Negative.

Positive cryoglobulin findings may be reported in clients with SLE. Cryoglobulins are also present in other conditions, such as rheumatoid arthritis, multiple myeloma, and leukemia.

Rheumatoid Factor (RF, RA Factor) (Serum): *Norms:* 1:20–1:80 positive for collagen diseases.

Even though RA factor is a serum test used to detect antibodies in clients with rheumatoid arthritis, positive findings are common in clients with collagen disease (e.g., SLE, scleroderma).

Synovial Fluid Analysis: Examination of synovial fluid might reveal positive LE cells and decreased complement levels in patients with SLE.

Hydroxyproline (Urine): Adult: 15–42 mg/24 h, 0.4–4.5mg/2 h. Child: Higher than adult.

Urine hydroxyproline levels increase with collagen breakdown such as with bone destruction. Levels are higher at night, in teenagers, and during the third trimester of pregnancy.

NURSING DIAGNOSES

- Deficient knowledge related to a lack of understanding of the laboratory test procedure, disease process, and/or outcome.
- Noncompliance with prescribed laboratory and diagnostic tests related to lack of adequate explanation.
- Fear related to disability (RA), kidney impairment (LE), and/or dependence on others.
- Impaired physical mobility related to stiff, swollen, painful joints secondary to rheumatoid arthritis.
- Situational low self-esteem related to dependence and/or role change.

NURSING IMPLICATIONS WITH RATIONALE

- Explain the purpose of the laboratory tests.
- Give an explanation concerning the test procedures and the need for the client's compliance. Explanation might be brief or in-depth, depending on the client's familiarity with the test.
- Inform the client of any food, fluid, or drug restrictions *(see Part I)*.
- Assess urinary output in clients with SLE.
- Assess the client's ability to ambulate. Elicit from the client the times of day when mobility is not as much of a problem.

- Listen to the client's expressed anxiety concerning tests and potential clinical problems. Clarification of test procedures might alleviate fear and anxiety and promote test compliance.
- Be supportive of the client and family members and answer questions or refer the questions to appropriate professionals.

Evaluation

- Determine if the test was correctly performed according to the procedure. Notify the laboratory and health care provider of any changes that occur during the test.
- Determine if the client and family members' fear and/or anxiety have been lessened or alleviated.
- Clarify or answer any additional questions the client and family members might have.
- Encourage the client to contact resources for additional information and support. Examples are Arthritis Foundation, Meals on Wheels, and others as related to the client's needs.
- Develop an activity and care plan with the client and family members.

Shock

Laboratory Tests	Diagnostic Tests
Electrolytes (Serum)	ECG/EKG
Lactic Acid (Serum)	Central Venous Pressure (CVP)
Anion Gap	Pulmonary Arterial Pressure (PAP)
Glucose (Blood/plasma)	Pulmonary Capillary Wedge Pressure
Osmolality (Serum)	(PCWP)
CBC (Hg, Hct, WBC, Platelets)	X-rays, Chest or Abdominal
Type and Cross Match (T&C) CT	
ABGs	
Enzymes (Cardiac)	
BUN	
Creatinine (Serum)	
Protein (Total) (Serum)	
Fibrin Degradation Products (Serum)	
Euglobulin Lysis Time (Plasma)	
PT and PTT	
Urinalysis (Specific Gravity)	
Urine Electrolytes	

Introduction

Laboratory and diagnostic assessment of shock is extremely important for evaluation and management of shock syndrome. Laboratory studies, ordered immediately, usually include electrolytes, lactic acid/lactate, glucose, osmolality, complete blood count (CBC), type and cross match, and arterial blood gases. Other laboratory tests used to determine the state and progression of shock include serum enzymes, especially if cardiogenic shock is likely, blood urea nitrogen (BUN), creatinine, total protein, prothrombin time, and urine electrolytes. Diagnostic tests performed to determine cardiac and circulatory status are electrocardiogram (ECG), central venous pressure (CVP) or pulmonary arterial pressure (PAP), and x-ray. Later computed tomography (CT) might be ordered.

Laboratory Tests

Electrolytes (Serum): Serum electrolytes—potassium, sodium, and calcium—are closely monitored during shock. Changes in electrolytes can occur quickly, such as in the levels of potassium and sodium. Table 17 shows the electrolytes associated with shock, with reasons for their decreases and increases.

Lactic Acid, Lactate (Blood): *Norms:* Adult: 0.5–2.0 mmol/l, 5–20 mg/dl.

Elevated blood lactic acid is related to cellular hypoxia. In shock, lactic acid/lactate levels increase greatly and quickly, >5 mmol/l or >25 mg/dl, before blood pressure (BP) falls and urine output decreases. Lactic acidosis occurs when blood lactic acid level is >2.5 mmol/l or >25 mg/dl. As lactic acid level increases, cells need more oxygen.

Anion Gap: 10–17 mEq/l.

Anion gap is an interrelationship between serum electrolytes in determining metabolic acid-base imbalances. An elevated anion gap >17 mEq/l is indicative of metabolic acidosis, a complication of shock. Formula for calculating anion gap is:

$$(sodium + potassium) - (chloride + CO_2) = mEq/l$$

Glucose (Blood, Plasma): *Norms:* Adult: Blood: 60–100 mg/dl. Plasma: 70–110 mg/dl. Child: 60–100 mg/dl. Newborn: 30–80 mg/dl.

During acute trauma and shock, blood/plasma glucose levels could rise to 200 mg/dl. After correction of shock, hypoglycemia could result. An elevated glucose level occurs as the result of an increase in epinephrine and steroid response because of tissue damage.

Osmolality (Serum): *Norms:* Adult: 280–300 mOsm/kg. Child: 270–290 mOsm/kg.

Serum osmolality is an indicator of body fluid concentration, mainly the vascular fluid. If shock is due to massive fluid loss, serum osmolality is increased, and fluid replacement is necessary. Care should be taken not to administer massive fluids for mild shock, because overhydration could result. In overhydration, a low serum osmolality occurs.

Complete Blood Count (CBC) (Blood): Abnormal hematology values in hemoglobin (Hgb/Hb), hematocrit (Hct), white blood cell count, and platelet count can

TABLE 17 ELECTROLYTE CHANGES

Electrolyte (Serum)	Reference Values	Comments
Potassium (K)	3.5–5.3 mEq/l	During shock, potassium leaves the cells because of tissue injury and hypoxia. If urinary output is adequate, potassium is excreted by the kidneys, thus causing a serum potassium loss, or hypokalemia. If kidney shutdown occurs during shock, potassium builds up in the vascular fluid, causing serum potassium excess, or hyperkalemia.
Sodium (Na)	135–145 mEq/l	Serum sodium level can be normal, decreased, or elevated. During cellular damage, potassium shifts out of the cells and sodium shifts in, contributing to the serum sodium loss, or hyponatremia. Also in massive tissue injury, sodium goes to the injured site. If the client is receiving liters of saline solutions and kidney shutdown occurs, serum sodium level is increased and hypernatremia occurs.
Calcium (Ca)	4.5–5.5 mEq/l	With massive tissue damage, calcium leaves the extracellular fluid and accumulates at the injured site, causing serum calcium deficit, or hypocalcemia. A calcium loss will increase cellular permeability, thus permitting electrolyte and fluid loss from cells.
Ionizing Calcium (iCa)	4.4–5.0 mg/dl, 2.2–2.5 mEq/l	Only ionized calcium can be used by the body. A decrease in iCa leads to tetany symptoms or neuromuscular irritability.
Chloride (Cl)	95–105 mEq/l	Chloride combines with sodium and potassium, and as these cations are lost, so is chloride. Result is hypochloremia.

occur in shock. Therefore a CBC is taken in early shock and is monitored for changes during treatment and recovery. Table 18 shows the changes that can occur with these four blood values in shock.

Type and Cross Match (T&C): Although method for type and cross match is more expedient today, blood sample for T&C should be obtained immediately when blood loss and shock are determined.

Arterial Blood Gases (ABGs): *Norms:* Adult: pH: 7.35–7.45; $PaCO_2$: 35–45 mm Hg; PaO_2: 75–100 mm Hg; HCO_3: 24–28 mEq/l; BE: +2 or −2.

715

TABLE 18 COMPLETE BLOOD COUNT

Hematology	Reference Values	Comments
Hgb	Male: 13.5–18.0 g/dl Female: 12–16 g/dl Child: 11–16 g/dl	Hemoglobin levels decrease after hemorrhage, but change may not occur until hours later.
Hct	Male: 40%–54% Female: 36%–46%	Hematocrit is an effective indicator of body fluid volume. If shock is due to a large fluid loss, increased hematocrit level occurs because of hemoconcentration. It usually takes 4–8 hours for the hematocrit to increase after fluid loss.
WBC	Adult: 5000–10,000 µl Child, 2 years old: 6000–17,000 µl	If WBC levels are slightly increased, the change could be due to tissue damage. If levels are markedly increased, the change could be due to infection.
Platelet count	Adult: 150,000–400,000 µl	Platelet count is monitored during and after blood loss and acute trauma. A low platelet count, thrombocytopenia, will cause bleeding. If platelet count is markedly decreased, hemorrhage might occur. Shock is intensified.

In shock, ABGs are helpful in evaluating respiratory and metabolic status. Normally metabolic acidosis occurs in shock as the result of tissue breakdown (release of acid metabolites from cells). Indicators of acidosis are pH <7.35, HCO_3 <24 mEq/l, PCO_2 of >45 mm Hg. If the pH is <7.35 and the HCO_3 is <24 mEq/l, *metabolic* acidosis is present. If the pH is <7.35 and the $Paco_2$ is >45 mm Hg, *respiratory* acidosis is present.

Enzymes: CPK/CK, LDH/lD, AST/SGOT (Serum): Norms: *See individual reference values in Part I.*

Cardiac enzyme levels are obtained when cardiac damage is suspected and in cardiogenic shock. After a myocardial infarction, serum CPK/CK rises first, then serum AST/SGOT, and last LDH/lD.

Blood Urea Nitrogen (BUN): Norms: Adult: 5–25 mg/dl.

BUN should be assessed during shock. A BUN of 30 to 40 mg/dl could be indicative of fluid loss and dehydration. If the BUN is >50 mg/dl and does not decrease substantially with the administration of IV fluids, kidney damage is highly suspected. Renal insufficiency or failure can result from prolonged shock.

Creatinine (Serum): Norms: Adult: 0.5–1.5 mg/dl. Older Child: 0.4–1.2 mg/dl. Infant to 6 Years: 0.3–0.6 mg/dl.

The laboratory test most effective in evaluating kidney function is serum creatinine. As kidney function diminishes, serum creatinine level rises. Creatinine level >3 mg/dl is indicative of kidney disorder.

Protein (Total) (Serum): Total protein count is composed mostly of albumin and globulins. With severe body fluid loss, elevated serum protein (total) level could be present because of hemoconcentration.

Fibrin Degradation Products (FDP) (Serum): *Norms:* Adult: 2–10 μg/ml.

FDP test indicates the activity of the fibrinolytic system. This test is performed when the client is hemorrhaging following a severe injury. An elevated FDP, >10 μg/ml, is usually indicative of DIC.

Euglobulin Lysis Time (Plasma): No lysis.

This test measures the fibrinogen activity by measuring the interval between clot formation and euglobulin precipitation. If clot lysis is less than 1 hour, pathologic fibrinolysis is occurring.

Prothrombin Time (PT) and Partial Thromboplastin Time (PTT) (Plasma): *Norms:* Adult: PT: 11–15 seconds; PTT: 60–70 seconds.

PT and PTT are ordered to evaluate clotting time. With prolonged PT and PTT times, bleeding can occur. These levels usually are monitored during shock.

Urinalysis/Specific Gravity (SG): In shock, clients frequently have a Foley catheter inserted, and so urine specific gravity can easily be checked. A specific gravity >1.026 is indicative of fluid volume deficit (dehydration). In certain renal diseases (e.g., glomerulonephritis, polynephritis), the specific gravity is <1.005.

Urine Electrolytes (Potassium and Sodium): *Norms:* Adult: Potassium: 40–80 mEq/24 h (average). Sodium: 40–220 mEq/l/24 h.

In renal failure the urine potassium and sodium levels could be increased (chronic failure) or decreased (acute failure). Urine electrolytes are frequently monitored.

Diagnostic Tests

Electrocardiography (ECG/EKG): ECG can detect cardiac changes occurring prior to or following shock. It is performed immediately in suspected cardiogenic shock.

Central Venous Pressure (CVP): *Norms:* Adult: 4–10 cm of H_2O.

CVP is monitored during shock to determine fluid imbalance. A decreased CVP is indicative of hypovolemia (fluid volume deficit), and an increased CVP is indicative of hypervolemia (fluid volume excess). As an indicator of left ventricular pressure, CVP is not as accurate as pulmonary arterial pressure (PAP) but is considered safer and accompanied by fewer complications.

Pulmonary Arterial Pressure (PAP) and Pulmonary Capillary Wedge Pressure (PCWP): *Norms:* Adult: PAP: 10–20 mm Hg mean, 20–30 mm Hg systolic, 10–15 mm Hg diastolic; PCWP: 4–12 mm Hg mean.

PAP indicates the pulmonary blood volume and the pulmonary vascular resistance. A low PAP is indicative of fluid volume deficit (hypovolemia) or vasodilation, and an elevated PAP is indicative of fluid volume overload or increased pulmonary vascular resistance, possibly due to pulmonary embolism. A decreased PCWP is indicative of fluid volume deficit (hypovolemia). An elevated PCWP can occur in fluid volume overload (hypervolemia) because of excess IV fluids or because of increased preload from fluid retention in cardiac failure. Increased afterload, vascular resistance to left ventricular ejection, will also increase PCWP.

X-Rays: Chest or abdominal x-rays at a suspected trauma site might be helpful in detecting cause of shock.

Computed Tomography (CT): Emergency CT might be ordered to determine cause of shock.

NURSING DIAGNOSES

- Noncompliance to prescribed laboratory and diagnostic tests related to a lack of understanding and adherence to the procedures.
- Anxiety related to fear of death and the unknown.
- Ineffective coping with disease process and laboratory and diagnostic test procedures.
- Deficient fluid volume related to loss of body fluid and blood, inadequate circulation, or body-fluid volume shift.
- Ineffective tissue perfusion related to ineffective blood circulation, loss of blood, or hypotension.
- Impaired patterns of elimination (renal) related to inadequate circulation and hypotension.
- Ineffective breathing patterns related to dyspnea, anxiety, pain, or impaired gas exchange secondary to trauma.

NURSING IMPLICATIONS WITH RATIONALE

- Explain the purpose of the laboratory and diagnostic tests briefly to the client and family members. A detailed explanation during a crisis might not be appropriate.
- Obtain a blood sample collection and send it to the laboratory immediately. Check that results are returned and report abnormal results.
- Monitor the client's intake and output and vital signs before and after laboratory and diagnostic tests and at specified times. Report changes immediately.
- Listen to the client's and family members' expressed anxiety and/or fear concerning the tests and the client's outcome from trauma.
- Assess for excess bleeding and apply pressure if appropriate. Report changes.
- Be supportive of the client and family members during and after the crisis.

Evaluation

- Determine if the test was correctly performed according to the procedure. Notify the laboratory of any changes that occur during the test.
- Check the client's urinary output and vital signs for changes and improvement.
- Determine if the client's and family members' anxiety and fear have been lessened or alleviated. Continue being supportive of the client and family members.
- Clarify or answer any additional questions the client and family members might have.

Neoplastic conditions

Laboratory Tests

ACTH (Plasma)
ADH (Serum)
Bence-Jones Protein (Urine)
Bilirubin (Serum)
Calcitonin (Serum)
Calcium (Serum)
Carcinoembryonic Antigen (Plasma)
Catecholamines (Plasma)
Ceruloplasmin (Serum
Cold Agglutinins (Serum)
Complements C_3, C_4 (Serum)
Copper (Serum)
Cortisol (Plasma)
C-Reactive Protein (Serum)
Cryoglobulins (Serum)
Cytology: sputum, gastric washing, colon, pleural fluid, bronchial secretions, urine, Pap smear, CSF
Enzymes: ACP, ALP, ALT/SGPT, AST/SGOT, GGTP, LDH, LAP
ESR (Blood)
Estradiol (E_2) (Serum)
Estrogen/Total (Serum and Urine)
FSH (Serum and Urine)
Gastrin (Serum)
Haptoglobin (Serum)
HCG (Serum, Urine)

Diagnostic Tests

X-rays: Chest, Bone, GI Series, Barium Enema, IVP, Bronchography
Mammography
Thermography
Lymphangiography
Thoracoscopy
Endoscopy: bronchoscopy, esophagogastroscopy, proctosigmoidoscopy, colonoscopy, colposcopy, cystoscopy, ERCP
Electronystagmography
Ultrasonography/Ultrasound
Nuclear Scans
Monoclonal Antibodies for Colon and Ovarian
CT
Angiography/Arteriography
Biopsy
Bone Marrow Aspiration
MRI

(*continued*)

Laboratory Tests	Diagnostic Tests
5-HIAA (Urine)	
Immunoglobins (Serum)	
17-KS (Urine)	
LH (Serum)	
Melanin (Urine)	
Occult Blood (Feces)	
PTH (Serum)	
PTT (Plasma)	
Platelet Count (Blood)	
Pregnanediol (Urine)	
Pregnanetriol (Urine)	
Prolactin (Serum)	
Prostate-Specific Antigen (PSA) (Serum)	
Protein Electrophoresis (Serum)	
Renin (Plasma)	
Serotonin (Plasma)	
Testosterone (Serum)	
Thyroid Antibodies (Serum)	
Uric Acid (Serum)	
WBC/leukocytes (Blood)	

Introduction

Numerous laboratory and diagnostic tests are performed to identify and to confirm the presence of cancer (i.e., carcinomas, sarcomas, leukemias, lymphomas). One test only is not sufficient to diagnose cancer. Although most laboratory tests are ordered to determine function of body organs and glands, there are many elevated and decreased test values associated with cancer. Usually diagnostic tests are necessary to confirm cancer site and diagnosis. In this section abnormal laboratory values, elevated or decreased, as they relate to cancer are given instead of the norms for the test. Laboratory tests are arranged in alphabetic order. Refer to Part I for the reference values of these laboratory tests.

A summarized chart of laboratory and diagnostic tests used for diagnosing specific cancers follows the brief description of the tests.

Laboratory Tests

Antidiuretic Hormone (ADH) (Serum): ADH may be elevated, >5 pg/ml in syndrome of secretion of inappropriate antidiuretic hormone (SIADH) as a result of ectopic secretion by bronchogenic carcinoma.

Adrenocorticotropic Hormone (ACTH) (Plasma): Decreased plasma ACTH could occur in clients with cancer of the adrenal gland, and elevated plasma ACTH could occur in clients with pituitary tumor. ACTH could be elevated with any tumor that secretes ACTH ectopically (e.g., bronchogenic carcinoma).

Bence-Jones Protein (Urine): Increased Bence-Jones protein >1.0 mg/dl is commonly found in the urine of clients with multiple myeloma, and increased levels are also associated with metastatic carcinoma, bone cancer, and leukemia.

Bilirubin: Total (Serum): Elevated serum total bilirubin >1.2 mg/dl could occur in clients with tumors of the liver or liver metastasis. Elevated bilirubin level could occur in pancreatic carcinoma secondary to common duct obstruction.

Calcitonin (hCT) (Serum): A high serum calcitonin level, >2000 pg/ml, indicates thyroid medullary carcinoma.

Calcium (Serum): Hypercalcemia, elevated serum calcium level >5.5 mEq/l or >11 mg/dl, occurs in 10% to 20% of all cancer clients. Metastatic tumors can cause bone destruction, which elevates the serum calcium level. Common causes of hypercalcemia are metastatic breast cancer, multiple myeloma, ectopic secretion of parathyroid hormone (PTH), and bony metastasis.

Carcinoembryonic Antigen (CEA) (Blood, Plasma): CEA has been extracted from tumors in the gastrointestinal (GI) tract. CEA has been frequently found in clients with cancer of the large intestine and pancreas. Plasma CEA might be elevated in other cancers (e.g., esophagus, stomach, lung, breast, bladder, kidney, cervix, testes, and leukemia). CEA is used to evaluate the effectiveness of cancer therapies and to monitor clients in remission for early signs of recurrence. CEA will be increased before clinical symptoms are evident.

Catecholamines (Plasma): *See Plasma Catecholamine in Part I.* *Epinephrine:* Supine: <50 pg/ml. *Norepinephrine:* Supine: 110–410 pg/ml.

Fractional analysis of catecholamine levels is helpful for identifying certain adrenal medullary tumors.

Ceruloplasmin (Cp) (Serum): Cp is produced in the liver and binds with copper. An elevated serum ceruloplasmin level >50 mg/dl could occur in clients with cancer of the bone, stomach, or lung and in clients with Hodgkin's disease.

Cold Agglutinins (CA) (Serum): Elevated serum CA, >1:16 to 1:32, might be present in lymphatic leukemia and multiple myeloma.

Complements C_3, C_4 (Serum): Elevated serum C_3 and C_4 could be found with malignant neoplasms of the esophagus, stomach, colon, rectum, pancreas, lungs, breast, cervix, ovary, prostate, and bladder.

Copper (Cu) (Serum): Elevated serum copper levels >140 μg/dl (male) might be present in cancer of the bone, stomach, large intestine, liver, and lung, and in Hodgkin's disease and leukemias.

Cortisol (Plasma): Plasma cortisol level could be elevated with cancer of the adrenal gland.

C-Reactive Protein (CRP) (Serum): Positive CRP titer might occur with cancer of the breast with metastasis. Clients with Hodgkin's disease might also have positive CRP titer.

Cryoglobulins (Serum): Positive cryoglobulin findings might be present in clients having Hodgkin's disease, lymphocytic leukemia, or multiple myeloma.

Cytology: Cells that have been sloughed from neoplasms/tumors can be found in body secretions. These secretions are obtained from sputum, gastric washing, colon, pleural fluid, bronchial tract, urine, Pap smear, and cerebrospinal (CSF) for cytologic examination.

Enzymes: When cancer affects organs that produce enzymes, enzyme values are checked. The enzyme *acid phosphatase (ACP)* is plentiful in the prostate gland, and an elevated serum ACP level usually indicates carcinoma of the prostate gland. If ACP is markedly elevated, metastasis to the bone is suspected. Also elevated serum ACP can be associated with multiple myeloma and Paget's disease. The enzyme *alkaline phosphatase (ALP),* produced by the bone and liver, is usually elevated in clients with cancer of the bone and liver. An elevated ALP might occur in clients with multiple myeloma. *Alanine aminotransferase (ALT/SGPT)* and *aspartate aminotransferase (AST/SGOT)* might be noted in clients with cancer of the liver. *Gamma-glutamyl (transpeptidase) transferase (GGT)* could be elevated in cancer of the liver, kidney, pancreas, prostate, breast, lung, and brain. Elevated *lactic dehydrogenase (LD/lDH)* might occur in clients with cancer of the lung, bone, intestines, liver, breast, cervix, testes, kidney, stomach, and melanoma of the skin. Serum LDH could be elevated in acute leukemia. *Leucine aminopeptidase (LAP)* is an enzyme produced by the liver. Elevated serum LAP could indicate cancer of the liver.

Erythrocyte Sedimentation Rate (ESR, Sed Rate) (Blood): Clients with Hodgkin's disease, multiple myeloma, and lymphosarcoma might have increased ESR.

Estradiol (E$_2$) (Serum): E$_2$ is useful in evaluating gonadal dysfunction. Elevated E$_2$ level in female, >500 pg/ml, may be present in ovarian tumor, and elevated E$_2$ level in male, >50 pg/ml, can indicate a testicular tumor.

Estrogen/Total (Serum and Urine-24-Hour): An elevated serum or urine estrogen test might indicate adrenocortical tumor, ovarian tumor, or some testicular tumor.

Follicle-Stimulating Hormone (FSH) (Serum and Urine): Decreased serum and urine FSH, <4 mU/ml (serum), or 4 IU/24 h (urine), could indicate tumor of the adrenal gland, testes, or ovary. Increased level could indicate FSH-producing pituitary tumor.

Gastrin (Serum): Elevated serum gastrin level, >200 pg/ml, might be present in clients with malignant neoplasm of the stomach.

Haptoglobin (Serum): Elevated haptoglobin level, >270 mg/dl, might be found in clients with cancer of the lung, large intestine, stomach, breast, and liver and in clients with Hodgkin's disease.

Hormones: Any hormone may be elevated with cancer, because many cancers secrete inappropriate hormones (ectopic hormone secretion) in response to bizarre differentiation of cancer cells.

Human Chorionic Gonadotropin (HCG) (Serum, Urine): Usually positive HCG levels indicate pregnancy, but they might indicate hydatidiform mole or choriocarcinoma.

5-Hydroxyindolacetic Acid (5-HIAA) (Urine): Elevated urine 5-HIAA, 10 to 100 mg/24 h, could indicate carcinoid tumors of the appendix and intestine. Usually these carcinoid tumor cells, which secrete excess serotonin, are of low-grade malignancy. When metastasis occurs, 5-HIAA could be >100 mg/24 h. Food and certain drugs could give false-positive results. Several random or spot urine specimens should be tested.

Immunoglobulins (Ig) (Serum): Clients with lymphocytic leukemia could have decreased serum IgG, IgA, IgM levels. Clients with lymphosarcoma might have an increased IgM level.

17-Ketosteroids (17-KS) (Urine): Elevated urine 17-KS, >25 mg/24 h (male), >15 mg/24 h (female), could be associated with neoplasms of the adrenal gland, testes, and ovary.

Luteinizing Hormone (LH) (Serum): In pituitary and testicular tumors, LH is elevated.

Melanin (Urine): This test is to verify the presence or progression of a melanoma. With metastatic melanoma, melanin metabolites are usually found in high concentration in the urine.

Occult Blood (Feces): Hidden blood in the stools could indicate cancer in the upper or lower GI tract. Orthotoluidine (Occultest) is considered more sensitive than the guaiac test.

Parathyroid Hormone (PTH): PTH is secreted ectopically by many carcinomas (i.e., squamous cell lung cancer [most common cause], renal carcinoma, pancreatic carcinoma, and ovarian carcinoma). Also PTH might be elevated in parathyroid carcinoma.

Partial Thromboplastin Time (PTT) (Plasma): Increased PTT could be present in clients with myelocytic and monocytic leukemias.

Platelet Count (Blood): Decreased platelet count, <100,000 mm^3, may occur in clients with cancer of the bone, gastrointestinal tract, and brain, and in multiple myeloma, lymphatic, myelocytic, and monocytic leukemias. An elevated platelet count, >400,000 mm^3, might occur in metastatic carcinoma. Many types of chemotherapy cause temporary thrombocytopenia.

Pregnanediol (Urine): Elevated urine pregnanediol, >7 mg/24 h may be present in choriocarcinoma of the ovary.

Pregnanetriol (Urine): Malignant neoplasm of the adrenal gland may have an elevated urine pregnanetriol, >2.4 mg/24 hours.

Prolactin (PRL) (Serum): In nonpregnant women and in men, an elevated prolactin level could indicate pituitary adenoma.

Prostate-Specific Antigen (PSA) Serum: Normal results: 0–4 ng/ml.

   PSA is slightly elevated in benign prostatic hypertrophy (BPH), 4–19 ng/ml; and in prostatic cancer the PSA level is greatly increased, 10–120 ng/ml.

Protein Electrophoresis (Serum): The following cancerous conditions could be reflected in protein fractions.

Protein	Decreased Level	Elevated Level
Albumin	Leukemia Liver cancer (primary or metastatic)	
Globulin		
β		Malignant hypertensive
γ	Lymphocytic leukemia Lymphosarcoma	Hodgkin's disease Chronic lymphocytic leukemia Multiple myeloma

Renin (Plasma): Clients with cancer of the kidney may have an elevated plasma renin level.

Serotonin (Plasma): 50–175 ng/ml.

The primary purpose of this test is to confirm the diagnosis of carcinoid tumors of the argentaffin cells in the gastrointestinal tract. Ectopic production of serotonin can result from oat cell carcinoma of the lung, pancreatic tumors, and thyroid cancer.

Testosterone (Serum): Increased testosterone in women after menopause can be caused by malignant neoplasm of the breast.

Thyroid Antibodies (TA) (Serum): Elevated serum TA titer could indicate carcinoma of the thyroid gland.

Uric Acid (Serum): Elevated serum-uric acid, >7.8 mg/dl, could occur in clients having lymphocytic, myelocytic, and monocytic leukemias, multiple myeloma, and in metastatic cancer (due to tumor lysis syndrome).

White Blood Cells (WBCs)/leukocytes (Blood): An elevated total WBC count frequently is present in lymphocytic, myelocytic, and monocytic leukemias. A differential WBC count is ordered to determine the cause of disease. With an elevated lymphocyte count, the disease entities could be chronic lymphocytic leukemia, Hodgkin's disease, or multiple myeloma. In monocytic leukemia, the monocyte count could be elevated. It is not uncommon to see the neutrophil count increased in myelocytic leukemia and Hodgkin's disease. Leukocytes may be decreased in many forms of cancer (immunosuppression occurs by unknown mechanism). Chemotherapy and radiation frequently cause severe, temporary, decreased WBCs.

Diagnostic Tests

X-Rays: X-rays are taken of various organs when malignant neoplasms and metastasis are suspected. Chest and bone x-rays are used to detect neoplasm in the lung and bone metastasis. Procedural x-rays taken of body organs include GI series, barium enema, intravenous pyelography (IVP), and bronchography.

Mammography: This is an x-ray examination of the breasts to detect cysts and tumors. Malignant tumors are irregular and poorly defined. They tend to be unilateral.

Thermography (Breast): Breast tumors cause increased metabolism, resulting in vascularity and increased breast-surface temperature. This test is used as a screening test; other diagnostic procedures are necessary to confirm breast cancer.

Lymphangiography, Lymphangiogram: This test is an x-ray examination of the lymphatic system (i.e., lymphatic vessels and lymph nodes). It is used to identify lymphoma (e.g., Hodgkin's disease) and metastasis to the lymph nodes. Lymphangiogram should not be performed on clients who are highly allergic to iodinated dye.

Electronystagmography (ENG): This test helps to determine if the problem or abnormality that occurs is in the brain stem or temporal lobe of the cerebral cortex such as a brain stem lesion.

Endoscopy: Endoscopes, rigid (metal) or flexible fiberoptic, are used for direct visualization of body organs and body cavities to detect any abnormalities. The endoscopes are named for the organ that they are designed to view (e.g., colonoscope [colon], gastroscope [stomach], bronchoscope [lungs], cystoscope [bladder], colposcope [vagina and cervix]). The following endoscopic examinations are performed to detect neoplasms of the lung: bronchoscopy and mediastinoscopy; the esophagus and stomach: esophagogastroscopy; the colon: colonoscopy; the duodenum and pancreas: endoscopic retrograde cholangiopancreatography (ERCP); the rectum and sigmoid: proctosigmoidoscopy; the vagina and cervix: colposcopy; and the bladder: cystoscopy. Peritoneoscopy is helpful in observing the peritoneum for effectiveness of treatment and recurrence of metastasis.

Thoracoscopy: This test can detect pleural or lung tumors and metastatic cancer in the lung or pleura area.

Ultrasonography, Ultrasound, Echography: This noninvasive test records echoes of sound from tissues of different densities. It is useful in detecting neoplasms of the brain, kidney, liver, pancreas, spleen, and thyroid. However, positive findings need to be confirmed by other diagnostic tests.

Nuclear Scans, Radioisotope Scan, Radionuclide Imaging. Nuclear scanning using radioactive isotopes or radionuclides is used to detect primary or metastatic cancer. If the radionuclide concentrates in the tumor, the involved area will show up as dark spot or hot spot on the scintigram. But if the tumor does not concentrate the radionuclide, then light-colored area or cold spot is recorded. Radioisotope scans are useful for detecting metastatic tumor of the bone, tumors of the brain, lung, liver, spleen, and thyroid gland.

Monoclonal Antibodies for Colon and Ovarian Cancers: The radionuclide, indium 111, is used to identify colon or ovarian cancer cells in areas of the body. The Inmonoclonal 111 antibodies attach to the cancer cells, which can be detected with the use of a gamma camera.

Computed Tomography (CT): CT is effective for detecting tumors of the brain, lung, liver, kidney, pancreas, and adrenals.

Angiography, Arteriography: Angiography is an examination of arteries leading to organs. This test is useful for detecting abnormal vascularization resulting from tumors. Cerebral angiography identifies brain tumors by the increased vascularization; pulmonary angiography can detect tumors of the lung; and renal angiography can identify kidney tumors.

Biopsy: Biopsy, excision of tissue, is a direct method for diagnosing cancer. Tissue specimens for microscopic examination can be obtained from the lung, liver, kidney, bone, thyroid, lymph nodes, skin, and bone marrow.

Bone Marrow Aspiration: Examination of the bone marrow detects abnormal cells. It is a useful test for diagnosing leukemias, lymphomas, and multiple myelomas.

Magnetic Resonance Imaging (MRI): MRI can detect small, primary, or metastatic tumors. It can distinguish solid masses from vascular structures better than CT. It is helpful in evaluating recurrent or residual masses. MRI is useful in supplementing CT.

A summary of laboratory and diagnostic tests used in diagnosing cancer is outlined in Table 19.

TABLE 19 TESTS USED TO DIAGNOSE SPECIFIC CANCERS

Cancer	Laboratory Tests	Diagnostic Tests
Leukemias	Bence-Jones protein	Bone marrow aspiration/biopsy
	CEA	
	Cold agglutinins	
	Cryoglobulins	
	PTT	
	Platelet count	
	Protein fraction	
	Uric acid	
	WBC	
Hodgkin's disease	Ceruloplasmin	Lymphangiography
	Copper	Lymph node biopsy
	CRP	Mediastinoscopy
	Cryoglobulins	
	ESR	
	Haptoglobin	
	Protein fraction	
	WBC	
Multiple myelomas	Bence-Jones protein	Bone marrow aspiration/biopsy
	Calcium	
	Cold agglutinins	
	Enzymes: ACP, ALP	
	Cryoglobulins	
	ESR	
	Melanin	
	Platelet count	
	Protein fraction	
	Uric acid	
	WBC	

TABLE 19 TESTS USED TO DIAGNOSE SPECIFIC CANCERS

Cancer	Laboratory Tests	Diagnostic Tests
Stomach	CEA	GI series
	Ceruloplasmin	Esophagogastroscopy
	C_3, C_4	
	Enzyme: LDH	
	Copper	
	Gastrin	
	Haptoglobin	
Colon	CEA	Barium enema
	C_3, C_4	Colonoscopy
	Copper	Proctosigmoidoscopy
	Enzyme: LDH	ERCP
	Haptoglobin	Biopsy
	5-HIAA	
	Occult stool	
Kidney, Bladder	C_3, C_4	IVP
	Enzymes: GGTP, LDH	Cystoscopy
	Renin	Ultrasound
		Nuclear scan
		CT
		Angiography
		Biopsy
Lung	ADH	Bronchography
	ACTH	Bronchoscopy
	Calcium	Nuclear scan
	CEA	CT
	Ceruloplasmin	Angiography
	Copper	Mediastinoscopy
	Cytology	Chest x-ray
	Enzymes: GGTP, LDH	MRI
	Haptoglobin	Thoracoscopy
Liver	Bilirubin	Ultrasound
	Ceruloplasmin	Nuclear scan
	Copper	CT
	Enzymes: ALP, LAP, ALT/ SGPT, AST/SGOT, GGTP	Biopsy
	Haptoglobin	
Reproductive	Calcium	Mammography
	CEA	Thermography
	C_3, C_4	Colposcopy
	CRP	Biopsy
	Enzymes: ACP, GGTP	Peritoneoscopy
	Estradiol	

(continued)

TABLE 19 TESTS USED TO DIAGNOSE SPECIFIC CANCERS
(continued)

Cancer	Laboratory Tests	Diagnostic Tests
	Estrogen	
	FSH	
	HCG	
	17-KS	
	LH	
	PAP smear	
	Pregnanediol	
	Testosterone	
Bone	Bence-Jones protein	X-ray
	Calcium	Biopsy
	Ceruloplasmin	
	Copper	
	Enzymes: ALP, LDH	
Brain	Enzyme: GGTP	Ultrasound
		Nuclear scan
		CT
		MRI
		Angiography
		Electronystagmography
Endocrine	ACTH	Ultrasound
	Calcitonin	Nuclear scan
	Cortisol	CT
	FSH	Biopsy
	17-KS	
	LH	
	Pregnanetriol	
	Prolactin	
	Thyroid antibodies	

NURSING DIAGNOSES

- Anxiety related to the unknown and pain.
- Deficient knowledge related to a lack of understanding of laboratory and diagnostic procedures, disease process, and/or outcome.
- Noncompliance to prescribed laboratory and diagnostic tests related to a lack of or inadequate explanation and/or anxiety about physical condition.
- Altered nutrition: less than body requirements related to anorexia, vomiting, reduced food intake secondary to treatment regimen for cancer.
- Risk for injury related to bleeding tendencies secondary to decreased platelet count.
- Risk for injury related to allergic reactions to contrast medium (dye) secondary to diagnostic tests (i.e., IVP, CT, with contrast medium, angiography).

- Activity intolerance related to diagnostic testing (e.g., angiography), pain (e.g., bone metastasis).
- Deficient fluid volume related to cellular catabolism, numerous laboratory and diagnostic tests, and/or treatment regimen.
- Ineffective coping with a disease process and laboratory and diagnostic procedures.
- Altered comfort related to the test procedure and pain secondary to neoplasm.
- Situational low self-esteem related to body changes, dependence, and/or role change.
- Ineffective family process related to numerous laboratory and diagnostic tests, hospitalization, and/or treatment.

NURSING IMPLICATIONS WITH RATIONALE

- Explain the purpose for the laboratory and diagnostic tests.
- Give detailed explanation concerning the test procedures and the need for client's compliance. Explanation might be brief or in-depth, depending on the client's familiarity with the test.
- Inform the client of any food, fluid, or drug restrictions. Each test should be checked for specific restrictions (see Parts I and II).
- Obtain specimen collection at specific times according to the procedures.
- Elicit from the client, client history, or family members information about any allergies, especially to contrast medium (dye), iodine, seafood.
- Monitor intake and output and vital signs before and after laboratory and diagnostic tests.
- Listen to the client's expressed anxiety or fear concerning the tests and potential clinical problems. Clarification of the test procedure might alleviate fear and anxiety and promote compliance. Assess communications for verbal or nonverbal expression of anxiety and fear.
- Assess the client's discomfort by eliciting from him or her the intensity, duration, and location of pain. Provide pain relief by positional changes and medication.
- Observe for bleeding caused by decreased platelet count and treatment regimen.
- Check laboratory results, and report the abnormal test results.
- Provide support to the client and family members during test procedure, treatment regimen, and in response to expressed fear and anxiety about physical condition and outcome.
- Repeat information to the client and family briefly and clearly if anxiety and/or fear level is determined to be high.

Evaluation

- Determine if the test was correctly performed according to the procedure. Notify laboratory and/or health care provider of any changes that occur during the test.
- Provide ongoing assessment before, during, and after procedure. Check the client's vital signs, intake and output, and for ecchymosis or bleeding site following laboratory or diagnostic procedure. Assess for changes and improvement.

- Determine if the client's and family members' fear and/or anxiety has been lessened or alleviated. Continue providing support measures.
- Clarify or answer any additional questions the client and family members might have.
- Encourage the client to seek health care assistance whenever any change in health status occurs (e.g., infection, bleeding, skin breakdown, elevated temperature, and others).
- Identify resources that would provide information, service, and support (e.g., American Cancer Association) to the client and family.
- Encourage the client and family members to participate in the decision-making process concerning plan of care and daily activities.
- Assist the family with the development of a care plan for health management and activities.

Hematologic conditions

Laboratory Tests

CBC
  RBC Count
  Hb (Hgb)
  Hct
  RBC Indices: MCV, MCH, MCHC, RDW
  WBC Count
  Differential WBC Count
Platelet Count
Platelet Aggregation
Platelet Antibody Test
Reticulocyte Count
Hb Electrophoresis
Erythrocyte Osmotic Fragility
Bleeding Time (Blood)
Coagulation Time (Blood)
Clot Retraction (Blood)
Fetal Hemoglobin
Fibrinogen (Plasma)
Fibrin Degradation Products (Serum)
Euglobulin Lysis Time
DIC Screening Tests
D-Dimer Test
Plasminogen (Plasma)

PT (Plasma)
PTT and APTT (Plasma)
Factors Assay (Coagulation Factors)
Blood Typing
Bone Marrow Aspiration
G-6-PD (Blood)
Haptoglobin (Serum)
Methemoglobin
Coomb's—Indirect (Serum)
Ferritin (Serum)
Iron (Serum)
IBC/TIBC (Serum)
Transferrin (Serum)
Bilirubin—Indirect (Serum)
Sickle Cell Screening Test
Heinz Bodies
Folic Acid (Serum)
Vitamin B_{12} (Serum)
ESR (Sed Rate) (Blood)
Urobilinogen (Urine)
Zinc Protoporphyrin (ZPP) (Blood)

Introduction

Laboratory tests for hematologic conditions described in this section are done to diagnose anemias such as microcytic (iron deficiency) and macrocytic (aplastic, hemolytic, pernicious), bleeding disorders, and blood cell changes.

For leukemias and multiple myeloma, see Neoplastic Conditions.

Laboratory Tests

Complete Blood Count (CBC): The six components of CBC include the RBC count; hemoglobin (Hb/Hgb); hematocrit (Hct); RBC (erythrocyte) indices: mean corpuscular volume (MCV), mean corpuscular hemoglobin (MCH), mean corpuscular hemoglobin concentration (MCHC), RBC distribution width (RDW); WBC; and differential WBC count. Usually a CBC is ordered to aid in the detection of anemias; to determine blood loss, hydration status, and as part of the routine hospital admission test; to evaluate blood cell status prior to surgery; and as part of a physical examination. The RBC count, Hb, Hct, and RBC index values are useful to determine the type of anemia *(see Part I on RBC indices)*.

The differential WBC is necessary for determining the type of infection. During an acute bacterial infection, the body's first line of defense is neutrophils. An increased number of lymphocytes occurs in chronic bacterial and acute viral infections. Monocytes increase in number late in acute bacterial infections but continue to function during the chronic phase.

Table 20 shows the norms for CBC tests and clinical problems associated with decreased and elevated levels.

Platelet Count: *Norms:* Adult: 150,000–400,000 µl (mm^3 or K/UL).

Thrombocytopenia (decreased platelet count) is associated with aplastic, iron deficiency, pernicious, folic acid deficiency, and sickle cell anemias. Thrombocytosis (elevated platelet count) occurs in polycythemia vera.

Platelet Aggregation and Platelet Adhesion (Blood): *Norms:* 3–5 minutes.

Platelet aggregation measures the ability of platelets adhering to one another. A decrease in platelet aggregation time will cause increased bleeding tendencies. Both platelet aggregation and platelet adhesion aid in diagnosing hereditary and acquired platelet diseases, such as von Willebrand's disease.

Platelet Antibody Test (Blood): Negative.

Platelet antibodies develop frequently as the result of platelet antigens from transfused blood. This can cause thrombocytopenia because of the destructrion of the platelets.

Reticulocyte Count: *Norms:* Adult: 25,000–75,000 µl, 0.5–1.5% of all RBCs. Elderly: 0.4–3.6%. Child: 0.5–2.0% of all RBCs.

Reticulocytes are immature, nonnucleated RBCs that are formed in the bone marrow. A decreased reticulocyte count might be present in pernicious, folic acid, and aplastic anemias. A persistently low count could be suggestive of bone marrow hypofunction or aplastic anemia. An elevated reticulocyte count could be present in hemolytic and sickle cell anemias and could be due to hemorrhage, hemolysis, or treatment of iron deficiency.

TABLE 20 HEMATOLOGIC CAUSES FOR ABNORMAL
CBC RESULTS

Type	Reference Value	Decreased Level	Elevated Level

RBC count	Adult:
	  Male: 4.5–6.0 μl
	  Female: 4.0–5.0 μl
	Elderly:
	  Male: 3.7–6.0 μl
	  Female: 4.0–5.0 μl
	Child: 3.8–5.5 μl
		Hemorrhage
		Anemias
		Hemodilution
		  (overhydration)
			Hemoconcentration
			  (dehydration)
			Polycythemia vera

Hb	Adult:
	  Male: 13.5–18.0 g/dl
	  Female: 12.0–16.0 g/dl
	Elderly:
	  Male: 11.0–17.0 g/dl
	  Female: 11.5–16.0 g/dl
	Infant: 10.0–15.0 g/dl
	Child: 11.0–16.0 g/dl
		Anemias:
		  Iron deficiency
		  Aplastic
		  Hemocytic
		Acute blood loss
		Hemodilution
			Hemoconcentration
			  (dehydration)
			Polycythemia vera

Hct	Adult:
	  Male: 40%–54%
	  Female: 36%–46%
	Elderly:
	  Male: 38%–42%
	  Female: 38%–41%
	Child, 1–3 years:
	  29%–40%
	Child, 4–10 years:
	  36%–38%
		Anemias:
		  Aplastic
		  Hemolytic
		  Folic acid
		    deficiency
		  Pernicious
		  Sickle cell
			Hemoconcentration
			  (dehydration)
			Polycythemia vera

RBC indices			

MCV	Adult: 80–98 μm³
	Elderly:
	  Male: 74–110 μm³
	  Female: 78–100 μm³
		Microcytic anemia:
		  Iron deficiency
			Macrocytic anemias:
			  Aplastic
			  Hemolytic
			  Pernicious

MCH	Adult: 27–31 pg
	Elderly:
	  Male: 24–33 pg
	  Female: 23–34 pg
		Microcytic,
		  hypochromic
		  anemia
			Macrocytic anemias

MCHC	Adult: 32%–36%
	  0.32–0.36 g/dl
	Elderly:
	  Male: 28%–36%
		Microcytic,
		  hypochromic
		  anemia
		Thalassemia	

TABLE 20 HEMATOLOGIC CAUSES FOR ABNORMAL
CBC RESULTS (*continued*)

Type	Reference Value	Decreased Level	Elevated Level
RDW	Female: 30%–36% 11.5–14.5 Coulter S		Anemias: Iron deficiency Folic acid deficiency Pernicious Sickle cell

WBC count	Adult: 5000–10,000 µl
	 Child, 2 years:
	  6000–17,000 µl
	 Elderly:
	  Male: 4200–16,000 µl
	  Female: 3100–10,000 µl
		Anemias:
		 Aplastic
		 Pernicious
			Anemias:
			 Hemolytic
			 Sickle cell

Differential WBC count			
Neutrophils	Adult: 50%–70% Elderly: 45%–75% Child: 35%	Anemias: Aplastic Folic acid deficiency Iron deficiency	Anemia: Acquired hemolytic
Basophils	Adult: 0.5%–1.0% Elderly, Average: 1%		Anemia: Acquired hemolytic
Lymphocytes	Adult: 25%–35% Elderly, Average: 30% Child: 38%–50%	Anemia: Aplastic	
Monocytes	Adult: 4%–6% Elderly, Average: 10%	Anemia: Aplastic	Anemias: Sickle cell Hemolytic

Hb/Hgb Electrophoresis: *Norms: See values in Part I.*
   This test detects abnormal types of Hb (i.e., Hb S [sickle cell anemia], in Hb C [hemolytic anemia], and Hb F [thalassemia]).

Erythrocyte Osmotic Fragility: *Norms:* Adult: 0.30–0.46%.
   This test determines the ability of RBCs to resist hemolysis (RBC destruction) in hypo-osmolar solutions. Osmotic fragility might be decreased in the anemias—iron deficiency, folic acid deficiency, sickle cell, thalassemia major and minor (Mediterranean anemia or Cooley's anemia)—and also in polycythemia vera. Elevated osmotic fragility might be present in acquired hemolytic anemia.

Bleeding Time: *Norms:* Adult: 1–6 minutes (Ivy's method), 1–3 minutes (Duke's method).

The bleeding time test is useful in determining abnormal function of platelets. A prolonged bleeding time could be due to decreased platelet count, increased platelet destruction, platelet abnormality, vascular abnormalities, disseminated intravascular coagulation (DIC) disease, aplastic anemia, and factor V, VII, and XI deficiencies.

Coagulation Time (CT), Lee-White Clotting Time (Blood): *Norms:* Adult: 5–15 minutes.

CT, frequently known as Lee-White clotting time, is one of the oldest tests of coagulation. A prolonged CT might be indicative of afibrinogenemia, hyperheparinemia, or severe coagulation factor deficiencies.

Clot Retraction (Blood): *Norms:* Adult: 1 h: half its size; 4 h: near completion; 24 h: completely shrunken. Child: same as adult.

Clot retraction (shrunken clot) test is useful for detecting platelet disorder (platelet deficit or platelet abnormality). A decreased clot retraction (>4 to 24 hours) could be indicative of thrombocytopenia (decreased platelets); thrombasthenia (platelet abnormality); or pernicious, folic-acid deficiency, or aplastic anemia.

Fetal Hemoglobin (Hb F) (Blood): Adult: 0.2%. Child: Newborn: 60–90%'; 1–5 mo: < 70%; 6–12 mo: < 5%; < 1 year: < 2%.

Elevated fetal hemoglobin is normal for an infant under 6 months old. After 6 months, hemoglobinopathy should be considered which could be minor or major thalassemias.

Fibrinogen (Plasma): *Norms:* 200–400 mg/dl.

Fibrinogen produces fibrin strands necessary for clot formation. A deficiency of fibrinogen results in bleeding. A low fibrinogen level may be due to DIC.

Fibrin Degradation Products (FDP) (Serum): *Norms:* Adult: 2–10 µg/ml.

The FDP test, also known as fibrin split products (FSP), indicates the activity of the fibrinolytic system. This test is frequently done in an emergency when the client is hemorrhaging. An increased FDP, >10 µg/ml, is usually indicative of DIC caused by severe injury or trauma.

Euglobulin Lysis Time (Fibrinolysis Time) Test: *Norms:* Adult: 1½–6 hours.

This test evaluates the activity of the fibrinolytic system by determining the time from clot formation to clot lysis. It is useful in differentiating between primary fibrinolysis (e.g., cancer of prostate) and DIC. The lysis time is short in primary fibrinolysis and normal or prolonged in DIC.

Disseminated Intravascular Coagulation (DIC) Screening Tests: This is a group of tests ordered for detecting the presence of DIC. Table 21 shows the screening tests used for suspected DIC.

D-Dimer Test (Blood): Negative for D-Dimer fragments; > 250ng/ml; 250 µg/l.

A fibrin degradation fragment, D-Dimer, occurs through fibrinolysis. This test confirms the presence of fibrin split products (FSPs) and is more specific for diagnosing disseminated intravascular coagulation (DIC) than FSPs.

TABLE 21 DISSEMINATED INTRAVASCULAR COAGULATION
SCREENING TESTS

Test	Positive Results
Platelet count	>400,000 µl
Bleeding time	>6 minutes
PT	>15 seconds
PTT	>60 seconds
APTT	>40 seconds
Factor I: fibrinogen	<100 mg/dl
Fibrin degradation products	>10 µg/dl
Euglobulin lysis time	1½–6 hours, or >6 hours
Plasminogen	<2.5 U/ml, <20 mg/dl

Plasminogen (Plasma): *Norms:* 2.5–5.2 U/ml; 7-16 mg/dl.

Plasminogen test is useful in evaluating the fibrinolytic process, a breakdown of fibrin clots in prevention of coagulation. The level is decreased in DIC, advanced liver disease, and thrombolytic therapy.

Prothrombin Time (PT): *Norms:* Adult: 11–15 seconds; 70–100%. Child: same as adult; INR: 2.0–3.0.

Prothrombin, factor II, is converted to thrombin by the action of thromboplastin, which is needed to form a clot. A prolonged PT time could be associated with afibrinogenemia, deficiencies of factors II, VII, and X. This test is useful for monitoring anticoagulant therapy.

Partial Thromboplastin Time (PTT), Activated Partial Thromboplastin Time (ATT) (Plasma): *Norms:* Adult: PTT: 60–70 seconds; APTT: 20–35 seconds.

The PTT is useful for detecting clotting factors and platelet disorders. APTT is more sensitive than PTT. PTT and APTT are commonly used to monitor heparin therapy.

Factor Assay (Coagulation Factors): Factor assay determines the concentration of specific coagulating factors in the blood. Prolonged clotting time occurs when values of factors I, II, V, VII, VIII, IX, X, and XI are decreased.

Blood Typing (Type and Cross Match): Blood typing and cross matching is necessary to provide compatible blood to recipients. Major and minor antigens can be detected through blood typing.

Bone Marrow Aspiration (Biopsy): Bone marrow specimen is useful for evaluating hematopoiesis. The size, shape, and number of RBCs, WBCs, and megakaryocytes (platelet precursors) are examined to diagnose hematologic disorders (i.e., aplastic anemia, leukemia, Hodgkin's disease, polycythemia vera, and multiple myeloma).

Glucose-6-Phosphate Dehydrogenase/G-6-PD (Blood): *Norms:* Adult (varies with method used): 8–18 IU/g Hb, 125–281 U/dl packed RBCs.

G-6-PD, an enzyme in RBCs, assists in glucose use in RBCs. A decreased amount of this enzyme causes hemolysis and hemolytic anemia.

Haptoglobin (Hp) (Serum): *Norms:* Adult: 60–270 mg/dl. Infant: 0–30 mg/dl, and then gradually increases.

Hp, a group of α_2-globulins, combines with free Hb during intravascular hemolysis. A decreased Hp level occurs in hemolytic anemia because of too much free Hb to bind. Also a decreased level could occur in pernicious, folic-acid deficiency, and sickle cell anemias.

Methemoglobin (Hb M) (Blood): *Norms*: <1.5% of total Hb; 0.06–0.24 g/dl; 9.2–37.0 μmol/l. Positive: >20–70%; >70% death.

Hb M occurs when the deoxygenated heme or iron portion of hemoglobin is oxidized to a ferric state; methemoglobinemia results. This problem can be due to chemicals, radiation, and certain drugs such as nitrites and nitrates.

Coombs Indirect (Serum): *Norms:* Negative.

This test detects free antibodies in the client's serum and identifies certain red cell antigens. It is done in cross matching blood for transfusion. Positive results mean incompatible cross-matched blood, anti-Rh antibodies, or acquired hemolytic anemia.

Ferritin (Serum): *Norms:* Male: 15–445 ng/ml. Female: 10–235 ng/ml.

Serum ferritin level is useful in evaluating the total storage of iron in the body. It can detect early iron deficiency anemia and anemias due to chronic disease.

Iron (Serum): *Norms:* Adult: 50–150 μg/dl. Infant: 40–100 μg/dl.

A decreased serum iron level frequently occurs in iron deficiency anemia. An elevated level might be present in hemolytic, pernicious, and folic acid deficiency anemias.

Iron-Binding Capacity (IBC) or Total Iron-Binding Capacity (TIBC) (Serum): *Norms:* Adult: 250–450 μg/dl. Infant: 100–350 μg/dl.

IBC is two to three times greater than the serum iron level. When serum iron is decreased, IBC is increased, and when serum iron is increased, IBC is decreased. A decreased IBC level is present in hemolytic, pernicious, and sickle cell anemias. An elevated IBC level is present in iron deficiency anemia.

Transferrin (Serum): *Norms:* 200–430 mg/dl; 2–4.3 g/l (SI units).

Transferrin is responsible for transporting iron to the bone marrow for the purpose of hemoglobin synthesis. A decrease in transferrin occurs in anemias of chronic diseases, and an elevated level occurs in iron deficiency anemia.

Bilirubin Indirect (Serum): *Norms:* Adult: 0.1–1.0 mg/dl.

An elevated indirect bilirubin is associated with transfusion reaction and with sickle cell, pernicious, and hemolytic anemias.

Sickle Cell Screening Test: *Norms:* Negative.

Hb S, a crescent- or sickle-shaped cell, is present in sickle cell disease when the RBC is deprived of oxygen. Hb electrophoresis is needed to confirm sickle cell anemia.

Heinz Bodies (Blood): Negative: Absence of Heinz Bodies; <30% Heinz Bodies present.

Heinz bodies are small, irregular, decomposed particles on the hemoglobin that are normally removed by the spleen. Heinz bodies can cause hemolytic anemia (hemolysis of red blood cells [RBCs]) or hemoglobinopathy.

Folic Acid Folate (Serum): *Norms:* Adult: 5–20 ng/ml, >2.5 ng/ml (RIA).

A decreased folic acid level is indicative of folic acid deficiency anemia. In pernicious anemia, the serum folic acid level might be elevated.

Vitamin B$_{12}$ (Serum): *Adult Norms:* 200–900 pg/ml, 132–703 pmol/l (SI Units).

Vitamin B$_{12}$ is essential for RBC maturation. A decreased Vitamin B$_{12}$ level is indicative of pernicious anemia.

Erythrocyte Sedimentation Rate (ESR/Sed Rate) (Blood): *Norms: See values in Part I.*

ESR, a nonspecific test, measures the rate at which RBCs settle in unclotted blood. A decreased ESR could be present in sickle cell anemia and polycythemia vera.

Urobilinogen (Urine): *Norms:* Adult: Random: 0.3–3.5 mg/dl; 24 hours: 0.05–2.5 mg/24 h.

Increased urine urobilinogen level could be present in hemolytic, pernicious, and sickle cell anemias.

Zinc Protoporphyrin (ZPP) Blood: *Adult and Child:* 15–77 μg/dl.

ZPP is a screening test to check for lead poisoning and iron deficiency. The test is positive for lead poisoning if the ZPP level is elevated.

NURSING DIAGNOSES

- Deficient knowledge related to a lack of understanding of laboratory procedures, disease process, and/or outcome.
- Noncompliance with prescribed laboratory tests related to a lack of adequate explanation.
- Risk for injury related to bleeding tendencies secondary to hematologic disorders.
- Ineffective tissue perfusion related to decreased hemoglobin-carrying oxygen.
- Ineffective coping with the disease process and laboratory test procedure.
- Situational low self-esteem related to dependence and/or role change.
- Ineffective family processes related to the client's chronic hematologic disorder.

NURSING IMPLICATIONS WITH RATIONALE

- Explain that the purpose for the laboratory tests is to identify the cause for the hematologic disorder.

- Give a detailed explanation concerning the test procedures and the need for the client's compliance. Explanation might be brief or in-depth, depending upon the client's familiarity with the test.
- Inform the client of any food, fluid, or drug restrictions. Each test should be checked for specific restrictions *(see Part I)*.
- Monitor the client's vital signs before, during, and after the laboratory test procedures. Check respiratory status and skin color, because oxygen deficit frequently results from a decreased hemoglobin.
- Listen to the client's expressed anxiety or fear concerning the tests and potential clinical problems. Clarification of the test procedure might alleviate fear and anxiety and promote compliance.
- Check laboratory results and report abnormal test reports.
- Be supportive of the client and family members during tests and treatment of hematologic disorders.

Evaluation

- Determine if the test was correctly performed according to the procedure. Notify the laboratory or health care provider of any changes that occur during the test.
- Check the client's vital signs and skin color for changes: improvement or deterioration.
- Determine if the client's and family members' fear or anxiety has been lessened or alleviated.
- Clarify or answer any additional questions the client and family members might have.
- Reinforce the importance of seeking health assistance when changes in health status occur.

PART FOUR

Therapeutic Drug Monitoring (TDM)*

4

Selected drugs are monitored by serum and urine for the purposes of achieving and maintaining therapeutic drug effect and for preventing drug toxicity. Drugs with a wide therapeutic range (window), the difference between effective dose and toxic dose, are not usually monitored. Drug monitoring is important in maintaining a drug concentration–response relationship, especially when the serum drug range (window) is narrow, such as with digoxin and lithium. Therapeutic drug monitoring (TDM) is the process of following drug levels and adjusting them to maintain a therapeutic level. Not all drugs can be dosed and/or monitored by their blood levels alone.

Drug levels are obtained at peak time and trough time after a steady state of the drug has been achieved in the client. Steady state is reached after four to five half-lives of a drug and can be reached sooner if the drug has a short half-life. Once steady state is achieved, the serum drug level is checked at the peak level (maximum drug concentration) and/or at trough/residual level (minimum drug concentration). If the trough or residual level is at the high therapeutic point, toxicity might occur. Careful assessment is needed by both physical and laboratory means.

TDM is required for drugs with a narrow therapeutic index or range (window); when other methods for monitoring drugs are noneffective, such as blood pressure (BP) monitoring; for determining when adequate blood

*Revised by Ronald J. LeFever, R.Ph., Pharmacy Services, Medical College of Virginia, Richmond, VA.

concentrations are reached; for evaluating a client's compliance to drug therapy; for determining whether other drugs have altered serum drug levels (increased or decreased) that could result in drug toxicity or lack of therapeutic effect; and for establishing a new serum-drug level when the dosage is changed.

Drug groups for TDM include analgesics, antibiotics, anticonvulsants, antineoplastics, bronchodilators, cardiac drugs, hypoglycemics, sedatives, and tranquilizers. To effectively conduct TDM, the laboratory must be provided with the following information: the drug name and daily dosage, time and amount of last dose, time blood was drawn, route of administration, and client's age. Without complete information, serum drug reporting might be incorrect.

Drug	Therapeutic Range	Peak Time	Toxic Level
Acetaminophen (Tylenol)	10–20 μg/ml	1–2½ hours	>50 μg/ml Hepatotoxicity: >200 μg/ml
Acetohexamide (Dymelor)	20–70 μg/ml (should be dosed according to blood glucose levels)	2–4 hours	>75 μg/ml
Alcohol	Negative		Mild toxic: 150 mg/dl Marked toxic: >250 mgl
Alprazolam (Xanax)	10–50 ng/ml	1–2 hours	>75 ng/ml
Amikacin (Amikin)	Peak: 20–30 μg/ml Trough: ≤10 μg/ml	Intravenously: ½ hour Intramuscular: ½–1½ hours	Peak: >35 μg/ml Trough: >10 μg/ml
Aminocaproic Acid (Amicar)	100–400 μg/ml	1 hour	>400 μg/ml
Aminophylline (see Theophylline)			
Amiodarone (Cordarone)	0.5–2.5 μg/ml	2–10 hours	>2.5 μg/ml
Amitriptyline (Elavil) + nortriptyline (parent and active metabolite)	110–225 ng/ml	2–4 hours (and up to 12 hours)	>500 ng/ml
Amobarbital (Amytal)	1–5 μg/ml	2 hours	>15 μg/ml Severe toxicity: >30 μg/ml

Drug	Therapeutic Range	Peak Time	Toxic Level
Amoxapine (Asendin)	200–400 ng/ml	1½ hours	>500 ng/ml
Amphetamine:			
Serum	20–30 ng/ml		0.2 μg/ml
Urine		Detectable in urine after 3 hours; positive for 24–48 hours	>30 μg/ml urine
Aspirin (see Salicylates)			
Atenolol (Tenormin)	200–500 ng/ml	2–4 hours	>500 ng/ml
Beta carotene	48–200 μg/dl	Several weeks	>300 μg/dl
Bromide	20–80 mg/dl		>100 mg/dl
Butabarbital (Butisol)	1–2 μg/ml	3–4 hours	>10 μg/ml
Caffeine	Adult: 3–15 μg/ml Infant: 8–20 μg/ml	½–1 hour	>50 μg/ml
Carbamazepine (Tegretol)	4–12 μg/ml	6 hours (range 2–24 hours)	>9–15 μg/ml
Chloral hydrate (Noctec)	2–12 μg/ml	1–2 hours	>20 μg/ml
Chloramphenicol (Chloromycetin	10–20 mg/l		>25 mg/l
Chlordiazepoxide (Librium)	1–5 μg/ml	2–3 hours	>5 μg/ml
Chlorpromazine (Thorazine)	50–300 ng/ml	2–4 hours	>750 ng/ml
Chlorpropamide (Diabinese)	75–250 μg/ml	3–6 hours	>250–750 μg/ml
Clonidine (Catapres)	0.2–2.0 ng/ml (Hypotensive effect)	2–5 hours	>2.0 ng/ml
Clorazepate (Tranxcnc)	0.12–1.0 μg/ml	1–2 hours	>1.0 μg/ml
Cimetidine (Tagamet)	Trough: 0.5–1.2 μg/ml	1–1½ hours	Trough: >1.5 μg/ml
Clonazepam (Klonopin)	10–60 ng/ml	2 hours	>80 ng/ml
Codeine	10–100 ng/ml	1–2 hours	>200 ng/ml

(continued)

Drug	Therapeutic Range	Peak Time	Toxic Level
Cyclosporine	100–300 ng/ml	3–4 hours	>400 ng/ml
Dantrolene (Dantrium)	1–3 µg/ml	5 hours	>5 µg/ml
Desipramine (Norpramin)	125–300 ng/ml	4–6 hours	>500 ng/ml
Diazepam (Valium)	0.5–2 mg/l 400–600 ng/ml therapeutic	1–2 hours	>3 mg/l >3000 ng/ml
Digitoxin (rarely administered)	10–25 ng/ml	Noticeable: 2–4 hours Peak: 12–24 hours	>30 ng/ml
Digoxin	0.5–2 ng/ml	PO: 6–8 hours IV: 1½–2 hours	2–3 ng/ml
Dilantin (see Phenytoin)			
Diltiazem (Cardizem)	50–200 ng/ml	2–3 hours	>200 ng/ml
Disopyramide (Norpace)	2–4 µg/ml	2 hours	>4 µg/ml
Doxepin (Sinequan)	150–300 ng/ml	2–4 hours	>500 ng/ml
Ethchlorvynol (Placidyl)	2–8 µg/ml	1–2 hours	>20 µg/ml
Ethosuximide (Zarontin)	40–100 µg/ml	2–4 hours	>150 µg/ml
Flecainide (Tambocor)	0.2–1.0 µg/ml	3 hours	>1.0 µg/ml
Fluoxetine	90–300 ng/ml	2–4 hours	>500 ng/ml
Flurazepam (Dalmane)	20–110 ng/ml	0.5–1 hour	>1500 ng/ml
Folate	>3.5 µg/ml	1 hour	
Gentamicin (Garamycin)	Peak: 6–12 µg/ml Trough: <2 µg/ml	IV: 15–30 minutes	Peak: >12 µg/ml Trough: >2 µg/ml
Glutethimide (Doriden)	2–6 µg/ml	1–2 hours	>20 µg/ml
Gold	1.0–2.0 µg/ml	2–6 hours	>5.0 µg/ml
Haloperidol (Haldol)	5–15 ng/ml	2–6 hours	>50 ng/ml
Hydromorphone (Dilaudid)	1–30 ng/ml	½–1½ hours	>100 ng/ml
Ibuprofen (Motrin, etc.)	10–50 µg/ml	1–2 hours	>100 µg/ml

Drug	Therapeutic Range	Peak Time	Toxic Level
Imipramine (Tofranil) + desipramine parent and active metabolite)	200–350 ng/ml	PO: 1–2 hours IM: 30 minutes	>500 ng/ml
Isoniazid (INH, Nydrazid)	1–7 µg/ml (dose usually adjusted based on liver function tests)	1–2 hours	>20 µg/ml
Kanamycin (Kantrex)	Peak: 15–30 µg/ml	PO: 1–2 hours IM: 30 minutes–1 hour	Peak: >35 µg/ml Trough: >10 µg/ml
Lead	<20 µg/dl Urine: <80 µg/24 hours		>80 µg/dl Urine: >125 µg/24 hours
Lidocaine (Xylocaine)	1.5–5 µg/ml	IV: 10 minutes	>6 µg/ml
Lithium	0.8–1.2 mEq/l	$^{1}/_{2}$–4 hours	>1.5 mEq/l
Lorazepam (Ativan)	50–240 ng/ml	1–3 hours	>300 ng/ml
Maprotiline (Ludiomil)	200–300 ng/ml	12 hours	>500 ng/ml
Meperidine (Demerol)	0.4–0.7 µg/ml	2–4 hours	>1.0 µg/ml
Mephenytoin (Mesantoin)	15–40 µg/ml	2–4 hours	>50 µg/ml
Meprobamate (Equanil, Miltown)	15–25 µg/ml	2 hours	>50 µg/ml
Methadone (Dolophine)	100–400 ng/ml	$^{1}/_{2}$–1 hour	>2000 ng/ml or >0.2 µg/ml
Methaqualone	1–5 µg/ml		>10 µg/ml
Methyldopa (Aldomet)	1–5 µg/ml	3–6 hours	>7 µg/ml
Methyprylon (Noludar)	8–10 µg/ml	1–2 hours	>50 µg/ml
Metoprolol (Lopressor)	75–200 ng/ml	2–4 hours	>225 ng/ml
Methotrexate	<0.1 µmol/l after 48 h	1–2 hours	1.0×10^6 at 48 h
Methsuximide	<1.0 µg/ml	1–4 hours	>40 µg/ml

(continued)

Drug	Therapeutic Range	Peak Time	Toxic Level
Mexiletine (Mexitil)	<0.5–2 µg/ml	2–3 hours	>2 µg/ml
Morphine	10–80 ng/ml	IV: immediately IM: $1/2$–1 hour SC: 1–$1^1/2$ hours	>200 ng/ml
Netilmicin (Netromycin)	Peak: 0.5–10 µg/ml Trough: <4 µg/ml	IV: 30 minutes	Peak: >16 µg/ml Trough: >4 µg/ml
Nifedipine (Procardia)	50–100 ng/ml	$1/2$–2 hours	>100 ng/ml
Nortriptyline (Aventyl)	50–150 ng/ml	8 hours	>200 ng/ml
Oxazepam (Serax)	0.2–1.4 µg/ml	1–2 hours	
Oxycodone (Percodan)	10–100 ng/ml	$1/2$–1 hour	>200 ng/ml
Pentazocine (Talwin)	0.05–0.2 µg/ml	1–2 hours	>1.0 µg/ml Urine: >3.0 µg/ml
Pentobarbital (Nembutal)	1–5 µg/ml	$1/2$–1 hour	>10 µg/ml Severe toxicity: >30 µg/ml
Phenmetrazine (Preludin)	5–30 µg/ml (Urine)	2 hours	>50 µg/ml (urine)
Phenobarbital (Luminal)	15–40 µg/ml	6–18 hours	>40 µg/ml Severe toxicity: >80 µg/ml
Phenytoin (Dilantin)	10–20 µg/ml	4–8 hours	>20–30 µg/ml Severe toxicity: >40 µg/ml
Pindolol (Visken)	0.5–6.0 ng/ml	2–4 hours	>10 ng/ml
Primidone (Mysoline)	5–12 µg/ml	2–4 hours	>12–15 µg/ml
Procainamide (Pronestyl)	4–10 µg/ml	1 hour	>10 µg/ml
Procaine (Novocain)	<11 µg/ml	10–30 minutes	>20 µg/ml
Prochlorperazine (Compazine)	50–300 ng/ml	2–4 hours	>1000 ng/ml
Propoxyphene (Darvon)	0.1–0.4 µg/ml	2–3 hours	>0.5 µg/ml
Propranolol (Inderal)	>100 ng/ml	1–2 hours	>150 ng/ml

Drug	Therapeutic Range	Peak Time	Toxic Level
Protriptyline (Vivactil)	50–150 ng/ml	8–12 hours	>200 ng/ml
Quinidine	2–5 µg/ml	1–3 hours	>6 µg/ml
Ranitidine (Zantac)	100 ng/ml	2–3 hours	>100 ng/ml
Reserpine (Serpasil)	20 ng/ml	2–4 hours	>20 ng/ml
Salicylates (Aspirin)	10–30 mg/dl	1–2 hours	Tinnitis: 20–40 mg/ml Hyperventilation: >35 mg/dl Severe toxicity: >50 mg/dl
Secobarbital (Seconal)	2–5 µg/ml	1 hour	>15 µg/ml Severe toxicity: >30 µg/ml
Theophylline (Theodur, Aminodur)	10–20 µg/ml	PO: 2–3 hours IV: 15 minutes (depends on smoking or nonsmoking)	>20 µg/ml
Thiocyanate	4–20 µg/ml		>60 µg/ml
Thioridazine (Mellaril)	100–600 ng/ml 1.0–1.5 µg/ml	2–4 hours	>2000 ng/ml >10 µg/ml
Timolol (Blocadren)	3–55 ng/ml	1–2 hours	>60 ng/ml
Tobramycin (Nebcin)	Peak: 5–10 µg/ml Trough: 1–1.5 µg/ml	IV: 15–30 minutes IM: ½–1½ hours	Peak: >12 µg/ml Trough: >2 µg/ml
Tocainide (Tonocard)	4–10 µg/ml	½–3 hours	>12 µg/ml
Tolbutamide (Orinase)	80–240 µg/ml	3–5 hours	>640 µg/ml
Trazodone (Desyrel)	500–2500 ng/ml	1–2 weeks	>4000 ng/ml
Trifluoperazine (Stelazine)	50–300 ng/ml	2–4 hours	>1000 ng/ml
Valproic Acid (Depakene)	50–100 µg/ml	½–1½ hours	>100 µg/ml Severe toxicity: >150 µg/ml
Vancomycin (Vanocin)	Peak: 20–40 µg/ml Trough: 5–10 µg/ml	IV: Peak: 5 minutes IV: Trough: 12 hours	Peak: >80 µg/ml
Verapamil (Calan)	100–300 ng/ml	PO: 1–2 hours IV: 5 minutes	>500 ng/ml

(continued)

Drug	Therapeutic Range	Peak Time	Toxic Level
Warfarin (Coumadin)	1–10 μg/ml (dose usually adjusted by 1 to 2.5 × control)	1$\frac{1}{2}$–3 days	>10 μg/ml

HIV drugs are primarily dosed based on the clients' viral load or CD4 counts. Many of these drugs have dosage adjustments for renal and/or hepatic impairment.

	Peak Time	Half-life
Combination HIV Drugs for Monitoring		
Antiretroviral Protease Inhibitors		
Lopinavir/ritonavir (Kaletra)	4 hours	5 to 6 hours
Nucleoside Analog Reverse Transciptase Inhibitors (NRTIs)		
Abacavir/lamivudine/ zidovudine (Trizivir)		
Lamivudine/zidovudine (Combivir)		
Single HIV Drugs for Monitoring		
Protease Inhibitors		
Amprenariv (Agenerase)	1–2 hours	7 to 9.5 hours
Indinavir (Crixivan)	0.8 hours	2 hours (hepatic impairment, 3 hours)
Antiretroviral		
Stavudine (Zerit)	1 to 1.5 hours	1.5 hours (8 hours in renal impairment)
Antiretroviral Protease Inhibitors		
Ritonavir (Norvir)	2 to 4 hours	3 to 5 hours
Guanosine Nucleoside Reverse Transciptase Inhibitor		
Abacavir (Ziagen)		1.5 hour
Nucleoside Reverse Transcriptase Inhibitor (NRTI)		
Didanosine (Videx)	0.25 to 1.5 hours	1.5 hour
Lamivudine (Epivir)		5 to 7 hours (dose adjustment in renal impairment)
Zidovudine (Retrovir)	0.5 to 1.5 hours	1 hour (1.4 to 2.9 hours in renal impairment)
Non-Nucleoside Reverse Transcriptase Inhibitor (NNRTI)		
Efavirenz (Sustiva)	3 to 5 hours	40 to 55 hours
Nevirapine (Viramune)	4 hours	25 to 30 hours

APPENDIX A

Abbreviations

ABG	Arterial blood gas
ACA	Anticardiolipin antibody
ACE	Angiotensin-converting enzyme
ACP	Acid phosphatase
ACTH	Adrenocorticotropic hormone
ADH	Antidiuretic hormone
AFB	Acid-fast bacillus
AFP	Alpha-fetoprotein
AGBM	Antiglomerular basement membrane antibody
A/G ratio	Albumin/globulin ratio
AHF	Antihemophilic factor
AIDS	Acquired immune deficiency syndrome
ALD	Aldolase
ALP	Alkaline phosphatase
ALT	Alanine aminotransferase (same as SGPT)
α-1-AT	Alpha-1-antitrypsin
AMA	Antimitochondrial antibody
ANA	Antinuclear antibodies
ANH	Atrial natriuretic hormone
Anti-DNA	Anti-deoxyribonucleic acid
APA	Antiphospholipid antibody
APTT	Activated partial thromboplastin time
ARC	AIDS-related complex

ASO	Antistreptolysin O
AST	Aspartate aminotransferase (same as SGOT)
BE	Base excess
BP	Blood pressure
BPH	Benign prostatic hypertropy
BUN	Blood urea nitrogen
C	Complement (e.g., complement C_3)
Ca	Calcium
CA	Cold agglutinins
cAMP	Cyclic adenosine monophosphate
CAT	Computed axial tomography
CBC	Complete blood count
CEA	Carcinoembryonic antigen
CHF	Congestive heart failure
CHO	Carbohydrate
CHS	Cholinesterase
Cl	Chloride
CO	Carbon monoxide
CO_2	Carbon dioxide
CMV	Cytomegalovirus antibody
Cp	Ceruloplasmin
CPK or CK	Creatine phosphokinase
CPK-BB	Creatine phosphokinase, brain
CPK-MB	Creatine phosphokinase, heart
CPK-MM	Creatine phosphokinase, skeletal muscle
Cr	Creatinine
CRF	Corticotropin-releasing factor
CRP	C-reactive protein
CSF	Cerebrospinal fluid
CT	Coagulation time
CT	Computed tomography
CTT	Computed transaxial tomography
Cu	Copper
DIC	Disseminated intravascular coagulation
E_1	Estrone
E_2	Estradiol
E_3	Estriol
E_4	Estetrol
EBV	Epstein-Barr virus
ECG (EKG)	Electrocardiogram
ECF	Extracellular fluid
EDTA	Ethylenediaminetetraacetate
EEG	Electroencephalogram
ELISA	Enzyme-linked immunosorbent assay
EMG	Electromyography

ERCP	Endoscopic retrograde cholangiopancreatography
ESR	Erythrocyte sedimentation rate
FBS	Fasting blood sugar
FDP	Fibrin degradation products
FSH	Follicle-stimulating hormone
FSP	Fibrin or fibrinogen-split product
FTA-ABS	Fluorescent treponemal antibody absorption
G-6-PD	Glucose-6-phosphate dehydrogenase
GGTP or GTP	Gamma-glutamyl (transferase) transpeptidase
GI series	Gastrointestinal series (upper)
GH	Growth hormone
HAA	Hepatitis-associated antigen
HAI or HI	Hemagglutination inhibition
HAV	Hepatitis A virus
Hb or Hgb	Hemoglobin
HB$_c$Ab	Hepatitis B core antibody
HB$_s$Ab	Hepatitis B surface antibody
HB$_s$Ag	Hepatitis B surface antigen
HBD	Hydroxybutyric dehydrogenase
HCG	Human chorionic gonadotropin
HCO$_3$	Bicarbonate
Hct	Hematocrit
hCT	Calcitonin
HDL	High-density lipoprotein
5-HIAA	5-Hydroxyindolacetic acid
HIV	Human immunodeficiency virus
Hp	Haptoglobin
HLA	Human leukocyte antigen
HPL	Human placental lactogen
HSV	Herpes simplex virus
HTLV-III	Human T-lymphotropic virus-III
IBC	Iron-binding capacity (see TIBC)
Ig	Immunoglobulin
IM	Intramuscular
INR	International normalized ratio
IV	Intravenous
IVP	Intravenous pyelography
K	Potassium
17-KS	17-Ketosteroid
KUB	Kidney, ureter, bladder
LAP	Leucine aminopeptidase
LAV	Lymphadenopathy-associated virus
LDH (LD)	Lactic dehydrogenase
LDL	Low-density lipoprotein
LE	Lupus erythematosus preparation

LH	Luteinizing hormone
L/S	Lecithin/sphingomyelin
MCH	Mean corpuscular hemoglobin
MCHC	Mean corpuscular-hemoglobin concentration
MCV	Mean corpuscular volume
Mg	Magnesium
MI	Myocardial infarction
5'NT	5'Nucleotidase
Na	Sodium
NPO	Nil per os (nothing by mouth)
17-OHCS	17-Hydroxycorticosteroid
P	Phosphorus
PA	Prealbumin antibody
PAP	Pulmonary arterial pressure
$PaCO_2$	Partial pressure of carbon dioxide
PCWP	Pulmonary capillary wedge pressure
pH	Negative logarithm of hydrogen ion concentration
PKU	Phenylketonuria
PaO_2	Partial pressure of oxygen
PPBS	Postprandial blood sugar (feasting blood sugar)
PRL	Prolactin
PSA	Prostate-specific antigen
PT	Prothrombin time
PTH	Parathyroid hormone
PTT	Partial thromboplastin time
RA	Rheumatoid arthritis
RAIU	Radioactive iodine uptake
RBC	Red blood cell (erythrocyte)
RDW	Red blood cell distribution width
RF	Rheumatoid factor
RIA	Radioimmunoassay
RPR	Rapid plasma reagin
SGOT	Serum glutamic oxaloacetic transaminase (same as AST)
SGPT	Serum glutamic pyruvic transaminase (same as ALT)
SIADH	Syndrome of inappropriate antidiuretic hormone
SLE	Systemic lupus erythematosus
SaO_2	Oxygen saturation
T_3	Triiodothyronine
T_4	Thyroxine
TA	Thyroid antibodies
TB	Tuberculosis
TBG	Thyroxine-binding globulin
TCA	Tricyclic antidepressants
TDM	Therapeutic drug monitoring
TIBC	Total iron-binding capacity (see IBC)

TRH	Thyrotropin-releasing hormone
T_3 RU	T_3 resin uptake
TSH	Thyroid-stimulating hormone
UA	Urinalysis
URI	Upper respiratory infections
VCT	Venous clotting time
VDRL	Venereal Disease Research Laboratory
VLDL	Very low-density lipoprotein
VMA	Vanillylmandelic acid
VS	Vital signs
WBC	White blood cell (leukocyte)
ZPP	Zinc protoporphyria

APPENDIX B

Laboratory Test Groups

Groups of laboratory tests, identified as panels, profiles, evaluations, and sequential analyzers (SMAs), are useful for diagnosing and assessing clinical problems. Tests are usually grouped as general tests for determining health status and organ and disease panels/profiles/evaluations. Laboratories, private or in health care institutions, develop test groups according to their equipment for analyzing laboratory values. The majority of these tests require either one 10-ml red-top tube, or two 10-ml red-top tubes of blood.

Today, the SMA group name is infrequently used. *Panel, profile,* and *chem* are the terms usually used to refer to groups of laboratory tests. Medicare may not pay for groups that have a large number of tests because of their cost. Laboratories and health care providers, including physicians, may select certain tests within the group to minimize cost and maximize medicare payments. Numerous tests may be performed from one tube of blood.

General laboratory test groups

General Health Panel

Albumin	Glucose
Alkaline phosphatase	LD/LDH
AST/SGOT	Potassium
Bilirubin (total)	Protein (total)

BUN	Sodium
Calcium	Triglyceride
Cholesterol	Uric acid
Creatinine	

Chemzyme Evaluation, or Profile 22

A/G ratio	Chloride
Albumin	Cholesterol
Alkaline phosphatase	CO_2 (content)
ALT/SGPT	Creatinine
AST/SGOT	Globulin
Bilirubin (total)	Glucose
BUN	LD/LDH
BUN/creatinine ratio	Phosphorus
Calcium	Potassium
Protein (total)	Triglyceride
Sodium	Uric acid

Chemistry Profile

Albumin	Creatinine
Alkaline phosphatase	Glucose
AST/SGOT	LD/LDH
Bilirubin (total)	Phosphorus
BUN	Protein (total)
Calcium	Uric acid

Profile 11

Albumin	CPK/CK
Alkaline phosphatase	LD/LDH
AST/SGOT	Phosphorus
Bilirubin (total)	Protein (total)
Calcium	Uric acid
Cholesterol	

Electrolytes (LYTES)

(Might be ordered with SMA 12, chemistry profile, or profile 11)

Chloride	Potassium
CO_2 content	Sodium

SMA 12-60

(Laboratory may select any 12 tests to program on their analyzer.)

Albumin	Cholesterol

Alkaline phosphatase
AST/SGOT
Bilirubin (total)
BUN
Calcium

Glucose
LD/LDH
Phosphorus
Protein (total)
Uric acid

Comprehensive Metabolic Panel/Profile

Albumin
Alkaline phosphatase
Aspartate transferase (AST, SGOT)
Bilirubin (total or direct)
Calcium
Chloride

Creatinine
Glucose
Potassium
Protein (total)
Sodium
Urea nitrogen (BUN)

Routine hematology and urine tests

Complete Blood Count (CBC)

WBC count and differential:
  Neutrophil
    band
    segment
  Basophils
  Eosinophils
  Lymphocytes
  Monocytes

Hematocrit
Hemoglobin
RBC count
RBC indices
MCV
MCH
MCHC
RDW

Urinalysis

Appearance
Bacteria
Casts
Color
Glucose
Ketones

pH
Protein
RBC
Specific gravity (SG)
WBC

Organ and disease panel/profile/evaluation

Anemia Panel/Profile/Evaluation

CBC with RBC indices
Folate/folic acid
Hemoglobin electrophoresis
Iron

Reticulocyte count
TIBC
Vitamin B_{12}

Arthritis Panel/Profile/Evaluation

ANA	ESR
ASO	Phosphorus
Calcium	Rheumatoid factor
CRP	Uric acid

Bone/Joint Panel/Profile/Evaluation

Albumin	Protein (total)
Alkaline phosphatase	Synovial fluid analysis
Calcium	Uric acid
Phosphorus	

Cardiac Panel/Profile/Evaluation

AST/SGOT	LDH/LD
CPK/CK	LDH isoenzymes
CPK isoenzymes	Potassium

Coagulation Panel/Profile/Evaluation

APTT	Factor assay
Bleeding time	FDP
Clot retraction	Platelet count
Coagulation time/clotting time	PT

Coma Panel/Profile/Evaluation

Alcohol	Electrolytes
Ammonia	Glucose
Blood gases (pH, $PaCO_2$, HCO_3)	Lactic acid
BUN	Osmolality (serum and urine)
Creatinine	Salicylate
Drug-abuse toxicology screen	

Coronary Risk Panel/Profile/Evaluation

Cholesterol (total)	Lipoprotein phenotyping
HDL	Phospholipids
LDL	Total lipids
VLDL	Triglycerides
Glucose	

Diabetes Mellitus Panel/Profile/Evaluation

BUN	Creatinine
Cholesterol	Electrolytes (K, Na, Cl, CO_2)

Glucose (fasting/2-hour feasting)
Glucose tolerance (*not* for high blood
  sugar)

Ketones (serum and urine)
Triglycerides

Drug Toxicology/Drug Abuse Panel/Profile/Evaluation

Acetaminophen
Amphetamines
Cocaine
Codeine
Meperidine (Demerol)
Meprobamate (Equanil)
Methadone
Morphine

Barbiturates
Benzodiazepines
Phenothiazines
Phenytoin (Dilantin)
Propoxyphene (Darvon)
Salicylates
Tricyclic antidepressants

Hepatic/Liver Panel/Profile/Evaluation

A/G ratio
Albumin
Alkaline phosphatase
ALT/SGPT
AST/SGOT
Bilirubin (total and direct)

Cholesterol
GGT/GGTP
LDH/LD
LDH isoenzymes
Protein (total)
PT

Hepatitis Panel/Profile/Evaluation

HB_cAb or Anti-HB_c (antibody to hepatitis B core antigen)
HB_eAb (hepatitis B e antibody) or
  Anti-HB_e (antibody to HB_eAg)
HB_eAg (hepatitis B e antigen)

HB_sAb (hepatitis B surface antibody)
  or Anti-HB_s (antibody to Hb_sAg)
HB_sAg (hepatitis B surface antigen)
Anti-HAV (antibody to hepatitis A
  virus [IgM])

Hypertension Panel/Profile/Evaluation

BUN
Creatinine
Cholesterol
Electrolytes (K, NA, Cl, CO_2)
Glucose

LDH/LD
Renin
T_4
Triglycerides
VMA

Lipid Panel/Profile/Evaluation

Cholesterol (total)
  HDL
  LDL

Lipids (total)
Phospholipids
Triglycerides

Neonatal Panel/Profile/Evaluation

Albumin
Bilirubin (total)
Blood type (ABO)
BUN

Calcium
Electrolytes (K, Na, Cl, CO_2)
Glucose
Rh typing

Pancreatic Panel/Profile/Evaluation

Amylase
Calcium

Glucose
Lipase

Parathyroid Panel/Profile/Evaluation

Alkaline phosphatase
Calcium (serum and urine)
Magnesium

Phosphorus
Protein (total)

Prenatal Panel/Profile/Evaluation

Atypical antibody screen
Blood type (ABO)
CBC with differential
Rh typing

Hepatitis B surface antigen (HBsAg)
RPR or VDRL
Rubella screen
Urinalysis

Pulmonary/Lung Panel/Profile/Evaluation

Blood gases (pH, $PaCO_2$, PaO_2, HCO_3)
CO_2 content
SaO_2

Renal Panel/Profile/Evaluation

Albumin
BUN
Creatinine (serum and 24-hour urine)
Creatinine clearance

Electrolytes (K, Na, Cl, CO_2)
Glucose
Protein (total and 24-hour urine)
Uric acid

Thyroid Panel/Profile/Evaluation

Calcitonin
Free thyroxine index (FTI or
    Free T_4)
T_4 RIA

T_3RIA
T_3 resin uptake
TSH
TA

APPENDIX C

Laboratory Test Values for Adults and Children

The laboratory tests and their reference values for adults and children are listed according to the laboratory sections that analyze the specimens. The personnel from the laboratory and nuclear medicine departments frequently work together in obtaining blood specimens to be tested by the radioimmunoassay (RIA) method. So that the client does not receive several venous punctures, the laboratory personnel will collect enough blood for all laboratory tests, including RIA.

Arterial blood gases are analyzed in either the pulmonary function laboratory, critical care units, or chemistry section of the laboratory. The cerebrospinal fluid tubes are distributed to the appropriate laboratory sections (i.e., hematology, chemistry, or microbiology).

Reference values differ from laboratory to laboratory, so nurses should refer to the published laboratory values used in their hospitals or private laboratories to check for any differences.

Hematology	Color-top tube	Reference Values	
		Adult	*Child*
Bleeding time		Ivy's method: 3–7 minutes	Same as adult
Carboxyhemoglobin (CO)—*See Chemistry*		Duke's method: 1–3 minutes	
Clot retraction	Red	1–24 hours	Same as adult
Coagulation time (CT)		5–15 minutes	Same as adult
		Average: 8 minutes	
D-Dimer test	Blue	Negative, Positive: >250 ng/ml	
Erythrocyte sedimentation rate (ESR)	Lavender	<50 years old (Westergren) Male: 0–15 mm/h Female: 0–20 mm/h >50 years old (Westergren) Male: 0–20 mm/h Female: 0–30 mm/h Wintrobe method: Male: 0–9 mm/h Female: 0–15 mm/h	Newborn: 0–2 mm/hour 4–14 years old: 0–10 mm/hour
Euglobulin lysis time	Blue	No lysis	Same as adult
Factor assay	Blue		
I Fibrinogen		200–400 mg/dl	
II Prothrombin		Minimum for clotting: 75–100 mg/dl Minimum hemostatic level: 10%–15% concentration	
III Thromboplastin		Variety of substances	
IV Calcium		4.5–5.5 mEq/l or 9–11 mg/dl	
V Proaccelerin labile factor		Minimum hemostatic level: 50%–150% activity; 5%–10% concentration	Same as adult
VI		Not used	
VII Proconvertin stable factor		Minimum hemostatic level: 65%–135% activity; 5%–15% concentration	
VIII Antihemophilic factor (AHF)		Minimum hemostatic level: 55%–145% activity; 30%–35% concentration	

Test	Tube Color	Reference Value	Pediatric/Other Values
IX Plasma thromboplastin component (PTC, Christmas factor)		Minimum hemostatic level: 60%–140% activity; 30% concentration	
X Stuart factor, Prower factor		Minimum hemostatic level: 45%–150% activity; 7%–10% concentration	
XI Plasma thromboplastin antecedent (PTA)		Minimum hemostatic level: 65%–135% activity; 20%–30% concentration	
XII Hageman factor		0% concentration	
XIII Fibrinase, fibrin stabilizing factor (FSF)		Minimum hemostatic level: 1% concentration	
Fetal Hemoglobin (Hb F)	Lavender Green	0.2%	Newborn: 60–90% 1–5 months: <70% 6–12 months: <5% >1 yr old: <2% Not usually done
Fibrin degradation products (FDP)	Blue	2 to 10 µg/ml	
Fibrinogen	Blue	200–400 mg/dl	Newborn: 150–300 mg/dl Child same as adult
Galactose-1-Phosphate Uridyl Transferase (GPUT)	Lavender	Negative Quantitative; 18.5–28.5 U/g; <5 µ/g in Hb Carrier of deficiency: 5–18 µ/g of Hb	
Hematocrit (Hct)	Lavender	Male: 40%–54%; 0.40–0.54 SI units Female: 36%–46%; 0.36–0.46 SI units	Newborn: 44%–65% 1–3 years old: 29%–40% 4–10 years old: 31%–43%
Hemoglobin (Hb or Hgb)	Lavender	Male: 13.5–17 g/dl Female: 12–15 g/dl	Newborn: 14–24 g/dl Infant: 10–17 g/dl Child: 11–16 g/dl
Hemoglobin Aic	Lavender Green	4.5–7.5% of Hb	
Hemoglobin electrophoresis	Lavender		
A$_1$		95%–98% total Hb	Newborn: 50%–80% total Hb
A$_2$		1.5%–4.0%	Infant: 2%–8% total Hb
F		<2%	Child: 1%–2% total Hb

Hematology	Color-top tube	Reference Values — Adult	Reference Values — Child
C	Lavender	0%	
D		0%	
S		0%	
Heinz Bodies	Lavender	Negative: <30% of Heinz bodies present	
Lymphocytes (T & B) assay	Lavender (2 tubes)	T cells: 60%–80%, 600–2400 cells/µl; B cells: 4%–16%; 50–250 cells/µl	
Methemoglobin	Lavender; Green	Normal: <1.5% total Hb; 0.06–0.24 g/dl; 9.2–37.0 Umol/l; Positive: >20–70%	
Osmotic fragility: erythrocyte		% Hemolysis (see below)	Same as adult
Partial thromboplastin time (PTT)	Blue	PPT: 60–70 seconds; APTT: 25–40 seconds	
Plasminogen	Blue	7–16 mg/dl	
Platelet aggregation and adhesion	Blue	Aggregation in 3–5 minutes	
Platelet Antibody Test	Blue	Negative	
Platelet count (thrombocytes)	Lavender	150,000–400,000 µl (mean, 250,000 µl) (mm³, K/Ul also) SI units: 0.15–0.4 × 10^{12}/l	Premature: 100,000–300,000 µl; Newborn: 150,000–300,000 µl

% Hemolysis (Osmotic fragility: erythrocyte)

% Saline (NaCl)	Fresh Blood (3 hours)	Incubated at 37°C (24-hour blood)
0.30	97–100	85–100
0.35	90–98	75–100
0.40	50–95	65–100
0.45	5–45	55–95
0.50	0–5	40–85
0.55	0	15–65
0.60	0	0–40

Test	Tube color	Reference value (adult)	Reference value (pediatric)
			Infant: 200,000–475,000 µl
Prothrombin time (PT)	Blue or black	11–15 seconds or 70%–100% Anticoagulant therapy: 2–2.5 times the control in seconds or 20%–30%	Same as adult
RBC indices (mil/µl)	Lavender	Male: 4.6–6.0 Female: 4.0–5.0	Newborn: 4.8–7.2 Child: 3.8–5.5
MCV (cuµ)		80–98	Newborn: 96–108 Child: 82–92
MCH (pg)		27–31	Newborn: 32–34 Child: 27–31
MCHC (%)		32–36	Newborn: 32–33 Child: 32–36
RDW (Coulter S)		11.5–14.5	
Reticulocyte count	Lavender	0.5%–1.5% of all RBCs	Newborn: 2.5%–6.5% of all RBCs Infant: 0.5%–3.5% of all RBCs Child: 0.5%–2.0% of all RBCs
		25,000–75,000 µl (absolute count)	
Sickle cell screening	Lavender	0	0
White blood cells (WBC)	Lavender	4,500–10,000 µl	Newborn: 9000–30,000 µl 2 years old: 6000–17,000 µl; 10 years: 4500–13,500 µl
White blood cell differential	Lavender		
Neutrophils		50%–70% of total WBCs	29%–47%
Segments		50%–65%	
Bands		0%–5%	
Eosinophils		0%–3%	0%–3%
Basophils		1%–3%	1%–3%
Lymphocytes		25%–35%	38%–63%
Monocytes		2%–6%	4%–9%

Reference Values

Hematology	Color-top tube	Adult	Child
Immunohematology (Blood Bank)			
Coombs direct	Lavender	Negative	Negative
Coombs indirect	Red	Negative	Negative
Cross matching	Red	Absence of agglutination (clumping)	Same as adult
Rh typing	Red	Rh+ and Rh−	Same as adult

Reference Values

Chemistry	Color-top tube	Adult	Child
Acetaminophen	Red	Therapeutic: 5–20 µg/ml; 31–124 µmol/l (SI units) Toxic: >50 µg/ml; >305 µmol/l (SI units) >200 µg/ml, possible hepatotoxicity	Therapeutic: same as adult
Acetone (ketone bodies) adult	Red	Acetone: 0.3–2.0 mg/dl; 51.6–344 µmol/l (SI units) Ketones: 2–4 mg/dl	Newborn: slightly higher than adult Infant and child: same as adult
Acid phosphatase (ACP)	Red	<2.6 ng/ml, 0–5 U/l	
Adrenocorticotropic Hormone (ACTH)	Lavender	7–10 AM: 8–80 pg/ml; 4 PM: 5–30 pg/ml; 10 PM to Midnight: <10 pg/ml	
Alanine aminotransferase (ALT, SGPT)	Red	10–35 U/l 4–36 U/l at 37°C (SI units)	Same as adult Infant: could be twice as high
Albumin	Red	3.5–5 g/dl	
Alcohol	Red	0%	
Aldolase (ALD)	Red	3–8 U/dl (Sibley-Lehninger) 22–59 mU/l at 37°C (SI units)	Infant: 12–24 U/dl Child: 6–16 U/dl

Test	Tube color	Value	Pediatric values
Aldosterone	Red or green	Fast: <16 ng/dl; 4–30 ng/dl (sitting position)	3–11 years: 5–70 ng/dl
Alkaline phosphatase (ALP)	Red	42–136 U/l	Infant: 40–300 U/l; Child: 40–115 U/l; Older child: 50–230 U/l
ALP[1]		20–130 U/l	
ALP[2]		20–120 U/l	
Alpha-1-antitrypsin	Red	78–200 mg/dl; 0.78–2.0 g/l	Newborn: 145–270 mg/dl; Infant and child: Same as adult
Alpha-fetoprotein (AFP)	Red	see table below	

Weeks of Gestation	Serum (ng/ml)	Amniotic Fluid (µg/ml)
14	7–50	11.0–32.0
15	7–60	5.5–31.0
16	10–72	5.7–31.5
17	11–90	3.8–32.5
18	14–94	3.6–28.0
19	24–112	3.7–24.5
20	31–122	2.2–15.0

Test	Tube color	Value	Pediatric values
Amikacin	Red	Therapeutic: Peak: 15–30 µg/ml; Trough: <10 µg/ml; Toxic: >35 µg/ml	
Amitriptyline (Elavil)		Therapeutic range: 125–200 ng/ml; Toxic level: >500 ng/ml	
Ammonia	Green	15–45 µg/dl; 11–35 umol/l (SI units)	Newborn: 64–107 µg/dl; Child: 21–50 µg/dl
Amylase		30–170 µ/l; Isoenzymes: S: 45–70%; P: 30–55%	
Angiotensin-converting enzyme (ACE)	Red or Green	11–67 U/l	
Anion gap	Green	10–17 mEq/l	
Antidiuretic hormone (ADH)	Lavender	1–5 pg/ml; 1–5 ng/l	Not usually performed

Reference Values

Chemistry	Color-top tube	Adult	Child
Arterial blood gases (*see Others*)			
Ascorbic acid (vitamin C)	Gray or red	0.6–2.0 mg/dl (plasma) 34–114 µmol/l (SI units, plasma) 0.2–2.0 mg/dl (blood) 12–114 µmol (SI units, serum)	0.6–1.6 mg/dl (plasma)
Aspartate aminotransferase (AST, SGOT)	Red	0–35 U/l Average: 8–38 U/l	Newborn: four times normal level Child: same as adult
Atrial natriuretic hormone (ANH)	Lavender	20–77 pg/ml 16–60 U/ml at 30°C 8–33 U/l at 37°C (SI units)	
Barbiturate		0	0
Phenobarbital		Therapeutic: 10–30 µg/ml Toxic: >60 µg/ml	15–30 µg/ml
Bilirubin (indirect)	Red	0.1–1.0 mg/dl 1.7–17.1 µmol/l (SI units)	
Bilirubin (total and direct)	Red	Total: 0.1–1.2 mg/dl; 1.7–20.5 µmol/l (SI units) Direct (conjugated): 0.1–0.3 mg/dl; 1.7–5.1 µmol/l (SI units)	Newborn, total: 1–12 mg/dl; 17.1–205 µmol/l (SI units) Child, total: 0.2–0.8 mg/dl
Blood urea nitrogen (BUN)	Red	5–25 mg/dl	Infant: 5–15 mg/dl Child: 5–20 mg/dl
Bromide	Green	0 Therapeutic: <80 mg/dl Toxic: >100 mg/dl	0
BUN/creatinine ratio	Red	10:1 to 20:1	
Calcitonin	Green or lavender	Male: <40 pg/ml Female: <25 pg/ml	Newborn: usually higher Child: <70 pg/ml
Calcium (Ca)	Red	4.5–5.5 mEq/l 9–11 mg/dl	Newborn: 3.7–7.0 mEq/l; 7.4–14 mg/dl Infant: 5.0–6.0 mEq/l; 10–12 mg/dl

Test	Tube Color	Reference Value	Other
Ionized Calcium (iCa)		2.3–2.8 mmol/l (SI units)	Child: 4.5–5.8 mEq/l; 9–11.5 mg/dl
Carbamazepine	Red	4.4–5.9 mg/dl 2.2–2.5 mEq/l 1.1–1.24 mmol/l Therapeutic: 4–12 µg/ml; 16.9–50.8 µmol/l (SI units) Toxic: >12–15 µg/ml; >50.8–69 µmol/l (SI units)	
Carbon dioxide combining power (CO$_2$)	Green	22–30 mEq/l, 22–30 mmol/l (SI units)	20–28 mEq/l
Carbon monoxide (CO)	Lavender	<2.5% saturation of Hb 2%–9% saturation of Hb (smokers)	Same as adult
Carboxyhemoglobin (may be done in hematology)			
Carotene	Red	60–200 mg/dl 0.74–3.72 µmol/l (SI units)	40–130 µg/dl
Catecholamines	Green or lavender	Positive for pheochromocytoma: >1000 pg/ml	
Epinephrine		Supine: <50 pg/ml Sitting: <60 pg/ml Standing: <90 pg/ml	
Norepinephrine		Supine: 110–410 pg/ml Sitting: 120–680 pg/ml Standing: 125–700 pg/ml	
Dopamine		Supine and standing: <87 pg/ml	
Ceruloplasmin (Cp)	Red	18–45 mg/dl	Infant: <23 mg/dl or normal Child: 30–65 mg/dl
Chlordiazepoxide (Librium)	Red	180–450 mg/l (SI units) Therapeutic Level: 1.0–5.0 µg/ml Toxic: >6 µg/ml	
Chloride (Cl)	Red	95–105 mEq/l 95–105 mmol/l (SI units)	Newborn: 94–112 mEq/l Infant: 95–110 mEq/l Child: 98–105 mEq/l Infant: 90–130 mg/dl

| | | Reference Values | |
Chemistry	Color-top tube	Adult	Child
Cholesterol	Red	Desirable level: <200 mg/dl Moderate risk: 200–240 mg/dl High risk: >240 mg/dl	2–19 years: Desirable level: 130–170 mg/dl; Moderate risk: 171–184 mg/dl; High risk: >185 mg/dl
Cholinesterase	Green	0.5–1.0 U (RBC) 3–8 U/ml (plasma) 6–8 IU/l (RBC)	Same as adult
Copper (Cu)	Red or green	8–18 IU/l at 37°C (plasma) Male: 70–140 µg/dl: 11–22 µmol/l (SI units) Female: 80–155 µg/dl; 12.6–24.3 µmol/l (SI units)	Newborn: 20–70 µg/dl Child: 30–190 µg/dl Adolescent: 90–240 µg/dl
Cortisol	Green	Pregnancy: 140–300 µg/dl 8 AM–10 AM: 5–23 µg/dl; 138–635 nmol/l (SI units) 4 PM–6 PM: 3–13 µg/dl; 83–359 nmol/l (SI units)	8 AM–10 AM: 15–25 µg/dl 4 PM–6 PM: 5–10 µg/dl
Creatine phosphokinase (CPK)	Red	Male: 5–35 µg/ml; 30–180 IU/l, 55–170 U/l at 37°C (SI units) Female: 5–25 µg/ml; 25–150 IU/l; 30–135 U/l at 37°C (SI units)	Newborn: 65–580 IU/l at 30°C Child: Male: 0–70 IU/l at 30°C Female: 0–50 IU/l at 30°C
Creatinine	Red	0.5–1.5 mg/dl 45–132.3 µmol/l (SI units)	Newborn: 0.8–1.4 mg/dl Infant: 0.7–1.7 mg/dl 2–6 years: 0.3–0.6 mg/dl, 24–54 µmol/l (SI units) 7–18 years: 0.4–1.2 mg/dl, 36–106 µmol/l (SI units)
Cryoglobulins	Red	Negative	
Diltiazem (Cardizem)	Red	Therapeutic: 50–200 ng/ml Toxic: >200 ng/ml	

Test	Tube	Reference values
Disseminated intravascular coagulation (DIC) screening test		*See Part III, Hematologic Conditions.*
Dexamethasone suppression test	Green	Cortisol: 8 AM: <10 µg/dl
Diazepam (Valium)	Red	Therapeutic: 400–600 ng/ml; 0.5–2.0 mg/l; Toxic: >1000 ng/ml; >3 mg/l
Digoxin	Red	Therapeutic: 0.5–2 ng/ml; 0.5–2 nmol/l (SI units) Toxic: >2 ng/ml; >2.6 nmol/l (SI units) Therapeutic: Infant: 1–3 ng/ml; 1–3 nmol/l (SI units) Toxic: >3.5 ng/ml
Doxepin (Sinequan)		Therapeutic range: 150–250 ng/ml Toxic level: >500 ng/ml
D-xylose absorption	Red	25–40 mg/dl/2h Elderly: same as adult 30 mg/dl/1h
Estetrol (E$_4$)	Red	Pregnancy: Serum

Weeks of Gestation	pg/ml
20–26	140–210
30	350
36	900
40	>1050

Test	Tube	Reference values
Estradiol (E$_2$)	Red	Female: Follicular: 20–150 pg/ml; Midcycle: 100–500 pg/ml; Luteal: 60–260 pg/ml; Postmenopausal: <30 pg/ml 3–10 pg/ml

Reference Values

Chemistry	Color-top tube	Adult	Child
Estriol/E₃	Red	Male: 15–50 pg/ml Pregnancy: Serum *Weeks of Gestation* *ng/dl* 25–28 25–165 29–32 30–230 33–36 45–370 37–38 75–420 39–40 95–450	
Estrone (E₁)	Red	Follicular phase: 30–100 pg/ml; Ovulatory phase: >150 pg/ml; Luteal phase: 90–160 pg/ml; Postmenopausal: 20–40 pg/ml Male: 10–50 pg/ml	1–10 years: <10 pg/ml

Estrogen	Red	Female:
		Early menstrual cycle:
		  60–200 pg/ml
		Midmenstrual cycle:
		  120–440 pg/ml
		Male: 40–155 pg/ml
			1–6 years: 3–10 pg/ml
			8–12 years: <30 pg/ml

Ethosuximide	Red	Therapeutic: 40–100 μg/ml; 283–708 μmol/l Toxic: >100 μg/ml; >708 μmol/l (SI units)	Therapeutic: 2–4 per/ mg/kg/day Toxic: same as adult or higher
Fasting blood sugar (FBS)	Gray or red	70–110 mg/dl (serum)	Newborn: 30–80 mg/dl
Feasting blood sugar (*See Postprandial blood sugar.*)		60–100 mg/dl (blood)	Child: 60–100 mg/dl
Ferritin	Red	Female: 10–235 ng/ml	Newborn: 20–200 ng/ml Infant: 30–200 ng/ml

Test	Tube color	Normal values	Child
		10–235 µg/l (SI units)	1–16 years: 8–140 ng/ml
		Male: 15–445 ng/ml; 15–445 µg/l (SI units)	
Folate (folic acid) (may be done by nuclear medicine)	Red	3–16 ng/ml (bioassay); >2.5 ng/ml (RIA; serum); 200–700 ng/ml (RBC)	Same as adult
Follicle-stimulating hormone (FSH)	Red	Pre-postovulation: 4–30 mU/ml; Midcycle: 10–90 mU/ml; Postmenopausal: 40–170 mU/ml; Male: 4–25 mU/ml	5–12 mU/ml
Gamma-glutamyl transferase (GGT)	Red	Male: 4–23 IU/l; Female: 3–13 IU/l; 4–33 U/l at 37°C (SI units)	
Gastrin	Red or lavender	Fasting: <100 pg/ml	Not usually done
Gentamicin	Red	Therapeutic: Peak: 5–10 µg/ml; Trough: <2 µg/ml; Toxic: >12 µg/ml	
Glucose-6-phosphate dehydrogenase (G-6-PD) (may be done in hematology)	Lavender or green	8–18 IU/gHb; 125–281 U/dl (packed RBC); 251–511 U/dl (cells); 1211–2111 mIU/ml (Packed RBC)	Same as adult
Glucose—fasting blood sugar (See *Fasting blood sugar.*)			
Glucagon	Lavender	50–200 pg/ml	
Glucose tolerance test (GTT)	Gray or red	(see table below)	

Time	Serum (mg/dl)	Blood (mg/dl)	Child (6 years or older)
Fasting	70–110	60–100	Same as adult
0.5 hour	<160	<150	
1 hour	<170	<160	
2 hour	<125	<115	
3 hour	Fasting level	Fasting level	

Chemistry	Color-top tube	Reference Values	
		Adult	*Child*
Growth hormone	Red	Male: <5 ng/ml Female: <10 ng/ml	<10 ng/ml
Haloperidol (Haldol)	Red	Therapeutic range: 3–20 ng/ml Toxic: >50 ng/ml	
Hexosaminidase	Red	Total: 5–20 U/l A: 55%–80%	
Human chorionic gonadotropin (HCG)	Red	Nonpregnant female: <0.01 IU/ml	

Pregnant (Weeks)   *Values*

1	0.01–0.04 IU/ml
2	0.03–0.10 IU/ml
4	0.10–1.0 IU/ml
5–12	10–100 IU/ml
13–25	10–30 IU/ml
26–40	5–15 IU/ml

Chemistry	Color-top tube	Reference Values	
Human immunosuppressive virus (HIV)	Red	Negative	
Human leukocyte antigen (HLA)	Green	Histocompatibility match	
Human placental lactogen (HPL)	Red or green	*Weeks of Gestation* *ng/ml*	

8–27	4.6 µg/ml
28–31	2.4–6.0 µg/ml
32–35	3.7–7.7 µg/ml
36–40	5.0–10.0 µg/ml

Chemistry	Color-top tube	Reference Values	
Imipramine (Tofranil)	Red	Therapeutic range: 150–300 ng/ml Toxic level: >500 ng/ml	
Immunoglobulins *(See Serology.)*	Red		
Insulin	Red	5–25 µU/ml	
International normalized ratio (INR)	Black	2.0–3.0	

Test	Tube color	Normal Values	Pediatric Values
Iron	Red	50–150 µg/dl; 10–27 µmol/l (SI units)	6 months–2 years: 40–100 µg/dl Newborn: 100–270 µg/dl Infant (6 months–2 years): 100–350 µg/dl Child: same as adult
Iron-binding capacity (IBC, TIBC)	Red	250–450 µg/dl	
Lactic acid	Green	Arterial blood: 0.5–2.0 mmol/l; <11.3 mg/dl Venous blood: 0.5–1.5 mmol/l; 8.1–15.3 mg/dl Critical: >5 mEq/l; >45 mg/dl	
Lactic dehydrogenase (LDH/LD)	Red	100–190 IU/l; 70–250 U/l	Newborn: 300–1500 IU/l Child: 50–150 IU/l
LDH isoenzymes LDH₁ LDH₂ LDH₃ LDH₄ LDH₅	Red	14%–26% 27%–37% 13%–26% 8%–16% 6%–16%	
Lactose tolerance test	Gray	20–50 mg/dl rise from fasting blood glucose	
Lead	Lavender or green	10–20 µg/dl 20–40 µg/dl (acceptable)	10–20 µg/dl 20–30 µg/dl (acceptable)
LE cells (Lupus) also in *Hematology*	Red or green	Negative	
Lecithin/sphingomyelin ratio (L/S; amniotic fluid)		1:1 before 35 weeks of gestation L: 6–9 mg/dl S: 4–6 mg/dl 4:1 after 35 weeks of gestation L: 15–21 mg/dl S: 4–6 mg/dl	
Leucine aminopeptidase (LAP)	Red	8–22 mU/ml, 12–33 IU/l; 75–200 U/ml	
Lidocaine	Red	Therapeutic: 1.5–5.0 µg/ml; 6.0–22.5 µmol/l (SI units) Toxic: >6 µg/ml	
Lipase	Red	20–180 IU/l; 114–286 U/l 14–280 mU/ml 14–280 U/l (SI units)	Infant: 9–105 IU/l at 37°C Child: 20–136 IU/l at 37°C

Chemistry	Color-top tube	Reference Values	
		Adult	Child

Chemistry	Color-top tube	Adult	Child
Lipoproteins (See Cholesterol, Phospholipids, and Triglycerides.)			
Lithium	Red	0 Therapeutic: 0.8–1.2 mEq/l Toxic: >2 mEq/l	0
Luteinizing hormone (LH)	Red or lavender	Pre-postovulation: 5–30 mIU/ml Midcycle: 50–150 mIU/ml Postmenopause: >35 mIU/ml Male: 5–25 mIU/ml	6–12 years: <10 mIU/ml; 13–18 years: <20 mIU/ml
Magnesium (Mg)	Red	1.5–2.5 mEq/l; 1.8–3.0 mg/dl	Newborn: 1.4–2.9 mEq/l Child: 1.6–2.6 mEq/l
Myoglobin	Red	12–90 μg/l; 12–90 ng/ml	
Nifedipine	Red	Therapeutic: 50–100 ng/ml Toxic: >100 ng/ml	

Nortriptyline (Aventyl)	Red	Therapeutic range:
		  50–150 ng/ml
		Toxic level:
		  >200 ng/ml	

5Nucleotidase (5N)	Red	<17 U/l	
Osmolality	Red	280–300 mOsm/kg PTH: 11–54 pg/ml	270–290 mOsm/kg
Parathyroid hormone (PTH)	Red	C Terminal PTH: 50–330 pg/ml; N-Terminal PTH: 8–24 pg/ml	
Pepsinogen I	Red	124–142 ng/ml	Premature: 20–24 ng/ml <1 year: 72–82 ng/ml 1–2 years: 90–106 ng/ml 3–6 years: 80–104 ng/ml 7–10 years: 77–103 ng/ml 11–14 years: 96–118 ng/ml
Phenothiazines (See Part 1.)			
Phenytoin (Dilantin)	Red	Therapeutic: 10–20 μg/ml; 39.6–79.3 μmol/l (SI units) Toxic: >20 μg/ml; >79.3 μmol/l (SI units)	Toxic: >15–20 μg/ml; 56–79 μmol/l (SI units)

Test	Tube color	Reference values
Phospholipids	Red	150–380 mg/dl
Phosphorus (P) (inorganic)	Red	1.7–2.6 mEq/l 2.5–4.5 mg/dl Newborn: 3.5–8.6 mg/dl Infant: 4.5–6.7 mg/dl Child: 4.5–5.5 mg/dl Same as adult
Postprandial blood sugar (feasting; PPBS)	Gray or red	<140 mg/dl 2 hours (plasma) <120 mg/dl 2 hours (blood) Older adult: <160 mg/dl 2 hours (plasma); <140 mg/dl 2 hours (blood)
Potassium (K)	Red	3.5–5.3 mEq/l 3.5–5.3 mmol/l (SI units) Infant: 3.6–5.8 mEq/l Child: 3.5–5.5 mEq/l
Primidone	Red	Therapeutic: 5–12 μg/ml; 23–55 μmol/l (SI units) Therapeutic: Child <5 years: 7–10 μg/ml; 30–45 μmol/l (SI units) Toxic: >12–15 μg/ml; >55–69 μmol/l (SI units) Toxic: >12 μg/ml; >55 μmol/l (SI units)
Procainamide	Red	Therapeutic: 4–8 μg/ml; 17–34 μmol/l (SI units) Toxic: >10 μg/ml; >102 μmol/l (SI units)
Progesterone	Red	Female: Follicular: 0.1–1.5 ng/ml Luteal: 2–28 ng/ml Pregnancy: First trimester: 9–50 ng/ml Second trimester: 18–150 ng/ml Third trimester: 60–260 ng/ml Male: <1.0 ng/ml
Prolactin (PRL)	Red or lavender	Nonpregnant: Follicular: 0–23 ng/ml; Luteal: 0–40 ng/ml; Postmenopausal: <12 ng/ml Pregnancy: First trimester: <80 ng/ml Second trimester: <160 ng/ml Third trimester: <400 ng/ml Male: 0.1–20 ng/ml Pituitary adenoma: >100–300 ng/ml

Reference Values

Chemistry	Color-top tube	Adult	Child
Propranolol (Inderal)	Red	Therapeutic: 50–100 ng/ml; 193–386 nmol/l (SI units)	
Prostate-specific antigen (PSA)	Red	Toxic: >150 ng/ml Normal: 0–4 ng/ml BPH: 4–19 ng/ml Prostate cancer: 10–120 ng/ml	
Protein	Red	6.0–8.0 g/dl	Premature: 4.2–7.6 g/dl Newborn: 4.6–7.4 g/dl Infant: 6.0–6.7 g/dl Child: 6.2–8.0 g/dl
Protein electrophoresis	Red	Albumin: 3.5–5.0 g/dl; 52%–68% of total protein Globulin: 1.5–3.5 g/dl; 32%–48% of total protein	Premature: 3.0–4.2 g/dl Newborn: 3.5–5.4 g/dl Infant: 4.4–5.4 g/dl Child: 4.0–5.8 g/dl
Quinidine	Red	Therapeutic: 2–5 µg/ml; 0.2–15.4 µmol/l (SI units) Toxic: >6 µg/ml; >18.5 µmol/l (SI units)	
Renin	Lavender	Normal sodium diet: supine 0.2–2.3 ng/ml upright 1.6–4.3 ng/ml. Restricted salt diet: upright: 4.1–10.8 ng/ml	3–5 years: 1.0–6.5 ng/ml; 5–10 years: 0.5–6.0 ng/ml
Salicylate	Red	0	0
Serotonin	Lavender	Therapeutic: 15–30 mg/dl Toxic: Mild: >30 mg/dl Severe: >50 mg/dl 50–175 ng/ml; 10–30 µg/dl; 0.29–1.15 µmol/l (SI units)	Toxic: >25 mg/dl
Sodium (Na)	Red	135–145 mEq/l 135–142 nmol/l (SI units)	Infant: 134–150 mEq/l Child: 135–145 mEq/l

Test	Tube color	Reference values	Pediatric/Additional values
T_3	Red	80–200 ng/dl	Newborn: 90–170 ng/dl Child: 6–12 years: 115–190 ng/dl
Testosterone	Red or green	Male: 0.3–1.0 µg/dl; 300–1000 ng/dl Female: 0.03–0.1 µg/dl; 30–100 ng/dl	Male adolescent: >0.1 µg/dl Male: 12–14 years old: >100 rg/dl
Theophylline	Red	Therapeutic: Adult: 5–20 µg/ml; 28–112 µmol/l (SI units) Elderly: 5–18 µg/ml Toxic: Adult: >20 µg/ml; >112 µmol/l (SI units) Elderly: same as adult	Therapeutic: Premature: 7–14 µg/ml Neonate: 3–12 µg/ml Child: same as adult Toxic: Premature: >14 µg/ml Neonate: >13 µg/ml Child: same as adult
Thyroid-binding globulin (TBG)	Red or green	10–26 µg/dl	
Tobramycin	Red	Therapeutic: Peak: 5–10 µg/ml Trough: <2 µg/ml Toxic: >12 µg/ml	
Thyroxine (T_4)	Red	4.5–11.5 µg/dl (T_4 by column) 5–12 µg/dl (T_4 RIA) 1.0–2.3 ng/dl (Thyroxine iodine)	Newborn: 11–23 µg/dl 1–4 months: 7.5–16.5 µg/dl 4–12 months: 5.5–14.5 µg/dl 1–6 years: 5.5–13.5 µg/dl 6–10 years: 5–12.5 µg/dl Newborn: 125–275 mg/dl
Transferrin	Red	200–430 mg/dl; 2–4.3 g/l (SI units) Pregnancy (full term): 300 mg/dl	
Transferrin percent saturation	Red	Male: 30%–50% Female: 20%–35%	
T_3 resin uptake (may be done by nuclear medicine)	Red	25–35 relative % uptake	Not usually done
Tricyclic antidepressants (See Part I.)			
Triglycerides	Red	10–150 mg/dl 0.11–2.09 mmol/l (SI units)	Infant: 5–40 mg/dl Child: 10–135 mg/dl
Uric acid	Red	Male: 3.5–8.0 mg/dl	2.5–5.5 mg/dl

Reference Values

Chemistry	Color-top tube	Adult	Child
Valproic acid	Red	Female: 2.8–6.8 mg/dl Therapeutic: 50–100 µg/ml; 347–693 µmol/l Toxic: >100 µg/ml; >693 µmol/l (SI units)	Therapeutic: same Toxic: same
Verapamil	Red	Therapeutic: 100–300 ng/ml; 0.08–0.3 µg/ml Toxic: >300 ng/ml; >0.3 µg/ml	
Vancomycin	Red	Therapeutic range: Peak: 20–40 µg/ml Trough: 5–10 µg/ml Toxic level: >40 µg/ml	
Vitamin A	Red	30–95 µg/dl; 1.05–3.0 µmol/l (SI units); 125–150 IU/dl	1–6 years: 20–43 µg/dl; 0.7–1.5 µmol/l (SI units); 7–12 years: 26–50 µg/dl; 13–19 years: 26–72 µg/dl
Vitamin B₁	Red	10–60 ng/ml; 5.3–8.0 µg/dl	
Vitamin B₆	Lavender	5–30 ng/ml; 20–120 nmol/l (SI units)	
Vitamin B₁₂	Red	200–900 pg/ml	Newborn: 160–1200 pg/ml
Vitamin C (See Ascorbic acid)			
Vitamin D₃	Red or green	1,23 dihydroxy: 20–76 pg/ml 25-hydroxy: 10–55 ng/ml	
Vitamin E	Red	5–20 µg/ml; 0.5–1.8 mg/dl; 12–42 µmol/l (SI units)	3–15 µg/ml; 0.3–1.0 mg/dl; 7–23 µmol/l (SI units)
Zinc	Navy-blue	60–150 µg/dl 11–23 µmol/l (SI units)	
Zinc	Urine	150–1250 µg/24 h	
Zinc proto-porphyrin (ZPP)	Green or lavender	15–77 µg/dl Average: <35 µg/dl; <0.56 µmol/l (SI units)	Same as adult

Serology	Color-top tube	Reference Values Adult	Reference Values Child
Adenovirus antibody	Red	Negative	Negative
Anticardiolipin antibody	Red	Negative	
Anti-DNA	Red	<1:85	<1:60 <1:70
Antiglomerular basement membrane antibody (AGBM)	Red	Negative	
Antimitochondrial antibody (AMA)	Red	Negative at 1:5 Positive: >1:160	
Antimyocardial antibody	Red	None detected	
Antinuclear antibodies (ANA)	Red	Negative at 1:20 dilution	Negative
Antiparietal cell antibody (APCA)	Red	Negative: <1:120 titer; Positive: 1:180 titer	
Antiscleroderma antibody	Gray	Negative: Borderline: 20–25 units; Positive: >25 units	
Antismooth muscle antibody (ASTHMA)	Red	Negative or <1:20; Positive: >1:20 titer	
Antistreptolysin O (ASO)	Red	100 IU/ml; <160 Todd U/ml	Newborn: similar to mother's 2–5 years: <100 IU/ml 12–19 years: <200 IU/ml; <200 Todd U/ml
Candida antibody test	Red	Negative; Positive: >1:8 titer	
Carcinoembryonic antigen (CEA) (may be done by nuclear medicine)	Red or lavender	<2.5 ng/ml (nonsmokers) <3.5 ng/ml (smokers)	Not usually done
Chlamydia test	Red	<1:16	
Cold agglutinins (CA)	Red	1:8 antibody titer	
Complement (total)	Red	75–160 U/ml; 75–160 kU/l (SI units)	Same as adult

Reference Values

Serology	Color-top tube	Adult	Child
Complement C$_3$	Red	Male: 80–180 mg/dl; 0.8–1.8 g/l (SI units) / Female: 76–120 mg/dl; 0.76–1.2 g/l (SI units)	Not usually done
Complement C$_4$	Red	15–45 mg/dl; 150–450 mg/l (SI units)	Not usually done
C-reactive protein (CRP)	Red	0	0
Cryoglobulins	Red	Up to 6 mg/dl	Negative
Cytomegalovirus (CMV) antibody	Red	Negative to <0.30	
Encephalitis virus antibody	Red	Titer: <1:10	
Enterovirus group	Red	Negative	
Febrile agglutinins	Red	Febrile group: titers *Brucella:* <1:20, Tularemia: <1:40, *Salmonella:* <1:40, *Proteus:* <1:40	Same as adult
FTA-ABS (fluorescent treponemal antibody absorption)	Red	Negative	Negative
Haptoglobin	Red	60–270 mg/dl; 0.6–2.7 g/l (SI units)	Newborn: 0–10 mg/dl; Infant: 1–6 months: 0–30 mg/dl, then gradual increase
Helicobacter pylori	Red	Negative	Negative
HB$_s$Ab	Red	Negative	Negative
HB$_c$Ab	Red	Negative	
Hepatitis A virus (HAV)	Red	None detected	
Hepatitis B surface antigen (HB$_s$Ag)	Red	Negative	Negative
Herpes simplex virus (HSV)	Red	<1:10	

	Specimen	Reference Values	Same as adult	
			1–3 years old	*7–11 years old*
Heterophile antibody	Red	<1:28 titer		
Immunoglobulins (Ig)	Red			
Total Ig		900–2200 mg/dl	400–1500 mg/dl	700–1700 mg/dl
IgG		800–1800 mg/dl	300–1400 mg/dl	600–1450 mg/dl
IgA		100–400 mg/dl	20–150 mg/dl	50–200 mg/dl
IgM		50–150 mg/dl	20–100 mg/dl	30–120 mg/dl
IgD		0.5–3 mg/dl		
Legionnaire antibody test	Red	Negative		
Lyme antibody test	Red	Titer <1:256	Same as adult	
Mumps antibody	Red	Negative or <1:8 titer		
Parvovirus B19 antibody	Red	Negative		
Prealbumin antibody	Red	17–40 mg/dl		
Rabies antibody test	Red	IFA: <1:16		
Rapid plasma reagin (RPR)	Red	Negative	Negative	
Rheumatoid factor (RF)	Red	<1:20 titer	Not usually done	
Rubella antibody detection (HAI or HI)	Red	<1:8 titer susceptible; 1:10–1:32 titer, past rubella exposure; 1:32–1:64 titer, immunity; >1:64 titer, definite immunity	Same as adult	
Thyroid antibodies (TA)	Red	Negative or <1:20 titer	Not usually done	
TORCH test	Red	Negative	Negative	
Toxoplasmosis antibody test	Red	No infection: <1:4; Infected: >1:256		
Venereal disease research laboratory (VDRL)	Red	Negative	Negative	

Reference Values

Microbiology	Adult	Child
Antibiotic susceptibility (sensitivity)	Sensitive to antibiotic Intermediate to antibiotic Resistant to antibiotic	Same as adult
Cultures (blood, sputum, stool, throat, wound, and urine)	No pathogen	Same as adult
Fungal organisms (mycotic infections)	No pathogen or under 8	Same as adult
Malarial smear	Negative	Negative
Occult blood (feces)	Negative	Negative
Parasites and ova (feces)	Negative	Negative
Trypsin (feces)	Negative at dilutions >1:10	
Rotavirus antigen (feces)	Negative	

Reference Values

Urine Chemistry	Adult	Child
Aldosterone	6–25 µg/24 h	Not usually done
Amino acid screen	200 mg/24 h	
Amylase	4–37 U/1/2h	Not usually done
Ascorbic acid tolerance (4-, 5-, or 6-hour sample)	Oral: 10% of administered amount IV: 30%–40% of administered amount	Not usually done
Bence-Jones protein	Negative to trace	Same as adult
Bilirubin and bile	Negative to 0.02 mg/dl	Same as adult
Calcium (Ca)	100–250 mg/24 h (average calcium diet) 2.50–6.25 mmol/24 h	Same as adult
Catecholamines	<100 µg/24 h <0.59 µmol/24 h (SI units) 0–14 µg/dl (random)	Lower level than adult—weight difference
Epinephrine	<20 ng/24 h	
Norepinephrine	<100 ng/24 h	
Cortisol	24–105 µg/24 h	
Creatinine clearance	85–135 ml/min	Similar to adult

Test	Values	Pediatric
Creatinine	Male: 20–26 mg/kg/24 h; 0.18–0.23 mmol/kg/24 h (SI units) Female: 14–22 mg/kg/24 h; 0.12–0.19 mmol/kg/24 h (SI units)	
Estriol (E_3)	Pregnant: | *Weeks of Gestation*	*mg/24 h*
---	---
25–28	6–28
29–32	6–32
33–36	10–45
37–40	15–60		<12 years: 1 µg/24 h >12 years: same as adult
Estrogens (total)	Preovulation: 5–25 µg/24 h Follicular phase: 24–100 µg/24 h Luteal phase (menstruation): 22–80 µg/24 Postmenopause: 0–10 µg/24 h Male: 4–25 µg/24 h	
Estrone (E_1)	Female: Follicular phase: 4–7 µg/24 h Ovulatory phase: 11–30 µg/24 h Luteal phase: 10–22 µg/24 h Post menopausal: 1–7 µg/24 h Follicular: 2–15 IU/24 h	
Follicle-stimulating hormone (FSH)	Luteal phase: 4–20 IU/24 h Menopause: >50 IU/24 h	<10 mIU/24 h (prepubertal)
Human chorionic gonadotropin (HCG)	Positive for pregnancy: no agglutination Negative for pregnancy: agglutination	Usually not done
17-Hydroxycorticosteroids (17-OHCS)	Male: 3–12 mg/24 h Female: 2–10 mg/24 h	Infant: <1 mg/24 h 2–4 years: 1–2 mg/24 h 5–12 years: 2–6 mg/24 h
5-Hydroxyindolacetic acid (5-HIAA)	Random: negative 24 hours: 2–10 mg/24 h	Usually not done
Hydroxyproline	14–42 mg/24 h 0.4–4.5 mg/2 h	Higher than adult
Ketone bodies (acetone)	Negative	Negative
17-Ketosteroids (17-KS)	Male: 5–25 mg/24 h	Infant: 1 mg/24 h

Reference Values

Urine Chemistry	Adult	Child

	Female: 5–15 mg/24 h
	>65 years: 4–8 mg/24 h
		1–3 years: <2 mg/24 h
		3–6 years: <3 mg/24 h
		7–10 years: <4 mg/24 h
		10–12 years:
		  Male: <6 mg/24 h
		  Female: <5 mg/24 h
		Adolescent:
		  Male: <3–15 mg/24 h
		  Female: <3–12 mg/24 h

Melanin	Negative	
Myoglobin	None detected	
Opiates	Negative	
Osmolality	50–1200 mOsm/kg Average: 200–800 mOsm/kg	Newborn: 100–600 mOsm/kg Child: same as adult
Phenylketonuria (PKU)	Not usually done	PKU: negative (positive when serum phenylalanine is 12–15 mg/dl) Guthrie: negative (positive when serum phenylalanine is 4 mg/dl)
Porphobilinogen	Random: negative 24 hour: 0–2 mg/24 h	Same as adult
Porphyrins Coproporphyrins	Random: 3–20 µg/dl 24 hours: 50–160 µg	0–80 µg/24 h
Uroporphyrins	Random: negative, 24 hours: <30 µg	10–30 µg/24 h
Potassium (K)	25–120 mEq/24 h 25–120 mmol/24 h (SI units)	17–57 mEq/24 h
Pregnanediol	Male: 0.1–1.5 mg/24 h Female: 0.5–1.5 mg/24 h (proliferative phase); 2–7 mg/24 h (luteal phase); 0.1–1.0 mg/24 h (postmenopausal)	0.4–1.0 mg/24 h

Pregnancy:

	Gestation Weeks	mg/24 h	Child
Pregnanetriol	10–19	5–25	
	20–28	15–42	
	29–32	25–49	
Protein	Male: 0.4–2.4 mg/24 h Female: 0.5–2.0 mg/24 h	Infant: 0–0.2 mg/24 h Child: 0–1.0 mg/24 h	
Sodium (Na)	0–5 mg/dl/24 h	Same as adult	
Uric acid	40–220 mEq/24 h	Same as adult	
Urinalysis	250–500 mg/24 h (low-purine diet)		
pH	4.5–8.0	Newborn: 5–7 Child: 4.5–8	
Specific gravity (SG)	1.005–1.030	Newborn: 1.001–1.020 Child: Same as adult	
Protein	Negative	Negative	
Glucose	Negative	Negative	
Ketones	Negative	Negative	
RBC	1-2/low-power field	Rare	
WBC	3–4	0–4	
Casts	Occasional hyaline	Rare	
Vitamin B$_1$	100–200 μg/24 h		

Reference Values

Others	Adult	Child
Urobilinogen	Random: 0.3–3.5 mg/dl 0.05–2.5 mg/24 h 0.5–4.0 Ehrlich units/24 h 0.09–4.23 μmol/24 h (SI units)	Same as adult
Vanillylmandelic acid (VMA)	1.5–7.5 mg/24 h 7.6–37.9 μmol/24 h (SI units)	Same as adult
Bleeding time	Ivy's method: 3–7 minutes	Same as adult

Reference Values

Others	Adult	Child
Arterial blood gases (ABGs)		
pH:	7.35–7.45	7.36–7.44
$PaCO_2$	35–45 mm Hg	Same as adult
PaO_2	75–100 mm Hg	Same as adult
HCO_3	24–28 mEq/l	Same as adult
BE	+2 to −2 (± 2 mEq/l)	Same as adult
Cerebrospinal fluid (CSF)		
Pressure	75–175 mm H_2O	50–100 mm H_2O
Cell count	0–8 mm^3	0–8 mm^3
Protein	15–45 mg/dl	15–45 mg/dl
Chloride	118–132 mEq/l	120–128 mEq/l
Glucose	40–80 mg/dl	35–75 mg/dl
Culture	No organism	No organism
Chloride (sweat)	<60 mEq/l	<50 mEq/l
Semen examination	60–150 millim/ml	Not usually
	Volume: 1.5–5.0 ml	done
	Morphology: >75% mature spermatozoa	
	Motility: >60% actively mobile spermatozoa	
Amyloid beta protein precursor (CSF)	Positive 450 units/l	
Viral culture (Blood, Biopsy, CSF, Sputum, Stool, Urine	Negative	

Bibliography

Abrams DI, Parker-Martin J, and Unger KW (1989). AIDS: Caring for the dying patient. *Patient Care, 23:* 22–36.

Abrams DI, Parker-Martin J, and Unger KW (1989). Psychosocial aspects of terminal AIDS. *Patient Care, 23:* 41–60.

Adam H (1989). Introduction. In: Adam H, ed. *Pediatric AIDS.* Report of the Twentieth Ross Round Table on Critical Approaches to Common Pediatric Problems. Columbus, OH: Ross Laboratories, pp 2–3.

AIDS in humans dates to 1930, researcher finds (2000, February 2). *The News Journal,* Wilmington, DE, p. A4.

Barrick B, Vogel S (1996). Application of laboratory diagnostics in HIV testing. *Nursing Clinics of North America, 31*(1): 41–45.

Bartholet J (2000, January 17). The years. *Newsweek,* 31–37.

Bishop ML, Duben-Engelkirk JL, Fody EP (1996). *Clinical Chemistry.* 3rd ed. Philadelphia: JB Lippincott.

Black JM, Matassarin-Jacobs E (1997). *Luckmann and Sorensen's Medical-Surgical Nursing.* 5th ed. Philadelphia: WB Saunders.

Brooks DJ, Beany RP, Thomas DGT (1986). The role of positron emission tomography in the study of cerebral tumors. *Seminars in Oncology, 13:* 83–93.

Brown CH (1989). *Handbook of Drug Therapy Monitoring.* Baltimore: Williams & Wilkins.

Bynum R (1999, August 31). Drop in deaths from AIDS slows. *The News Journal,* Wilmington, DE, p. A5.

Cassetta RA (1993). AIDS: Patient care challenges nursing. *The American Nurse, 25:* 1, 24.

Cassetta RA (1993). The new faces of the epidemic. *The American Nurse, 25:* 16.

CDC revises AIDS definition (1993). *The American Nurse, 25:* 20.

Chernecky CC, Krech RL, Berger BJ (1993). *Cholesterol Uptake In Laboratory Tests and Diagnostic Procedures.* Philadelphia: WB Saunders. 1: 7, 8.

Chernecky CC, Berger BJ, eds (2001). *Laboratory Tests and Diagnostic Procedures.* 3rd ed. Philadelphia: WB Saunders.

Cholesterol Uptake (1988). 1(6): 7, 8.

Clinical Laboratory Tests. 2nd ed. (1995). Springhouse, PA: Springhouse.

Cose E (2000, January 17). A cause that crosses the color line. *Newsweek,* p 49.

Cowley G (2000, January 17). Fighting the disease: What can be done. *Newsweek.* p 38.

Crandall BF, Kulch P, Tabsh K (1994). Risk assessment of amniocentesis between 11 and 15 weeks: Comparison to later amniocentesis controls. *Prenatal Diagnosis, 14:* 913–939.

C-Sections recommended for HIV positive pregnant women (1999, October/November). *AWHONN Lifelines, 3*(5): 17.

Curry JC (1994). Interpreting laboratory data. In: Murma RD, Lyons BA, Borucki MJ, Pollard RB, eds. *HIV Manual for Health Care Professionals.* Norwalk, CT: Appleton & Lange, pp 111–122.

Curry NS (1995). Renal imaging and congenital lesions. In: Sutton D, Young JWR. *A Concise Textbook of Clinical Imaging.* 2nd ed. St. Louis: CV Mosby.

DeLorenzo L (1993). The changing face of AIDS. *The Nursing Spectrum, 2:* 19.

Deprest JA, Gratacos E (1999). Obstetrical endoscopy. *Curr Opin Obstet Gynecol, 11*(2): 195–203.

DeVita VT Jr, Hellman S, Rosenberg SA (1992). *AIDS: Etiology, Diagnosis, Treatment and Prevention.* 3rd ed. Philadelphia: JB Lippincott.

Dunn AM (2001). Children with HIV/AIDS. In: Kirton CA, Talotta D, and Zwolski K., eds. *Handbook of HIV/AIDS Nursing.* St. Louis: CV Mosby, pp 380–420.

Epstein JD (1998, September, 19). Dupont AIDS drug gets FDA approval. *The News Journal,* Wilmington, DE, pp A1, A8.

Erasmus JJ, Patz EF (1999, December). Positron emission tomography imaging in the thorax. *Clinics in Chest Medicine, 20*(4): 715–724.

Facione NC (1999). Breast cancer screening in relation to access to health services. *Oncology Nursing Forum, 26*(4) 689–696.

Fahey JL, Nishanian P (1997). Laboratory diagnosis and evaluation of HIV infection. In: Fahey JL, Flemmig DS (eds). *AIDS/HIV Reference Guide for Medical Professionals.* 4th ed. Baltimore: Wilkins and Wilkins, pp 232–242.

Farrell J (1982). Arthroscopy. *Nursing '82, 12: 73–75.*

Fischbach FT (2000). *A Manual of Laboratory Diagnostic Tests.* 6th ed. Philadelphia: JB Lippincott.

Fisher M, Prichard JW, Warach S (1995). New magnetic resonance techniques for acute ischemic stroke. *Journal of the American Medical Association, 274*(11): 908–911.

Flachskampf F (1995). Recent progress in quantitative echocardiography. *Current Opinion in Cardiology, 10*(6): 634–639.

Flake KJ (2000). HIV testing during pregnancy: Building the case for voluntary testing. *AWHONN Lifelines,* 4 C: 13–16.

Flaskerud JH (1992). Psychosocial aspects. In: Flaskerud JH, Unguarski PJ, eds. *HIV/AIDS: A Guide to Nursing Care.* 2nd ed. Philadelphia: Saunders, pp 239–274.

Flemmig DS, Johiro AK (1997). HIV counseling and testing. In: Fahey JL, Flemmig DS, eds. *AIDS/HIV Reference Guide for Medical Professionals.* 4th ed. Baltimore: Wilkins and Wilkins, pp 57–74.

Food and Drug Administration (1995). Mammography quality deadline. *FDA Medical Bulletin, 25*(1): 3.

Froelicher ES (1994). Usefulness of exercise testing shortly after acute myocardial infarction for predicting 10 year mortality. *American Journal of Cardiology, 74:* 318–323.

Garza D, Becan-McBride K (1999). *Phlebotomy Handbook: Blood Collection Essentials,* 5th ed. Stamford, CT: Appleton and Lange.

Ge J, Erbel R (1995). Novel techniques of coronary artery imaging. *Current Opinion in Cardiology, 10*(6): 626–633.

Gefter WB (1988). Chest applications of magnetic resonance imaging: An update. *Radiologic Clinics of North America, 26:* 573–586.

Gerberding JL (1992). HIV transmission to providers and their patients. In: Sande MA, Volberding PA, eds. *The Medical Management of AIDS.* 3rd ed. Philadelphia: WB Saunders, pp 54–64.

Goldstein RA, Mullani NA, Wong WH (1986). Positron imaging of myocardial infarction with rubidium-82. *Journal of Nuclear Medicine, 27:* 1824–1829.

Gorman C (1997, January 6; 1996, December 30). The disease detective. *Time, 148*(29): 56–62, 63.

Grady C (1992). HIV disease: Pathogens and treatment. In: Flaskerud JH, Unguarski PJ, eds. *HIV/AIDS: A Guide to Nursing Care.* 2nd ed. Philadelphia: WB Saunders. pp 30–53.

Grady C (1992). Ethical aspects. In: Flaskerud JH, Unguarski PJ, eds. *HIV/AIDS: A Guide to Nursing Care.* 2nd ed. Philadelphia: WB Saunders, pp 424–439.

Grossman CB (1996). *Magnetic Resonance Imaging and Computed Tomography of the Head and Spine,* 2nd ed. Baltimore: Wilkins and Wilkins.

Guzman ER, Rosenberg JC, Houlihan C (1994). A new method using vaginal ultrasound and transfundal pressure to evaluate the asymptomatic incompetent cervix. *Obstetrics and Gynecology, 83*(2): 248–252.

Handbook of Diagnostic Tests, 2nd ed. (1999). Springhouse, PA: Springhouse Corp.

Haney DQ (2000, January 31). Virus levels linked to AIDS transmission. *The News Journal,* Wilmington, DE, p A3.

Hardick M, Beck M, eds. (1989). *Manual of Gastrointestinal Procedures.* 2nd ed. New York: Society of Gastroenterology Nurses and Associates, Inc.

Hardy CE, Helton GJ, Kondo C, et al. (1994). Usefulness of magnetic resonance imaging for evaluating great-vessel anatomy after arterial switch operation for D-transposition of the great arteries. *American Heart Journal, 128:* 326–332.

Henry JB (1996). *Todd-Sanford-Davidsohn: Clinical Diagnosis and Management by Laboratory Methods,* 19th ed. Philadelphia: WB Saunders.

HIV/AIDS Surveillance Reports (1999, June). Atlanta: Centers for Disease Control and Prevention, 11(1).

Hochrein MA, Sohl L (1992). Heart smart: a guide to cardiac tests. *American Journal of Nursing, 92*(12): 22–25.

Hyman RA, Gorey MT (1988). Imaging strategies for MR of the brain. *Radiologic Clinics of North America, 26:* 471–502.

Intermountain Thoracic Society (1984). *Clinical Pulmonary Function Testing, a Manual of Uniform Laboratory Procedures.* 2nd ed.

Iskandrian AE, Chaudhry FA (2000, July). Stress echocardiography and stress nuclear testing, Part I. *Echocardiography: A Journal of CV Ultrasound and Allied Technology, 17*(5): 463–469.

Itchhaporia D, and Cerqueira, MD (1995). New agents and new techniques and nuclear cardiology. *Current Opinion in Cardiology, 10*(6): 650–655.

IV Persantine Thallium Imaging: Protocol (1990). Delaware: DuPont-Merck Pharmaceutical Co.

Jacobs DS (1994). *Laboratory Test Handbook.* 3rd ed. St. Louis: CV Mosby.

Jaffe MS (1996). *Medical–Surgical Nursing Care Plans: Nursing Diagnoses & Interventions.* 3rd ed. Stamford, CT: Appleton & Lange.

Jasper ML (2000). Antepartum fetal assessment. In Mattson S, Smith JE (eds). *Core Curriculum for Maternal Newborn Nursing,* 2nd edition. Philadelphia: WB Saunders, pp 127–160.

Johnson D, Silverstein-Currier J, Sanchez-Keeland L (1999). Building barriers to HIV: Protecting women through contraception and infection prevention. *Advance for Nurse Practitioners, 7*(5): 40–44.

Johnson LL, Lawson MA (1996). New imaging techniques for assessing cardiac function. *Critical Care Clinics, 12*(4): 919–937.

Kanal E, Shaibani A (1994). Firearm safety in MR imaging environment. *Radiology, 193:* 875–876.

Kaplan A, Jack R, Opheim KE, et al (1995). *Clinical Chemistry. Interpretation and Techniques.* 4th ed. Baltimore: Williams & Wilkins.

Kee JL (2000). *Fluids and Electrolytes With Clinical Applications.* 6th ed. New York: Delmar Publishers.

Kee JL (2001). *Handbook: Laboratory and Diagnostic Tests with Nursing Implications.* 4th ed. Upper Saddle River, NJ: Prentice-Hall.

Kee JL, Hayes ER (2000). *Pharmacology: A Nursing Process Approach.* 3rd ed. Philadelphia: WB Saunders.

Keeys, MU (1994). Nuclear cardiology stress testing. *Nursing 94, 24*(1): 63, 64.

Khoshnevis R, Wilson JM, Ferguson JJ (1994). Noninvasive imaging of the cardiovascular system with electron beam tomography. *Current Opinion in Cardiology, 9*(6): 729–739.

Kirton CA (2001). Immunizations in HIV care. In: Kirton CA, Talotta D, and Zwolski K, eds. *Handbook of HIV/AIDS Nursing.* St. Louis: CV Mosby.

Knoben JE, Anderson PO (1993). *Clinical Drug Data.* 7th ed. Hamilton, IL: Drug Intelligence Publications.

Kramer DM (1984). Basic principles of magnetic resonance imaging. *Radiologic Clinics of North America, 22*(4): 765–778.

Kryger MH, Roth T, Dement W, eds. (2000). *The Principals and Practice of Sleep Medicine.* Philadelphia: WB Saunders.

Kurytka D (1996). Advances in HIV/AIDS care. *The Nursing Spectrum, 5*(26): 6.

Locher AW (1996, July/August). Ethics, women with HIV, and procreation: Implications for nursing practice. *Journal of Obstetric, Gynecologic and Neonatal Nursing, 25*(6): 465–469.

Lopez M, Fleisher T, deShazo RD (1992). Use and interpretation of diagnostic immunologic laboratory tests. *Journal of the American Medical Association, 268*(20): 2970–2990.

Marwick TH (1995). Recent advances in stress echocardiography. *Current Opinion in Cardiology, 10*(6): 619–625.

Masland T, Norland R (2000, January 17). 10 Orphans. *Newsweek,* 42–45.

Maule WF (1994). Screening for colorectal cancer by nurse endoscopists. *New England Journal of Medicine, 330*(3): 183–184.

McClatchey KD, ed. (1994). *Clinical Laboratory Medicine.* Baltimore: Williams & Wilkins.

McLelland R, Pisano ED, Braeuning MP (1995). Breast imaging. In: Sutton D, Young JWR. *A Concise Textbook of Clinical Imaging.* 2nd ed. St. Louis: CV Mosby.

Mellico KD (1993). Interpretation of abnormal laboratory values in older adults. Part I. *Journal of Gerontological Nursing, 19*(1): 39–45.

Mennemeyer ST, Winkelman JW (1993). Searching for inaccuracy in clinical laboratory testing using medicare data: Evidence for prothrombin time. *Journal of the American Medical Association, 269:* 1030–1033.

Mettler FA (1996). *Essentials of Radiology.* Philadelphia: WB Saunders.

Miller WF, Scacci R, Fast LR (1987). *Laboratory Evaluation of Pulmonary Function.* Philadelphia: JB Lippincott.

Moran BA (2000). Maternal infections. In: Mattson S and Smith JE, eds. *Core Curriculum for Maternal-Newborn Nursing,* 2nd ed. Philadelphia: WB Saunders, pp. 419–448.

Moulton-Barrett R, Triadafilopoulos G, Michener R, et al (1993). Serum C-bicarbonate in the assessment of gastric *Heliobacter pylori* urease activity. *American Journal of Gastroenterology, 88*(3): 369–373.

Myers MC, Page MD (1996). Caring for the laboring woman with HIV infection on AIDS. In: Martin EJ, ed. *Intrapartum Management Modules,* 2nd ed. Baltimore: Wilkins and Wilkins, pp 451–486.

Nanda NC, Miller A, Puri VK, PoHoey F, Tiemann K, et al. (2000, July). Assessment of myocardial perfusion by power contrast imaging using a new echo contrast agent. *Echocardiography: A Journal of CV Ultrasound and Allied Technology, 17*(5): 457–460.

National Committee for Clinical Laboratory Standards (1995). *How to Define, Determine and Utilize Reference Intervals in the Clinical Laboratory, Approved Guidelines,* NCCLS Document C-28-A, *25*(4).

National Multiple Sclerosis Society (1987). MRI—no mystique. *Inside, 5*(4): 24–27.

Noble D (1993). Controversies in the clinical chemical laboratory. *Analtyical Chemistry, 84*(6): 797–800.

Norris MKG (1993). Evaluating serum triglyceride levels. *Nursing 93, 23*(5): 31.

Nursing Diagnoses: Definitions and Classification 2001–2002. North American Nursing Diagnosis Association (NANDA), Philadelphia.

Nyamath A, Flemmig DS (1997). Prevention consideration for women. In: Hahey JL and Flemmig DS, eds. *AIDS/HIV Reference Guide for Medical Professionals,* 4th ed. Baltimore: Wilkins and Wilkins, pp 232–242.

Olds SB, London ML, Ladewig PAW (2000). *Maternal-Newborn Nursing: A Family and Community-Based Approach.* 6th ed. Upper Saddle River, NJ: Prentice-Hall Health.

Pagana KD, Pagana TJ (1999). Mosby's Diagnostic and Laboratory Test References, 4th ed. St. Louis: CV Mosby.

Parris NB (1992). Infection control. In: Flaskerud JH, Unguarski PJ, eds. *HIV/AIDS: A Guide to Nursing Care.* 2nd ed. Philadelphia: WB Saunders, pp 397–423.

Pasquale MJ (1992). *Application of Radionuclide Stress Tests.* Wilmington, DE: Cardiac Diagnostic Center.

Peterson KJ, Solie CJ (1994). Interpreting laboratory values in chronic renal insufficiency. *American Journal of Nursing, 94*(5): 56B, 56E, 56H.

Peterson KL, Nicod P (1997) *Cardiac Catherization Methods, Diagnosis, and Therapy.* Philadelphia, PA: WB Saunders.

Physicians' Current Procedural Terminology (cpt 98) (1998). Chicago: American Medical Association.

Pizzo PA, Wilfert CM (1991). *Pediatric AIDS: The Challenge of HIV Infection in Infants, Children and Adolescents.* Baltimore: Williams & Wilkins.

Population Information Program, Center for Communications Programs (1989). *Population Reports: AIDS Education—A Beginning.* Issues in World Health. Baltimore: The Johns Hopkins University, xvii: 1–32.

Porembka, DT (1996). Transesophageal echocardiography. *Critical Care Clinics, 12*(4): 875–903.

Purvis A (1997, January 6; 1996, December 30). The global epidemic. *Time, 148*(29): 76–78.

Rakel RE (1996). *Saunders Manual of Medical Practice.* Philadelphia: WB Saunders.

Ravel R (1995). *Clinical Laboratory Medicine.* 6th ed. Chicago: Year Book.

Reed JD, Soulen RL (1988). Cardiovascular MRI: Current role in patient management. *Radiologic Clinics of North America, 26:* 589–600.

Renkes J (1993). GI endoscopy: Managing the full scope of care. *Nursing 93, 23*(6): 50–55.

Romancyzuk AN, Brown JP (1994). Folic acid will reduce risk of neural tube defects. *American Journal of Maternal Child Nursing, 19*(6): 331–334.

Rotello LS, Radin EJ, Jastremski MS, et al. (1994). MRI protocol for critically ill patients. *American Journal of Critical Care, 3*(3): 187–190.

Saag MS (1992). AIDS testing: Now and in the future. In: Sande MA, Volberding PA, eds. *The Medical Management of AIDS.* 3rd ed. Philadelphia: WB Saunders, pp 33–53.

Sacher RA, McPherson RA, eds. (1995). *Widmann's Clinical Interpretation of Laboratory Tests.* 11th ed. Philadelphia: FA Davis.

Sayad DE, Clarke GD, Peshock RM (1995). Magnetic resonance imaging of the heart and its role in current cardiology. *Current Opinion in Cardiology, 10*(6): 640–649.

Selig PM (1996). Pearls for practice. Management of anticoagulation therapy with international normalized ratio. *Journal of the American Academy of Nursing Practitioner, 8*(2): 77–80.

Sherman D, Sherman N (2001). HIV/AIDS and pregnancy. In: Kirton CA, Talotta D, and Zwolski K. *Handbook of HIV/AIDS Nursing.* St. Louis: CV Mosby, pp 361–379.

Sipes C (1995, January/February). Guidelines for assessing HIV in women. *MCN: The American Journal of Maternal Child Nursing, 20*(1): 29–33.

Smith S, Forman D (1994). Laboratory analysis of cerebrospinal fluid. *Clinical Laboratory Science, 7*(4): 32, 38.

Soothill PW (1999). Fetal blood sampling before labor. In: James DK, Steer PJ, Weiner CP, Gonick B, eds. *High Risk Pregnancy: Management Options,* 2nd ed. Philadelphia: WB Saunders, pp 225–233.

Stephenson J (2000, July 12). AIDS in South Africa takes center stage. *Journal of the American Medical Association, 284*(2): 165–167.

Strimike C (1996). Understanding intravascular ultrasound. *American Journal of Nursing, 96*(6) 40–43.

Stringer M, Librizzi R (1994). Complications following prenatal genetic procedures. *Nursing Research, 43*(2): 184–186.

Sutton D (1995). Angiography. In Sutton D, Young JWR. *A Concise Textbook of Clinical Imaging.* 2nd ed. St Louis: CV Mosby.

Talotta D (2001). Health care worker risk reduction in HIV/AIDS care. In: Kirton CA, Talotta D, Zwolski K. *Handbook of HIV/AIDS Nursing.* St Louis: CV Mosby, pp 430–451.

Tannenbaum I (1993). Women and HIV. *RN, 56:* 34–40.

TB Facts for Health Care Workers (1993). Atlanta, GA: Department of Health and Human Services, Public Health Service, Centers for Disease Control and Prevention, National Center for Prevention Services, Division of Tuberculosis Elimination.

Te-Chuan C, Ceaser JH (1993). Ambulatory electrocardiogram: Clinical applications. In Fowler NO, ed. *Noninvasive Diagnostic Methods in Cardiology.* Philadelphia: FA Davis, pp 321–333.

Thomas C (1994, January 2). Salvation through condoms: A trojan horse. *The Sunday News Journal,* p H-4.

Thompson E, Detwiler DS, Nelson CM (1996). Dobutamine stress echocardiography: A new noninvasive method for detecting ischemic heart disease. *Heart & Lung, 25*(2): 87–97.

Thompson L (1995). Percutaneous endoscopic gastrostomy. *Nursing 95, 25*(4): 62–63.

Thrall JH, Ziessman HA (1995). *Nuclear Medicine.* St Louis: CV Mosby.

Tietz NW, ed. (1995). *Clinical Guide to Laboratory Tests.* 3rd ed. Philadelphia: WB Saunders.

Tokars JI, Martone WJ (1992). Infection control considerations in HIV infection. In Wormser GP, ed. *AIDS and Other Manifestations of HIV Infection.* 2nd ed. New York: Raven, pp 54–145.

Topol EJ, Holmes DR, Rogers WJ (1991). Coronary angiography after thrombolytic therapy for acute myocardial infarction. *Annual of Internal Medicine, 114:* 877–885.

Ungvarski PJ (1992). Clinical manifestations of AIDS. In: Flaskerud JH, Unguarski PJ, eds. *IIIV/AIDS. A Guide to Nursing Care.* 2nd ed. Philadelphia: Saunders, pp 54–145.

Vannier MW, Marsh JL (1996). Three-dimensional imaging, surgical planning, and image-guided therapy. *Radiologic Clinics of North America, 34*(3): 545–561.

Wallach J (1996). *Interpretation of Diagnostic Tests.* 6th ed. Boston: Little, Brown.

Ward JW, Drotman DP (1992). Epidemiology of HIV and AIDS. In: Wormser GP, ed. *AIDS and Other Manifestations of HIV Infection.* 2nd ed. New York: Raven, pp 1–15.

Washington JA (1993). Laboratory diagnosis of infectious diseases. *Infectious Disease Clinics of North America, 7*(2): 13.

Weisse AB (1995). TE echocardiography: Its clinical role. *Hospital Practice.* Oct 15, 30(10): 11, 12.

Wilde P, Hartnell GC (1995). Cardiac imaging. In: Sutton D, Young JWR. *A Concise Textbook of Clinical Imaging.* 2nd ed. St. Louis: CV Mosby.

Williams L (1993). AIDS update. *The Nursing Spectrum, 2:* 7.

Williamson MR (1996). *Essentials of Ultrasound.* Philadelphia: WB Saunders.

Wofson AB, Paris PM (1996). *Diagnostic Testing in Emergency Medicine.* Philadelphia: WB Saunders.

Womack C, Thomas JD (1996). Easing the way through an MRI. *RN, 59*(10): 34–37.

Wong ND, Vo W, Abrahamson D, et al (1994). Detection of coronary artery calcium by ultra-fast computed tomography and its relation to clinical evidence of coronary artery disease. *American Journal of Cardiology, 73:* 223–227.

Wormser GP, Horowitz H (1992). Care of the adult patient with HIV infection. In: Wormser GP, ed. *AIDS and Other Manifestations of HIV Infection.* 2nd ed. New York: Raven, pp 173–200.

Yang EY, Adzick NS (1998). Fetoscopy. *Seminar Laparoscopic Surgery, 5*(1): 31–39.

Young SW (1984). *Nuclear Magnetic Resonance Imaging.* New York: Raven.

Zaret BL, Wackers FJ (1993). Nuclear cardiology. *New England Journal of Medicine, 329*(12): 855–863.

Zubal IG (1996). The evolution of imaging devices: A constant challenge with combining progress. In *Yearbook of Nuclear Medicine.* St. Louis: CV Mosby.

Zwolski K (2001). HIV immunopathogenesis. In: Kirton CA, Talotta D, Zwolski K. *Handbook of HIV/AIDS Nursing.* St. Louis: CV Mosby, pp 3–25.

INDEX